Evidence-based Ophthalmology

Evidence-based Ophthalmology

Edited by

Richard Wormald
Consultant Ophthalmologist, Moorfields Eye Hospital,
Honorary Senior Lecturer, London School of Hygiene and Tropical Medicine and Coordinating Editor, Cochrane Eyes and Vision
Group, London, UK

Liam Smeeth
Senior Lecturer in Clinical Epidemiology, London School of Hygiene and Tropical Medicine, General Practitioner, London and
Editor, Cochrane Eyes and Vision Group, London, UK

Katherine Henshaw
Review Group Coordinator, Cochrane Eyes and Vision Group, London, UK

With research by Anupa Shah
Trial Search Coordinator, Cochrane Eyes and Vision Group, London, UK

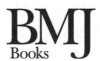

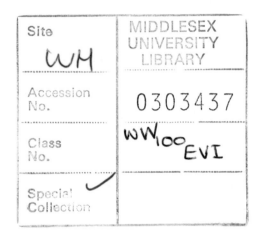
© BMJ Publishing Group 2004
BMJ Books is an imprint of the BMJ Publishing Group

First published in 2004
by BMJ Books, BMA House, Tavistock Square,
London WC1H 9JR

www.bmjbooks.com

British Library Cataloguing in Publication Data
A catalogue record for this book is available from the British Library

ISBN 0 7279 1443 X

Typeset by SIVA Math Setters, Chennai, India
Printed and bound by MPG Books, Bodmin, Cornwall

Contents

Contributors

Section editors

James Acheson
Moorfields Eye Hospital
and National Hospital for Neurology and Neurosurgery
London, UK

Bill Aylward
Moorfields Eye Hospital
London, UK

Linda Ficker
No address supplied

Clare Gilbert
International Centre for Eye Health
London School of Hygiene and Tropical Medicine
London, UK

Emma Hollick
Moorfields Eye Hospital
London, UK

Carlos Pavesio
Moorfields Eye Hospital,
London, UK

Jugnoo S Rahi
Clinical Senior Lecturer in Ophthalmic Epidemiology,
Centre for Paediatric Epidemiology and Department of
Ophthalmology,
Institute of Child Health and Great Ormond Street Hospital
and Department of Epidemiology, Institute of Ophthalmology,
London, UK

Bernd Richter
Cochrane Metabolic and Endocrine Disorders Group
Medizinische Einrichtungen
Heinrich-Heine Universitaet
Germany

Gary Rubin
Division of Rehabilitation Research
Institute of Ophthalmology
London, UK

Aziz Sheikh
Professor of Primary Care Research and Development
Department of Community Health Sciences
University of Edinburgh
Edinburgh, UK

Arun D Singh
Wills Eye Hospital
Oncology Service
Philadelphia
Pennsylvania, USA

Michael J Wearne
Department of Ophthalmology
Eastbourne District Hospital
Eastbourne, UK

Other contributors

David F Anderson
Moorfields Eye Hospital
London, UK

Heather Baldwin
St Thomas' Hospital
London, UK

Michael Bearn
Department of Ophthalmology
Cumberland Infirmary
Carlisle, UK

Kostas G Boboridis
Department of Ophthalmology
Oculoplastic Service
AHEPA University Hospital
Aristotle University of Thessaloniki
Greece

Fion Bremner
National Hospital for Neurology and Neurosurgery
and Moorfields Eye Hospital
London, UK

Lorraine Cassidy
The Royal Victoria Eye and Ear Hospital, Dublin, Ireland and
The Adelaide and Meath Hospital Incorporating the National
Children's Hospital
University of Dublin, Trinity College, Dublin, Ireland

David G Charteris
Moorfields Eye Hospital
London, UK

Michael Clarke
Children's Eye Clinic and Orthoptic Department
Claremont Wing
Royal Victoria Infirmary
Newcastle-upon-Tyne, UK

Kay Dickersin
Center for Clinical Trials and Evidence-based Healthcare
Brown University Medical School
Providence, Rhode Island
USA

Jonathan GF Dowler
International Centre for Eye Health
London School of Hygiene and Tropical Medicine
London, UK

Graham Duguid
Western Eye Hospital
London, UK

Henry Ejere
International Health Division
Liverpool School of Tropical Medicine
Liverpool, UK

Jennifer Evans
International Department of Epidemiology
and Eye Health
Institute of Ophthalmology
London, UK

Hazel Everitt
Primary Medical Care
Aldermoor Health Centre
Aldermoor Close
Southampton, UK

Eric Ezra
Moorfields Eye Hospital
London, UK

Ian Flitcroft
Department of Ophthalmology
Mater Misericordiae Hospital and the Children's
University Hospital
Dublin, Ireland

Lawrence Gnanaraj
Department of Ophthalmology
Royal Victoria Infirmary
Newcastle upon Tyne, UK

Simon J Hickman
NMR Research Unit
Institute of Neurology
University College London
and
Department of Neuro-ophthalmology
Moorfields Eye Hospital
London, UK

Santosh G Honavar
Division of Plastic and Orbital Surgery
LV Prasad Eye Institute
Banjara Hills
Hyderabad, India

Andrew S Jacks
Centre for Defence Medicine
Selly Oak Hospital
Birmingham, UK

Nicholas P Jones
The Royal Eye Hospital
Manchester, UK

PT Khaw
Wound Healing Research Unit
Glaucoma Unit and Department of Pathology
Moorfields Eye Hospital and Institute of Ophthalmology
London, UK

JK Kirwan
Portsmouth NHS Trust
Portsmouth, UK

Eva Kohner
St Thomas' Hospital
London, UK

Alistair Laidlaw
St Thomas's Hospital
London, UK

Sarit Lesnik-Oberstein
Moorfields Eye Hospital
London, UK

Martin Leyland
Royal Berkshire Hospital NHS Trust
Reading, Berkshire, UK

Christian J Lueck
The Canberra Hospital
Canberra, Australia

Denise Mabey
St Thomas' Hospital
London, UK

Vincenzo Maurino
Moorfields Eye Hospital
London, UK

Gawn G McIlwaine
Princess Alexandra Eye Pavilion
Edinburgh, UK

Jodhbir S Mehta
Moorfields Eye Hospital
London, UK

Jane Moseley
The Medicines and Healthcare Products Regulatory Agency
London, UK

Philip I Murray
Academic Unit of Ophthalmology
Division of Immunity and Infection
University of Birmingham and Midland Eye Centre
Birmingham, UK

Christopher G Owen
Department of Community Health Sciences
St George's Hospital Medical School
London, UK

Vinidh Paleri
Department of Otolaryngology – Head and Neck Surgery
Freeman Hospital
Newcastle upon Tyne, UK

Maria Papadopoulos
Glaucoma Unit
Moorfields Eye Hospital
London, UK

Ian G Rennie
Department of Ophthalmology and Orthoptics
Royal Hallamshire Hospital
Sheffield, UK

Sarah Richardson
Department of Ophthalmology Orthoptics
Royal Victoria Infirmary
Newcastle upon Tyne, UK

Andrew K Robson
Department of Otolaryngology – Head and Neck Surgery
Cumberland Infirmary
Carlisle, UK

Alonso Rodriguez
Cornea and External Disease Department
Moorfields Eye Hospital
London, UK

Paul A Rundle
Department of Ophthalmology and Orthoptics
Royal Hallamshire Hospital
Sheffield, UK

Anupa Shah
Cochrane Eyes and Vision Group
London, UK

Rajiv Shah
Moorfields Eye Hospital
London, Uk

Paul Sullivan
Moorfields Eye Hospital
London, Uk

Ahmed Toosy
NMR Research Unit
Institute of Neurology
University College London
London, UK and
Department of Neuro-Ophthalmology
Moorfields Eye Hospital
London, UK

Adnan Tufail
Corneal and External Diseases
Moorfields Eye Hospital
London, UK

Stephanie L Watson
Corneal and External Diseases
Moorfields Eye Hospital
London, UK

Silvia Wengrowicz
Department of Endocrinology
Hospital de la Santa Creu i Sant Pau
Autonomous University of Barcelona
Spain

Charles P Wilkinson
Greater Baltimore Medical Center and Johns Hopkins University
Baltimore
Maryland
USA

Cathy Williams
Bristol Eye Hospital and Departments of Child Health
and Ophthalmology
University of Bristol
Bristol, UK

Preface

In an ideal world, every clinician would have easy access to up to date information on the safety and effectiveness of all treatments offered to their patients. But the volume of medical literature is immense, and growing rapidly. Therefore a systematic and unbiased method for summarising and disseminating the evidence is necessary. Hence the efforts of the international Cochrane Collaboration and its Database of Systematic Reviews and others such as the Centre for Reviews and Dissemination in York, UK and the Agency for Healthcare Research and Quality in the US.

Ophthalmology has a long way to go before the implementation of evidence-based practice is established but in this, ophthalmology is similar to many other surgically dominated subjects. There are many who vociferously reject its principles, particularly in the valuation of experimental versus experiential dogma. The traditional practice of medicine is based on the individual, and opinion, but modern practice requires a more solid foundation. In order to form opinions and make judgements, clinicians require access to reliable sources of evidence.

This book does not describe the whole of the evidence base and the chapters do not have the rigour of systematic reviews but they illustrate where reviews have been conducted, which trials have been identified, and, perhaps more important, where the gaps in the evidence exist. It is inevitable that by the time this text is published, it will be out of date. Despite this, there is a wealth of information that has the potential to change our practice, not just because trial findings contradict what is common practice, but because it might help generate a more inquisitive approach to our routine clinical activity.

Richard Wormald
Liam Smeeth

Evidence-based Ophthalmology CD Rom

Features
Evidence-based Ophthalmology PDF eBook

- Bookmarked and hyperlinked for instant access to all headings and topics
- Fully indexed and searchable text – just click "Search Text" button

PDA Edition sample chapter

- A chapter from Evidence-based Ophthalmology, adapted for use on handheld devices such as *Palm* and *Pocket PC*
- Click on the underlined text to view an image (or images) relevant to the text concerned
- Uses Mobipocket Reader technology, compatible with all PDA devices and also available for Windows
- Follow the on-screen instructions on the relevant part of the CD Rom to install Mobipocket for your device
- Full title available for purchase as a download from http://www.pda.bmjbooks.com

BMJ Books catalogue

- Instant access to BMJ Books full catalogue, including an order form
  Also included – a direct link to the Evidence-based Ophthalmology update website

Instructions for use

The CD Rom should start automatically upon insertion, on all Windows systems. The menu screen will appear and you can then navigate by clicking on the headings. If the CD Rom does not start automatically upon insertion, please browse using "Windows Explorer" and double-click the file "BMJ_Books.exe".

Tips

The viewable area of the PDF ebook can be expanded to fill the full screen width, by hiding the bookmarks. To do this, click and hold on the divider in between the bookmark window and the main window, then drag it to the left as required. By clicking once on a page in the PDF ebook window, you "activate" the window. You can now scroll through pages using the scroll-wheel on your mouse, or by using the cursor keys on your keyboard.

Note: the Evidence-based Ophthalmology PDF eBook is for search and reference only and cannot be printed. A printable PDF version as well as the full PDA edition can be purchased from http://www.bmjbookshop.com

Troubleshooting

If any problems are experienced with use of the CD Rom, we can give you access to all content via the internet. Please send your CD Rom with proof of purchase to the following address, with a letter advising your email address and the problem you have encountered:

Evidence-based Ophthalmology eBook access
BMJ Bookshop
BMA House
Tavistock Square
London
WC1H 9JR

Evidence-based Ophthalmology update website

Updates and further information on the book can be found at
http://www.evidbasedophth.com

Glossary

Ab	antibiotic
ABMD	anterior basement membrane dystrophy
AC	anterior chamber
AC/A ratio	accommodative convergence: accommodation
ACO	anterior capsule opacification
ACV	aciclovir
AION	anterior ischaemic optic neuropathy
AKC	atopic keratoconjunctivitis
AMD	age-related macular degeneration
AU	anterior uveitis
BCL	bandage soft contact lens
BENT	Between nine and twelve o'clock
BK	bacterial keratitis
BMD	bone mineral density
BRVO	branch retinal vein occlusion
BSS	balanced salt solution
BSV	binocular single vision
C3F8	perfluoropropane
CCC	continuous curvilinear capsulorhexis
CCT	clinical controlled trial
CDMS	clinically definite multiple sclerosis
CEVG	Cochrane eyes and vision group
CF	count fingers visual acuity
CG	congenital glaucoma (primary and secondary)
CI	confidence interval
CMO	cystoid macular oedema
CMV	cytomegalovirus
CMV-R	cytomegalovirus retinitis
CNV	choroidal neovascularisation
COMS	Collaborative Ocular Melanoma Study
CP	convex surface anterior
CPC	cumulative probability of cure
CRVO	central retinal vein occlusion
CSF	cerebrospinal fluid
CTON	chlamydial ophthalmia neonatorum
CVST	cortical venous sinus thrombosis
DEC	diethylcarbamazine
DM	diabetes mellitus
DS	dioptre sphere
DVD	dissociated vertical deviation
EBM	evidence-based medicine
ECCE	extracapsular cataract extraction
EKC	epidemic keratoconjunctivitis
ELBW	extremely low birth weight
ERM	epiretinal membrane
FAZ	foveal avascular zone
5-FU	5-fluorouracil
FFA	fundus fluorescein angiogram
FTMH	full-thickness macular hole
FU	follow up
GA	gestational age
GCA	giant cell arteritis
GON	gonococcal ophthalmia neonatorum
HAART	highly active antiretroviral therapy
HELP	heparin-induced extracorporeal LDL/fibrinogen precipitation
HIV	human immunodeficiency virus
HM	hand motion vision
HRT	hormone replacement therapy
HSM	heparin-surface-modified
HSV	herpes simplex virus
ICCE	intracapsular cataract extraction
IDDM	insulin-dependent diabetes mellitus
IDU	idoxuridine
IIH	idiopathic intracranial hypertension
ILM	internal limiting membrane
IM	intramuscular
IOL	intraocular lens
IOP	intraocular pressure
IU	international units
IVIG	intravenous immunoglobulin
IVMP	intravenous methylprednisolone
KTP	potassium titanyl phosphate
LBW	low birth weight
LEC	lens epithelial cell
LHON	Leber's hereditary optic neuropathy
LMWH	low molecular weight heparin
LP	light perception
LPS	lumboperitoneal shunting
LR	laser-ridge
+ M	with antiglaucoma medications
– M	without antiglaucoma medications
MIC	minimum inhibitory concentration
MK	microbial keratitis
MMC	mitomycin-C
MS	multiple sclerosis
Nd:YAG	neodymium yttrium–aluminium–garnet
NG	*Neisseria gonorrhoeae*
NLP	no light perception
NNH	number needed to harm
NNT	number needed to treat
Non/CT/GON	Non-chlamydial/non-gonococcal ophthalmia neonatorum
NPDR	non-proliferative diabetic retinopathy
NSAID	non-steroidal anti-inflammatory drug
NSC	national screening committee
NTG	normal tension glaucoma
NVD	new vessels disc
NVE	new vessels elsewhere
OCT	optical coherence tomography
ON	ophthalmia neonatorum
ONSF	optic nerve sheath fenestration
ONTT	optic neuritis treatment trial
OR	odds ratio

OSSN	ocular surface squamous neoplasia		RDS	respiratory distress syndrome
PAC	perennial allergic conjunctivitis		RE	Reese-Ellsworth
PC	convex surface posterior		RGP	rigid gas permeable
PCO	posterior capsular opacification		ROP	retinopathy of prematurity
PDR	proliferative diabetic retinopathy		RR	relative risk
PERG	pattern electroretinogram		RVO	retinal vein occlusion
PGC	primary congenital glaucoma		SAC	seasonal allergic conjunctivitis
PHE	periodic health examination		SF6	sulphur hexafluoride
PK	penetrating keratoplasty		SK	suppurative keratitis
PMMA	polymethylmethacrylate		SLE	slit lamp examination
PPC	primary posterior capsulotomy		SSD	statistically significant difference
PPV	pars plana vitrectomy		STD	sexually transmitted disease
PRP	panretinal photocoagulation		TCA	traumatic corneal abrasion
PTK	phototherapeutic keratectomy		TGF-β2	transforming growth factor-β2
PVC	posterior vitreous cortex		TMA	tissue plasminogen activator
PVD	posterior vitreous detachment		TTPH	taut thickened posterior hyaloid
PVD-I	povidone-iodine		UCVA	uncorrected visual acuity
PVR	proliferative vitreoretinopathy		VA	visual acuity
RAPD	relative afferent pupil defect		VKC	vernal keratoconjunctivitis
RAST	radioallergosorbent test		VKH	Vogt-Koyanagi-Harada disease
RCE	recurrent corneal erosion		WHO	World Health Organization
RCT	randomised controlled trial		YAG	yttrium–aluminium–garnet

Section I

The basics

1 Finding the evidence

Kay Dickersin

Introduction

For more than a decade healthcare practitioners have been discussing the merits of evidence-based medicine. But what is evidence? Most use this term to mean the best available research evidence. And when one wants to know how well a particular diagnostic, therapeutic or preventive intervention works, the preferred type of research is that using randomised controlled trials (RCTs). The Canadian Task Force on Preventive Health Care, which formally introduced the concept of "levels of evidence", has assigned RCTs the highest level of evidence (see Tables 1.1 and 1.2).[1] Other types of research evidence, for example, controlled observational studies and case series, are considered to be at a lower level, and expert opinion is lowest of all. What this means is that reviewers should give the greatest weight to evidence from RCTs and progressively less to studies that are likely to produce less valid or reliable results.

Systematic reviews, even when they include only randomised controlled trials, are a type of observational study. Instead of studying human participants, however, the systematic review includes research studies. As in human studies, if the population gathered for study is biased or not generalisable, the integrity of the entire project is brought into question. Having a predefined, well-constructed, comprehensive search for eligible studies is one of the ways in which a systematic review differs from a traditional narrative review.

One of the most challenging aspects of performing a search for studies for a systematic review is the requirement for comprehensiveness. If we could assume that identified studies were a random sample of all relevant studies, the absence of unidentified studies would not cause a problem. Unfortunately, evidence indicates that those studies with the potential for being missed by a standard search (for example, studies that are unpublished) are systematically different from those that are more likely to be found.

Thus, an entire area of research has grown up around how best to identify studies, and in particular clinical trials, for systematic reviews. Along the way we have learned

Table 1.1 Canadian Task Force grades of recommendations

Grade	Description
A	Good evidence to support the recommendation that the condition be specifically considered in a PHE
B	Fair evidence to support the recommendation that the condition be specifically considered in a PHE
C	Poor evidence regarding inclusion or exclusion of a condition in a PHE, but recommendations may be made on other grounds
D	Fair evidence to support the recommendation that the condition be specifically excluded from consideration in a PHE
E	Good evidence to support the recommendation that the condition be specifically excluded from consideration in a PHE

PHE, periodic health examination

Table 1.2 Canadian Task Force quality of published evidence

Grade	Description
I	Evidence from at least one properly randomised controlled trial (RCT)
II-1	Evidence from well-designed controlled trials without randomisation
II-2	Evidence from well-designed cohort or case-control analytical studies, preferably from more than one centre or research group
II-3	Evidence from comparisons between times or places with or without the intervention; dramatic results in uncontrolled experiments could also be included here
III	Opinions of respected authorities, based on clinical experience, descriptive studies or reports of expert committees

some important facts: a comprehensive search to identify published research is surprisingly hard to do, and a search for unpublished studies is even harder. This chapter will outline what we know about both of these challenges and how to use what we know to ensure comprehensive reviews.

Searching for published studies

Electronic databases

Anyone who has embarked on research in a new area knows that it is not easy to gather "from scratch" all of the state-of-the-art literature. Electronic searching of bibliographic databases is used more and more for searching the extant literature, in part because it is easier than going to a library, but also because, over time, it is increasingly what we know best. What is not generally known is just how much of the literature each of these databases covers, and what might be missed if searches are limited so that they produce manageable numbers of citations.

There are probably hundreds or even thousands of bibliographic databases available for searching. Prominent English language databases include MEDLINE, EMBASE, Healthstar, CINAHL (Cumulative Index of Nursing and Allied Health Literature), PsycLIT, CancerLIT, BIOSIS, AMI (Australasian Medical Index), SciSearch and Dissertation Abstracts. In addition, there are databases for the Japanese literature, the Latin-American literature, the Chinese literature and many others. These databases each only cover a fraction of the literature, and sometimes there are large overlaps in coverage. Well over 20,000 biomedical periodicals are being published around the world, yet MEDLINE, one of the primary bibliographic resources, includes only about 4600 of these.[2]

While journals from a diverse group of countries and representing numerous languages are included in MEDLINE, the majority are US-based and in English. This would not be a problem if one could assume that publishing in English or in a US journal was a random decision. Egger has shown that at least for investigators in German-speaking countries, there is a tendency to publish statistically significant positive results in international English language journals and negative results in German language journals.[3] Furthermore, there is reasonable evidence that journals tend to publish articles from their home countries,[4] although there is no direct evidence as yet that there is an author or editorial bias favouring submission or acceptance of articles from a home country over others. Thus, limiting a search to articles in English or in journals accessible through the investigator's library may introduce bias to a review.

Limiting a search to a single or a few databases may result in a failure to identify any publications if the topic is not covered well by the journals in the database. For example, studies of complementary and alternative medicine have only recently been considered part of mainstream US medicine, and represent a small proportion of articles in MEDLINE-indexed journals.[5]

Even when studies are included in MEDLINE, they may be difficult to find. Most investigators know that a broad search using a few terms may be more likely to find most of the relevant records, but at the same time it may also retrieve thousands of citations. Use of additional indexing terms that narrow the search and reduce the number of retrieved citations runs the risk of missing relevant articles. Studies in the 1980s and early 1990s indicated that it was particularly difficult at that time to identify reports of RCTs in MEDLINE.[6]

The Cochrane Collaboration is an international organisation that aims to help people make well-informed decisions about health care by preparing, maintaining and promoting the accessibility of systematic reviews of the effects of healthcare interventions. It has developed methods to overcome some of the difficulties in producing a comprehensive search. The Collaboration has developed an electronic, centralised register of studies potentially eligible for systematic reviews of healthcare interventions. This database, called CENTRAL, includes published and unpublished controlled trials, in any language, from any country, performed at any point in time.[7] CENTRAL is available as part of the *Cochrane Library*, which is available through libraries and by subscription. As of the end of 2002, CENTRAL included over 345 378 citations to controlled clinical trials – about 120 000 more than contained in MEDLINE.

Members of the Collaboration, including review groups such as the Cochrane Eyes and Vision Group, contribute trials they have identified to CENTRAL. In turn, the review groups use CENTRAL to create their own "specialised registers" that they use to help their reviewers find the best evidence for the group's systematic reviews. Review groups use all the methods described in this chapter, and more, to identify trials that are potentially relevant for their reviews.

Handsearching

Studies have repeatedly shown that even using multiple databases and the best search strategies, searching of electronic databases does not identify all relevant published studies for a systematic review.[8,9] There are a number of reasons for this. First, not all study reports are included in at least one of the existing electronic databases. For example, conference abstracts and letters to journal editors often contain information about trial results, but are not centrally electronically indexed. In many cases, the only way to find trial reports presented solely in abstracts is by handsearching conference proceedings.

Systematic reviews that fail to include data from conference abstracts may be excluding results that are different from the types of data appearing in full reports. Indeed, less than half (44·8%) of conference abstracts and other short reports ever reach full publication.[10] Furthermore, there appears to be an association between statistically significant results and full publication (relative risk (RR) = 1·51; 95% confidence interval (CI) 1·27–1·79), although no such association was detected between direction of results (i.e. favouring the experimental arm) and full publication (RR = 0·97; 95% CI 0·81–1·18). In addition, McAuley has shown that results presented in the "grey" literature, including conference abstracts, tend more often to be "negative" than results published in full journal reports.[11]

A second reason why searching of electronic databases tends not to identify all relevant studies for a systematic review is that most electronic databases are not indexed with systematic reviewers in mind, that is, indexing is not done to ensure comprehensiveness of a search. And, although there are almost always explicit rules for application of the index terms, these rules are not always followed by the indexers. Studies of MEDLINE and EMBASE searching conducted in the past have shown that on average MEDLINE searches identify 77% of the randomised trials that they index,[12] and in one study at least EMBASE identified 85% of controlled trials.[9] Other databases almost certainly have similar or worse problems. The percentage of total relevant citations retrieved by MEDLINE is probably improved today because of newer indexing terms that became available in the 1990s and a massive "retagging" effort the National Library of Medicine has undertaken in collaboration with the United States in Cochrane Center Providence, to ensure that all citations in the MEDLINE database are assigned the newer terms.[7] Still, recent studies have shown that even with these improvements, an additional handsearch of the literature is warranted.[13]

Thus, the Cochrane Collaboration has elected to handsearch journals, conference proceedings and other documents to ensure comprehensive systematic reviews. As of March 2001, over 2100 periodicals have been or are being handsearched, page by page, from 1948 onward.[7] This handsearching has contributed to CENTRAL citations to thousands of abstracts that might otherwise not be accessible through electronic means. On average, as of Issue 1 2001 of the *Cochrane Library*, 10% of the trials in Cochrane reviews are referenced to abstracts, dissertations or other "grey" sources only.[14]

Perusal of reference lists

Perusal of reference lists is a common method used to search for relevant studies for systematic reviews. Used less often, SciSearch, the Institute for Scientific Information's electronic database for citation searching, provides a similar opportunity.[15] The major problem with either approach is that citation is subjective and may be biased. Several studies have shown a tendency of investigators to cite articles supporting effectiveness of an intervention,[16,17] or conversely, articles failing to support effectiveness.[18] This is not to say that reference lists should not be searched, rather one should not consider that an electronic search supplemented by a search of reference lists would lead to comprehensive identification of all relevant work.

Searching for unpublished studies

Up to now, we have assumed that all important research can be accessed through the published literature, but this is not true. A systematic review of studies following all initiated research approved by local ethics committees showed that 25–50% of all initiated studies are never published in full.[19] Follow up of clinical trials funded by the National Institutes of Health showed that a lower percentage remained unpublished (only 7%).[20]

Failure to publish is a problem because, as several studies have now shown, publication is associated with positive or statistically significant study outcomes. That is, there is a publication bias such that investigators are less likely to publish study findings if the results are "negative".[19] Those who perform systematic reviews without making an effort to identify unpublished data thus run the risk of overestimating a beneficial effect.[21] Publication bias is not only a matter of selective publication of entire research studies, but also relates to selective publication of outcomes. We currently have no estimates of how often this happens, but suffice to say that the tendency for preferential reporting of statistically significant results in journal articles contributes to the problem.

Good methods for identifying unpublished studies and outcomes have not been developed. There is some evidence that publication bias may be associated with industry funding sources,[22] and that information of this type may be particularly hard to come by.[23] Cochrane reviewers have specifically reported on the difficulties of obtaining unpublished information for their reviews, regardless of funding source.[24,25] Hetherington and colleagues tried writing to 42 000 perinatal researchers internationally to identify unpublished trials conducted in the past, but this effort was essentially unfruitful.[26]

There is widespread agreement that the best way to ensure comprehensive identification of clinical trials, regardless of funding source, is through prospective registration at study initiation. Though progress has been made in this area,[27] coverage tends to favour government supported trials, with industry trials less well identified.[28]

The Cochrane Collaboration is only beginning to address how best to identify and include all trials in its databases, regardless of publication status. Until a comprehensive register of all initiated studies exists, individual reviewers will need to assess the likelihood that publication bias could influence their findings.

Conclusion

It is perhaps presumptuous to think we can have truly evidence-based medicine if finding the evidence is so difficult. The Cochrane Collaboration has made a concerted effort to ensure that resources are available to assist with the process, but some problems remain, especially those related to identification of unpublished results. Interestingly, very little parallel effort has taken place related to ensuring complete identification of the evidence for systematic reviews of observational and epidemiological data.[29] This fact lends further support to the decision of the Cochrane Collaboration to focus on summarising evidence on interventions using the highest possible evidence, preferably randomised controlled trials.

References

1. Canadian Task Force on Preventive Health Care. http://www.ctfphc.org, accessed on 26 May 2003.
2. US National Library of Medicine *MEDLINE Fact Sheet*, 2000. http://www.nlm.nih.gov/pubs/factsheets/medline.html, accessed on 26 May 2003.
3. Egger M, Zellweger-Zahner T, Schneider M, Junker C, Lengeler C, Antes G. Language bias in randomised controlled trials published in English and German. *Lancet* 1997;**350**:326–9.
4. Joyce J, Rabe Hesketh S, Wessely S. Reviewing the reviews: the example of chronic fatigue syndrome. *JAMA* 1998;**280**:264–6.
5. Barnes J, Abbot NC, Harkness EF, Ernst E. Articles on complementary medicine in the mainstream medical literature: an investigation of MEDLINE, 1966 through 1996. *Arch Int Med* 1999;**159**:1721–5.
6. Dickersin K, Scherer R, Lefebvre C. Identifying relevant studies for systematic reviews. *BMJ* 1994;**309**:1286–91.
7. Dickersin K, Manheimer E, Wieland LS *et al.* Development of a Centralized Register of Controlled Clinical Trials: The Cochrane Collaboration's CENTRAL Database. *Eval Health Professions* 2002;**25**:38–64.
8. Avenell A, Handoll HH, Grant AM. Lessons for search strategies from a systematic review, in the *Cochrane Library*, of nutritional supplementation trials in patients after hip fracture. *Am J Clin Nutr* 2001;**73**:505–10.
9. Suarez Almazor ME, Belseck E, Homik J, Dorgan M, Ramos Remus C. Identifying clinical trials in the medical literature with electronic databases: MEDLINE alone is not enough. *Control Clin Trials* 2000;**21**:476–87.
10. Scherer RW, Langenberg P. Full publication of results initially presented in abstracts (Cochrane Methodology Review). In: Cochrane Collaboration: *Cochrane Library*. Issue 1. Oxford: Update Software, 2002.
11. McAuley L, Pham B, Tugwell P, Moher D. Does the inclusion of grey literature influence estimates of intervention effectiveness reported in meta-analyses? *Lancet* 2000;**356**:1228–31.
12. Dickersin K, Scherer R, Lefebvre C. Identification of relevant studies for systematic reviews. *BMJ* 1994;**309**:1286–91.
13. Hopewell S, Clarke M, Lusher A, Lefebvre C, Westby M. A comparison of handsearching versus electronic searching to identify reports of randomized trials. *Stat Med* 2002;**21**:1625–34.
14. Mallett S, Hopewell S, Clarke M. Grey literature in systematic reviews: The first 1000 Cochrane systematic reviews. In: *4th Symposium on Systematic Reviews: Pushing the Boundaries*, 2–4 July 2002, Oxford, UK. Abstract no 5.
15. Pao ML. Perusing the literature via citation links [published erratum]. *Comput Biomed Res* 1993;**26**:143–56.
16. Gotzsche PC. Reference bias in reports of drug trials. *BMJ (Clin Res Ed)*.1987;**295**:654–6.
17. Ravnskov U. Cholesterol lowering trials in coronary heart disease: frequency of citation and outcome. *BMJ* 1992;**305**:15–19.
18. Hutchinson BG, Oxman AD, Lloyd S. Comprehensiveness and bias in reporting clinical trials. *Can Fam Physician* 1995;**41**:1356–60.
19. Dickersin K. How important is publication bias? A synthesis of available data. *AIDS Educ Prev* 1997;**9**(Suppl 1):15–21.
20. Dickersin K, Min YI. NIH clinical trials and publication bias. *Online J Curr Clin Trials* 1993;Doc No 50.
21. Simes RJ. Publication bias: the case for an international registry of clinical trials. *J Clin Oncol* 1986;**4**:1529–41.
22. Easterbrook PJ, Berlin JA, Gopalan R, Matthews DR. Publication bias in clinical research. *Lancet* 1991;**337**:867–72.
23. Herxheimer A. Data on file cited in pharmaceutical advertisements: What are they? The International Congress on Biomedical Peer Review and Global Communications, September 1997, Prague, Czech Republic, 1997.
24. Hadhazy V, Ezzo J, Berman B. How valuable is effort to contact authors to obtain missing data in systematic reviews? *7th Annual Cochrane Colloquium Abstracts*, October 1999, Rome, Italy, 1999.
25. Walters EH, Walters JA. Many reports of RCTs give insufficient data for Cochrane reviewers. *BMJ* 1999;**319**:257.
26. Hetherington J, Dickersin K, Chalmers I, Meinert CL. Retrospective and prospective identification of unpublished controlled trials: lessons from a survey of obstetricians and pediatricians. *Pediatrics* 1989;**84**:374–80.
27. McCray AT. Better access to information about clinical trials. *Ann Intern Med* 2000;**133**:609–14.
28. Manheimer E, Anderson D. Survey of public information about ongoing clinical trials funded by industry: evaluation of completeness and accessibility. *BMJ* 2002;**325**:528–31.
29. Dickersin K. Systematic reviews in epidemiology: Why are we so far behind? *Int J Epidemiol* 2002;**31**:6–12.

2 Synthesising the evidence

Jennifer Evans

The output of the biomedical publication industry is huge. It has been estimated that individual clinicians would need to read nearly 17 articles a day to keep up to date with original articles published in their field.[1] When we prepare systematic reviews we aim to combine the available evidence into a whole in order to understand better and, hopefully, to answer a clinical question.

Systematic reviews avoid bias and improve precision

The main aim of a systematic review is to avoid bias and to improve precision. *Bias* is a broad term encompassing all the possible types of systematic error that may lead to incorrect conclusions being drawn from observational and experimental studies. In this context we can view the systematic review as an observational study of the experimental studies on a particular topic. Since systematic reviews are conducted retrospectively, they are prone to the effects of bias.

When we talk about *precision*, we are referring to random or biological variation. The main way that we can improve precision, or reduce random error, is to increase the size of the study. Within systematic reviews, it is often possible, and desirable, to pool the results of the studies included in the review to obtain an overall measure of treatment effect. This statistical pooling is termed *meta-analysis*. The pooled estimate will be more precise than individual estimates from the contributing studies.

Steps involved in doing a systematic review

Box 2.1 sets out the steps involved in conducting a systematic review. These structured steps have been developed in order to minimise bias and improve precision. It is important to see a systematic review as a research project in its own right. As in primary research, a protocol should be prepared, setting out all the work that is to be done. The protocol should state clearly the problem to be addressed, and define the population, interventions and outcome measures to be used. Inclusion and exclusion criteria should be described and the analysis strategy should be developed in detail. The purpose of this detailed protocol

---

Box 2.1 Steps in conducting a systematic review (Source: adapted from Egger and Smith, 2001[2])

1 Formulate review question.

2 Define inclusion and exclusion criteria:
- participants
- interventions and outcomes
- study designs and methodological quality.

3 Locate studies (see Chapter 1).

4 Select studies:
- have eligibility checked by more than one observer
- develop strategy to resolve disagreements
- keep log of excluded studies, with reasons for exclusions.

5 Assess study quality:
- consider assessment by more than one observer
- use simple checklists rather than quality scales
- always assess concealment of treatment allocation, blinding and handling of patient attrition
- consider masking of observers to authors, institutions and journals.

6 Extract data:
- design and pilot data extraction form
- consider data extraction by more than one observer
- consider masking of observer to authors, institutions and journals.

7 Analyse and present results:
- tabulate results from individual studies
- examine forest plot
- explore possible sources of heterogeneity
- consider meta-analysis of all trials or subgroups of trials
- perform sensitivity analyses, examine funnel plots
- make list of excluded studies available to interested readers.

8 Interpret results:
- consider limitations, including publication and related biases
- consider strength of evidence
- consider applicability
- consider numbers needed to treat to benefit/harm
- consider economic implications
- consider implications for future research.

is to prevent decisions about the conduct of the review being influenced by the results.

Location and appraisal of relevant studies

The individual studies that are included in the systematic review form the "data" to be collected. A major task of the reviewer is to identify all the studies that might be relevant to the review (see Chapter 1). Having identified the potentially relevant studies, the reviewer has to decide whether or not to include them in the review. It is important that this process is independent of the results of the study. The best way to ensure this is to have clear criteria for inclusion and exclusion. Another method is to have studies selected independently by at least two people. Masking the study results and identity of the authors is very time-consuming and empirical studies of their usefulness have been contradictory.[3,4] Each study also has to be appraised critically in order to assess how likely it is that its results are biased.

Data extraction

Data extraction should be done with as much care as would be taken for data collection in a primary research study. In many cases it will be necessary to contact study authors for clarification. Double data entry and other common sense checks to ensure the accuracy of the data entered into the review are useful.

Individual patient data

In some situations it is feasible and desirable to obtain individual patient data from all studies that contribute to the review. This is particularly useful in studies where time to an event is the outcome of interest. The reviewer can also perform simple checks on the data to improve the validity of the review and can explore appropriate subgroups in more depth. What the reviewer cannot do is pool the data ignoring the studies from which the data have been drawn. The methods of combining the results of the studies are similar to those where individual patient data are not available.

Ways of presenting data

There are several different ways of presenting data drawn from individual studies. Table 2.1 summarises the advantages and disadvantages of the different measures.

Deeks *et al.* have set out criteria for use when deciding which measure of effect to use, including consistency, mathematical properties and ease of interpretation.[5] In general people find it easier to interpret a risk than an odds ratio. Conveniently, the odds ratio is a good estimate of the risk ratio when events are rare, which is often the case in healthcare studies. In these situations, the odds ratio can be analysed and the risk ratio can be interpreted. However, in situations when events are common, odds ratios will overestimate the benefits and harms of a treatment.

Graphical presentation

The forest plot is the traditional way of presenting the data in a systematic review. Figure 7.1 on page x shows an example of a forest plot, in which the results of individual studies are plotted horizontally with a line representing the confidence intervals. All the studies are plotted one after another and, if appropriate, a combined estimate is presented at the bottom of the diagram. The order in which the studies are plotted can be varied, but often they are presented chronologically.

When not to combine data from different studies

A statistical synthesis, or meta-analysis, is not always recommended in a review. If the studies give very different results then a summary measure will hide the different results and will be meaningless. It is possible to do a statistical test to measure the level of heterogeneity, although this test is not very powerful. In some situations, the reviewer might decide that a summary measure is not indicated because of important differences between the individual studies. However, these judgements may vary from reviewer to reviewer and might explain differences that are sometimes found between different reviews of the same research.

Interpreting data that has not been combined

A common pitfall in interpreting data is counting positive studies. For example, if none of the contributing studies is statistically significant, this is commonly interpreted as evidence of no effect. However, if the results were to be combined, the overall pooled estimate could be statistically significant. It is always important to look at the level of the effect in each contributory study. In situations when pooling is not advisable the results need to be discussed in a way that avoids counting positive studies.

Table 2.1 Effect measures

Type of outcome measure	Type of effect measure	Synonyms/ acronyms	Calculation	Advantages	Disadvantages
Binary, for example disease vs disease free	Odds ratio	–	Odds of event in intervention group/odds of event in control group	Convenient mathematical properties	Difficult to interpret; differs from relative risk if outcome is common. Tends to overestimate both beneficial and harmful effects of treatment
	Risk ratio	Relative risk	Risk of event in intervention group/risk of event in control group	More intuitively comprehensible than odds ratio	Constrained when considering good outcomes and common events, for example if the event rate in the control group is 66% then the observed risk ratio cannot exceed 1·5 [5]
	Risk difference	Absolute risk reduction	Risk of event in intervention group minus risk of event in control group	Useful measure of clinical significance	Measure constrained, for example if meta-analysis produces risk difference of 25% this cannot be applied to situations where the initial risk is less than 25%
	Number needed to treat for one person to benefit	NNT	1/risk difference	Useful measure of clinical significance	Cannot pool directly but can be derived from other statistics in the meta-analysis
Continuous, for example biological measure such as intraocular pressure	Difference in means		Mean in treatment group minus mean in control group	–	–
	Standardised difference		Mean in treatment group divided by standard deviation minus mean in control group divided by standard deviation	Useful when different measurement scales have been used in different studies	–
Time to event	Hazard ratios	–		–	Meta-analysis usually requires individual patient data

Fixed effect versus random models for combining data

Broadly, there are two models for pooling study results. Fixed effect models weight the summary statistics according to some attribute, usually size, of the contributing studies (inverse variance, Mantel-Haenszel and Peto). Random effects models include an estimate of between-study variation in the estimate of the overall effect (DerSimonian and Laird). There is no consensus on which model is better and they will give the same results unless there is considerable heterogeneity, in which case the random effects model will give a more conservative estimate of effect size.[5]

Sensitivity analyses

Sensitivity analyses aim to evaluate the extent to which the results of the review are dependent upon key assumptions. Usually this involves excluding or including a group of trials of lesser quality.

Subgroup analyses

Subgroup analyses are subject to bias. For this reason it is recommended that the subgroups of interest be set out before the review is started. *Post hoc* analyses are particularly difficult to interpret because significant differences may have arisen due to chance. However, some would argue that one role of the systematic review is to explore possible differences of effect in different populations.

Statistical issues relating to eyes

There are particular statistical issues in randomised controlled trials relating to eyes because each individual has two eyes and the outcome of the two eyes is related, i.e. not statistically independent. As statistical methods assume statistical independence, in general, the analysis of studies where the results from both eyes are included is not straightforward. An analogous situation is the case of cluster-randomised trials, where the extra variation introduced by the clustering needs to be taken into account when calculating the confidence intervals. Currently the methods for dealing with the meta-analysis of such data are not well developed. One strategy commonly used in surgical trials is to apply the intervention to one eye only, in which case the problem does not arise.

Summary

The statistical pooling (meta-analysis) of study results forms a very small part of the process of synthesising the evidence. It reduces the effect of random error and therefore improves the precision of the estimate of the effect of an intervention. The value of systematic reviews lies in the efforts put into locating and appraising all the available evidence, in order to reduce the effects of bias.

References

1. Davidoff F, Haynes B, Sackett D, Smith R. Evidence-based medicine. *BMJ* 1995;**310**:1085–6.
2. Egger M, Smith GD. Principles of and procedures for systematic reviews. In: Egger M, Smith GD, Altman DG, eds. *Systematic Reviews in Health Care: Meta-analysis in context.* London: BMJ Publishing Group, 2001, pp. 23–42.
3. Moher D, Pham B, Jones A *et al.* Does quality of reports of randomised trials affect estimates of intervention efficacy reported in meta-analyses? *Lancet* 1998;**352**:609–13.
4. Berlin JA. Does blinding of readers affect the results of meta-analyses? *Lancet* 1998;**350**:185–6.
5. Deeks JJ, Altman DG, Bradburn MJ. Statistical methods for examining heterogeneity and combining results from several studies in meta-analysis. In: Egger M, Smith GD, Altman DG, eds. *Systematic Reviews in Health Care: Meta-analysis in context.* London: BMJ Publishing Group, 2001, pp. 285–312.

3 Evidence in practice

Richard Wormald

Introduction

A common concern about the emergence of evidence-based medicine (EBM) is the suggestion that medicine will be reduced to an automated "recipe book" method and the potential for skill and excellence in clinical practice will be lost. It is true that modern demands of clinical governance require the achievement of uniformly high standards of care. One of the means of implementing and maintaining standards of governance is through the development of clinical guidelines. Clearly, these need to be based on good quality evidence.

Evidence-based practice is in fact the converse of restrictive recipe book care. The culture of EBM has emerged with a shift in the paradigm of medical teaching from a factual basis, learnt by rote, to one of enquiry and thinking in terms of probabilities; moving from certainties to measures of uncertainty. Thus, the clinician challenges established dogma and strives for new answers to old problems. This approach protects the clinician from professional boredom and means that a blind eye is not turned on observations that do not fit the factual paradigm. It allows for progress.

None of these prescriptions limit the freedom of the clinician to strive for individual excellence in the diagnosis, prognosis and offer of therapies to their patients who understand the trade-off of risk and benefit for any given treatment. Archie Cochrane's view was simple: if the taxpayer was to fund public health services, then finance should be provided only for interventions whose effectiveness was beyond doubt.[1]

Evidence may be applied in three main domains: individual patient care, policy making and research prioritisation.

Individual patient care

Modern clinical practice requires the setting of clinical standards for governance and this is achieved through guideline development. Guidelines are used for setting local standards for the delivery of care. These standards can then be the subject of regular audit to ensure the guidelines are being followed.

Guideline development should be an evidence-based process and organisations such as the Scottish Intercollegiate Guideline Network (SIGN)[2] have refined the process with graded levels of evidence for each guideline. Guideline development also feeds back to research prioritisation when evidence is absent. Systematic reviews are valuable in providing accessible unbiased summaries of evidence for those developing clinical guidelines.

Evidence may sometimes contradict current practice. The use of antibiotic ointment and an eye pad remains standard management for corneal abrasion. A few trials have examined the effectiveness of this measure and have failed to show any benefit (see Chapter 21). So why is this evidence not applied? There is much debate on what factors actually influence and change practice. A key issue remains the need for clinicians to be aware of the evidence. The importance of dissemination of research findings is critical. The Cochrane Collaboration, the numerous agencies for setting standards of care and publications such as *Clinical Evidence* are all dedicated to tackling this issue.

Bedside EBM, as advocated by David Sackett,[3] means asking questions relevant to the individual patient during a ward round and using live online searches to seek answers to those questions. This approach is probably not compatible with the accelerated rounds used by surgeons but it is an important training methodology that teaches training clinicians to question the evidence base for every clinical situation.

Patients or consumers of health care are increasingly aware of the importance of evidence in guiding their choice of treatment. Consumer networks are becoming increasingly vocal and demand access to evidence in lay terminology that allows them to make informed choices.

Policy making

Major decisions are made by institutions such as academies, colleges and non-governmental organisations, as well as ministries of health, which require reliable information or good evidence as their basis. Such decisions often follow rather than precede changes in practice. Thus, standards are set based on what is observed to be common practice and therefore acceptable by consensus. How then do changes occur? Often, a new treatment option emerges with much marketing support from the manufacturers or having been pioneered by individuals who have influence and reputation in the profession. Acceptance of the new intervention as an important advance occurs and those who fail to adopt the change are in danger of being regarded as obsolete and outdated. Sometimes trials are then undertaken to justify the change in practice that has already occurred.

This probably describes the process of change from intracapsular to extracapsular cataract extraction in the 1980s. The shift was an expensive and challenging adventure for ophthalmologists in the more advanced economies but presented insurmountable obstacles to those in poorer parts of the world. The evidence indicates that there is not much difference in risk of adverse outcome between the two techniques compared to the impact of any cataract surgery versus none (see Chapter 32).[4] Forcing experts in the old technique to change may actually have done harm by reducing the throughput of operations and causing poorer outcomes as a result of a long learning curve for the new technique. Ironically, it is not uncommon for the extracapsular procedure to be performed without the implantation of an intraocular lens where patients cannot afford to purchase the lens. When funds are insufficient, an operation that was previously superseded by the intracapsular technique (an improvement because of the absence of posterior capsular opacification (PCO)), is almost inevitable in an extracapsular procedure without an intraocular lens. It was the intraocular lens, whether in the anterior or posterior chamber, that had the critical influence on outcome. Good quality trial evidence on the longer term outcomes of cataract surgery and PCO rates in the developing world setting where there are no Nd:YAG lasers is still lacking.

There are worse examples where irrevocable harm has been done. Diethylcarbamazine (DEC) was widely distributed in regions where onchocerciasis was endemic on the basis that it was known to be a powerful microfilaricide. Death of microfilaria in the eye caused uveitis (the Mazzotti reaction) but it took years to realise that DEC actually precipitated blindness by causing an inflammatory optic neuropathy.

These examples illustrate the importance of the use of evidence in informing policy. This includes organisation of care as well as specific interventions. It embraces decisions on public health policy, sanitation and health promotion. When evidence is found to be absent, new studies are needed before change in practice is implemented.

Research prioritisation

Within the NHS, there is a debate on the value of evidence and the extent to which research is useful in guiding practice. Although there are some who feel that scarce healthcare resources should not be wasted on research but should be committed only to patient care, most

recognise the value of evidence that guides practice. But research resources are seriously limited and providers of funding need guidance on the evidence that is most needed.

Critically important in making funding decisions is consideration of what is already known and what is not known about the effectiveness of interventions. The description of the evidence base needs a scientific and unbiased method, which is provided by systematic reviews.

It is the policy of the UK's Medical Research Council[5] to require applicants to include the results of a systematic review of the effectiveness of an intervention in their application for funding for a new trial. Not only does the review provide the detailed summary of the existing knowledge but it educates the applicant about the pitfalls and difficulties encountered by previous research. The exact knowledge deficit in terms of the reference population, the types of intervention and the most relevant and reliable way of measuring outcome can be determined.

The WHO has adopted the SAFE strategy as part of the VISION 2020 initiative to eliminate blinding trachoma by the year 2020.[6] This is an example of a policy preceding the systematic description of the evidence base. However, this pragmatic policy has helped focus resources. Systematic reviews of each of the components will identify the key questions in implementing this strategy. None of the interventions yet have sound evidence on which any acceptably precise estimate of effectiveness and cost effectiveness can be made (see Chapter 20). The WHO and other international non-governmental organisations can use systematic reviews of these questions to make decisions about priorities in funding new research to fill the existing gaps in the evidence base for their policies.

Quality of evidence

Randomised controlled trials (RCTs) and systematic reviews of RCTs are considered to provide the highest level of evidence. This is because the process of randomisation, innate in the design of a properly conducted RCT, is the best way of controlling for both known and unknown confounding factors that may determine differences between control and intervention arms of a study. Thus, observed differences in outcome can be attributed to the intervention alone.

Observational studies can deal only with known confounders in the design and/or analysis. When no such confounding is present, observational studies and RCTs may produce the same results, as has been observed by Benson and Hartz.[7] Because so many factors may be present that consciously or unconsciously influence clinicians in the conduct of studies of effectiveness of new interventions, clinician scientists need to adopt the scepticism of laboratory scientists in attributing cause and effect before believing and implementing the findings of such studies.

It is for this reason that the Cochrane Collaboration, the BMJ's *Clinical Evidence* and the authors of this book have decided to deal only with RCTs. It leaves out a huge body of lesser evidence that may or may not influence our practice but there must be doubt of the value of summarising studies of effectiveness other than those that use the optimum design.

A systematic method is needed for judging the quality of trials selected for summary. This is an evolving art but current policies advise considering allocation concealment, masking of participants and observers of outcome, completeness of follow-up in the randomisation groups and intention to treat analysis.[8]

Many now agree that there is no satisfactory method for giving trials a single trial quality score. A trial may be excellent in all but one critical domain and hence score well despite being fundamentally flawed. Thus each domain should be considered independently. More can be read about these issues on the Cochrane website at http://www.cochrane.org.

Limitations of trial evidence

There are two important areas where RCTs fail to inform clinicians. The first concerns the external validity of trials. Strict inclusion and exclusion criteria employed in many studies mean that the effectiveness of interventions on population subgroups excluded from studies remains unknown. Inevitably, vulnerable subgroups such as pregnant women and children often remain in an evidence vacuum.

In addition, it is recognised that participants in RCTs fare better, even in the control or placebo arm, than in the real world. Thus an important addition to the armoury of evidence is the outcome study, where a large representative and unselected or sequential series of interventions are monitored for their outcome. Good examples of this are the national surveys of cataract surgery outcome conducted by the Royal College of Ophthalmologists.[9] These studies are important in establishing standards for care that reflect reality more closely than RCTs.

The second concern is that trials cannot inform the clinician of rare but serious adverse events. Trials are rarely large enough to answer these important questions and follow-up is seldom long enough to detect late but serious complications. For drugs there are mechanisms for reporting such events to a central authority but no such mechanisms are uniformly in place for surgical techniques. An example of this is the concern that has arisen about the long-term safety of mitomycin in the control of wound healing in glaucoma surgery. Surveillance systems are developing, such as the BOSU for monitoring rare but important adverse outcomes.[10] There is no doubt that better and more reliable information systems are required to deal with this issue but one might expect with the development of reliable methods of information retrieval, systematic audit of outcomes will help.

Conclusion

The importance of the emergence of evidence-based medicine is freeing the evolution of clinical practice from the dangerous biases of the medical market and fashion to a protocol-driven scientific process. Contrary to the fears of limiting clinical freedom, evidence-based practice releases clinicians from the factual paradigm to understanding the importance of probability and levels of uncertainty. This opens the mind of the clinician to question continually the basis of their practice and to the possibility of progress.

Enormous challenges remain and there are many areas of our practice that present significant difficulties to clinical researchers who wish to fill the gaps in the evidence revealed in the following chapters; not least, the huge difficulty in finding funding for clinical research.

At least two of the annual meetings of the international Cochrane Collaboration have been addressed by the host country's minister of health. On both such occasions, the ministers have agreed that the importance and value of evidence to inform health policy is essential but that it rarely happens. We hope that this wisdom will eventually prevail on those who provide funding for clinical research.

References

1. Cochrane AL. *Effectiveness and Efficiency. Random Reflections on Health Services.* London: Nuffield Provincial Hospitals Trust, 1972.
2. Scottish Intercollegiate Guideline Network. http://www.sign.ac.uk
3. Sackett DL, Straus SE. Finding and applying evidence during clinical rounds: the "evidence cart". *JAMA* 1998;**280**:1336–8.
4. Snellingen T, Evans JR, Ravilla T, Foster A. Surgical interventions for age-related cataract. In: Cochrane Collaboration: *Cochrane Library.* Issue 2. Oxford: Update Software, 2002.
5. *MRC guidelines for good clinical practice in clinical trials: 1998.* London: Medical Research Council, 1998, Appendix 2:2.4.
6. Cook JA. Trachoma and the safe strategy. *J Community Eye Health* http://www.jceh.co.uk/journal/32_1.asp
7. Benson K, Hartz AJ. A comparison of observational studies and randomized controlled trials. *N Engl J Med* 2000;**342**:1878–86.
8. Juni P, Altman DG, Egger M. Systematic reviews in health care: Assessing the quality of controlled clinical trials. *BMJ* 2001;**323**:42–6.
9. Desai P, Minassian DC, Reidy A. National cataract surgery survey 1997–8: a report of the results of the clinical outcomes. *Br J Ophthalmol* 1999;**83**:1336–40.
10. Foot B, Stanford M, Rahi J, Thompson J. The British Ophthalmological Surveillance Unit: an evaluation of the first 3 years. *Eye* 2003;**17**:9–15.

Section II

Primary care

Aziz Sheikh, Editor

Primary care: mission statement

Why does this section focus on primary care?

There are two main reasons for focusing on primary care. Firstly, primary care clinicians are, in many parts of the world, the first port of call for those suffering from ocular symptoms. Eye-related consultations represent a significant proportion of the general practitioners workload, representing an estimated 1 in 20 of all general practitioner consultations in economically developed countries such as Britain. Only a small minority of these consultations are for conditions that may require subsequent referral for specialist assessment and treatment and these conditions are covered in other sections of this book. The majority of patients can, however, safely be diagnosed and treated within a primary care setting and it is the management of these commonly encountered external ocular conditions that forms the focus of this section. Secondly, as health systems in many parts of the world increasingly begin to focus on ways of preventing visual impairment, there is an emerging body of evidence, drawn from primary care, evaluating the role of screening interventions for ocular problems.

The main aim of this section is to describe and critically appraise the available evidence from trials from the Cochrane Eyes and Vision Group Register and published systematic reviews of randomised controlled trials of treatments for bacterial, viral and allergic conjunctivitis and screening interventions for visual impairment in older people. Contributors have also highlighted areas in which evidence is lacking and identified key questions that have yet to be addressed in relation to the management of these primary care problems.

4 Allergic conjunctivitis

Christopher G Owen, Katherine Henshaw, Liam Smeeth, Aziz Sheikh

Background

Primary eye care physicians can expect between 2 and 5% of all consultations to be related to eye conditions.[1] Fifteen percent of these are caused by allergic conjunctivitis,[2] which may or may not be accompanied with rhinitis (so called allergic rhinoconjunctivitis).[3] Half of these cases are likely to be diagnosed with seasonal allergic conjunctivitis (SAC),[4] which is a type 1, IgE mediated hypersensitivity to grass or tree pollen (the allergen). Hence, most are seen when pollens are present in the atmosphere (typically between April and August in the UK). Cases may present severely in the rare event of excessive allergen exposure. Perennial allergic conjunctivitis (PAC) has a similar immunology to SAC, except that the allergens, such as house dust mite (*Dermatophagoides pteronyssinus*), animal dander and moulds, are present all year round. These conditions do not affect the cornea (i.e. are non-sight threatening), and affect approximately a fifth of the population,[5–7] including both genders. Racial and geographical differences in prevalence remain unclear.[7] Symptoms associated with this condition, such as ocular itching and redness, often accompanied with tearing and nasal congestion, are treated by avoidance of offending antigens (although this is not always possible), topical mast cell stabilisers and topical antihistamines (with and without a vasoconstrictor).[8] Systemic antihistamines can be used in association with other atopic symptoms. Ophthalmic specialists treat serious sight threatening atopic conditions such as vernal keratoconjunctivitis (VKC) and atopic keratoconjunctivitis (AKC), as these may require surgical or topical steroid intervention.

Questions

What is the comparative efficacy of topical mast cell stabilisers and topical antihistamines (with and without a decongestant) in providing symptomatic relief from allergic conjunctivitis (SAC and PAC)?

Limitations of this chapter

The efficacy of oral antihistamines in the treatment of allergic conjunctivitis, and the use of steroids and NSAIDs for more serious conditions, such as VKC and AKC, are not considered, although these are both the subject of ongoing Cochrane reviews. In addition, the treatment of foreign body induced giant capillary conjunctivitis is not considered, as this is often complicated by the contact lens/prosthetic used.

Question

Do topical mast cell stabilisers (sodium cromoglycate, nedocromil sodium and lodoxamide) confer benefit over placebo in providing symptomatic relief from allergic conjunctivitis?

The evidence

A systematic review of all double-masked, randomised, placebo-controlled crossover and non-crossover trials comparing topical mast cell stabilisers with placebo in the management of allergic conjunctivitis, identified from the Cochrane Eyes and Vision Group Register, was performed. The authors were unaware of any previous systematic review.

Sodium cromoglycate

Eighteen double-masked studies that compared use of topical sodium cromoglycate with placebo were found. Eight studies recorded subjective symptoms whilst using treatment and placebo interventions, including ocular itching, burning, soreness and lacrimation. Five studies reported an improvement in a variety of subjective symptoms whilst using topical sodium cromoglycate preparations, and the remaining three trials found no difference in symptoms between treatment groups. Symptoms were scored and reported in different ways, with insufficient data for formal meta-analysis (this was also true of studies that contained clinician assessment of ocular signs).

Ascertainment of preferred treatment in crossover trials and overall assessment of perceived treatment benefit in non-crossover trials was more consistently reported. The characteristics of these six small trials are detailed in Table 4.1[9–14]; note that the largest study found less difference in preference between treatment groups. Overall, a random effects estimate (due to considerable heterogeneity between estimates; $P<0.001$) showed that those using topical sodium cromoglycate preparations were 17 times more likely (95% CI 4–78) to perceive benefit than those using placebo (Figure 4.1). Heterogeneity between estimates may be explained by differences in sample ages, timing of the study and/or active preparations used (see Table 4.1). The combined estimate may overestimate the beneficial effect of sodium cromoglycate, as studies that reported no differences in subjective symptoms between treatment groups did not have sufficient data for inclusion. No important side effects with the active treatment were reported, although one historic study that used phenylethanol reported stinging on installation both in treatment and placebo groups.[11]

Nedocromil sodium

We found five double-masked, randomised controlled trials that compared use of topical nedocromil sodium and placebo (over at least one month) for the treatment of SAC (Table 4.2).[15–19] To facilitate masking, placebo drops were coloured yellow with riboflavin (0·005%) in all studies, to make them indistinguishable from the active preparation. Subjective symptoms (including itching and overall eye condition) were less in those using nedocromil sodium compared to those using placebo. The differences were statistically significant in three of these studies,[15,17,18] and of borderline significance in the remaining two studies.[16,19] Heterogeneity in the approaches to subjective recording of symptoms and presentation of results did not allow for a formal meta-analysis (this was also true of clinician-based assessment of treatment efficacy). Patient-perceived total and moderate effectiveness of treatment was reported in all studies (see Table 4.2). A fixed effects estimate (as differences between estimates were not statistically significant; $P=0.27$) showed that those using nedocromil sodium were 1·8 times more likely (95% CI 1·3–2·6) to be moderately or totally controlled than those using placebo (Figure 4.2).

The patient-perceived benefit of nedocromil sodium compared to placebo appears less than the benefit of sodium cromoglycate over placebo. However, the estimate associated with nedocromil sodium is derived from studies with more participants (compare Table 4.1 with Table 4.2), is consistent between studies, and is associated with narrower confidence intervals. Apart from an unpleasant taste immediately after instillation of the active treatment, no other important side effects were reported.

Lodoxamide tromethamine

Only one randomised controlled trial of four weeks' duration compared the use of lodoxamide tromethamine 0·1% with placebo for the treatment of allergic conjunctivitis in adults.[20] Those using lodoxamide (n = 14) reported significantly less symptoms of lacrimation, burning–itching,

photophobia and lid swelling compared to those using placebo (n = 13). Fewer patients treated with lodoxamide (n = 2/14) compared to the placebo group (n = 11/13) complained of symptoms requiring additional pharmacological treatment. Three other studies using conjunctival provocation tests to a variety of allergens showed greater short-term symptomatic relief in those using lodoxamide compared to placebo. Cytological assessment in these three provocation studies found fewer inflammatory cells in the tear fluid of the lodoxamide-treated group. Alas, due to heterogeneity in methods and presentation of results, a meta-analysis of these studies could not be performed. No side effects associated with the active treatment were reported.

Comment

Although these studies consistently report improvement in symptoms of SAC in those using different topical mast cell stabilisers versus placebo, there was no evidence from randomised controlled trials to support the use of one type of mast cell stabiliser over another. Hence, treatment preferences can only be based on convenience of use (with reduced frequency of instillation for nedocromil preparations) and laboratory studies.

Question

Do topical antihistamines (levocabastine hydrochloride, azelastine hydrochloride, emedastine, antazoline sulphate) confer benefit over placebo in providing symptomatic relief from allergic conjunctivitis?

The evidence

The authors were unaware of any systematic review comparing the use of topical antihistamine preparations with placebo for the treatment of allergic conjunctivitis. In total, nine double-masked, randomised controlled trials (both crossover and non-crossover designs) on the Cochrane Vision Group database were identified; six studies compared treatment with levocabastine with placebo, one study compared azelastine hydrochloride with placebo, one study compared emedastine with placebo, and one other study from the 1970s compared antazoline phosphate with placebo (Table 4.3).[21–29]

Experimental[25] and laboratory studies[30] have shown rapid modes of action of antihistamines, especially in comparison to mast cell stabilisers. Hence, most studies used short-term conjunctival provocation tests to a variety of allergens, sometimes performed outside the pollen season, to establish the relative efficacy of topical antihistamines and placebo (see Table 4.3). A variety of symptoms and signs,

Table 4.1 Studies reporting the patient-perceived benefit of topical sodium cromoglycate versus placebo, included in the meta-analysis.

Reference	Type of trial	Setting	Sample age	Time of year	Patient inclusion criteria	Patient exclusion criteria	Active treatment	Length of trial	Number that preferred placebo	Number that preferred active
Greenbaum, 1977[9]	RCT	St Joseph's Hospital and McMaster University, Ontario, Canada	Mean 29 yrs, 14–52 yrs	Ragweed Aug 1976	Ragweed allergic conjunctivitis, symptomatic for 2 yrs, with allergic rhinitis, skin prick positive to ragweed pollen	Perennial symptoms or autumn seasonal symptoms excluded	4% SCG	1 mon	8/14	15/15
Hechanova, 1984[10]	RCT	Makati Medical Centre, Philippines	Mean 35, 5–71 yrs	Not stated	Bilateral chronic allergic conjunctivitis	Other ophthalmic pathology, contact lens wearers, topical or systemic steroids, systemic antihistamines	4% SCG	4 wks	4/19	17/19
Lindsay, 1979[11]	RCT	Bangor Hospital, Northern Ireland, UK	All ages	Grass pollen Apr – Sept (mostly May – July)	On a "hayfever register", history of eye symptoms and hayfever rhinitis, positive skin test to grass pollens	Other eye diseases, contact lens wearers, topical or systemic steroids	2% SCG, 0·01% benzalkonium chloride, 0·4% phenylethanol	4 wks	12/33	18/20
Nizami, 1981[12]	Crossover RCT	Private patients, Torronto, Canada	Mean 28 yrs	Ragweed Aug 1980	Eye symptoms and allergic rhinitis for 2 yrs, skin prick positive to ragweed pollen	Those with perennial symptoms or on other influential medications excluded	2% SCG	1 wk	2/26	22/26

(Continued)

Table 4.1 *(Continued)*

Reference	Type of trial	Setting	Sample age	Time of year	Patient inclusion criteria	Patient exclusion criteria	Active treatment	Length of trial	Number that preferred placebo	Number that preferred active
Ruggieri, 1987[13]	RCT	Istituto di Oftalmologia, University of Rome, Italy	Mean 19 yrs, 6–40 yrs	Feb 1983 – Apr 1984	Active bilateral VKC or conjunctivitis due to a seasonal allergen	Other eye disease, purulent conjunctivitis, contact lens wearers, systemic corticosteroids or antihistamines	4% SCG ointment	4 wks	1/14	13/15
van Bijsterveld, 1984[14]	Crossover RCT	Department of Ophthalmology, Utrecht State University, The Netherlands	Mean 38.6 yrs, 9–73 yrs	Not stated	Diagnosis of chronic conjunctivitis not due to infection or trauma	Not stated	Topical SCG	4 wks	15/58	23/57

VKRC, vernal keratoconjunctivitis; SCG, Sodium cromoglycate; wks, weeks; mon, months; yrs, years

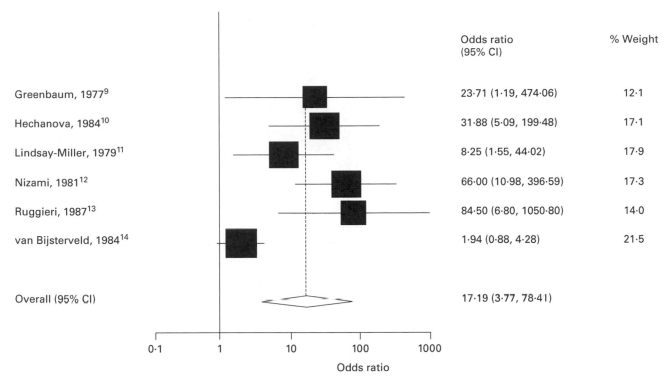

	Odds ratio (95% CI)	% Weight
Greenbaum, 1977[9]	23·71 (1·19, 474·06)	12·1
Hechanova, 1984[10]	31·88 (5·09, 199·48)	17·1
Lindsay-Miller, 1979[11]	8·25 (1·55, 44·02)	17·9
Nizami, 1981[12]	66·00 (10·98, 396·59)	17·3
Ruggieri, 1987[13]	84·50 (6·80, 1050·80)	14·0
van Bijsterveld, 1984[14]	1·94 (0·88, 4·28)	21·5
Overall (95% CI)	17·19 (3·77, 78·41)	

Figure 4.1 Odds ratio of perceived benefit of using sodium cromoglycate compared to placebo.
The box area of each study is proportional to the inverse of the variance, with horizontal lines showing 95% confidence intervals of the odds ratio. Study authors are indicated on the y-axis in alphabetical order. The pooled estimate based on a random effects model is shown by a dashed line vertical line with an estimate on the right of the line indicating benefit from sodium cromoglycate. The diamond shows the 95% CI of the pooled estimate. The statistical weight given to each study is indicated.

including itching, redness, burning and swelling, were graded using scales ranging from 0 (none) to 3 (severe),[22,24,25,29] to 0 (none) to 6 (severe)[23] or visual analogue subjective scales.[27] Formal meta-analysis was not possible, as most studies did not tabulate the mean scores and error associated with these scores. Often, P values associated with the difference between treatment groups were given (these are summarised in Table 4.3), but this does not allow the degree of benefit to be gauged. Despite this, most studies showed improvement in symptoms post provocation and improvement of symptoms of allergic conjunctivitis, especially itching (the hallmark symptom of allergic conjunctivitis) in those treated with antihistamines compared to those given placebo. There was no evidence from the randomised, controlled trials identified to support the use of one type of antihistamine over another.

Question

Are topical mast cell stabilisers (sodium cromoglycate, nedocromil sodium, lodoxamide) different from topical antihistamines (levocabastine hydrochloride, azelastine hydrochloride, emedastine, antazoline sulphate) in providing symptomatic relief from allergic conjunctivitis?

The evidence

The authors were not aware of any systematic review meta-analysis comparing the use of topical mast cell stabilisers with topical antihistamine preparations for the treatment of allergic conjunctivitis. Eight double-masked randomised, controlled trials comparing the use of topical mast cell stabilisers (five studies of sodium cromoglycate,[31–35] one of lodoxamide[36] and two of nedocromil sodium[37,38]) with one type of topical antihistamine (levocabastine) were identified on the Cochrane Eyes and Vision Group Register. Two were short-term trials comparing the response to conjunctival provocation to a variety of grass pollens 15 minutes after treatment with nedocromil sodium and levocabastine,[37] and after 18 days of treatment with sodium cromoglycate, and four hours with levocabastine,[31] in studies with 24 to 50 participants, respectively. Six trials established the longer term response to treatment with mast cell stabilisers and levocabastine in studies ranging from 14 days[36] to four months in duration,[32] with 37[33] to 110[34] study participants. Placebo drops were used to facilitate masking between treatment groups requiring different daily dosage, for example, sodium cromoglycate four times daily (qds), levocabastine twice daily (bd), ensuring an equivalent daily instillation of drops. No trials were found comparing topical

Table 4.2 Studies reporting the patient-perceived benefit of topical nedocromil sodium versus placebo, included in the meta-analysis

Reference	Setting	Sample age	Time of year	Patient inclusion criteria	Patient exclusion criteria	Active treatment	Length of trial	Number that preferred placebo	Number that preferred active
Blumenthal, 1992[15]	Multi-centre study, USA	Mean 32 yrs, 12–62 yrs	Ragweed Aug 1976	Previous seasonal allergic conjunctivitis, skin test reaction to ragweed	Women of childbearing age not using contraception, absent or minimal symptoms during previous ragweed season, not using medication for seasonal allergic conjunctivitis, evidence of perennial allergic conjunctivitis, other ocular disease	Nedocromil sodium 2%, benzalkonium chloride 0·01%, disodium edetate 0·05%, sodium chloride 0·55%, purified water	8 wks	26/71	36/69
Leino, 1990[16]	5 centres in Finland	Mean 22 yrs, 7–60 yrs	Not stated	History of seasonal allergic conjunctivitis to birch pollen for the past 2 seasons, patients with concomitant rhinitis included	Additional eye diseases, contact lens wearers, systemic or topical corticosteroids or systemic antihistamines, hyposensitization in the last year, pregnant or lactating women	Nedocromil sodium 2%, benzalkonium chloride 0·01%, disodium edetate 0·05%, sodium chloride 0·55%, purified water	4–6 wks	22/62[†]	37/64[†]
Melamed, 1994[17]	Multi-centre study, USA	Mean 32 yrs, 13–60 yrs	Grass pollen Apr – Sept (mostly May – July)	History of seasonal allergic conjunctivitis for the past 2 seasons, skin test reaction to ragweed, patients receiving immunotherapy included	Women of childbearing age not using contraception, asymptomatic or mildly symptomatic during the previous ragweed pollen season, not requiring medications to control their allergic conjunctivitis, perennial conjunctivitis, other conjunctival pathology	Nedocromil sodium 2%, benzalkonium chloride 0·01%, disodium edetate 0·05%, sodium chloride 0·55%, purified water	9 wks	14/38	26/42

(Continued)

Table 4.2 (*Continued*)

Reference	Setting	Sample age	Time of year	Patient inclusion criteria	Patient exclusion criteria	Active treatment	Length of trial	Number that preferred placebo	Number that preferred active
Moller, 1994[18]	4 paediatric clinics in Sweden	Mean 12 yrs, 6–16 yrs	Ragweed Aug 1980	History of seasonal allergic conjunctivitis for the past 2 seasons to birch pollen, confirmed by RAST test and/or a positive skin prick test	Other eye disorders, contact lens wearers, known sensitivity to constituents of active or placebo drops, use of other ophthalmic medications, systemic corticosteroids or antihistamines, hyposensitization treatment during the last year	Nedocromil sodium 2%, benzalkonium chloride 0·01%, disodium edetate 0·05%, sodium chloride 0·55%	4 wks	49/70	52/76
Stockwell, 1994[19]	Bristol Eye Hospital, UK	> 6 yrs	Feb 1983 – Apr 1984	Symptomatic hay fever conjunctivitis	Additional eye disease, contact lens wearers, systemic steroids, pregnant or lactating women	Nedocromil sodium 2%, benzalkonium chloride 0·01%, edetate sodium (EDTA) 0·05%, sodium chloride 0·55%	4 wks	19/32	24/32

† Intention to treat analysis; wks = weeks; yrs = years; RAST = radioallergosorbent test

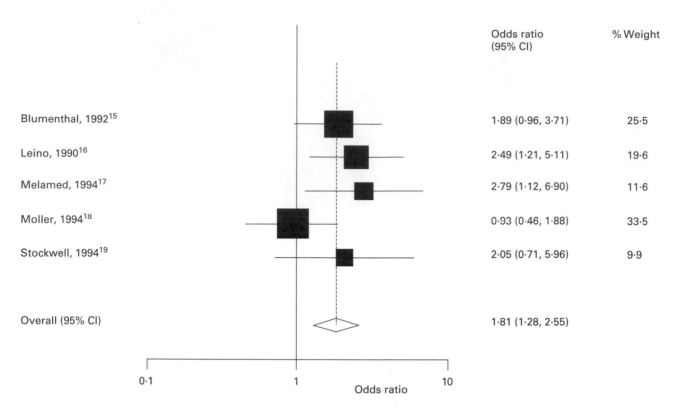

	Odds ratio (95% CI)	% Weight
Blumenthal, 1992[15]	1·89 (0·96, 3·71)	25·5
Leino, 1990[16]	2·49 (1·21, 5·11)	19·6
Melamed, 1994[17]	2·79 (1·12, 6·90)	11·6
Moller, 1994[18]	0·93 (0·46, 1·88)	33·5
Stockwell, 1994[19]	2·05 (0·71, 5·96)	9·9
Overall (95% CI)	1·81 (1·28, 2·55)	

Figure 4.2 Odds ratio of perceived benefit of using sodium nedocromil sodium 2% compared to placebo. The box area of each study is proportional to the inverse of the variance, with horizontal lines showing 95% confidence intervals of the odds ratio. Study authors are indicated on the y-axis in alphabetical order. The pooled estimate based on a fixed effects model is shown by a dashed, vertical line with an estimate on the right of the line indicating benefit from nedocromil sodium 2%. The diamond shows the 95% CI of the pooled estimate. The statistical weight given to each study is indicated.

mast cell stabilisers with antihistamine and vasoconstrictor preparations.

A variety of subjective symptom scores, such as itching, tearing and burning, as well as signs (for example, redness) were graded using scales from 0 (none) to 3 (severe)[31,32,34,36,37] or visual analogue scales.[33,35] These were used either as separate scores or summed to give overall symptom scores. As with earlier comparisons, formal meta-analysis was not possible, as most studies did not tabulate the mean scores and error associated with these measures. Despite this, differences in scores between treatment groups were reported as not being statistically significant in the six longer term studies. A statistically significant reduction in itching and redness ($P < 0.05$) in those treated with antihistamines was reported in the two short-term provocation studies.[31,37] Mean scores were tabulated in one of these studies allowing the comparative benefit of topical antihistamine over sodium cromoglycate to be gauged.[31] The benefit of antihistamine use in short studies was confirmed in interim results (at two weeks) from one of the longer studies (four

weeks).[34] Patient-perceived excellent or good treatment efficacy was reported in four of the six longer term studies (these are summarised in Table 4.4). A fixed effect estimate (as there was little heterogeneity between estimates; $P = 0.44$) showed that those using levocabastine were 1·32 times more likely (95% CI 0·81–2·16) to perceive good treatment efficacy than those using mast cell stabilisers (Figure 4.3). However, this difference was not statistically significant. Removal of one study that compared nedocromil sodium with levocabastine (instead of sodium cromoglycate) slightly increased the perceived benefit of levocabastine over sodium cromoglycate (odds ratio 1·75, 95% CI 0·94–3·24) but this, again, was not statistically significant. The use of concomitant medications (such as systemic antihistamines, ocular and nasal medications) amongst treatment groups as a rescue medication in cases of severe symptoms, was not routinely reported and hence could not be analysed further. Despite concerns about the sedative effect with systemic use of antihistamines, there were no side effects associated with topical use.

Table 4.3 Studies comparing topical antihistamines with placebo

Reference	Type of trial	Setting	Sample age	Time of year	Patient inclusion criteria	Patient exclusion criteria	Active treatment	Length of trial	No. in placebo, active grp (No. of subjects)	Subjective assessment (placebo v active)
Abelson, 1994[21]	RCT btn eyes, CPT	Harvard Medical School, Schepens Eye Research Institute, Boston, USA	Mean 33 yrs, 18–63 yrs	Not stated	History of symptoms of clinically active allergic conjunctivitis, positive skin or RAST test for allergic disease, consenting/able adults aged 18 to 65 years, either sex, any race, a successful challenge inducing at least moderate itching and redness	Bacterial or viral ocular infection, dry-eye syndrome, blepharitis, follicular conjunctivitis, iritis, preauricular lymphadenopathy, pregnant or nursing women, women of childbearing potential using inadequate contraceptive methods, allergy to levocabastine, contact lens wearers, using any type of topical agent (in the last 2 weeks) or systemic medication that might interfere with test parameters, signs and symptoms of allergic conjunctivitis prior to entry into the study	Levocabastine 0·05%	4 hrs	47 eyes, 47 eyes (47)	Reduced itching $P \leq 0{\cdot}007$ at 4 hrs, hyperaemia $P \leq 0{\cdot}045$, chemosis $P \leq 0{\cdot}002$ in active grp
Buscaglia, 1996[22]	Crossover RCT, CPT	University of Genoa, Italy	18–55 yrs	Outside the pollen season	Parietaria judacia sensitive subjects with seasonal allergic rhinoconjunctivitis, history of pollen allergy for at least 2 previous seasons, no symptoms at other times, positive skin prick and RAST test for specific pollen	No other ocular diseases, contact lens wearers, allergy to drugs under study, women of child bearing potential, lactating women, no topical or systemic drugs for at least 1 month prior to study	Levocabastine 0·5 mg/ml	0·5–6 hrs	10,10 (10)	Reduced total symptom score $P < 0{\cdot}002$ after 30 mins in active grp

(*Continued*)

Table 4.3 (Continued)

Reference	Type of trial	Setting	Sample age	Time of year	Patient inclusion criteria	Patient exclusion criteria	Active treatment	Length of trial	No. in placebo, active grp (No. of subjects)	Subjective assessment (placebo v active)
Donshik, 2000[23]	RCT	Multi-centre study, USA	Mean 36 yrs, 14–69 yrs	July–Nov 1994	At least 14 years of age, good health, history of seasonal allergic conjunctivitis during the ragweed season, skin prick positive to ragweed within the last 2 years, moderate ocular itching	Uncontrolled systemic or ocular diseases or illness, known sensitivity to any of the study medications, active ocular infection, history of ocular trauma or surgery, pregnancy or nursing status, women of childbearing age not using reliable contraception, involvement in another trial within 30 days prior to the study, ophthalmic medications and any topical or systemic histamine preparations for at least 5 days prior to the study	Levocabastine hydrochloride 0·05%	6 wks	75, 75 (150)	Reduced itching $P<0.05$ at 1, 3, 5 wks, and lid swelling at 1 wk in active grp. Placebo more effective than active at 3 wks $P=0.04$, no other difference
Pipkorn, 1985[24]	RCT	Sahlgrens Hospital, Göteborg, Sweden	Mean 29 yrs, 18–47 yrs	May 1984	At least a 2 year history of hay fever during the birch pollen season, with conjunctival and rhinitis symptoms, skin prick positive to birch pollen	Clinical or biochemical evidence of renal, hepatic, gastrointestinal or other disease requiring medication, patients < 16 yrs, pregnant women, women seeking pregnancy	Levocabastine 0·5 mg/ml	4 wks	Not stated (37)	Reduced itching $P<0.05$, runny eyes $P<0.05$, redness $P<0.05$, overall symptoms $P<0.05$ at 4 wks in active grp

(Continued)

Table 4.3 (Continued)

Reference	Type of trial	Setting	Sample age	Time of year	Patient inclusion criteria	Patient exclusion criteria	Active treatment	Length of trial	No. in placebo, active grp (No. of subjects)	Subjective assessment (placebo v active)
Stokes, 1993[25]	RCT btn eyes, CPT	St Thomas' Hospital, London, UK	Mean 43 yrs, 23–62 yrs	Not stated	Healthy, non-atopic volunteers	History of perennial allergy, concurrent medication with any topical eye medication, steroids, anti-inflammatory drugs or antihistamines, a history of conjunctivitis within 2 weeks of the study, keratitis, glaucoma, contact lens wearers, pregnant, nursing women	Levocabastine 0·5 mg/ml	30 mins	16, 16 (16)	Reduced total severity score (redness, swelling, overall) $P=0\cdot002$ in active grp
Zuber, 1988[26]	RCT, CPT	Centre Hospitalier Universitaire, Lausanne, Switzerland	Mean 30 yrs, 12–37 yrs	Jan – Feb	Asymptomatic patients with seasonal rhinoconjunctivitis caused by hypersensitivity to grass pollens, skin prick and RAST test positive to a mixture of grass pollens	Non-seasonal rhinoconjunctivitis, any other eye disease, taking medications, contact lens wearers	Levocabastine 0·5 mg/ml	24 hrs	Not stated (11)	Greater conjunctival provocation needed to elicit itching and redness in the placebo group compared to those treated with levocabastine 24 hrs before provocation

(Continued)

Table 4.3 *(Continued)*

Reference	Type of trial	Setting	Sample age	Time of year	Patient inclusion criteria	Patient exclusion criteria	Active treatment	Length of trial	No. in placebo, active grp (No. of subjects)	Subjective assessment (placebo v active)
Horak, 1996[27]	Cross-over RCT, CPT	Vienna, Austria	20–30 yrs	Outside the pollen season	History of allergic conjunctivitis caused by dactylis grass pollen with a positive skin prick test, RAST and conjunctival provocation test	Not stated	Azelastine hydrochloride 0·05%	4 hrs	24, 24 (24)	Reduced itching P=0·0007 in active grp
Discepola, 1999[28]	Cross-over RCT btn eyes, CPT	Not stated	Not stated	Not stated	History of allergic conjunctivitis, positive diagnostic skin test, repeated ocular reaction to weed, grass or animal dander	Not stated	Emedastine 0·05%	20 mins	18,18 (18)	Reduced itching P<0·05 at 3,10, 20 mins in active grp
Miller, 1975[29]	RCT btn eyes, CPT	Kennedy Memorial Hospital, Philadelphia, USA	12–67 yrs	Not stated	History of ragweed pollen sensitivity, with current signs and symptoms of allergic conjunctivitis	Narrow angle glaucoma, known hypersensitivity or idiosyncrasy to drugs under study. Patients receiving corticosteroids within 30 days prior to the study, those on salicylates or antihistamines (topical or systemic) within 3 dys	Antazoline phosphate and naphazoline hydrochloride	24–72 hrs	Not stated (Not stated)	Reduced inflammation P<0·01, photophobia P<0·05 in active grp

RAST, radioallergosorbent test; btn between; CPT, conjunctival provocation test; mins, minutes; hrs, hours; dys, days; wks, weeks; mon, months; yrs, years; grp, group

Table 4.4 Studies reporting perceived good or excellent treatment efficacy with topical mast cell stabilisers (MCS) versus antihistamines, included in the meta-analysis

Reference	Setting	Sample age	Time of year	Patient inclusion criteria	Patient exclusion criteria	Active treatments	Length of trial	Number with good treatment efficacy with MCS	Number with good treatment efficacy with anti-histamines
Frostad, 1993[32]	Allergologisk Poliklinikk, Oslo, Norway	Median 30 yrs, 19–51 yrs	Hay fever season	History of conjunctivitis due to birch and grass pollen, positive skin prick and RAST test to birch and grass pollen in the last year, over 18 yrs of age	Conjunctivitis due to other causes, participation in a hypcsensitisation programme, concurrent disease or therapy likely to complicate treatment efficacy, treatment with investigational drug 1 month prior to trial, contact lens wearer, poor compliance, pregnant or nursing women	SCG 20mg/dl (qds), levocabastine 0·5 mg/dl (bd)	4 mon	25/34†	32/37†
Vermeulen, 1994[34]	Multi-centre, South Africa	6–15 yrs	Not stated	1 year history of seasonal allergic rhinoconjunctivitis, skin prick and RAST test positive	Medications which could interfere with evaluation of the study drugs (oral antihistamines, vasoconstrictors, corticosteroids)	SCG 2% (qds), levocabastine 0·05% (bd), both with nasal spray	4 wks	34/57†	38/53†
Wihl, 1991[35]	3 centre study in Malmö, Hässleholm, Örebro, Sweden	Median 25 yrs, 17–52 yrs	April 1989	History of seasonal allergic conjunctivitis during the tree and grass pollen seasons, for at least 1 year, positive skin prick and RAST test to birch and thimothy grass allergens, current allergic rhinitis, aged > 15 yrs	Not stated	SCG (qds), levocabastine (bd)	10 wks	26/29	29/32

(Continued)

Table 4.4 *(Continued)*

Reference	Setting	Sample age	Time of year	Patient inclusion criteria	Patient exclusion criteria	Active treatments	Length of trial	Number with good treatment efficacy with MCS	Number with good treatment efficacy with anti-histamines
Richard, 1998[36]	7 centre study, France	Mean 31 yrs, 6–67 yrs	Not stated	History of allergic conjunctivitis and symptomatic for at least 24 hrs, positive skin prick or RAST test, personal or family history of allergy	Hypersensitivity to any constituents of study eyedrops, other conjunctivitis, medications (including topical ocular preparations, corticoids, antihistamines, nasal sodium cromoglycate, local vasoconstrictors), which could influence the results of the study (unless washed-out), contact lens wearers, monocular patients, pregnant or lactating women	Lodoxamide 0·1% (qds), levocabastine 0·05% (bd) + vehicle (bd)	14 dys	30/46	28/47

Intention to treat analysis, dys, days; wks, weeks; yrs, years; SCG, sodium cromoglycate, RAST, radioallergosorbent test; qds, four times daily; bd, twice daily

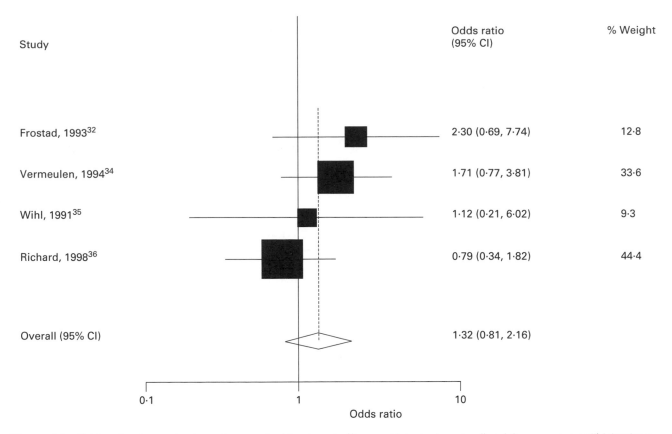

Figure 4.3 Odds ratio of perceived good or excellent treatment efficacy with topical mast cell stabilisers versus antihistamines. The box area of each study is proportional to the inverse of the variance, with horizontal lines showing 95% confidence intervals of the odds ratio. Study authors are indicated on the y-axis in alphabetical order. The pooled estimate based on a fixed effects model is shown by a dashed line vertical line with an estimate on the right of the line indicating benefit from topical antihistamines. The diamond shows the 95% CI of the pooled estimate. The statistical weight given to each study is indicated.

Comment

Evidence from randomised control trials may show that topical antihistamines may have a quicker mode of action than mast cell stabilisers in protecting against symptoms of allergic conjunctivitis, but that there is little difference in treatment efficacy in studies of two weeks' or longer duration. However, the relevance of acute ocular provocation studies to chronic environmental allergen exposure in the pollen season is yet to be clarified.

Summary

Despite differences in reported subjective outcomes from different studies, evidence from randomised controlled trials confirms the benefit of topical sodium cromoglycate and antihistamines over placebo preparations for the treatment of SAC. There is insufficient evidence to support the use of one class of active medication over another, hence treatment preferences should be based on convenience of use (with reduced frequency of instillation for some preparations), risk of side effects and costs. Although we found limited evidence to suggest that topical antihistamines may have a faster mode of action than mast cell stabilisers (especially sodium cromoglycate) there was little difference in treatment efficacy beyond two weeks. Larger trials, with standardised methods and results presentation, are needed to distinguish between different topical treatments, before the increased expense of newer topical preparations can be fully justified. The use of oral antihistamines and topical steroids for the treatment of allergic conjunctivitis are the topic of ongoing Cochrane reviews.

Acknowledgements

Our thanks to Anupa Shah (Cochrane Eyes and Vision Group), who identified the references used in this chapter.

References

1. Featherstone PI, James C, Hall MS, Williams A. General practitioners' confidence in diagnosing and managing eye conditions: a survey in south Devon. *Br J Gen Pract* 1992;**42**:21–4.
2. Manners T. Managing eye conditions in general practice. *BMJ* 1997;**315**:816–17.
3. Johansson SG, Hourihane JO, Bousquet J *et al.* A revised nomenclature for allergy. An EAACI position statement from the EAACI nomenclature task force. *Allergy* 2001;**56**:813–24.
4. Freissler KA, Lang GE, Lang GK. Allergic diseases of the lids, conjunctiva, and cornea. *Curr Opin Ophthalmol* 1997;**8**:25–30.
5. Dart JK, Buckley RJ, Monnickendan M, Prasad J. Perennial allergic conjunctivitis: definition, clinical characteristics and prevalence. A comparison with seasonal allergic conjunctivitis. *Trans Ophthalmol Soc UK* 1986;**105**:513–20.
6. Buckley RJ. Allergic eye disease – a clinical challenge. *Clin Exp Allergy* 1998;**28**(suppl 6):39–43.
7. Austin JB, Kaur B, Anderson HR *et al.* Hay fever, eczema, and wheeze: a nationwide UK study (ISAAC, international study of asthma and allergies in childhood). *Arch Dis Child* 1999;**81**:225–30.
8. Leibowitz HM. The red eye. *N Engl J Med* 2000;**343**:345–51.
9. Greenbaum J, Cockcroft D, Hargreave FE, Dolovich J. Sodium cromoglycate in ragweed-allergic conjunctivitis. *J Allergy Clin Immunol* 1977;**59**:437–9.
10. Hechanova MG. A double-blind study comparing sodium cromoglycate eye ointment with placebo in the treatment of chronic allergic conjunctivitis. *Clin Trials J* 1984;**21**:59–66.
11. Lindsay-Miller AC. Group comparative trial of 2% sodium cromoglycate (Opticrom) with placebo in the treatment of seasonal allergic conjunctivitis. *Clin Allergy* 1979;**9**:271–5.
12. Nizami RM. Treatment of ragweed allergic conjunctivitis with 2% cromolyn solution in unit doses. *Ann Allergy* 1981;**47**:5–7.
13. Ruggieri ML, Scorcia G. Double-blind group comparative trial of sodium cromoglycate eye ointment and placebo in the treatment of allergic eye diseases. *Ann Allergy* 1987;**58**:109–12.
14. van Bijsterveld OP. A double-blind crossover study comparing sodium cromoglycate eye drops with placebo in the treatment of chronic conjunctivitis. *Acta Ophthalmol (Copenh)* 1984;**62**:479–84.
15. Blumenthal M, Casale T, Dockhorn R *et al.* Efficacy and safety of nedocromil sodium ophthalmic solution in the treatment of seasonal allergic conjunctivitis. *Am J Ophthalmol* 1992;113:56-63.
16. Leino M, Carlson C, Jaanio E *et al.* Double-blind group comparative study of 2% nedocromil sodium eye drops with placebo eye drops in the treatment of seasonal allergic conjunctivitis. *Ann Allergy* 1990;**64**:398–402.
17. Melamed J, Schwartz RH, Hirsch SR, Cohen SH. Evaluation of nedocromil sodium 2% ophthalmic solution for the treatment of seasonal allergic conjunctivitis. *Ann Allergy* 1994;**73**:57–66.
18. Moller C, Berg IM, Berg T, Kjellman M, Stromberg L. Nedocromil sodium 2% eye drops for twice-daily treatment of seasonal allergic conjunctivitis: a Swedish multicentre placebo-controlled study in children allergic to birch pollen. *Clin Exp Allergy* 1994;**24**:884–7.
19. Stockwell A, Easty DL. Group comparative trial of 2% nedocromil sodium with placebo in the treatment of seasonal allergic conjunctivitis. *Eur J Ophthalmol* 1994;**4**:19–23.
20. Cerqueti PM, Ricca V, Tosca MA, Buscaglia S, Ciprandi G. Lodoxamide treatment of allergic conjunctivitis. *Int Arch Allergy Immunol* 1994;**105**:185–9.
21. Abelson MB, George MA, Schaefer K, Smith LM. Evaluation of the new ophthalmic antihistamine, 0·05% levocabastine, in the clinical allergen challenge model of allergic conjunctivitis. *J Allergy Clin Immunol* 1994;**94**:458–64.
22. Buscaglia S, Paolieri F, Catrullo A et al. Topical ocular levocabastine reduces ICAM-1 expression on epithelial cells both in vivo and in vitro. *Clin Exp Allergy* 1996;**26**:1188–96.
23. Donshik PC, Pearlman D, Pinnas J et al. Efficacy and safety of ketorolac tromethamine 0·5% and levocabastine 0·05%: a multicenter comparison in patients with seasonal allergic conjunctivitis. *Adv Ther* 2000;**17**:94–102.
24. Pipkorn U, Bende M, Hedner J, Hedner T. A double-blind evaluation of topical levocabastine, a new specific H1 antagonist in patients with allergic conjunctivitis. *Allergy* 1985;**40**:491–6.
25. Stokes TC, Feinberg G. Rapid onset of action of levocabastine eye-drops in histamine-induced conjunctivitis. *Clin Exp Allergy* 1993;**23**:791–4.
26. Zuber P, Pecoud A. Effect of levocabastine, a new H1 antagonist, in a conjunctival provocation test with allergens. *J Allergy Clin Immunol* 1988;**82**:590–4.
27. Horak F, Berger U, Menapace R, Schuster N. Quantification of conjunctival vascular reaction by digital imaging. *J Allergy Clin Immunol* 1996;**98**:495–500.
28. Discepola M, Deschenes J, Abelson M. Comparison of the topical ocular antiallergic efficacy of emedastine 0·05% ophthalmic solution to ketorolac 0·5% ophthalmic solution in a clinical model of allergic conjunctivitis. *Acta Ophthalmol Scand Suppl* 1999;**228**:43–46.
29. Miller J, Wolf EH. Antazoline phosphate and naphazoline hydrochloride, singly and in combination for the treatment of allergic conjunctivitis – a controlled, double-blind clinical trial. *Ann Allergy* 1975;**35**:81–6.
30. Dechant KL, Goa KL. Levocabastine. A review of its pharmacological properties and therapeutic potential as a topical antihistamine in allergic rhinitis and conjunctivitis. *Drugs* 1991;**41**:202–24.
31. Abelson MB, George MA, Smith LM. Evaluation of 0·05% levocabastine versus 4% sodium cromolyn in the allergen challenge model. *Ophthalmol* 1995;**102**:310–16.
32. Frostad AB, Olsen AK. A comparison of topical levocabastine and sodium cromoglycate in the treatment of pollen-provoked allergic conjunctivitis. *Clin Exp Allergy* 1993;**23**:406–9.
33. Odelram H, Bjorksten B, af Klercker T, Rimas M, Kjellman NI, Blychert LO. Topical levocabastine versus sodium cromoglycate in allergic conjunctivitis. *Allergy* 1989;**44**:432–6.
34. Vermeulen J, Mercer M. Comparison of the efficacy and tolerability of topical levocabastine and sodium cromoglycate in the treatment of seasonal allergic rhinoconjunctivitis in children. *Pediatr Allergy Immunol* 1994;**5**:209–13.
35. Wihl JA, Rudblad S, Kjellen H, Blychert LA. Levocabastine eye drops versus sodium cromoglycate in seasonal allergic conjunctivitis. *Clin Exp Allergy* 1991;**21**(suppl 2):37–8.
36. Richard C, Trinquand C, Bloch-Michel E. Comparison of topical 0·05% levocabastine and 0·1% lodoxamide in patients with allergic conjunctivitis. Study Group. *Eur J Ophthalmol* 1998;**8**:207–16.
37. Hammann C, Kammerer R, Gerber M, Spertini F. Comparison of effects of topical levocabastine and nedocromil sodium on the early response in a conjunctival provocation test with allergen. *J Allergy Clin Immunol* 1996;**98**:1045–50.
38. Kremer B, Tundermann A, Goldschmidt O. Onset of action, effectiveness and tolerance of levocabastine and nedocromil in topical therapy of seasonal allergic rhinoconjunctivitis. The Deutsche Rhinitis-Studiengruppe. *Arzneimittelforschung* 1998;**48**:924–30.

5 Acute bacterial conjunctivitis

Aziz Sheikh

Background

Acute "red eye" is one of the commonest reasons for consultation with primary care physicians in the developed world, accounting for up to 5% of all clinical encounters.[1-3] In the majority of cases an acute bacterial conjunctivitis is diagnosed,[4-7] the pathogens most frequently responsible being *Streptococcus pneumoniae, Haemophilus influenzae* and *Staphylococcus aureus.*[7-9] The condition affects both sexes, all ages, and all races.[1] Generally considered to be a self-limiting disorder, antibiotics are nevertheless usually prescribed in the belief that they speed recovery, reduce the risk of developing sight-threatening complications and reduce the rate of reinfection.[10-11] Guidelines on the management of conjunctivitis recommend their routine use where bacterial infection is suspected,[12-14] with distinct regional preferences in the topical agent to be used.[15]

Question

What is the efficacy of antibiotic treatment in the management of acute bacterial conjunctivitis?

The evidence

A systematic review of the efficacy of antibiotics in the management of acute bacterial conjunctivitis is published in the *Cochrane Library.*[16] This review includes double-blind randomised placebo controlled trials. The main outcome measures of interest were time to clinical and microbiological remission.

Three trials, studying a total of 527 patients, satisfied the review inclusion criteria. Two of the eligible trials were based in the United States,[17,18] with the third recruiting patients from the United States, Mali and Morocco.[19] Studies were heterogeneous with respect to age groups of patients studied, diagnostic inclusion criteria adopted by the trials, and for antibiotic treatments used (polymyxin 10 000 U/g and bacitracin 500 U/g; norfloxacin 0·3%; and ciprofloxacin 0·3%), all of which involved topical preparations. However, there was no evidence of statistical heterogeneity as revealed by the results of chi-square tests.[16] The three trials included used different combinations of outcome measures, and focused upon clinical cure, microbiological cure, or a combination of these. Clinical and microbiological outcomes were assessed "early" (days two to five post-intervention) and "late" (days six to ten post-intervention).

Meta-analysis showed acute bacterial conjunctivitis frequently to be a self-limiting condition as clinical remission (defined as clinical cure or significant clinical improvement) occurred by days two to five in 64% (95% CI 57–71) of those treated with placebo. Treatment with topical antibiotics was associated with significantly better rates of early clinical remission (days two to five: RR 1·31, 99% CI 1·11–1·55) (Figure 5.1) and suggested that the benefit was maintained for late clinical remission (days six to ten: RR 1·27, 95% CI 1·00–1·61). Antibiotic treatment was associated with improved rates of microbiological remission, defined as pathogen eradication or reduction (days two to five: RR 1·71, 99% CI 1·32–2·21; days six to ten: RR 1·71, 99% CI 1·26–2·34) (Figure 5.2). No serious outcomes were reported in either the active or the placebo arms of these trials.

Implications for practice

This review confirms the commonly held belief that acute bacterial conjunctivitis is, indeed, usually self-limiting. The meta-analysis showed topical antibiotic treatment to be clearly associated with significantly better rates of early (days two to five) clinical and microbiological remission than is treatment with placebo, and strongly suggests that this benefit is maintained for late (days six to ten) clinical remission. No serious adverse events were noted in the 527 patients enrolled in the three antibiotic–placebo controlled trials included in this review, suggesting that important sight-threatening complications occur infrequently. But in view of the probable rarity of such adverse events the possibility of Type II errors cannot be entirely excluded.

Implications for research

The outcome measures adopted in the trials included in this review do not distinguish patient-oriented outcomes

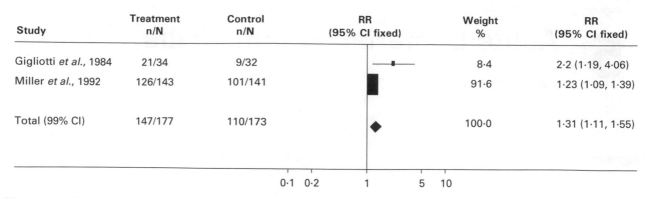

Study	Treatment n/N	Control n/N	RR (95% CI fixed)	Weight %	RR (95% CI fixed)
Gigliotti *et al.*, 1984	21/34	9/32		8·4	2·2 (1·19, 4·06)
Miller *et al.*, 1992	126/143	101/141		91·6	1·23 (1·09, 1·39)
Total (99% CI)	147/177	110/173		100·0	1·31 (1·11, 1·55)

Figure 5.1 Early clinical remission. n, number of subjects in clinical remission; N, number of subjects tested; CI, confidence interval; RR, relative risk.

Study	Treatment n/N	Control n/N	RR (95% CI fixed)	Weight %	RR (95% CI fixed)
Gigliotti *et al.*, 1984	24/34	6/32		8·2	3·76 (1·77, 8·00)
Leibowitz *et al.*, 1991	132/140	22/37		46·4	1·59 (1·21, 2·08)
Miller *et al.*, 1992	53/76	32/67		45.4	1·46 (1·09, 1·95)
Total (99% CI)	209/250	60/136		100·0	1·71 (1·32, 2·21)

Figure 5.2 Early microbiological remission. For abbreviations see above.

(such as mean interval from treatment to relief of symptoms) from doctor-oriented outcomes (such as clinical and microbiological remission rates). Despite the self-limiting nature of acute bacterial conjunctivitis, and concerns regarding antibiotic safety[15] and resistance,[20,21] it is surprising that none of the trials attempted to determine the cost-effectiveness of topical antibiotic treatment, or assessed the impact of treatment upon re-infection rates. Such a pragmatic trial is clearly warranted and should ideally be based in primary care where the overwhelming majority of patients presenting with acute bacterial conjunctivitis are managed.[22]

Acknowledgements

I thank Professor Brian Hurwitz, the Cochrane Eyes and Vision Group and the Systematic Reviews Training Unit for their assistance in preparing the original review. I am supported by the NHS R&D National Primary Care Post Doctoral Training Programme.

References

1. American Optometric Association. *Optometric clinical practice guideline: care of the patient with conjunctivitis.* San Francisco: AOA, 1995.
2. McCormick A, Flemming D, Charlton J. *Morbidity statistics from general practice. Fourth national study 1991–2.* London: HMSO, 1995.
3. Britt H, Miles DA, Bridges-Webb C, Neary S, Charles J, Traynor V. A comparison of country and metropolitan general practice. *Med J Aust* 1999;**159**(Suppl 1):S31.
4. Heggie AD. Incidence and etiology of conjunctivitis in navy recruits. *Military Medicine* 1990;**155**:1–3.
5. Dart J. Eye disease at a community health centre. *BMJ* 1986;**293**: 1477–80.
6. Fitch CP, Rapoza PA, Owens S *et al.* Epidemiology and diagnosis of acute conjunctivitis at an inner-city hospital. *Ophthalmology* 1989;**96**:1215–20.

7. Gigliotti F, Williams WT, Hayden FG *et al.* Etiology of acute conjunctivitis in children. *J Pediatr* 1981;**98**:531–6.

8. Mahajan VM. Acute bacterial infections of the eye: their aetiology and treatment. *Br J Ophthalmol* 1983;**67**:191–4.

9. Perkins RE, Kundsin RB, Pratt MV, Abrahamsen I, Leibowitz HM. Bacteriology of normal and infected conjunctiva. *J Clin Microbiol* 1975;**1**:147–9.

10. McDonnell PJ. How do general practitioners manage eye disease in the community? *Br J Ophthalmol* 1988;**72**:733–6.

11. Morrow GL, Abbott RL. Conjunctivitis. *Am Fam Physician* 1998;**57**:735–46.

12. Donahue SP, Khoury JM, Kowalski RP. Common ocular infections: a prescriber's guide. *Drugs* 1996;**52**:528–9.

13. Canadian Ophthalmological Society. *Eye conditions, disorders and treatments.* http://www.eyesite.ca/info/04ae-condconj.html (accessed 25 Feb 2000).

14. British Medical Association and Royal Pharmaceutical Society of Great Britain. *British National Formulary.* London: BMA, 1999, p 38.

15. Doona M, Walsh JD. Use of chloramphenicol as topical eye medication: time to cry halt? *BMJ* 1995;**310**:1217–18.

16. Sheikh A, Hurwitz B, Cave J. Antibiotics for acute bacterial conjunctivitis (Cochrane Review). In: Cochrance Collaboration: *Cochrane Library.* Issue 2. Oxford: Update Software, 2003.

17. Gigliotti H, Hendley JO, Morgan J, Michaels R, Dickens M, Lohr J. Efficacy of topical antibiotic therapy in acute conjunctivitis in children. *J Pediatr* 1984;**104**:623–6.

18. Leibowitz HM. Antibacterial effectiveness of ciprofloxacin 0·3% ophthalmic solution in the treatment of bacterial conjunctivitis. *Am J Ophthalmol* 1991;**112**:29s–33s.

19. Miller IM, Wittreich J, Vogel R. The safety and efficacy of topical norfloxacin compared with placebo in the treatment of acute, bacterial conjunctivitis. *Eur J Ophthalmol* 1992;**2**:58–66.

20. Chaudhry NA, Flynn HW, Murray TG, Tabandeh H, Mello MO, Miller D. Emerging ciprofloxacin-resistant *Pseudomonas aeurginosa. Am J Ophthalmol* 1999;**128**:509–10.

21. Goldstein MH, Kowlaski RP, Gordon YJ. Emerging fluoroquinolone resistance in bacterial keratitis: a 5-year review. *Ophthalmology* 1999;**106**:1313–18.

22. Sheikh A, Hurwitz B. Topical antibiotics for acute bacterial conjunctivitis: a systematic review. *Br J Gen Pract* 2001;**51**:475–7.

6 Viral conjunctivitis

Hazel Everitt

Background

Viral conjunctivitis is an extremely common ocular disorder, accounting for an estimated 20–30% of all eye related primary care consultations in the UK.[1-3] Cases may present sporadically or as part of an epidemic. Epidemic keratoconjunctivitis (EKC) is usually due to adenovirus infection and acute haemorrhagic conjunctivitis (AHC) is most commonly due to picornavirus infection.[4]

Presentation

Symptoms and signs may include watery discharge, a foreign body sensation, lacrimation, eye discomfort, redness and oedema of the eyelids, sub-conjunctival haemorrhage, conjunctival follicles and palpable pre-auricular lymphadenopathy.[4] Secondary bacterial infection is not uncommon.

Diagnosis

Diagnosis is usually made on clinical grounds, viral cultures rarely being used because of expense, time considerations, and the low sensitivity of the tests commonly employed. Discriminating viral from bacterial conjunctivitis on clinical grounds is often difficult, however, and many cases diagnosed clinically as presumed bacterial conjunctivitis are probably in fact viral in origin. In one study, 50% of cases diagnosed by ophthalmologists as presumed acute bacterial conjunctivitis did not have a bacterial aetiology on culture.[2]

Prognosis

Viral conjunctivitis is generally a self-limiting condition – acute symptoms typically lasting for between four to seven days before resolution gradually occurs over the following one to three weeks.

Treatment options

Numerous treatments have been used in an attempt to give symptomatic relief, shorten duration of illness and reduce infectivity; these treatments include artificial tears, cold compresses, and topical decongestants, antibiotics, antiviral agents, corticosteroids, interferon, non-steroidal anti-inflammatory drugs (NSAIDs) and povidone-iodine.[5]

Question

Does treatment for viral conjunctivitis confer benefit (where benefit is defined in terms of either reducing symptoms, shortening duration of illness or reducing infectivity)?

We will examine the evidence for interferon, antiviral agents, topical corticosteroids and topical NSAIDS separately.

Question

Does interferon treatment for viral conjunctivitis confer benefit?

The evidence

We found no systematic reviews. We found five published randomised controlled trials investigating the role of topical interferon.

Wilhelmus *et al.* undertook a double-blind trial comparing topical human fibroblast interferon with placebo for patients with acute conjunctivitis.[6] Of the 50 patients studied, tear-film cultures proved to be positive in only 13 (26%). Outcome data were available for 37 patients. After one week of therapy, the interferon group showed significantly greater improvement in the symptoms and signs severity score than the controls for affected left (mean difference in severity score day 0 to day 7 was 9·4 for interferon and 6·6 for placebo group $P = 0·02$) but not right eyes ($P = 0·5$). Transient ocular irritation occurred more often in the treatment group than the control group (81% v 33%, $P = 0·001$).

Reilly *et al.* compared interferon with placebo eye drops in 34 patients recruited during an outbreak of EKC.[7] Twenty of the 34 patients had positive viral cultures; 26 patients completed the study end-point. There was no significant difference between the groups in duration of symptoms. Summary statistics were not provided.

Adams *et al.* conducted a double-blind placebo controlled trial investigating the role of interferon alpha-2 for the treatment of adenoviral conjunctivitis in 14 patients.[8] No difference was found in either duration or severity of illness between the treatment and placebo groups. No summary statistics were available for these outcome measures.

Stansfield *et al.* undertook a double-blind placebo controlled trial of human leucocyte interferon (HLI) in 15 subjects with acute haemorrhagic conjunctivitis (AHC).[9] They described no difference in the "clinical course" of the illness between the two groups. The use of HLI did, however, appear to reduce the spread of AHC to other household members (secondary cases); three secondary cases were noted in the placebo group and none in the HLI group (*P* = 0·02).

Sundmacher *et al.* randomised 14 patients with virologically confirmed adenoviral conjunctivitis to either interferon alfa or placebo (albumin) eye drops.[10] The authors reported "no clinically relevant therapeutic effect" for interferon but suggested that interferon may exert a prophylactic effect on uninflamed fellow eyes; no summary data were presented.

Question

Do antiviral agents for viral conjunctivitis confer benefit?

The evidence

We found no systematic review. We found three randomised controlled trials that evaluated the use of antiviral agents.

Dudgeon *et al.* conducted a double-blind trial comparing 5-iodo-2-deoxyuridine (IDU) with placebo in 70 patients with presumed adenoviral conjunctivitis.[11] Adenovirus infection was proven in 35 patients. There was no difference in the severity or duration of symptoms between the two groups. No summary statistics were available.

A UK study compared amantadine with placebo in a conjunctivitis outbreak in a hospital for those with learning difficulties.[12] Fifty per cent of subjects had positive viral cultures. The main outcome measures of interest were visual acuity (VA), the period of incapacity, and time required to attend hospital. Data on VA were available for only five patients in each group. The authors suggested that there was a marked difference between the amantadine

and placebo groups in 'incapacity' but no summary statistics were presented.

Pavan-Langston *et al.* compared two antiviral agents: adenine arabinoside (Ara A) and IDU in 22 eyes (15 subjects).[13] The average duration of symptoms was 17 days in the Ara A treated group and 16 days in the IDU treated group. The authors concluded that neither treatment had an apparent effect on the course or severity of the conjunctivitis. No summary data were presented.

Question

Do topical corticosteroids for viral conjunctivitis confer benefit?

The evidence

We found no systematic review. We found one double-blind randomised controlled trial. Ward *et al.* comparing topical trifluridine, topical dexamethasone and artificial tears in 74 military personnel with viral keratoconjunctivitis.[14] Laboratory verification showed positive viral cultures in only 11 of the 74 patients in the study. No significant difference was found between the three groups in duration of symptoms. Mean duration of symptoms was 11 days in the control group (artificial tears), 11 days in trifluridine group and 10 days in dexamethasone group (*P* = 0·56).

Question

Do topical NSAIDS for viral conjunctivitis confer benefit?

The evidence

We found no systematic review but we found two trials. In an open trial, Kosrirukvongs studied the effect of topical NSAID eye drops combined with antibiotic eye drops for AHC.[15] One hundred patients were randomised to either topical antibiotic alone (control group) or topical antibiotic and piroxicam eye drops. Seventy-five patients completed the study. Baseline comparison of symptoms showed pain to be a more common presenting feature in the control group (60·3%) than in the piroxicam group (36·6%). Mean recovery time for the piroxicam group was significantly reduced (4·9 (SD 4·4) versus 5·2 (SD 3·8); *P* = 0·003). Foreign body sensation, pain and tearing (lacrimation) were also relieved significantly more quickly in the piroxicam group. However, there was no significant difference in resolution of clinical signs and it does not appear that the difference in pain between the groups at recruitment was controlled for in the statistical analysis. A burning sensation in the eyes was noted significantly more frequently in the topical piroxicam group than the control group (89·5% *v* 41·2%; *P*<0·001).

Shuley *et al.* reported a double-blind trial of 117 patients diagnosed clinically with viral conjunctivitis.[16] Patients were randomised to keterolac 0·5% eye drops four times a day or artificial tears. The 105 subjects were assessed three to four days post-randomisation. No significant difference was found in the change in symptom or sign scores or in the patients' opinion of the usefulness of treatment between the groups, except for eye redness (which showed greater improvement in the artificial tears group, *P* = 0·012). Stinging with application of the drops was noted significantly more often in the keterolac group than in the placebo group (59·2% *v* 18·8%; *P*<0·001).

Discussion

Viral conjunctivitis is a common self-limiting condition for which various treatments have been investigated. Research into viral conjunctivitis is hampered by difficulties in obtaining confirmatory virological evidence of viral infection.

The evidence for the treatment of viral conjunctivitis is limited. The published RCTs are, in general, of poor quality and insufficiently powered to reliably detect a difference.[6–10,13–15] Additionally, confirmation of the clinical diagnosis by virological methods has proved difficult.

On the basis of this limited evidence it appears that none of the treatments studied to date confer benefit in the management of viral conjunctivitis.

Implications for practice

There is insufficient evidence for any of the treatments to evaluate their usefulness for viral conjunctivitis. The evidence suggests that topical antiviral agents and interferon do not significantly alter the course of the disease. The two trials of topical NSAIDs have yielded conflicting results, one suggesting some benefit from piroxicam[15] and the other showing no benefit from keterolac.[16] However, neither trial showed a significant difference in the resolution of clinical signs and both indicate that a stinging sensation is more common with topical NSAIDs.

Implications for research

Larger, more rigorous trials are needed to clarify whether any of the treatments may be of benefit. Until more sensitive virological tests are developed, pragmatic trials studying those with a clinical diagnosis of viral conjunctivitis are likely to represent the most appropriate way forward.

References

1. Sheldrick JH, Wilson AD, Vernon SA, Sheldrick CM. Management of ophthalmic disease in general practice. *Br J Gen Pract* 1993;**43**: 459–62.
2. Mahajan VM. Acute bacterial infections of the eye: their aetiology and treatment. *Br J Ophthalmol* 1983;**67**:191–4.
3. Wilson A. The red eye: a general practice survey. *J R Coll Gen Pract* 1987;**37**:62–4.
4. Donahue S, Khoury J, Kowalski R. Common ocular infections: a prescriber's guide. *Drugs* 1996;**52**:527–39.
5. Isenberg SJ, Apt L, Valenton M *et al.* A controlled trial of povidone-iodine to treat infectious conjunctivitis in children. *Am J Ophthalmol* 2002;**134**:681–8.
6. Wilhelmus K, Dunkel E, Herson J. Topical human fibroblast interferon for acute adenoviral conjunctivitis. *Graefe's Arch Clin Exp Ophthalmol* 1987;**225**:464.
7. Reilly S, Dhillon B, Nkanza K *et al.* Adenovirus type 8 keratoconjunctivitis – an outbreak and its treatment with topical human fibroblast interferon. *J Hyg Camb* 1986;**96**:557–75.
8. Adams C, Cohen E, Albrecht J, Laibson P. Interferon treatment of adenoviral conjunctivis. *Am J Ophthalmol* 1984;**98**:429–32.
9. Stansfield S, De La Pena W, Koenig S *et al.* Human leucocyte interferon in the treatment and prophylaxis of acute haemorrhagic conjunctivitis. *J Infect Dis* 1984;**149**:822–3.
10. Sundmacher R, Wigand R, Cantell K. The value of exogenous interferon in adenovirus keratoconjunctivitis. *Graefe's Arch Clin Exp Ophthalmol* 1982;**218**:139–40.
11. Dudgeon J, Bhargava S, Ross C. Treatment of adenovirus infection of the eye with 5-iodo-2-deoxyuridine. *Br J Ophthalmol* 1969; **53**:533.
12. Marmion V. Treatment of adenovirus type 8 keratoconjunctivitis. *Trans Ophthalmol Soc UK* 1972;**92**:619–23.
13. Pavan-Langston D, Dohlman CH. A double blind clinical study of adenine arabinosine therapy of viral keratoconjunctivitis. *Am J Ophthalmol* 1972;**74**:81–8.
14. Ward J, Siojo L, Waller S. A prospective masked clinical trial of trifluridine, dexamethasone and artificial tears in the treatment of epidemic keratoconjunctivitis. *Cornea* 1993;**12**:216–21.
14. Kosrirukvongs M. Topical piroxicam and conjunctivitis. *J Med Assoc Thail* 1997;**80**:287–92.
15. Shiuey Y, Ambati B, Adamis AP. A randomized, double-masked trial of topical ketorolac versus artificial tears for treatment of viral conjunctivitis. *Ophthalmology* 2000;**107**:1512–17.

7 Screening older people for impaired vision

Liam Smeeth

Background

There are a number of factors that make visual impairment among older people an attractive target for screening. Visual impairment is common, causes substantial disability, is easy to diagnose, and many people's vision could be improved with treatment. A recent survey in the United Kingdom found bilateral visual acuity of less than 6/12 in around 30% of people aged 65 or more,[1] over 70% of which was considered potentially remediable. Only 12% of older people with a cataract causing impaired vision were in touch with eye care services and only one-third of those with substantial uncorrected refractive error had seen an optometrist in the past 12 months.[1] Comparable results have been found in other surveys undertaken in other developed countries.[2–5] Visual impairment has been reported as having physical, psychological and social ramifications. For example, functional status, social contacts and quality of life are lower.[6–12] Furthermore, visual impairment has been shown to be strongly associated with depression[10,13] falls and hip fractures.[14–17]

In practice, screening for visual impairment is only likely to be one part of a broader package of screening measures, an approach commonly referred to as a multidimensional screening assessment.[18] Most forms of assessment include some attempt to assess vision.

Question

What is the effectiveness of mass screening for visual impairment in unselected older people (65 and over) in a community setting, either alone or as part of a regular multidimensional assessment programme?

The evidence

A systematic review of randomised controlled trials of mass screening of older people for visual impairment is included in the *Cochrane Library*.[19] The review included all randomised controlled trials of population based screening for visual impairment (using any screening method) in a community setting in people aged 65 or over. The outcomes used were the risk of visual impairment (however measured) in the population at the end of the trial. Although screening for visual impairment may have other beneficial effects, such as reducing falls or improving quality of life, any such improvement would be a result of improving vision.

The review found five randomied trials that included a total of 3494 participants.[20–24] All trials were of multidimensional screening with vision screening as one component. There were no trials that primarily assessed visual screening. Allocation concealment was adequate in all trials. Because of the nature of the intervention, it would not have been possible to mask either recipients or providers of care to their allocation.

The results in all five trials were similar (Figure 7.1). There was no evidence of heterogeneity of effect between the five trials. The pooled relative risk for self-reported visual problems at the time of outcome assessment (range two to four years after the screening assessment) comparing the intervention and control groups was 1·03 (95% CI 0·92–1·16). The pooled odds ratio was 1·04 (95% CI 0·89–1·22).

Discussion

Given that visual impairment is common, disabling, frequently unreported, and often treatable, the lack of improvement in vision seen in these trials is somewhat surprising. A screening procedure alone would not be expected to lead to improvements in vision. Such improvements would be dependent on subsequent interventions to improve vision. The trial reports did not include information about whether screening improved the detection of treatable visual impairment or about the subsequent management of the visual problems detected. In addition, the use of questions about vision both for the initial screening assessment and for the outcome assessment may have affected the results. The sensitivity of questions about vision for the detection of visual impairment is typically around 30% when compared to formal acuity

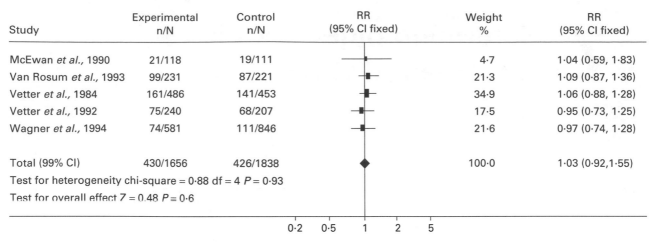

Study	Experimental n/N	Control n/N	RR (95% CI fixed)	Weight %	RR (95% CI fixed)
McEwan *et al.*, 1990	21/118	19/111		4·7	1·04 (0·59, 1·83)
Van Rosum *et al.*, 1993	99/231	87/221		21·3	1·09 (0·87, 1·36)
Vetter *et al.*, 1984	161/486	141/453		34·9	1·06 (0·88, 1·28)
Vetter *et al.*, 1992	75/240	68/207		17·5	0·95 (0·73, 1·25)
Wagner *et al.*, 1994	74/581	111/846		21·6	0·97 (0·74, 1·28)
Total (99% CI)	430/1656	426/1838		100·0	1·03 (0·92,1·55)

Test for heterogeneity chi-square = 0·88 df = 4 *P* = 0·93

Test for overall effect *Z* = 0·48 *P* = 0·6

Figure 7.1 The effect of screening older people for visual impairment[19]

testing.[25] Although the specificity is generally much higher, the low sensitivity of the tests used means that many people's visual impairment would not have been detected by screening.

Implications for practice and policy

The aim of population screening of older people for visual impairment is to identify people with potentially treatable visual impairment that is hitherto undetected and to offer interventions to improve vision. The evidence from randomised controlled trials undertaken to date does not currently support the inclusion of questions about vision in regular multidimensional assessment programmes for unselected older people in a community setting. Although a reduction of 8% in the number of older people with visual impairment cannot be excluded, even this figure is disappointingly low.

Implications for research

In practice, screening for visual impairment is highly likely to be one part of a broader screening package. A large randomised trial of screening older people for visual impairment as part of a broader screening assessment, which overcomes the possible limitations of the trials undertaken to date, is warranted. A trial funded by the United Kingdom Medical Research Council is currently underway, and results will be available in late 2003. Further details are available from the chapter author.

References

1. Reidy A, Minassian DC, Vafidis G *et al*. Prevalence of serious eye disease and visual impairment in a north London population: population based, cross sectional study. *BMJ* 1998;**316**:1643–6.
2. Klein R, Klein BE, Linton KL, De MD. The Beaver Dam eye study: visual acuity. *Ophthalmology* 1991;**98**:1310–15.
3. Wormald RP, Wright LA, Courtney P, Beaumont B, Haines AP. Visual problems in the elderly population and implications for services. *BMJ* 1992;**304**:1226–9.
4. Klaver CC, Wolfs RC, Vingerling JR, Hofman A, de Jong PT. Age-specific prevalence and causes of blindness and visual impairment in an older population: the Rotterdam Study. *Arch Ophthalmol* 1998;**116**:653–8.
5. van der Pols JC, Bates CJ, McGraw PV *et al*. Visual acuity measurements in a national sample of British elderly people. *Br J Ophthalmol* 2000;**84**:165–70.
6. Scott IU, Schein OD, West S, Bandeen-Roche K, Enger C, Folstein MF. Functional status and quality of life measurement among ophthalmic patients. *Arch Ophthalmol* 1994;**112**:329–35.
7. Salive ME, Guralnik J, Glynn RJ, Christen W, Wallace RB, Ostfeld AM. Association of visual impairment with mobility and physical function. *J Am Geriatr Soc* 1994;**42**:287–92.
8. Rudberg MA, Furner SE, Dunn JE, Cassel CK. The relationship of visual and hearing impairments to disability: an analysis using the longitudinal study of aging. *J Gerontol* 1993;**48**:M261–5.
9. Dargent-Molina P, Hays M, Breart G. Sensory impairments and physical disability in aged women living at home. *Int J Epidemiol* 1996;**25**:621–9.
10. Carabellese C, Appollonio I, Rozzini R *et al*. Sensory impairment and quality of life in a community elderly population. *J Am Geriatr Soc* 1993;**41**:401–7.
11. West SK, Munoz B, Rubin GS *et al*. Function and visual impairment in a population-based study of older adults. The SEE project. *Invest Ophthalmol Vis Sci* 1997;**38**:72–82.
12. Wulsin LR, Jacobson AM, Rand LI. Psychosocial correlates of mild visual loss. *Psychosom Med* 1991;**53**:109–17.
13. Rovner BW, Zisselman PM, Shmuely-Dulitzki Y. Depression and disability in older people with impaired vision: a follow-up study. *J Am Geriatr Soc* 1996;**44**:181–4.
14. Grisso JA, Kelsey JL, Strom BL *et al*. Risk factors for falls as a cause of hip fracture in women. The Northeast Hip Fracture Study Group. *N Engl J Med* 1991;**324**:1326–31.

15. Felson DT, Anderson JJ, Hannan MT, Milton RC, Wilson MC, Kiel DP. Impaired vision and hip fracture, the Framingham study. *J Am Geriatr Soc* 1989;**37**:495–500.

16. Tinneti ME, Speechley M, Ginter SF. Risk factors among elderly persons living in the community. *N Engl J Med* 1988;**319**:1701–7.

17. Dargent-Molina P, Favier F, Grandjean H *et al.* Fall-related factors and risk of hip fracture: the EPIDOS prospective study. *Lancet* 1996;**348**:145–9.

18. Fletcher A. Multidimensional assessment of elderly people in the community. *Br Med Bull* 1998;**54**:945–60.

19. Smeeth L, Iliffe S. Community screening for visual impairment in the elderly (Cochrane Review). In: Cochrane Collaboration *Cochrane Library.* Issue 2. Oxford: Update Software, 2003.

20. Vetter NJ, Jones DA, Victor CR. Effect of health visitors working with elderly patients in general practice: a randomised controlled trial. *BMJ* 1984;**288**:369–72.

21. McEwan RT, Davison N, Forster DP, Pearson P, Stirling E. Screening elderly people in primary care: a randomized controlled trial. *Br J Gen Pract* 1990;**40**:94–7.

22. Vetter NJ, Lewis PA, Ford D. Can health visitors prevent fractures in elderly people? *BMJ* 1992;**304**:888–90.

23. van Rossum E, Frederiks CM, Philipsen H, Portengen K, Wiskerke J, Knipschild P. Effects of preventive home visits to elderly people. *BMJ* 1993;**307**:27–32.

24. Wagner EH, LaCroix AZ, Grothaus L *et al.* Preventing disability and falls in older adults: a randomised controlled trial. *Am J Public Health* 1994;**84**:1800–6.

25. Smeeth L. Assessing the likely effectiveness of screening older people for impaired vision in primary care. *Fam Pract* 1998;**15**(Suppl 1): 24–9.

Section III

Paediatrics and ocular motility

Jugnoo S Rahi, Clare Gilbert, Editors

Paediatrics and strabismus: mission statement

Why does this section focus on ophthalmic disorders specific to children? First, because anatomical and physiological changes occur throughout childhood in the developing visual system. Therefore, the nature and impact of visual loss in children differs from adults, with visual impairment in childhood having important consequences for all aspects of a child's development, their education and their care by family and professionals. Second, many visually impairing paediatric disorders are specific to children and those that are not often have different functional effects in children compared to adults. Third, as a high proportion of visually impaired children have other significant sensory, motor or learning impairments, visual loss needs to be considered in this broader context.

There are particular difficulties in undertaking clinical trials of childhood eye diseases. Most visually impairing disorders are individually rare, necessitating large, collaborative multi-centre studies that are difficult and expensive to undertake. Although many disorders are present from early childhood, visual maturation is not complete until much later. Therefore important outcomes can only be reliably determined through long-term follow-up, which is difficult to achieve. Finally, there a number of ethical considerations about children's participation in trials, which are the subject of ongoing debate, that do not arise with adult subjects able to consent to participation themselves. Although these potential obstacles are important, they only partly account for the limited extent to which paediatric ophthalmic practice is currently based on evidence from high-quality randomised controlled trials.

The aims of this section are to describe the available evidence from trials (from the Cochrane Eyes and Vision Group (CEVG) register and published systematic reviews of trials), as well as to highlight the areas where evidence is lacking, and to identify the important questions that have yet to be addressed.

The section comprises chapters on those disorders most commonly encountered in paediatric ophthalmic practice (amblyopia and strabismus) as well as on the major, and preventable or treatable, visually impairing disorders congenital cataract, retinopathy of prematurity, congenital glaucoma and ophthalmia neonatorum). Other important disorders affecting children are addressed in the sections on adnexal disease (lacrimal obstruction), uveitis (toxoplasma and toxocara infection) and oncology (retinoblastoma).

8 Congenital and infantile cataract

Jugnoo S Rahi

Background

Definition

As their clinical management is the same, the terms congenital cataract and infantile cataract are generally used interchangeably to describe visually significant lens opacity during the first year of life,[1] although standard disease classification systems distinguish between these and further subcategories of cataract in infancy.[2]

Frequency

Despite being a treatable cause of visual loss, bilateral congenital cataract accounts for 15% of the world's blind children, being important in both industrialised and developing countries.[1] Currently, of every 10 000 children born in industrialised countries each year about three will be diagnosed as having congenital/infantile cataract by their first birthday. A further one will be diagnosed by age 15 years.[3,4] The frequency is likely to be higher in some developing countries where specific causes of cataract, such as prenatal rubella infection or recessively inherited disease, are more common.[5]

Aetiology

The pattern of underlying or associated causes varies throughout the world.[2,6,7] Idiopathic cataract accounts for a substantial proportion in most populations.

Prevention of congenital cataract

Prevention of visual impairment due to congenital cataract is now an international priority.[4] There has been limited research on modifiable environmental risk factors. Thus, primary prevention is currently limited to avoidance, where possible, of known teratogens especially prevention of prenatal rubella infection through immunisation, and to provision of pre-conceptional genetic counselling of couples at known risk. It would not be appropriate for the effectiveness of these strategies to be evaluated in an intervention trial. Thus to date, treatment (secondary prevention) has been the focus of clinical practice and research on congenital cataract.

Question

What is the most effective way of screening newborn and young infants for congenital cataract?

The evidence

We found no randomised controlled trials (RCTs) that have specifically addressed either the issue of the most effective method of screening or who is the optimal health professional to undertake screening.

Comment

Early diagnosis of congenital cataract is essential in ensuring that treatment, together with parental advice and support, can be provided promptly. Consequently in many industrialised countries routine examination of the red-reflex of newborn children is an established practice. Recent observational research in the United Kingdom, which is likely to reflect the situation in other similar settings, indicates the need for improvements in this established national practice, in particular in the training of those responsible.[5] There is increasing interest in establishing the optimal age at which the clinical screening examination should be carried out, the best health professional to undertake it and, in some countries, the additional value of routine mydriasis for the examination. These questions are not easily addressed through trials. However, there is good scope for investigating them using other approaches.

Question

What are the benefits (overall functional vision, cosmesis and quality of life) of treating newborn and young infants with unilateral congenital cataract?

The evidence

We found no RCTs that have addressed this question.

Comment

Managing children with congenital cataract is a complex, long-term process requiring considerable input from parents, who are responsible for the occlusion and optical correction, as well as high healthcare expenditure. As the overall functional consequences of untreated unilateral cataract may not be considerable, there is disagreement[8] about whether the potential benefits to the affected child and family of undertaking treatment outweigh the potential disadvantages. Recent work suggests that the risk of visual impairment through loss of vision in the normal eye may be higher than previously thought.[9] Research to characterise the disability associated with unilateral cataract would be helpful to this debate.

Question

What is the optimal occlusion regime for the management of amblyopia in congenital cataract?

The evidence

We found no RCTs that have addressed this question.

Comment

Visual loss in congenital/infantile cataract is mainly due to amblyopia.[10] This arises in a number of ways[7,11]: stimulus/form deprivation during the sensitive period of visual development; competition between the two eyes in unilateral or asymmetric bilateral cases; inadequate correction of refractive error (aphakia); or stimulus/form deprivation due to posterior capsular opacification. Although no randomised clinical trials have been undertaken, there has been considerable clinical and experimental work on occlusion treatment for amblyopia in general (see Chapter 12, Unilateral amblyopia). This has informed the development of postoperative occlusion regimes for cataract based on objective measures of visual function.[11–13]

Question

In children with bilateral cataract present from birth does "very early" surgery (for example, before four to six weeks of age), compared with 'later' surgery, result in better long-term visual functions (acuity, stereo-vision, contrast sensitivity)?

The evidence

We found no RCTs that have addressed this question.

Comment

In clinical observational studies of children with unilateral cataract, visual outcomes have been better in children undergoing surgery by six to eight weeks of age than those who have been operated on later.[14–16] This "critical period" for treatment has been extrapolated to bilateral disease, despite less investigation of the correlation between visual outcome and timing of surgery. As long-term observational data become available, there is increasing concern about an association between aphakic glaucoma and very early surgery.[17,18] Together, these issues underpin current interest in establishing the optimal timing for surgery.[11]

Question

In children with bilateral cataract present from birth does "very early" surgery (for example, before four to six weeks of age), compared with 'later' surgery, increase the risk of vision threatening complications, in particular aphakic glaucoma, in the long-term?

The evidence

We found no RCTs that have addressed this question.

Comment

There is limited information available about the long-term outcomes in children treated with modern surgical techniques. However, recent observational studies indicate that aphakic glaucoma, often developing some years after surgery, may be a particularly important visually disabling problem in the long term, perhaps affecting up to a quarter of all treated children.[11,18] It has been suggested that the risk is higher amongst those undergoing very early surgery, for example, within the first month of life.[2,7,11,18–20] Some have suggested, from early findings of observational clinical studies, that primary intraocular lens (IOL) implantation may be protective against the development of aphakic glaucoma.[20,21] Thus, as discussed below, the long-term risk of aphakic glaucoma would be an important outcome in any treatment trial, but essential in those comparing early versus later surgery and those comparing surgery with and without primary IOL implantation.

Questions

What is the optimal surgical procedure for:

- bilateral congenital cataract
- unilateral congenital cataract.

Does cataract extraction combined with primary IOL implantation, compared with cataract extraction without IOL implantation, result in:

● better overall visual function?
● reduced risk of aphakic glaucoma?
● increased risk of significant myopic shift?

The evidence

We found three published randomised controlled trials which have included children with known/assumed congenital/infantile cataract (Table 8.1). These trials are described below.

1   A trial in India comparing lensectomy and anterior vitrectomy in one eye with lens aspiration and primary posterior capsulotomy in the other eye of children under 10 years with bilateral cataract, mostly assumed to be congenital/infantile.[22] The two procedures were found to be equally effective in terms of visual acuity three years postoperatively. However, secondary procedures to restore vision were required much more frequently in eyes undergoing aspiration. The main purpose of this trial was to determine which of the two most common procedures for congenital cataract are preferable in settings where opportunities for long-term follow up of patients are limited and where the necessary maintenance and technical support for vitrectomy equipment may not be available. Thus the findings are particularly relevant to the many developing countries throughout the world where congenital cataract is major cause of visual impairment and blindness.[8]

2   A trial in children with congenital cataract (mainly bilateral) aged less than five years in India, all undergoing lens aspiration, posterior capsulorhexis and anterior vitrectomy, in which implantation of both haptic and optic of the IOL in the capsular bag was compared with optic placement behind the capsular bag (optic "capture").[23] Short-term follow up showed no difference in visual outcome (fixation and following) in the two groups of eyes or in IOL centration assessed clinically, but optic "capture" was associated with greater postoperative inflammation. The main purpose of this trial was to ascertain whether optic capture would reduce clinically significant posterior capsular opacification, a common complication of IOL implantation.[21] The findings of this trial do not support adoption of optic capture for this purpose.

3.   A trial in India of children aged 2–14 years, with unspecified type/causes of cataract, undergoing cataract extraction, compared the use of unmodified polymethylmethacrylate (PMMA) IOLs with heparin-surface-modified IOLs.[24] Short-term findings indicated that the use of modified IOLs reduced postoperative uveitis and its sequelae. The findings support the use of heparin-surface-modified IOLs in children to avoid/reduce the risk of complications of postoperative uveitis, which is generally much more pronounced in children than adults.[7]

A fourth published trial (not shown in the table) compared limbal versus par plana approaches for lensectomy, anterior vitrectomy, primary capsulectomy and IOL implantation in children with developmental or traumatic cataract aged three years (unilateral) or five years (bilateral) to 10 years in Iran.[25] There were no differences between the groups in visual outcome or complications at one year. Given age-related anatomical changes in the infant eye, with the pars plana approaching adult dimensions around the age of two years, the findings of this study are not directly applicable to the management of children younger than this.

Comment

Despite significant improvements in the surgical, optical and visual rehabilitation techniques available during the past few decades, there is no consensus regarding optimal surgical treatment.[11,26] Initial advances, over the past few decades, in surgical instrumentation and technique, led first to lens aspiration and subsequently to lensectomy with vitrectomy becoming the two surgical procedures of choice, with aphakic correction using contact lenses or glasses. The importance of peri and/or postoperative attention to the posterior capsule, to avoid the amblyogenic effect of capsular opacification, is well recognised.[11,21] This may be particularly important in determining choice of surgical procedure in those developing countries where patients are unable to reattend hospital for long-term follow up, or where there is limited access to YAG laser treatment for capsular opacification.[22,27]

Currently, in industrialised countries, and increasingly in many developing countries,[27] the most topical questions regarding the management of congenital cataract relate to the use of intraocular lenses (IOL) in infants and young children. Cataract extraction combined with primary posterior chamber IOL implantation has been increasingly adopted in *older* children, mainly those with acquired cataract, for example, due to trauma or drugs. Medium to longer-term outcome data are becoming available.[12,20,28–42] Whilst there is burgeoning interest in primary posterior chamber IOL implantation for children under two years, short-term outcomes in this age group are not yet widely available and, where reported, are based on relatively small numbers of children.[20,30,31,34–36,43] Thus there is considerable

Table 8.1   Summary of published randomised controlled trials in children with congenital/infantile cataract

Authors	Study design and setting	Subjects	Interventions compared	Outcomes reported
Eckstein *et al.*, 1999[22]	Randomised (eye) trial India	Children <10 years with bilateral cataract, mostly assumed congenital/infantile n = 65 children	Lensectomy and anterior vitrectomy versus lens aspiration and posterior capsulotomy	3 years postop: acuity, complications, and reoperation rates
Vasavada and Trivedi, 2000[23]	Randomised (eye) trial India	Children <5 years with congenital cataract n = 28 children	IOL placement in the capsular bag versus IOL optic placement behind capsular bag following lens aspiration, posterior capsulorhexis and anterior vitrectomy	At 16 months postop (range 5 to 24 months): visual fixation/following, squint, synechiae, IOL deposit, IOL centration
Basti *et al.*, 1999[24]	Randomised (eye) trial India	Children aged 2 to 14 years, some assumed congenital/infantile n = 90 children	Unmodified PMMA IOL versus heparin-surface-modified PMMA IOL following extracapsular cataract extraction +/− posterior capsulotomy and anterior vitrectomy	At 6 months (maximum): posterior capsular opacification, synechiae, IOL deposits, anterior chamber activity

uncertainty[8,21] about the mooted potential long-term benefits of primary IOL implantation in children aged 2 years and younger, in terms of quality and degree of visual rehabilitation, especially in unilateral disease.[8,32,44] Equally, there are important unanswered questions about long-term risks, in particular postoperative glaucoma[20,43,45–47] and major postoperative refractive changes.[20,21,48,49] As these issues regarding safety and efficacy are age-dependent, they cannot be addressed by studies of older children with cataract. Thus, there is a pressing need for standardised outcome data in young children to inform practice and plan future trials.

Implications for practice

Currently, the evidence base for the management of congenital/infantile cataract is drawn mainly from observational clinical studies. These support important differences in the management of unilateral and bilateral disease. A secular trend of improved visual outcomes with earlier detection and treatment supports continued screening of young infants for congenital cataract. However, emerging questions about the impact of timing of surgery on the risk of late complications, in particular aphakic glaucoma, indicate the need for life-long follow up of treated children. There is considerable uncertainty about the benefits of primary intraocular lens implantation in infants, suggesting that, if undertaken, it should be restricted to selected patients without other risk factors for postoperative complications.

Implications for research

Published randomised controlled trials to date have addressed some questions but do not offer insights into the most important emerging issues. Standardised longer-term outcome data are required about young children (aged up to two years) undergoing intraocular lens implantation as a basis for planning necessary future trials. Given the rarity of the disorder, such trials will need to be collaborative, involving many centres, and will require a range of primary outcomes, such as visual function, complications and vision-related quality of life, to be evaluated in the long term.

References

1. Foster A, Gilbert C. Epidemiology of visual impairment in children. In: Taylor D, ed. *Paediatric Ophthalmology, 2nd edn.* London: Blackwell Science, 1997: pp. 3–12.
2. Lambert SR, Drack AV. Infantile cataracts. *Surv Ophthalmol* 1996;**40**:427–58.
3. Rahi JS, Dezateux C, for the British Congenital Cataract Interest Group. Congenital and infantile cataract in the United Kingdom: underlying or associated factors. *Invest Ophthalmol Vis Sci* 2000;**41**:2108–14.
4. Gilbert CE, Foster A. Blindness in children: control priorities and research opportunities. *Br J Ophthalmol* 2001;**85**:1025–7.
5. Rahi JS, Dezateux C, for the British Congenital Cataract Interest Group. National cross-sectional study of detection of congenital and infantile cataract in the United Kingdom: role of screening and surveillance. *BMJ* 1999;**318**:362–5.
6. Jain IS, Pillay P, Gangwar DN, Dhir SP, Kaul VK. Congenital cataract: etiology and morphology. *J Pediatr Ophthalmol Strabismus* 1983;**20**:238–42.
7. Lambert SR. Lens. In: Taylor D, ed. *Paediatric Ophthalmology, 2nd edn.* London: Blackwell Science, 1997: pp. 445–77.
8. Taylor DSI, Wright LA, Amaya L, Cassidy L, Nischal K, Russell-Eggitt IM. Should we aggressively treat unilateral congenital cataracts? *Br J Ophthalmol* 2001;**85**:1120–6.
9. Rahi JS, Logan S, Timms C, Russell-Eggitt I, Taylor DSI. Risk, causes and outcomes of visual impairment after loss of vision in the non-amblyopic eye: a population-based study. *Lancet* 2002;**360**:597–602.
10. Wiesel TN. Postnatal development of the visual cortex and the influence of environment. *Nature* 1982;**299**:583–91.
11. Taylor D. Congenital cataract: the history, the nature and the practice. The Doyne Lecture. *Eye* 1998;**12**:9–36.
12. Cassidy L, Rahi JS, Nischal K, Russell-Eggitt IM, Taylor DSI. Outcome of lens aspiration and intra-ocular lens implantation in children aged 5 years and under. *Br J Ophthalmol* 2001;**85**:540–2.
13. Harrad R. Modulation of amblyopia therapy following early surgery for unilateral congenital cataracts. *Br J Ophthalmol* 1995;**79**:793.
14. Birch EE, Swanson WH, Stager DR, Woody M, Everett M. Outcome after very early treatment of dense congenital unilateral cataract. *Invest Ophthalmol Vis Sci* 1993;**34**:3687–99.
15. Birch EE, Stager DR, Leffler J, Weakley D. Early treatment of congenital unilateral cataract minimizes unequal competition. *Invest Ophthalmol Vis Sci* 1998;**39**:1560–6.
16. Lloyd IC, Dowler JGF, Kriss A *et al.* Modulation of amblyopic therapy following early surgery for unilateral congenital cataracts. *Br J Ophthalmol* 1995;**79**:802–6.
17. Abrahamsson M, Fabian G, Andersson AK, Sjostrand J. A longitudinal study of a population based sample of astigmatic children. I. Refraction and amblyopia. *Acta Ophthalmol* 1990;**68**:428–34.
18. Russell-Eggitt IM, Zamiri P. Review of aphakic glaucoma after surgery for congenital cataract. *J Cataract Refract Surg* 1997;**23**:664–8.
19. Asrani SG, Wilensky JT. Glaucoma after congenital cataract surgery. *Ophthalmology* 1995;**102**:863–7.
20. Ahmadieh H, Javadi MA. Intra-ocular lens implantation in children. *Curr Opinion Ophthalmol* 2001;**12**:30–4.
21. Lloyd IC. Intra-ocular lens implantation in infants. *Clin Exp Ophthalmol* 2000;**28**:338–40.
22. Eckstein M, Vijayalakshmi P, Gilbert C, Foster A. Randomised clinical trial of lensectomy versus lens aspiration and primary capsulotomy for children with bilateral cataract in south India. *Br J Ophthalmol* 1999;**83**:524–9.
23. Vasavada AR, Trivedi RH. Role of optic capture in congenital cataract and intra-ocular lens surgery in children. *J Cataract Refract Surg* 2000;**26**:824–31.
24. Basti S, Aasuri MK, Reddy MK *et al.* Heparin surface modified intra-ocular lenses in pediatric cataract: prospective randomised study. *J Cataract Refract Surg* 1999;**25**:782–7.
25. Ahmadieh H, Javadi MA, Ahmady M *et al.* Primary capsulotomy, anterior vitrectomy, lensectomy, and posterior chamber lens implantation in children: limbal versus pars plana. *J Cataract Refract Surg* 1999;**25**:768–75.
26. Wilson ME, Bluestein E, Wang X-H. Current trends in the use of intra-ocular lenses in children. *J Cataract Refract Surg* 1994;**20**:579–83.
27. Yorston D, Wood M, Foster A. Results of cataract surgery in young children in east Africa. *Br J Ophthalmol* 2001;**85**:267–71.
28. Burke JP, Willshaw HE, Young JDH. Intra-ocular lens implants for uniocular cataracts in childhood. *Br J Ophthalmol* 1989;**73**:860–4.
29. Basti S, Ravishankar U, Gupta S. Results of a prospective evaluation of three methods of management of pediatric cataracts. *Ophthalmology* 1996;**103**:713–20.
30. Knight-Nanan D, O'Keefe M, Bowell R. Outcome and complications of intra-ocular lenses in children with cataract. *J Cataract Refract Surg* 1996;**22**:730–6.
31. Markham RHC, Bloom PA, Chandna A, Newcomb EH. Results of intra-ocaulr lens implantation in paediatric aphakia. *Eye* 1992;**6**:493–8.
32. Awner S, Buckley EG, DeVaro JM, Seaber JH. Unilateral pseudophakia in children under 4 years. *J Pediatr Ophthalmol Strabismus* 1996;**33**:230–6.
33. Ainsworth JR, Cohen S, Levin AV, Rootman DS. Pediatric cataract management with variations in surgical technique and aphakic optical correction. *Ophthalmol* 1997;**104**:1096–101.
34. Sinskey RM, Stoppel JO, Amin P. Long-term results of intra-ocular lens implantation in pediatric patients. *J Cataract Refract Surg* 1993;**19**:405–8.
35. Young TL, Bloom JN, Ruttum M, Sprunger DT, Weinstein JM, on behalf of the AAPOS research committee. The IOLAB, Inc pediatric intra-ocular lens study. *J AAPOS* 1999;**3**:295–302.
36. Zwaan J, Mullaney PB, Awad A, Al-Mesfer S, Wheeler DT. Pediatric intaocular lens implantation. *Ophthalmology* 1998;**105**:112–19.
37. Wheeler DT, Mullaney PB, Abdulaziz Awaz, Al-Mesfer S, Al-Nahdi T, Zwaan J. Pediatric IOL implantation: the KKESH experience. *J Pediatr Ophthalmol Strabismus* 1997;**34**:341–6.
38. Kora Y, Inatomi M, Fukado Y, Marumori M, Yaguchi S. Long-term study of children with implanted intra-ocular lenses. *J Cataract Refract Surg* 1992;**18**:485–8.
39. Menzo JL, Taboada JF, Ferrer E. Complications of intra-ocular lenses in children. *Trans Ophthalmol Soc UK* 1985;**104**:546–52.
40. Crouch ER, Pressman SH. Posterior chamber intra-ocular lenses: long-term results in pediatric cataract patients. *J Pediatr Ophthalmol Strabismus* 1995;**32**:210–18.
41. Simons BD, Siatkowski RM, Schiffman JC, Flynn J, Capo H, Munoz M. Surgical technique, visual outcome, and complications of pediatric intra-ocular lens implantation. *J Pediatr Ophthalmol Strabismus* 1999;**36**:118–24.
42. Gimbel HV, Basti S, Ferensowicz M, DeBroff BM. Results of bilateral cataract extraction with posterior chamber intraocular lens implantation in children. *Ophthalmology* 1997;**104**:1737–43.
43. Lambert SR, Buckley EG, Plager DA, Medow NB, Wilson ME. Unilateral intra-ocular lens implantation during the first six months of life. *J AAPOS* 1999;**3**:344–9.
44. Ellis FD. Intra-ocular lenses in children. *J Pediatr Ophthalmol Strabismus* 1992;**29**:71–2.
45. Brady KM, Atkinson CS, Kilty LA, Hiles DA. Glaucoma after cataract extraction and posterior chamber lens implantation in children. *J Cataract Refract Surg* 1997;**23**:669.
46. Lambert SR, Lynn M, Drews-Botsch C *et al.* A comparison of grating visual acuity, strabismus and reoperation outcomes among children with aphakia and pseudophakia after unilateral cataract surgery during the first six months of life. *J AAPOS* 2001;**5**:70–5.
47. O'Keefe M, Fenton S, Lanigan B. Visual outcomes and complications of posterior chamber intraocular lens implantation in the first year of life. *J Cataract Refract Surg* 2002;**27**:2006–11.
48. Young JDH. Paediatric pseudophakia – choosing the implant power. *Br J Ophthalmol* 1999;**83**:258–9.
49. Filtcroft DI, Knight-Nanan D, Bowell R, Lanigan B, O'Keefe M. Intraocular lenses in children: changes in axial length, corneal curvature, and refraction. *Br J Ophthalmol* 1998;**83**:265–9.

9 Congenital glaucoma

Maria Papadopoulos, PT Khaw

Background

Definition

Congenital glaucoma encompasses a diverse group of conditions that have one common feature – raised intraocular pressure (IOP). Many different classifications exist, but it can be classified simply as (i) primary, characterised by a specific developmental abnormality of the anterior chamber angle (isolated trabeculodysgenesis) and (ii) secondary, due to various ocular or systemic developmental anomalies or diseases that raise IOP. In primary congenital glaucoma (PCG), although the underlying defect is present at birth (hence, congenital), the age at which glaucoma manifests can vary. It typically presents in the neonatal or infantile period and so is synonymous with primary infantile glaucoma.

Incidence

Primary congenital glaucoma is the commonest glaucoma in infancy.[1] It has a reported incidence of 1 in 10 000 to 20 000 live births in Western countries.[2,3] The incidence rises in the Middle East to 1 in 8200 live births in Palestinian Arabs[4] and 1 in 2500 live births in Saudi Arabians.[5] The highest reported incidence in the literature is 1 in 1250 in Slovakian Gypsies.[6] Parental consanguinity, especially cousin–cousin marriages, is thought to be responsible for the higher prevalence of PCG in certain ethnic and religious groups.[4,6–8]

Secondary congenital glaucoma is much rarer and can be associated with phakomatoses such as Sturge-Weber syndrome (up to 60% of glaucoma is congenital onset)[9] and Klippel-Trenaunay-Weber syndrome. Anterior segment dysgenesis is associated with glaucoma in 50% of cases but rarely in infancy, as is also the case with aniridia.[9]

Genetics

Most cases of PCG appear to be sporadic.[10] Autosomal recessive inheritance with variable penetrance ranging from 40–100% is reported in familial cases.[11] The GLC3A locus on the short arm of chromosome 2 (2p21) is thought to account for 85–90% of all familial cases, specifically mutations of the *CYP1B1* gene.[12] With regard to anterior segment dysgenesis, two loci, REIG1 at 4q25 and REIG2 at 13q14 have been implicated.[13] Aniridia has been associated with the *PAX6* gene at 11p13.[13]

Treatment and prognosis

The prognosis of congenital glaucoma is poor if untreated or sub-optimally treated.[14] As PCG is a relatively rare condition, it is prone to misdiagnosis and sub-optimal treatment, leading to irreversible visual impairment. The preservation of a lifetime of vision for these patients depends on early, accurate diagnosis followed by appropriate successful treatment. To maximise visual outcome, the two objectives are first to control IOP at a level where progression is unlikely, and second to prevent or minimise amblyopia. This chapter deals with the surgical treatment of congenital glaucoma to control IOP. Based on observational data, there is consensus that the definitive treatment for IOP control is surgical. However, the approach to management varies throughout the world and somewhat reflects our understanding of the mechanisms underlying raised IOP. The different surgical procedures have varying indications and potentially good success rates, especially when performed at referral centres.[3,15–18] The procedure of choice is largely determined by corneal clarity, the age of the patient and the surgeon's experience, but may further be influenced by the degree of optic nerve damage, race, history of previous surgery, other ocular pathology such as cataract and the state of the fellow eye.

In PCG, the IOP is raised, owing to a developmental defect in the trabecular meshwork that reduces aqueous outflow.[19] Therefore, surgery has centred on incising the trabecular meshwork *ab interno* (goniotomy) and *ab externo* (trabeculotomy) or providing an alternative drainage channel (trabeculectomy). Drainage implant surgery is typically the treatment of choice for refractory congenital glaucoma. Rarely, cyclodestruction may play a role.

Question

In children with PCG, does goniotomy compared with trabeculotomy provide better long-term IOP control?

Table 9.1   Summary of prospective studies

Authors	Study	Procedure	Glaucoma	No. of patients	Success	% success
Senft et al., 1989[20]	Prospective randomised controlled	Surgical v Nd:YAG laser goniotomy (1 operation)	PCG	10 (20 eyes)	IOP ≤ 22 mmHg + M or Δ% > 25%	40% both procedures (mean FU = 9·5 months)
Luntz and Livingston, 1977[21]	Prospective case series	Trabeculotomy (≥1 operation)	CG	47 (75 eyes)	IOP ≤18 mmHg − M	85% after 1 operation 93·4% after ≥1 operation (minimum FU = 12 months)
Agarwal et al., 1997[22]	Prospective randomised double blind	0·2 mg/ml v 0·4mg/ml MMC trabeculotomy– trabeculectomy (1 operation)	CG	16 (30 eyes)	IOP ≤20 mm Hg − M IOP ≤20 mmHg + M excluding oral carbonic anhydrase inhibitors No further surgery	86·7% both groups 60% 0·2 mg/ml MMC 86·7% 0·4 mg/ml MMC 3 patients (6 eyes, 40%) 0·4 mg/ml group dropped out after 6 months
Elder, 1994[23]	Prospective case series	Trabeculotomy– trabeculectomy (1 operation)	CG	9 (16 eyes)	IOP ≤20 mmHg − M	93·5% 12 months Cumulative chance success
Coleman et al., 1997[24]	Prospective case series	Ahmed implant	CG	21 (24 eyes)	IOP ≤21 mmHg + M No further glaucoma surgery No vision threatening complications	78% 12 months (69–87%, 95% CI) 60·6% 24 months (47–73%, 95% CI) Cumulative chance success

PCG, primary congenital glaucoma; CG, congenital glaucoma (primary and secondary); MMC, mitomycin-C; IOP, intraocular pressure; + M, with antiglaucoma medications; − M, without antiglaucoma medications; FU, follow up; CI, confidence interval

The evidence

We found no randomised, controlled trials comparing goniotomy with other surgical techniques. One small randomised trial compared surgical goniotomy with Nd:YAG goniotomy in 10 Saudi Arabian patients less than a year old with bilateral, symmetrical PCG and clear corneas[20] (see Table 9.1). The first eye of each patient was selected for either surgical or Nd:YAG laser goniotomy in a randomised, double masked fashion. The fellow eye underwent the alternative treatment. The main outcomes were IOP and the per cent of IOP change (IOP/initial IOP, Δ%). Success was defined as IOP ≤22 mmHg with antiglaucoma medications or a Δ% > 25%. Mean follow-up was 9·5 months. There was a strong positive correlation (r = 0·81) of the per cent of IOP change between two treatments. However, only four eyes (40%) in each group met the criteria for success. The response to laser was generally found to mirror the surgical outcome of the contralateral eye.

Comment

This is a small, preliminary study with short-term outcomes. By allocating the alternative procedure to the fellow eye, the patients were thought to act as "his/her own control", which may be problematic if the outcome in the two eyes is not completely independent. The overall success rate of 40% for either incisional or laser goniotomy is comparable with results of retrospective studies following one goniotomy,[16,25] which usually increases to 70–90% when repeated.[17,26–28] That the outcome of either procedure was usually similar in the same patient supports observations from retrospective studies that success is dictated more by the severity of the disease than by surgical procedure.[1,29] Given the lack of long-term results for laser goniotomy, this evidence is insufficient to warrant a change from surgical goniotomy.

A prospective case series of trabeculotomies performed in 47 white and black American children (75 eyes) with congenital glaucoma has been reported[21] (see Table 9.1). Intraocular pressure was controlled in 85% of patients after the first trabeculotomy, increasing to 93·4% when repeated. There was no relationship between successful outcome and corneal diameter, age of onset, preoperative IOP and race.

Question

In children with secondary congenital glaucoma, does goniotomy, trabeculotomy or trabeculectomy provide the best long-term pressure control?

The evidence

We found no randomised, controlled trials of trabeculotomy, nor randomised, controlled trials comparing trabeculotomy–trabeculectomy with other surgical techniques. In a small prospective, randomised, double-blind study, four-minute intraoperative 0·2 mg/ml mitomycin-C (MMC) was compared to 0·4 mg/ml MMC enhanced trabeculotomy–trabeculectomy[22] (see Table 9.1). It was performed in 16 Indian patients (30 eyes), aged seven years or younger, with congenital glaucoma. Success was defined as IOP control ≤20 mmHg at final follow-up including antiglaucoma medications but without further surgery. After a follow-up of six months, the 0·4 mg/ml group had a 40% drop out rate (three patients, six eyes). The decrease in IOP six months after surgery between the two groups was not statistically significant (Student's t test, $P = 0.64$). Surgical success without medications was achieved in 60% of patients who had received 0·2 mg/ml MMC and 86·6% in those with 0·4 mg/ml at final follow up of 18 months (chi-squared test, $P = 0.21$). With medications the success rate was 86·7% in both groups.

Comment

Full details of randomisation were not provided beyond stating that patients were "systematically randomised" and the two groups could only be accurately compared for six months. The success rates reported in both arms of the trial are comparable to those reported in previous observational studies.[30–32] However, there is no evidence that adjunctive 0·4 mg/ml MMC is superior to 0·2 mg/ml MMC in trabeculotomy–trabeculectomy.

A prospective case series evaluating trabeculotomy–trabeculectomy in nine Palestinian Arab children (16 eyes) less than one year old with congenital glaucoma has reported a cumulative probability of successful IOP control of 93·5% at 24 months[23] (see Table 9.1).

Question

In refractory congenital glaucoma, is MMC trabeculectomy or drainage implant surgery the procedure of choice for the control of IOP?

The evidence

We found no randomised, controlled trials of drainage implants.

Comment

In a prospective case series, the Ahmed valve implant was evaluated in 21 consecutive patients (24 eyes) of mixed ethnicity, in people aged less than 18 years (mean 4·8 years). Fifty-four per cent were described as having "congenital glaucoma" and all patients had either previously failed glaucoma surgery or other surgery was considered inappropriate[24] (see Table 9.1). Cumulative probabilities of success were 78% at 12 months and 60·6% at 24 months. Race, sex, age, aphakia and number of previous surgeries were not associated with increased failure (cox regression, $P \geq 0.15$). These findings are similar to other observational studies of unenhanced Baerveldt and Molteno implants without antifibrosis regimens in paediatric patients.[33–35] However, longer term follow-up has demonstrated an association with age and the number of previous intraocular operations.[36]

Implications for practice

Currently, clinical practice is based largely on observational data derived mainly from retrospective case series with varying diagnoses, ages, criteria for inclusion and follow-up. The criteria for successful outcome have often varied and included the level of IOP (measured with various anaesthetics and instruments), number of operations, the use of antiglaucoma medications and visual criteria.

Implications for research

The limited data available from RCTs fails to address the major issues such as, "What is the best primary procedure for IOP control in primary or secondary congenital glaucoma?" or "What is the procedure of choice to control IOP in refractory congenital glaucoma?" Furthermore, trabeculotomy–trabeculectomy in theory provides two major outflow pathways and so may be expected to be more successful than either procedure alone, but the clinical benefit is unclear from studies and warrants further study. Another useful study would be the comparison of conventional 180° trabeculotomy to 360° suture trabeculotomy.[37] Clinical data regarding concentration, duration of exposure and safety of antimetabolites in paediatric patients would also be worthwhile. The answers to these questions will probably be found in multi-centre studies, possibly performed in areas of high incidence of this condition, such as the Middle East.

References

1. Shaffer RN, Weiss DI. *Congenital and Paediatric Glaucomas*. St Louis: CV Mosby, 1970.
2. François J. Congenital glaucoma and its inheritance. *Ophthalmologica* 1980;**181**:61–73.
3. McGinnity FG, Page AB, Bryars JH. Primary congenital glaucoma: twenty years experience. *Ir J Med Sci* 1987;**156**:364–5.
4. Elder MJ. Congenital glaucoma in the West Bank and Gaza Strip. *Br J Ophthalmol* 1993;**77**:413–16.
5. Jaafar MS. Care of the infantile glaucoma patient. In: Reinecke RD, ed. *Ophthalmology Annual*. New York: Raven Press, 1988: pp. 15–37.
6. Gencik A. Epidemiology and genetics of primary congenital glaucoma in Slovakia. Description of a form of primary congenital glaucoma in gypsies with autosomal-recessive inheritance and complete penetrance. *Dev Ophthalmol* 1989;**16**:115.
7. Debnath SC, Teichmann KD, Salamah K. Trabeculectomy versus trabeculotomy in congenital glaucoma. *Br J Ophthalmol* 1989;**73**:608–11.
8. Turaçli ME, Aktan SG, Sayli BS, Akarsu N. Therapeutic and genetical aspects of congenital glaucoma. *Int Ophthalmol* 1992;**16**:359–62.
9. Ritch R, Shields MB, Krupin T. *The Glaucomas, 2nd edn*. St. Louis: Mosby, 1996.
10. Merin S, Morin D. Heredity of congenital glaucoma. *Br J Ophthalmol* 1972;**56**:414–17.
11. Sarfarazi M, Stoilov I. Molecular genetics of primary congenital glaucoma. *Eye* 2000;**14**:422–8.
12. Stoilov I, Akarsu AN, Sarfarazi M. Identification of three different truncating mutations in cytochrome P4501B1 (CYP1B1) as the principle cause of primary congenital glaucoma (Buphthalmos) in families linked to the GLC3A locus on chromosome 2p21. *Hum Mol Genet* 1997;**6**:641–7.
13. Craig JE, Mackey DA. Glaucoma genetics: where are we? where will we go? *Curr Opin Ophthalmol* 1999;**10**:126–34.
14. Duke-Elder S. *System of Ophthalmology*. St Louis: CV Mosby, 1969: pp. 548–65.
15. Fulcher T, Chan J, Lanigan B, Bowell R, O'Keefe M. Long term follow up of primary trabeculectomy for infantile glaucoma. *Br J Ophthalmol* 1996;**80**:499–502.
16. Haas JS. Symposium: Congenital glaucoma. End results of treatment. *Trans Am Acad Ophthalmol Otolaryngol* 1955;**59**:333–41.
17. Russell-Eggitt IM, Rice NSC, Jay B, Wyse RKH. Relapse following goniotomy for congenital glaucoma due to trabecular dysgenesis. *Eye* 1992;**6**:197–200.
18. Quigley HA. Childhood glaucoma. Results with trabeculotomy and study of reversible cupping. *Ophthalmology* 1982;**89**:219–25.
19. Anderson DR. The development of the trabecular meshwork and its abnormality in primary congenital glaucoma. *Trans Am Ophthalmol Soc* 1981;**79**:481–5.
20. Senft SH, Tomey KF, Traverso CE. Neodymium-YAG laser goniotomy *v* surgical goniotomy. *Arch Ophthalmol* 1989;**107**:1773–6.
21. Luntz MH, Livingston DG. Trabeculotomy *ab externo* and trabeculectomy in congenital and adult-onset glaucoma. *Am J Ophthalmol* 1977;**83**:174–9.
22. Agarwal HC, Sood NN, Sihota R, Sanga L, Honavar SG. Mitomycin-C in congenital glaucoma. *Ophthalmic Surg Lasers* 1997;**28**:979–85.
23. Elder MJ. Combined trabeculotomy–trabeculectomy compared with primary trabeculectomy for congenital glaucoma. *Br J Ophthalmol* 1994;**78**:745–8.
24. Coleman AL, Smyth RJ, Wilson MR, Tam M. Initial clinical experience with the Ahmed glaucoma valve implant in pediatric patients. *Arch Ophthalmol* 1997;**115**:186–91.
25. Shaffer RN. Prognosis of goniotomy in primary infantile glaucoma (trabeculodysgenesis). *Trans Am Ophthalmol Soc* 1982;**80**:321–5.
26. Broughton WL, Parks MM. An analysis of treatment of congenital glaucoma by goniotomy. *Am J Ophthalmol* 1981;**91**:566–72.
27. Douglas DH. Reflections on buphthalmos and goniotomy. *Trans Ophthalmol Soc UK* 1970;**90**:931–7.
28. Barsoum-Homsy M, Chevrette L. Incidence and prognosis of childhood glaucoma. A study of 63 cases. *Ophthalmology* 1986;**93**:1323–7.
29. Anderson DR. Trabeculotomy compared to goniotomy for glaucoma in children. *Ophthalmology* 1983;**90**:805–6.
30. Mandal AK, Naduvilath TJ, Jayagandan A. Surgical results of combined trabeculotomy–trabeculectomy for developmental glaucoma. *Ophthalmology* 1998;**105**:974–82.
31. Turut P, Ribstein G, Milazzo S, Madelain J. L'intervention combinée trabéculotomie trabéculectomie dans le glaucome congénital primitif. *Bull Soc Ophtalmol Fr* 1988;**88**:1021–4.
32. Mullaney PB, Selleck C, Al-Awad A, Al-Mesfer S, Zwaan J. Combined trabeculotomy and trabeculectomy as an initial procedure on uncomplicated congenital glaucoma. *Arch Ophthalmol* 1999;**117**:457–60.
33. Netland PA, Walton DS. Glaucoma drainage implants in pediatric patients. *Ophthalmic Surg* 1993;**24**:723–9.
34. Fellenbaum PS, Sidoti PA, Heuer DK, Minckler DS, Baerveldt G, Lee PP. Experience with the Baerveldt implant in young patients with complicated glaucomas. *J Glaucoma* 1995;**4**:91–7.
35. Muñoz M, Tomey KF, Traverso C, Day SH, Senft SH. Clinical experience with the Molteno implant in advanced infantile glaucoma. *J Pediatr Ophthalmol Strabismus* 1991;**28**:68–72.
36. Molteno ACB, Dempster AG, Carne A. Molteno implants: the principles of bleb management. *Aust NZ J Ophthalmol* 1999;**27**:350–2.
37. Beck AD, Lynch MG. 360° trabeculotomy for primary congenital glaucoma. *Arch Ophthalmol* 1995;**113**:1200–2.

10 Retinopathy of prematurity

Clare Gilbert

Background

Definition

Retinopathy of prematurity (ROP) is a vasoproliferative disease of premature, low birth weight (LBW) babies, which occurs as a result of aberrant vascularisation of the immature retina. The disease is classified by severity (stages I–V); by site (zones 1–3); and by extent (clock hours 1–12). A further constellation of signs, characterised by vascular incompetence and breakdown of blood-ocular barriers ("plus" disease), denotes an active process.[1,2] Threshold disease is defined as five continuous clock hours, or a total of eight clock hours, stage III ROP in zones 1 and 2, in the presence of "plus" disease. Cicatricial changes, which are sequelae of resolved disease, are also described.

Blindness due to ROP

Retinopathy of prematurity is responsible for up to 15% of all causes of blindness in children in industrialised countries. However, the proportion of blindness in children due to ROP has changed over time – during the 1950s up to 50% of blind children were blind from ROP (the "first epidemic"). Controlling the use of unmonitored supplemental oxygen led to a decline in the incidence of ROP blindness in the 1960s and 1970s.

Natural history

The first signs of ROP usually develop four to six weeks after birth, and stage III disease is unlikely to occur before six weeks after birth. However, the onset and development of ROP are governed predominantly by postmenstrual age (i.e. in more premature babies the disease is likely to start at a later postnatal age than in less preterm babies). Stage I and II ROP resolve spontaneously in the majority of babies. However, eyes progressing to Stage III "threshold" disease have an almost 50% risk of progressing to retinal detachment and loss of vision. Progression to threshold disease can occur over a matter of one to two weeks, particularly in babies with disease in zone 1.

Incidence/prevalence

The proportion of preterm babies with advanced ROP (i.e. stage III or more) increased during the 1980s (the "second epidemic") due to the increased survival of very preterm, extremely low birth weight babies (ELBW) (i.e. less than 1000 g at birth), but there is evidence that the proportion affected is declining again despite increasing survival rates among extremely premature, ELBW babies.[3] The overall impact of these two factors on the incidence of advanced ROP at the population level (i.e. increased survival of ELBW babies combined with a lower proportion being affected by ROP) is difficult to gauge, requiring long-term population-based data that are not readily available. The proportion of premature babies developing the different stages of ROP varies depending on the population being studied. The proportion of ELBW babies developing the early stages of ROP is very high but spontaneous regression occurs in the majority. In the UK approximately 8–10% of babies <1500 g at birth develop stage III disease[4] and recent data suggest that approximately 2% of babies examined develop disease needing treatment.[5]

Aetiology

Recent studies are all in agreement that the major risk factors for advanced ROP in industrialised countries are prematurity and low birth weight: the majority of babies developing stage III ROP have a birth weight of <900 g and are extremely premature (less than 29 weeks gestational age (GA)). Other risk factors include fluctuation in blood oxygen levels during the first few weeks of life, being small for GA, intraventricular haemorrhage, factors that influence the condition termed "oxygen radical disease of neonatology" (for example, blood transfusions), and certain maternal risk factors.[6] A wide range of other risk factors have been explored, often with conflicting results.

Treatment options

The CRYO-ROP clinical trial showed that ablation of the avascular retinal periphery with cryotherapy almost halved the rate of unfavourable outcomes in eyes with threshold disease.[7] Since this study was published, laser has become a more popular method of treatment for a variety of reasons, and case series report very high rates of regression following treatment. However, stage III ROP in zone 1 carries a much worse prognosis than disease in zones 2 or 3, and many ophthalmologists treat these eyes before threshold disease has been reached. Despite earlier treatment the anatomical and functional results remain poorer than for disease in more peripheral retina. Complex vitreoretinal surgery for stage V gives uniformly poor functional and anatomical results,[8] but some surgeons achieve good results for stage IV (sub-total retinal detachment).[9]

Prognosis

Many follow-up studies have been undertaken of babies with ROP and on eyes following treatment. These studies show that babies with stage III disease are at higher risk of a range of long-term sequelae compared to babies of similar GA and BW without ROP (for example, refractive errors, strabismus).[10] Long-term follow-up is required so that amblyogenic factors can be identified and managed.

Screening for ROP

Given the availability of an effective treatment for threshold ROP it is imperative that the population of babies at risk is examined at the right time so that those needing treatment can be identified and treated promptly. Industrialised countries such as the UK and the USA have different screening criteria[4,11] and there is debate about whether criteria should be changed in light of the lower risk in more mature babies.[12–14] In Canada this discussion is based on a multi-centre study of over 16 000 babies screened for ROP.[12]

Retinopathy of prematurity in middle and low income countries

Retinopathy of prematurity in babies in middle-income countries and in urban centres in developing countries presents a very different picture from that currently seen in industrialised countries. The proportion of blindness in children due to ROP is much higher in many middle countries than is now the case in industrialised countries[15] and the BWs and GAs of babies with stage III threshold disease to stage V disease are also different: reports from ophthalmologists running screening programmes in several countries in Latin America report threshold disease in babies with BWs in the range 600–2000 g (mean 1100 g) and many have a GA of more than 30 weeks.[16] It would appear that in these countries, where neonatal outcomes are often poor, the population of babies at risk is different, which has implications for screening programmes.

Issues

Clinical trials of interventions in preterm babies are complicated by the fact that the organs of very premature babies are still differentiating as well as growing – the time of onset of the interventions as well as the dose, duration, and cessation (for example, abrupt versus gradual) of the intervention may all be relevant variables. Questions relate to interventions designed to prevent ROP (primary prevention) or designed to delay progression once ROP has developed (secondary) or designed to restore function (tertiary prevention). As in all clinical trials, potential benefit needs to be weighed against possible adverse outcomes.

Primary prevention

Question

What interventions are effective at preventing ROP in premature, LBW babies, and does the time of onset of the intervention, its duration, dose and mode of cessation have any bearing on the outcome?

The evidence

Trials in this area can be grouped under studies where the main outcome was prevention of ROP, and those where ROP was a secondary outcome. Many of the latter have been reviewed by the Cochrane Neonatal group,[17–30] while others have been subject to other meta-analysis.[31] The findings of the systematic reviews are summarised in Tables 10.1 and 10.2.

Oxygen

Seven trials were evaluated in three Cochrane systematic reviews.[17–19] Although many of the studies were carried out several years ago, they confirm the historical association between high and prolonged exposure to oxygen as a risk factor for ROP. However, the studies do not address the issue of what is the optimum level of exposure to oxygen during the early neonatal period (the first week after birth), or the late neonatal period (weeks two to four after birth).

Vitamin E

Six trials of vitamin E supplementation have been evaluated in one review.[31] Three trials concluded that vitamin E reduced the severity but not the incidence of ROP, and three showed no effect. There were differences in study design between the trials, for example, some trials were designed to maintain physiological levels of vitamin E while others aimed to achieve serum levels higher than this. All the trials were undertaken before the International Classification of ROP was described, which makes their

Table 10.1 Primary prevention of ROP: trials where ROP was the main, or one of the main outcomes

Intervention – oxygen	No. of trials	Main outcome(s)	Impact on ROP	Ref
Restricted versus liberal oxygen exposure, trials in which ambient oxygen concentrations were targeted to achieve a lower *v* a higher blood oxygen range	5	Mortality, and incidence and severity of ROP	Restricted oxygen use associated with a significant reduction in the incidence and severity of ROP	17
Gradual *v* abrupt discontinuation of oxygen	1 small trial	ROP	Gradual weaning was associated with a significantly lower risk of ROP	18
Early *v* late discontinuation of oxygen	1 small trial	Mortality and ROP	No significant differences	19
Intervention – vitamin E				
Vitamin E prophylaxis (vitamin E is an anti-oxidant), trials to reduce retinopathy of prematurity: a reappraisal of published trials	6	Incidence of all stages of ROP and of stage III "plus" disease Adverse effects were not analysed in this meta-analysis	• No difference in incidence of all stages of ROP but the pooled odds ratio showed a significant reduction of stage III 'plus' in the supplemented group (OR 0·44; CI 0·21–0·81; $P<0.02$) • Some trials showed an increased rate of adverse effects such as necrotising enterocolitis in supplemented babies	30
Intervention – light				
Early light reduction (light may increase oxidative stress to the developing retina), trials comparing reduced light exposure to premature babies within the first 7 days following birth	4 + 1 quasi-randomised trial	Any acute ROP and poor ROP outcome	Preliminary report from the Cochrane review states that "decreasing light exposure in premature infants is very unlikely to reduce the incidence of ROP"	31
Intervention – D-penecillamine				
D-Penicillamine (used to prevent hyperbilirubinaemia), trials where D-Penicillamine was administered to infants <2000 g at birth within 24 hours of birth *v* no treatment	2	Acute or severe ROP	• Significant reduction in acute ROP (RR 0·09; CI 0·01–0·71). • Severe stages could not be analysed • Further trials are warranted with particular attention to adverse effects	20

interpretation difficult. The meta-analysis did not include an assessment of whether there are increased risks of adverse effects in supplemented infants. The author of the meta-analysis argues that a large, well-conducted clinical trial is warranted to address issues of potential benefit as well as side effects.

Lighting levels

One Cochrane review summarises four clinical trials of early light reduction. Preliminary results suggest that lower ambient lighting is of no benefit in preventing ROP.[20]

D-Penicillamine

Two trials were summarised in one Cochrane systematic review.[22] While the trials showed a reduction in acute

ROP, the review concluded that further studies of D-penicillamine are warranted, paying attention to possible side effects.

Surfactants

Five Cochrane systematic reviews have evaluated 36 trials of surfactant: two reviews looked at trials for prevention of respiratory distress syndrome (RDS)[22,23] and three reviewed trials in which surfactants were used to treat RDS.[24–26] Trials suggest that there is no difference between treated and untreated babies in the proportion developing ROP. However, the positive impact on mortality means that the actual number of babies surviving who are at risk of ROP will be greater with surfactant use. Another Cochrane

Table 10.2   Primary prevention of ROP: trials where ROP was a secondary outcome

Intervention – prevention of respiratory distress syndrome with surfactants and factors that promote surfactant maturation (inositol)	No. of trials	Main outcome(s)	Impact on ROP	Ref
• Prophylactic *natural* surfactant extract: intratracheal natural surfactant given prophylactically to high risk preterm babies at or shortly after birth to prevent RDS. Control babies given surfactant if they developed RDS	8	Multiple, for example, respiratory distress syndrome, pneumothorax, patent ductus arteriosus, mortality	No differences in rates of ROP but reduced mortality and other respiratory outcomes	21
• Prophylactic *synthetic* surfactant: surfactant given prophylactically to high risk preterm babies at or shortly after birth to prevent RDS. Control babies given surfactant if they developed RDS	7	As above	No differences in rates of ROP but reduced mortality and other respiratory outcomes	22
Intervention – treatment of respiratory distress syndrome with surfactants				
• Early *v* delayed selective surfactant: early admin via endotracheal tube within 2 hours of birth for babies intubated for RDS. Delayed administration of surfactant for babies with established RDS	4	As above	No differences in rates of ROP but reduced mortality and other respiratory outcomes	23
• Natural surfactant extract *v* synthetic surfactant: trials comparing natural or synthetic surfactant to prevent RDS or for treatment of established RDS	11	As above	No differences in rates of ROP but reduced mortality	24
• Synthetic surfactant for respiratory distress syndrome: comparison of surfactant treatment and routine management *v* routine management alone	6	As above	No differences in rates of any ROP or of severe ROP, but reduced mortality	25
Intervention – inositol				
• Inositol for respiratory distress syndrome (inositol is an essential nutrient that promotes maturation of several components of surfactant): trials comparing inositol supplementation with placebo or no intervention	3	Bronchopulmonary dysplasia, mortality; intraventricular haemorrhage, ROP	Mortality and rates of threshold and stage IV ROP significantly reduced (RR 0·09; CI 0·01–0·67); reduction in any stage of ROP (RR 0·53; CI 0·29–0·97)	26
Intervention – vitamin A				
• Vitamin A supplementation (vitamin A promotes epithelial cell differentiation and is an anti-oxidant): trials comparing vitamin A supplementation with standard regimes	7	Mortality; oxygen requirements; nosocomial infections; ROP (2 trials)	Trend towards a reduction in ROP; reduced oxygen requirements	33

(Continued)

Table 10.2 (Continued)

Intervention – prevention of respiratory distress syndrome with surfactants and factors that promote surfactant maturation (inositol)	No. of trials	Main outcome(s)	Impact on ROP	Ref
Intervention – steroids:				
• Early postnatal (<96 hours) corticosteroids for preventing chronic lung disease in preterm infants	19	Multiple, for example, chronic lung disease (CLD), mortality, pneumothorax	No significant effect on ROP; mortality and CLD reduced but increased adverse effects	27
• Moderately early (7–14 days) postnatal corticosteroids for preventing chronic lung disease in preterm infants	7	As above	No significant effect on ROP, mortality and CLD reduced but increased adverse effects	28
• Delayed (>3 weeks) postnatal corticosteroids for chronic lung disease in preterm infants	9	Multiple, including mortality, failure to extubate, necrotising enterocolitis, hypertension, hyperglycaemia, severe ROP	Increase in severe ROP of borderline significance in survivors given steroids	29

review evaluated three trials of inositol (an essential nutrient that promotes maturation of several components of surfactant) and found lower rates of ROP, particularly of stages needing treatment or stage IV (reported in two of the three trials).[27]

Prenatal steroids

Many of the trials to determine whether prenatal steroids given to women at high risk of premature birth would result in improved neonatal outcomes were conducted several years ago; several meta-analyses have been undertaken, as well as long-term cohort studies. The findings of these earlier trials showed a protective effect, and they are now given routinely. Many women at high risk of preterm birth are currently given weekly steroid therapy from 24 weeks gestation.

Postnatal steroids

Three Cochrane reviews have evaluated 35 trials of different steroid regimens given at different intervals after premature birth to prevent or treat chronic lung disease, as it has been suggested that steroids and surfactant may act synergistically. Trials of early and moderately early steroid treatment have not demonstrated any significant effect on ROP, but adverse effects were more common.[28,29] There is a suggestion that late steroids may increase the risk of ROP.[30] Concern has been raised about possible adverse effects of antenatal and postnatal steroids (for example, sepsis), and in very preterm babies, brain growth retardation and increased rates of cerebral palsy in treated infants. The current consensus seems to be that there is a limit to which medical interventions can accelerate cerebral maturation and/or prevent brain injury in babies born at 23–25 weeks gestation.[32]

Others

A Cochrane review of seven trials of vitamin A supplementation suggests that this intervention is associated with a trend towards a reduction in ROP.[33] There have been a few other small trials where ROP has been a secondary outcome. These include two different interventions for clinically significant patent ductus arteriosus: surgical intervention within 24 hours of birth compared with no surgical intervention,[34] and a placebo controlled trial of indometacin.[35] The results of both studies showed a non-significant increase in the proportion of babies developing ROP in the intervention groups.

Comment

A very large number of clinical trials have been undertaken, usually to investigate neonatal outcomes other than ROP, which means that many are underpowered to detect significant findings with respect to ROP. The findings of some of the systematic reviews are conclusive (for example, that surfactants improve neonatal outcomes but do not influence the incidence of ROP), whereas others suggest that more studies are needed (for example, vitamin E supplementation; treatment with D-penicillamine; treatment with inositol). An important area that has not been subject to recent clinical trials relates to optimum oxygen concentrations during the first few weeks of life. Such trials would be challenging and pose ethical issues, and would probably best be undertaken after reliable, non-invasive means of measuring ocular oxygen levels had been developed and used to explore optimum ocular oxygenation in case-control studies.

Secondary prevention

Several interventions have been evaluated in clinical trials to determine whether they alter the progression or prognosis in babies with established ROP.

Question

Does supplemental oxygen halt the progression of established retinopathy of prematurity?

The evidence

We found one multi-centre randomised controlled trial, the STOP-ROP trial,[36] which was designed to determine whether higher levels of oxygen after ROP had developed had a beneficial effect on disease progression. This trial is summarised in Table 10.3. The results of the STOP-ROP trial were essentially negative, but secondary analysis suggested that babies without "plus" disease at baseline fared better than those with these features.

Question

Does peripheral retinal cryotherapy prevent unfavourable outcomes in babies with threshold ROP?

The evidence

One small clinical trial,[37] and one very large multi-centre study with long-term follow up[7,38–42] have addressed whether cryotherapy prevents unfavourable outcomes in babies with threshold ROP. The details of the trials are summarised in Table 10.4.

Question

Is earlier treatment (i.e. for high risk pre-threshold disease) more effective than treatment of threshold disease, with fewer adverse effects?

The evidence

One small trial has been undertaken,[43] and another large multi-centre trial is currently being undertaken in the USA (the ETROP trial).[44] These trials are summarised in Table 10.5. At the moment there is no evidence from clinical trials that earlier treatment (i.e. before threshold disease is reached) gives better results than treatment of threshold disease. Hopefully the ETROP trial will provide answers to this question.

Question

Is laser as effective as cryotherapy, and is one form of laser more effective than another? Does the method of delivery of the laser, or the density of the laser treatment, affect the outcome?

The evidence

Three small trials have addressed whether laser is as effective as cryotherapy.[45–50] These trials are summarised in Table 10.6. Two trials have compared the method of delivery and density of laser treatment[51,52] and these are summarised in Table 10.7. Other important outcomes relate to the comparison of adverse effects between the two treatment modalities, and methods of reducing stress during treatment.[53]

Comment

Both cryotherapy and laser are highly effective and prevent unfavourable outcomes in babies with threshold disease. The available evidence suggests that the type of laser is not important; confluent placing of burns in the avascular retina may give better results than sparser applications. Laser is associated with fewer operative complications than cryotherapy. The results of the large trial to explore whether earlier treatment gives more favourable results are awaited.

Table 10.3 Does supplemental oxygen halt the progression of established retinopathy of prematurity?

Design	No. of studies	Quality	Intervention	Participants	Main outcomes	Findings/comments	Ref
Prospective randomised multi-centre study in USA – the STOP-ROP study	1	High	Target pulse oximetry: 89–94% (conventional arm) or 96–99% (supplemental arm) for at least 2 weeks	649 babies with established pre-threshold ROP in at least one eye and median pulse oximetry of <94%	• Rate of progression to threshold disease • Adverse effects	• Rates of progression: 48% in conventional arm 41% in supplemental arm (OR 0·72; CI 0·52–1·01) • Subgroup analysis suggests that babies without "plus" disease at baseline may respond better to supplemental oxygen • Supplemented babies had slightly higher rates of adverse effects (exacerbation of lung disease, prolonged oxygen requirements and hospitalisation) • Sample size: initial target was 880 babies, but enrolment was curtailed, which reduced the power of the study • Possible bias: only 649/1213 eligible babies were enrolled in the study	36

Table 10.4 Does peripheral retinal cryotherapy prevent unfavourable outcomes in babies with threshold ROP?

Design	Quality	Intervention	Participants	Main outcome	Findings/comments	Ref
Prospective randomised trial	First, small	Peripheral retinal ablation with cryotherapy v no treatment	17 babies with symmetrical threshold disease randomised to cryotherapy or no treatment	• Regression of disease • Time interval not stated	• Treated eyes: 71% resolved • Untreated eyes: 41% resolved • Not statistically significant	37
Prospective randomised multi-centre study in USA (the CRYO-ROP study)	High	Peripheral retinal ablation of eyes with threshold ROP with cryotherapy v no treatment	• 291 babies randomised • Some had bilateral threshold disease others had asymmetrical disease • Interim analysis – data available on 172 babies at 3 months	Structural results at 3 months clearly defined as favourable or unfavourable (interim analysis)	• Cryotherapy associated with a highly statistically significant reduction in unfavourable outcomes in treated babies • Recruitment stopped early	7
			• As above • 273 of 291 babies randomised with follow up data 3 months after randomisation	Structural results at 3 months clearly defined as favourable or unfavourable (analysis of all those randomised)	• Cryotherapy associated with a highly statistically significant reduction in unfavourable outcomes in treated babies • Zone 1 disease had a poorer outcome	38
			• 246 of the original 291 babies were examined at one year	Structural and functional results	• Benefit of cryotherapy maintained at one year in terms of structural outcome (45·8% reduction in unfavourable outcome in treated eyes) and functional outcome (50·6% control eyes blind v 31·9% of treated eyes) • Treated eyes were more myopic than untreated eyes	39

(Continued)

Table 10.4 (Continued)

Design	Quality	Intervention	Participants	Main outcome	Findings/comments	Ref
			• 236 of the original 291 babies were examined at 3½ years. • Visual acuity data available on 212 children	Structural and functional results at 3½ years	• Treated eyes had significantly lower rates of unfavourable visual acuity outcomes (19% and 20% reductions) and a 42.5% reduction in unfavourable structural outcomes • Disease in zone 1 had worse outcomes than disease in zone 2	40
			234 of the original 291 babies were examined at 3½ years	Snellen visual acuity and structural outcome at 5½ years	• Treated eyes had significantly lower rate of unfavourable outcomes in terms of visual acuity and structural outcomes • Concerns raised that cryo may have an adverse effect on visual acuity	41
			247 of the original 291 babies were examined at 10 years	Snellen near and distance visual acuity and structural outcome at 10 years	• Treated eyes had significantly lower rate of unfavourable outcomes in terms of visual acuity and structural outcomes than untreated eyes • No difference in % of eyes with visual activity 20/40 or better between treated and control eyes	42

Table 10.5 Is earlier treatment (i.e. for high risk, pre-threshold disease) more effective than treatment of threshold disease, with fewer adverse effects?

Design	No. of studies	Quality	Intervention	Participants included/ excluded	Main outcome	Other outcome(s)	Findings/comments	Ref
Prospective multi-centre randomised study	1	Too small	Immediate laser treatment (argon or diode) or treatment delayed until threshold reached	19 infants with bilateral (2) or unilateral (17) ROP (international classification not used and enrolment criteria not very clear)	Regression of disease after one or more treatments	–	• 16% of early treated eyes progressed compared with 18% of deferred group • Not statistically significant • Some eyes probably treated unnecessarily	43
Prospective randomised multi-centre study in USA (ETROP study)	1	Will be high	Immediate treatment or treatment delayed until threshold reached	• Babies with high risk pre-threshold ROP • Study designed to recruit 370 infants over 3 years	Disease regression and visual acuity at 9 months	• Myopia • Amblyopia • Strabismus	Ongoing	44

Table 10.6 Is laser as effective as cryotherapy and is one form of laser more effective than another?

Design	No. of studies	Quality	Intervention	Participants	Main outcomes	Findings/comments	Ref
Prospective randomised study	1	Very small study	Eyes randomised to cryotherapy or diode laser	14 infants with symmetrical threshold ROP and 5 babies with unilateral threshold disease (total 19 babies)	• Treatment complications • Findings at follow up (1–15 months)	• More complications during treatment with cryo and more obvious chorioretinal scars at follow up • One eye in each treatment group had an unfavourable outcome • Study too small for meaningful conclusions	45
				• 12 of the 19 babies examined at 34–52 months	• Structural outcome • Visual acuity • Refractive error	• There was a tendency for laser treated eyes to have better outcomes but the numbers are too small for meaningful conclusions	46
Prospective randomised study	1	Very small study	Eyes randomised to cryotherapy or diode laser	6 infants with symmetrical threshold ROP	• Structural outcome at 8–19 weeks	• One eye treated with cryotherapy progressed to stage IV despite retreatment • Study too small for meaningful conclusions	47
Prospective randomised study	1	Very small study	• Eyes randomised to cryotherapy or laser (argon or diode) • Allocation to laser type was not random	Babies with threshold ROP in one or both eyes (65 recruited in total; 55 had bilateral ROP)	• Structural outcome at 3 months in those treated with argon laser	• Initial report on 28 eyes in 18 babies. • 3/12 cryo treated eyes and 1/16 laser treated eyes had unfavourable outcomes • Study too small for meaningful conclusions	48
					• Structural outcome at 3 or more months in eyes treated with diode laser	• 28 babies treated with diode compared with 24 eyes treated with cryo • Unfavourable outcome in 3/28 laser treated eyes v 4/24 cryo treated eyes • Study small	49
					• Visual acuity and refractive error at 4·3–7·6 years in babies with bilateral ROP	• Data available on 25/55 babies recruited • All outcomes were better for laser treated eyes but follow up was incomplete	50

Table 10.7 Does the method of delivery of the laser or the density of the laser treatment affect the outcome?

Design	No. of studies	Quality	Intervention	Participants	Main outcomes	Findings/comments	Ref
Prospective randomised study	1	Small study	Eyes randomised to transpupillary or trans-scleral diode laser	25 infants with bilateral symmetrical threshold ROP	Regression of acute disease and incidence of adverse effects	• Only one eye treated with trans-scleral laser failed to regress • No adverse effects were noted apart from retinal and preretinal haemorrhage, which occurred with both treatments	51
Mixed design: retrospective non-randomised study and prospective randomised trial	1	Small study	Confluent burns (56 eyes) or non-confluent diode laser burns (51 eyes) for threshold ROP	107 eyes from 58 babies: 12 in retrospective study and 46 in trial, data pooled	Rates of progression, postoperative complications, retreatment rates at 3–12 months	• Eyes treated with confluent burns had a significantly lower rate of progression and needed fewer retreatments • No difference in complication rates • Weakness: data pooled and some differences in the groups at baseline	52

Tertiary prevention

Question

Does complex vitreoretinal surgery give better anatomical and/or functional results than no treatment?

The evidence

We found no trials that have been undertaken for stage IV or stage V disease.

Comment

There is no evidence that surgical treatment of advanced stages of ROP is of benefit.

Implications for practice

The body of evidence is overwhelmingly supportive of the short and long-term benefits of peripheral retinal ablation for acute, severe ROP, and there is weaker evidence that confluent laser burns give optimal results with fewer side effects. There is no evidence from trials that surgery for stage IV and V ROP give better results than the natural history. There is little new conclusive evidence from clinical trials concerning interventions that can prevent ROP or modify its natural history. However, many of the interventions investigated to explore other neonatal outcomes have given positive results, so increasing the survival, and hence the population, of babies requiring screening.

Implications for research

Although there is a large body of literature on many aspects of the epidemiology of ROP there are still many unanswered questions. Further clinical trials are warranted to determine the following.

- What are optimum oxygen concentrations during the first few weeks of life to prevent ROP? Are the levels required during the early neonatal period the same as during the late neonatal period, and are optimum levels maturity-dependant?[54]
- Are there other interventions that can prevent the development of ROP, or halt its progress, particularly those which reduce oxidative stress, such as use of vitamin E?

- What are the benefits and risks of treating pre-threshold disease compared with treating threshold disease, particularly for disease in zone 1?
- Are there other approaches to inhibiting angiogenesis that are safe and effective in this group of vulnerable babies?
- Does surgery for stage IV ROP give better long-term anatomical and functional results than the natural history?

References

1. Patz A. An international classification of retinopathy of prematurity. II: The classification of retinal detachment. *Arch Ophthalmol* 1987;**105**:905–12.
2. Committee for the Classification of Retinopathy of Prematurity. An international classification system of retinopathy of prematurity. *Arch Ophthalmol* 1984;**102**:1130–4.
3. Gilbert C. Retinopathy of prematurity: the second "lull"? Editorial. *Br J Ophthalmol* 2001;**85**:1017–19.
4. Royal College of Ophthalmologists Joint Working party. *Retinopathy of Prematurity: guidelines for screening and treatment.* London: Royal College of Ophthalmologists, 1995.
5. Haines L, Fielder AR, Pollock JI, Scrivener R, Wilkinson AR. Retinopathy of prematurely in the UK 1: the organisation of services for screening and treatment. *Eye* 2002;**16**:33–8.
6. Fielder A. Retinopathy of prematurity. In: Taylor D, ed. *Paediatric Ophthalmology, 2nd edn.* Oxford: Blackwell Science, 1997.
7. Cryotherapy for Retinopathy of Prematurity Co-operative Group. Multicenter trial of cryotherapy for retinopathy of prematurity. Preliminary results. *Arch Ophthalmol* 1988;**106**:471–9.
8. Quinn GE, Dobson V, Barr CC *et al.* Visual acuity of eyes after vitrectomy for retinopathy of prematurity: follow-up at 5 1/2 years. The Cryotherapy for Retinopathy of Prematurity Co-operative Group. *Ophthalmol* 1996;**103**:595–600.
9. Trese MT, Droste PJ. Long term postoperative results of a consecutive series of stages 4 and 5 retinopathy of prematurity. *Ophthalmology* 1998;**105**:992–7.
10. Hebbandi SB, Bowen JR, Hipwell GC, Ma PJ, Leslie GI, Arnold JD. Ocular sequelae in extremely premature infants at 5 years of age. *J Paediatr Child Health* 1997;**33**:339–42.
11. Fierson WM, Palmer EA, Biglan AW *et al.* Screening examination of premature infants for retinopathy of prematurity. *Pediatrics* 1997;**100**: 273–4.
12. Lee SK, Normand C, McMillan D, Ohlsson A, Vincer M, Lyons C. Evidence for changing guidelines for routine screening for retinopathy of prematurity. *Arch Pediatr Adolesc Med* 2001;**155**:387–95.
13. Wright K, Anderson ME, Walker E, Lorch V. Should fewer premature infants be screened for retinopathy of prematurity in the managed care era? *Pediatrics* 1998;**102**:31–4.
14. Goble RR, Jones HS, Fielder AR. Are we screening too many babies for retinopathy of prematurity? *Eye* 1997;**11**:509–14.
15. Gilbert C, Rahi J, Eckstein M, O'Sullivan J, Foster A. Retinopathy of prematurity in middle-income countries. *Lancet* 1997;**350**:12–14.
16. Report of workshop on Prevention of Blindness due to ROP in children in Mexico. London: London School of Hygiene and Tropical Medicine, 2001 (unpublished document).
17. Askie LM, Henderson-Smart DJ. Restricted versus liberal oxygen exposure for preventing morbidity and mortality in preterm or low birth weight infants (Cochrane Review). In: Cochrane Collaboration: *Cochrane Library.* Issue 2. Oxford: Update Software, 2002.
18. Askie LM, Henderson-Smart DJ. Gradual versus abrupt discontinuation of oxygen in preterm or low birth weight infants (Cochrane Review). In: Cochrane Collaboration: *Cochrane Library.* Issue 2. Oxford: Update Software, 2002.

19. Askie LM, Henderson-Smart DJ. Early versus late discontinuation of oxygen in preterm or low birth weight infants (Cochrane Review). In: Cochrane Collaboration: *Cochrane Library.* Issue 2. Oxford: Update Software, 2002.

20. Phelps DL, Lakatos L, Watts JL. D-Penicillamine for preventing retinopathy of prematurity in preterm infants (Cochrane Review). In: Cochrane Collaboration: *Cochrane Library.* Issue 2. Oxford: Update Software, 2002.

21. Soll RF. Prophylactic natural surfactant extract for preventing morbidity and mortality in preterm infants (Cochrane Review). In: Cochrane Collaboration: *Cochrane Library.* Issue 2. Oxford: Update Software, 2002.

22. Soll RF. Prophylactic synthetic surfactant for preventing morbidity and mortality in preterm infants (Cochrane Review). In: Cochrane Collaboration: *Cochrane Library.* Issue 2. Oxford: Update Software, 2002.

23. Yost CC, Soll RF. Early versus delayed selective surfactant treatment for neonatal respiratory distress syndrome (Cochrane Review). In: Cochrane Collaboration: *Cochrane Library.* Issue 2. Oxford: Update Software, 2002.

24. Soll RF, Blanco F. Natural surfactant extract versus synthetic surfactant for neonatal respiratory distress syndrome (Cochrane Review). In: Cochrane Collaboration: *Cochrane Library.* Issue 2. Oxford: Update Software, 2002.

25. Soll RF. Synthetic surfactant for respiratory distress syndrome in preterm infants (Cochrane Review). In: Cochrane Collaboration: *Cochrane Library.* Issue 2. Oxford: Update Software, 2002.

26. Howlett A, Ohlsson A. Inositol for respiratory distress syndrome in preterm infants (Cochrane Review). In: Cochrane Collaboration: *Cochrane Library.* Issue 2. Oxford: Update Software, 2002.

27. Halliday HL, Ehrenkranz RA. Early postnatal (< 96 hours) corticosteroids for preventing chronic lung disease in preterm infants (Cochrane Review). In: Cochrane Collaboration: *Cochrane Library.* Issue 2. Oxford: Update Software, 2002.

28. Halliday HL, Ehrenkranz RA. Moderately early (7–14 days) postnatal corticosteroids for preventing chronic lung disease in preterm infants (Cochrane Review). In: Cochrane Collaboration: *Cochrane Library.* Issue 2. Oxford: Update Software, 2002.

29. Halliday HL, Ehrenkranz RA. Delayed (> 3 weeks) postnatal corticosteroids for chronic lung disease in preterm infants (Cochrane Review). In: Cochrane Collaboration: *Cochrane Library.* Issue 2. Oxford: Update Software, 2002.

30. Raju TN, Langenberg P, Bhutani V, Quinn GE. Vitamin E prophylaxis to reduce retinopathy of prematurity: a reappraisal of published trials. *J Pediatr* 1997;**131**:844–50.

31. Phelps DL, Watts JL. Early light reduction for preventing retinopathy of prematurity in very low birth weight infants (Cochrane Review). In: Cochrane Collaboration: *Cochrane Library.* Issue 2. Oxford: Update Software, 2002.

32. Hack M, Fanaroff AA. Outcomes of children of extremely low birthweight and gestational age in the 1990s. *Semin Neonatol* 2000;**5**:89–106.

33. Darlow BA, Graham PJ. Vitamin A supplementation for preventing morbidity and mortality in very low birthweight infants (Cochrane Review). In: Cochrane Collaboration: *Cochrane Library.* Issue 2. Oxford: Update Software, 2002.

34. Cassady G, Crouse DT, Kirklin JW *et al.* A randomized controlled trial of very early prophylactic ligation of the ductus arteriosus in babies who weighed 1000 g or less at birth. *N Engl J Med* 1989;**320**:1511–16.

35. Peckham GJ, Miettinen OS, Ellison RC *et al.* Clinical course to 1 year of age in premature infants with patent ductus arteriosus: results of a multicenter randomized trial of indomethacin. *J Pediatr* 1984;**105**:285–91.

36. The STOP-ROP Multicentre Study Group. Supplemental Therapeutic Oxygen for Prethreshold Retinopathy of Prematurity (STOP-ROP): a randomized controlled trial. I: primary outcomes. *Pediatrics* 2000;**105**:295–310.

37. Tasman W. Management of retinopathy of prematurity. *Ophthalmology* 1985;**92**:995–9.

38. Cryotherapy for Retinopathy of Prematurity Co-operative Group. Multicenter trial of cryotherapy for retinopathy of prematurity. Three-month outcome. *Arch Ophthalmol* 1990;**108**:195–204.

39. Cryotherapy for Retinopathy of Prematurity Co-operative Group. Multicenter trial of cryotherapy for retinopathy of prematurity. One year outcome – structure and function. *Arch Ophthalmol* 1990;**108**:1408–16.

40. Cryotherapy for Retinopathy of Prematurity Co-operative Group. Multicenter trial of cryotherapy for retinopathy of prematurity. 3 1/2 year outcome – structure and function. *Arch Ophthalmol* 1993;**111**:339–44.

41. Cryotherapy for Retinopathy of Prematurity Co-operative Group. Multicenter trial of cryotherapy for retinopathy of prematurity. Snellen visual acuity and structural outcome at 5 1/2 tears after randomisation. *Arch Ophthalmol* 1996;**114**:417–24.

42. Cryotherapy for Retinopathy of Prematurity Co-operative Group. Multicenter Trial of Cryotherapy for Retinopathy of Prematurity: ophthalmological outcomes at 10 years. *Arch Ophthalmology* 2001;**119**:1110–18.

43. Vander JF, Handa J, McNamara JA *et al.* Early treatment of posterior retinopathy of prematurity: a controlled trial. *Ophthalmology* 1997;**104**:1731–5.

44. Good WV, Hardy RJ. The multicenter study of Early Treatment for Retinopathy of Prematurity (ETROP). *Ophthalmology* 2001;**108**:1013–14.

45. Hunter DJ, Repka MX. Diode laser photocoagulation for threshold retinopathy of prematurity. *Ophthalmology* 1993;**100**:238–44.

46. White JE, Repka MX. Randomized comparison of diode laser photocoagulation versus cryotherapy for threshold retinopathy of prematurity: 3 year outcome. *J Paediatr Ophthalmol Strabismus* 1997;**34**:83–7.

47. Iverson DA, Trese MT, Orgel IK, Williams GA, Mich RO. Laser photocoagulation for threshold retinopathy of prematurity. *Arch Ophthalmology* 1991;**109**:1342–3 (letter).

48. McNamara JA, Tasman W, Brown G, Federman JL. Laser photocoagulation for Stage 3+ retinopathy of prematurity. *Ophthalmology* 1991;**98**:576–80.

49. McNamara JA, Tasman W, Vander JF, Brown GC. Diode laser photocoagulation for retinopathy of prematurity. Preliminary results. *Arch Ophthal* 1992;**110**:1714–16.

50. Connolly BP, McNamara JA, Sharma S, Regillo CD, Tasman W. A comparison of laser photocoagulation with transcleral cryotherapy in the treatment of threshold retinopathy of prematurity. *Ophthalmology* 1998;**105**:1628–31.

51. Seiberth V, Linderkamp O, Vardarli I. Transscleral *v* transpupillary diode laser photocoagulation for the treatment of threshold retinopathy of prematurity. *Arch Ophthalmol* 1997;**115**:1270–5.

52. Banach MJ, Ferrone PJ, Trese MT. A comparison of dense versus less dense diode laser photocoagulation patterns for threshold retinopathy of prematurity. *Ophthalmology* 2000;**107**:324–7.

53. Saunders RA, Miller KW, Hunt HH. Topical anaesthesia during infant eye examinations: does it reduce stress? *Ann Ophthalmol* 1993;**25**:436–9.

54. Tin W, Wariyar U. Giving small babies oxygen: 50 years of uncertainty. *Semin Neonatol* 2002;**7**:361–8.

11 Ophthalmia neonatorum

Jane Moseley

Background

Gonococcal ophthalmia neonatorum (GON) is a recognised cause of visual loss[1] that may cause between 4000 and 30 000 new cases of blindness annually.[2,3]

Other causes of neonatal purulent conjunctivitis include *Chlamydia trachomatis*, *Staphylococcus aureus*, Streptococcus *pneumoniae* and, to a lesser extent, *H. influenzae*, *B. catarrhalis*, *E. coli* and *klebsiella pneumoniae*. Attention has focused on *Neisseria gonorrhoeae* and chlamydia because of ocular morbidity and because of the opportunity for prevention of perinatal ocular infection afforded by prophylaxis at birth. The relative proportions of ophthalmia neonatorum (ON) due to these organisms vary. *Chlamydia trachomatis* may cause up to 54% of ophthalmia neonatorum in Europe and the United States and up to 33% in African countries. *Neisseria gonorrhoeae* accounts for 0–9% in Europe and the United States series, but up to 43% for some African cohorts.[4–23]

The incidence of gonococcal ophthalmia depends on mother to infant transmission rates and the prevalence of gonorrhoea in the population. The rate of perinatal transmission from infected mothers in Kenya has been recorded at 42%.[22] However, since the mid-1990s there has been an increase in the number of new cases of gonorrhoea in England and Wales, Sweden, the United States and Eastern Europe. Estimates of the number of new adult gonorrhoea infections in 1999 ranged from 120 000 (Australia and New Zealand) to 27·7 million new cases for South and South East Asia.[24,25] Antibiotic resistance patterns differ by country and are changing year on year.

Chlamydial ophthalmia neonatorum

Chlamydial ophthalmia neonatorum (CTON) may cause up to 8000 cases of blindness per year.[2] Perinatal transmission rates in the order of 35% in Kenya and Florida have been recorded.[5,16,22]

Control of ophthalmia neonatorum

Perinatal prophylaxis is one of four possible strategies for control of ophthalmia neonatorum (see Box 11.1).[26] This chapter will review the trial-based evidence for efficacy and toxicity of perinatal prophylaxis of gonococcal, chlamydial

---

This chapter reflects the author's personal opinion and not MHRA policy.

> **Box 11.1 Control strategies for ON**
>
> - Primary sexually transmitted disease (STD) prevention in sexually active subjects
> - STD screening in mothers
> - Prophylaxis in the newborn
> - Case identification and treatment in the newborn

and all-cause purulent conjunctivitis in the newborn. Further, treatment options for confirmed cases of ophthalmic neonatorum are considered.

There is worldwide variation in guidelines and practice for prophylaxis and treatment of ophthalmia neonatorum. National STD management guidelines published in 1998 in the United States[27] and Canada[28] recommended tetracycline 1%, silver nitrate 1% or erythromycin 0·5% for gonococcal ophthalmia neonatorum prophylaxis. In 2001, the WHO[29] recommended tetracycline 1% or silver nitrate 1%. However, prophylaxis has been discontinued in many European countries. Lately, the use of silver nitrate as agent of choice for prophylaxis has been questioned.[3]

Question

What is the evidence for the effecacy of interventions for preventing ophthalmia neonatorum?

The evidence

Five randomised controlled trials were identified[30–34] (see Table 11.1). Only Bell *et al*.[30] and Wahlberg[31] included an intervention-free arm.

Prophylaxis versus no prophylaxis

Bell *et al*.[30] found the following frequencies of non-gonococcal conjunctivitis: 14% with silver nitrate prophylaxis, 16% with topical erythromycin and 22% with no prophylaxis, by two months of observation. The hazard ratio (95% confidence interval) of conjunctivitis for silver nitrate compared to no prophylaxis was 0·61 (0·39–0·97). Only the reduction in conjunctivitis associated with silver

Table 11.1 Randomised controlled trials on efficacy of prophylaxis for conjunctivitis in the newborn

Authors	Intervention (no. randomised)	Outcome	Result	Comment
Bell *et al.*, 1993[30] USA	• Erythromycin ointment 0·5% (222) • Silver nitrate 1% (221) • Prophylaxis (226) • Not at risk of gonococcal conjunctivitis	Hazard of non-gonococcal conjunctivitis with cytological or biochemical confirmation	• Compared to no prophylaxis, silver nitrate had a lower rate of conjunctivitis 14% *v* 22% at 2 months (hazard ratio 0·61, 95% CI 0·39–0·97) • Erythromycin also had lower rate of conjunctivitis 16% *v* 22% (hazard ratio 0·69, 95% CI 0·44 to 1·07)	• 2577 potentially eligible, 758 enrolled: 669 randomised, 39 of whom lost to follow up, 4 given incorrect allocation, 29 received additional treatment • Double-blind • Low risk population
Isenberg *et al.*, 1994[32] USA	100 neonates received povidone-iodine solution 2·5% in one eye and either silver nitrate 1% (52 eyes) or erythromycin 0·5% ointment (48 eyes) in the contralateral eye	% reduction in no. of colony-forming units and no. of species pre and 2–4 hours post-installation of prophylaxis	• Povidone resulted in greater reduction in no. of species (*P*<0·002) and no. of colony-forming units (*P*<0·05) than erythromycin • Povidone was not as effective in reducing no. of colony-forming units but had a greater reduction in no. of species compared to silver nitrate	• Eye as unit of randomisation • Microbiologist masked to intervention
Brussieux *et al.*, 1991[34] France	• Silver nitrate 1% (475) • Topical oxytetracycline (425)	% with conjunctivitis culture positive rates in those with conjunctivitis at week 1 and weeks 3/4	• Marginal benefit of oxytetracycline compared to silver nitrate in week 1 • Silver nitrate: 7·1% – minimal ocular signs and 5·4% – severe conjunctivitis in first week *v* 4·8% (*P*=0·02) and 2·8% (*P*=0·05) with oxytetracycline • No gonococci isolated • 1 confirmed *Chlamydia trachomatis* conjunctivitis with oxytetracycline	• Only 195/425 of the oxytetracycline group and 212/475 of the silver nitrate group were analysed in the 2nd phase
Hammerschlag *et al.*, 1980[33] USA	• Erythromycin ointment (24) • Silver nitrate 1% (33)	Conjunctivitis with positive chlamydial culture in 60 infants born to mothers with confirmed *Chlamydia trachomatis*.	12 (33%) of 36 infants receiving silver nitrate developed conjunctivitis compared to none of 24 infants receiving erythromycin *P*=0·001.	• Masking unknown • Subgroup of larger randomised population • sparse report

(Continued)

Table 11.1   (Continued)

Authors	Intervention (no. randomised)	Outcome	Result	Comment
Wahlberg, 1982[31] Sweden	• Silver nitrate 1% (105) • Hexarginum 10% (225) • Physiological saline placebo (214) • Not at risk of gonococcal conjuctivitis	• Gonococcal culture results in infants with week 1 discharge • Chlamydial culture in 15 infants with persistent discharge and sample of 250 healthy infants	• No gonococcal positive conjunctivitis out of 156 neonates with purulent discharge in week one • 2/15 infants with persistent discharge and none of the 250 healthy infants were chlamydia positive	• Treatment groups not identified for culture positive results • Selection of sub-samples not transparent • All mothers with gonococcus cultures excluded

nitrate prophylaxis achieved the pre-specified statistical significance levels when compared with no prophylaxis. The protective effect appeared to be greatest in the first two weeks. The investigators followed up the 109 identified conjunctivitis cases; 61 of 69 untreated cases resolved quickly. There was no association of the need for treatment with prophylactic regimen. The Bell *et al.* study featured many desirable qualities of good clinical trial design. In an attempt to improve completeness of follow-up, the investigators excluded mothers aged under 16 years, those who were living far away, those without telephone access, those who were non-English language speaking or those who had social problems. Mothers were also excluded if they had positive gonococcus cultures in their current pregnancy. A consequence of this was that the population in question was possibly at a lower risk of STDs in general.

In Wahlberg's study, the prophylactic effect compared to placebo was not estimable (allocation status of the two chlamydial conjunctivitis cases not stated). In this low-risk population (only 1/165 mothers tested for chlamydia were positive), there were two cases in 627 infants observed (0·3%).

Different prophylactic regimens

None of the other three randomised studies provided strong evidence of a difference between prophylactic agents. The study by Brussieux *et al.*[34] compared silver nitrate to topical oxytetracycline prophylaxis. There was weak evidence of a prophylactic benefit in terms of reduction of mild conjunctivitis with oxytetracycline in the first week of life, but this difference was not statistically significant by the third week. Staphylococcus aureus, staphylococcus epidermidis and streptococci were the most frequently cultured isolates. Although there were major losses to follow-up in the second phase, these were evenly distributed across groups. The study, in 1994, of providone-iodine, silver nitrate and erythromycin used the eye as the unit of randomisation and presented the results as within, as opposed to between, treatments.

Toxicity

Bell *et al.*[30] identified a higher proportion of neonates with lid staining in those receiving silver nitrate but no other differences in external ocular findings between prophylactic groups at two days. Wahlberg[31] observed short-term modest adverse reactions of pain registration, discharge, transient, decreased scanning behaviour and maternal eye contact associated with silver nitrate and hexarginum compared to placebo. A short-term or medium-term effect of silver nitrate on nasolacrimal obstruction is not evident.[30,35]

Non-randomised studies

Table 11.2 provides the incidence and attack rate* for different categories of ophthalmia neonatorum by intervention and study.

In the first of two studies conducted in Kenya, Laga 1988[36] used untreated historical controls from the same hospital prior to the trial for comparisons. Forty-one per cent completed the 30-day follow-up in the tetracycline group compared to 46% in the silver nitrate group. Cultures were conducted only if infants were symptomatic. Both treatment groups (tetracycline and silver nitrate) had a significantly lower incidence of all-cause ON and of non-chlamydial/non-gonococcal ON (NonCT/GON) compared to prophylaxis-free historical controls. There was a trend to lower incidences of CTON or GON rates compared to these controls. The only demonstrable between-treatment difference was a lower all-cause ON incidence with tetracycline compared to silver nitrate ($P<0·05$). Maternal gonococcal infection rates were 6·6% and 6·4% in the silver nitrate and tetracycline groups respectively. Use of historical controls

---

*The percentage of cases amongst offspring of women with confirmed infection

Table 11.2   Non-randomised studies of efficacy of prophylaxis for conjunctivitis in the newborn

Author	Category of ON	Intervention (no. treated) Incidence (attack rate)			Control
Laga et al.,1988[36]		Silver nitrate 1%	Tetracycline 1%		Historical controls;
Kenya		(1233)	(1499)		No prophylaxis
	GON	0·4% (7·0%)	0·1% (3·%)		2·7 (42%)
	CTON	0·7% (10·1%)	0·5% (7·2%)		6·2 (31.3%)
	NonCT/GON	6·2%	4·5%		9·4
Isenberg et al., 1995[37]		Silver nitrate 1% (929)	Erythromycin 0·5% (1112)	Povidone 2·5% (1076)	
Kenya	GON	0·8%	1·0%	0·4%	
	CTON	10·5%	7·4%	5·5%	
	NonCT/GON	6·8	6·8	6·6	
Chen, 1992[38]		Silver nitrate (1082)	Tetracycline (1156)	Erythromycin (1163)	No prophylaxis
Taiwan	GON	0	0	0	0
	CTON	1·7%	1·3%	1·5%	1·6%
	NonCT/GON	3·9	4·2	5·8	6·5
Hammerschlag et al., 1989[39]		Silver nitrate % (3804)	Tetracycline % (4468)	Erythromycin % (4159)	
USA	GON	0·3	0·07	0·1	
	CTON	0·4% (20%)	0·2 %(11%)	0·3% (14%)	
	Non CT/GON				

GON, gonococcal ophthalmia; CTON, chlamydia ophthalmia; NonCT/GON, non-chlamydial and non-gonococcal ophthalmia

lessens the confidence that the intervention rather than unknown factors is responsible for the benefits observed.

In the second study based in Kenya,[37] mothers were instructed to return if the infant developed clinical signs of conjunctivitis. All-cause ON rate was 15·2%, which compares favourably with previously published literature for Kenya (23% in the absence of prophylaxis). Additionally, the rate of GON in the study population was 0·8% (previously published GON rates in the absence of prophylaxis were 2·3% and 7·3%). Povidone solution had a significantly lower all-cause ON compared to erythromycin ($P < 0·01$) and tetracycline ($P < 0·001$). A similar pattern was present for CTON ($P < 0·008$, $P < 0·001$). It needs to be borne in mind that literature-based controls are a poor basis for comparison as they cannot exclude many alternative factors that may account for any difference.

In the study by Chen,[38] infants were followed up at one and four weeks and if symptomatic. No details were provided on losses to follow-up. In Taiwan, there was no apparent difference in incidence of CTON with prophylaxis compared to no prophylaxis, although the all-cause incidence of ON and nonCT/GON compared favourably with no prophylaxis. No difference was detected between interventions regarding incidence of all-cause ON.

In Hammerschlag et al.'s[39] study in a high-risk inner-city USA population, "most" infants were seen twice between two and 16 weeks. There was no difference in either GON or CTON attack rates between silver nitrate, erythromycin or tetracycline. Thirty-seven per cent of CTON infants born to chlamydia-infected mothers also had extraocular chlamydia culture-positive sites. Ten per cent of those without CTON also had nasopharyngeal chlamydial infection. Of the eight cases of GON, seven mothers had received no prenatal care. The rate of maternal gonorrhoea in a subpopulation registered for antenatal care was 2·7%: there were no GON cases following maternal treatment in this subpopulation.

Comment

Risk

An ideal prophylactic agent for ON should have an overwhelmingly positive risk benefit profile as it will be given in many instances to healthy infants. Adverse effects of silver nitrate appear to be mild and short term.

Benefits: prophylaxis versus no prophylaxis

Only one randomised controlled trial comparing silver nitrate and erythromycin to no prophylaxis in a low-risk population in the United States provides evidence of a modest prophylactic benefit of silver nitrate in non-gonococcal conjunctivitis although 63% of confirmed conjunctivitis cases required no treatment. Large non-randomised controlled studies from a higher risk population suggest that prophylaxis lowers all-cause ON rates irrespective of intervention in African and Taiwanese populations. This reduction may be accounted for by a decrease in non-chlamydial/non-gonococcal infection. The poor performance of the interventions studied in preventing chlamydial conjunctivitis compared to no prophylaxis in Taiwan is noteworthy although there were lower incidences and attack rates for chlamydial and gonococcal conjunctivitis in a high-risk population following prophylaxis that used historical controls as a basis for comparison.

Prophylaxis measures for gonococcal ON must recognise that major shifts in the patterns of antimicrobial susceptibility are occurring and that these shifts vary by region. The picture is also changing annually. In this situation, older studies are of limited value. High rates of gonococcal tetracycline resistance together with decreasing susceptibility to erythromycin have been reported in some countries. Extraocular neonatal chlamydial infection is unlikely to be prevented by ocular prophylaxis at birth. The thresholds of GON risk and the level of resources at which prophylaxis becomes an acceptable control strategy are unknown. A comparison of different strategies in different world regions is unavailable.

Benefits: different prophylactic agents

There is a suggestion that povidone solution may be more efficacious in preventing chlamydia ON compared to topical silver nitrate or erythromycin prophylaxis but this is based mainly on non-randomised evidence. Topical oxytetracycline was associated with fewer mild ocular signs in neonates than silver nitrate.

Question

What is the most efficacious treatment of ophthalmia neonatorum?

The evidence

Five randomised controlled trials were identified for this question: two examining treatment of gonococcal ON and three examining chlamydial ON.

Treatment of GON

Fransen et al.[40] provide a report of trials of intramuscular (IM) kanamycin plus different topical preparations (saline,

gentamicin or erythromycin). The cumulative probability of cure (CPC) was greater when topical gentamicin was added to 75 mg of IM kanamycin (CPC: 86%) than when topical saline was added (CPC: 60%) at the same kanamycin dose. There appeared to be little difference between the topical regimens when the 150 mg IM kanamycin was examined (CPC rates: > 80%). Further details of these studies are given in Table 11.3.

Laga et al.[41] provided the second report of a randomised controlled trial in GON. Kanamycin 75 mg IM plus gentamicin or topical tetracycline was compared with 125 mg IM ceftiaxone plus ocular washes. The completers-only analysis showed that there was no significant difference in recurrence rates of 3/42 and 3/36 respectively.

Comment

Both European[42] and American[43] regulatory authorities have published guidelines on standards of efficacy required in order to license agents to treat *Neisseria gonorrhoeae* (NG). Whilst ON is not specially included, other indications require eradication of infection in 95% or more cases with documented cultures before and after treatment. Notably, active or historical controls are considered acceptable because of the established morbidity of the disease. Prior to clinical trials in GON, *in vitro* studies in at least 200 NG isolates less than two years previously in four areas should be available, which demonstrate susceptibility to the agent at clinically relevant levels in plasma or tissues. Agents in single dose treatment of NG should be present at four times the MIC_{95}* for more than eight hours. In trials, all isolates should be tested for susceptibility and subjects should have at least a single follow-up two days after the predicted concentration of the drug falls below the inhibitory level. In the case of the studies above, the cure rates have not quite achieved the standard of 95%. These studies may also not reflect current Kenyan antibiotic resistance patterns. The results may not be valid for other regions of the world. The dosing regimen would also need to be tailored to the special neonatal population such as on a per kg basis and trials monitored for safety and tolerability.

Treatment of CTON

In the trial by Heggie et al.,[44] sulfacetamide drops appear ineffective compared to oral erythromycin estolate for 14 days (persistence rates of only 7%). There is also a trend to higher relapse rates with topical erythromycin therapy in

---

*MIC is the minimal inhibitory concentration and the lowest concentration that prevents the growth *in vitro* of a specific microbe over a defined period under standardised conditions. the MIC_{50} inhibits 50% of strains and the MIC_{90} inhibits 90% of strains.

Table 11.3   Randomised controlled trials on efficacy of treatment for conjunctivitis in the newborn

Authors	Intervention	No. study ON type	Outcome	Result	Comment
Fransen et al., 1984[40] Kenya	1. IM 75 mg kanamycin + topical gentamicin 2. IM 75 mg kanamycin + topical saline 3. IM 150 mg kanamycin + topical gentamicin 4. IM 150 mg kanamycin + topical saline 5. IM 150 mg kanamycin + topical erythromycin	117 GON	The cumulative probability of cure on day 3 and 30 days post-treatment, i.e. the number of cases cured divided by the number cases treated in GON	Ratio of cumulative probability of cure between treatments, considering all defaulters as failures 1. 86% v 2. 60% at 30 days (P=0·03) 3. v 4. 86% v 89·5% (not significant) 5. CPC min 80%	• Baseline groups comparable, including proportion of penicillinase-producing gonococci
Laga et al., 1986[41] Kenya	125 mg IM stat of ceftriaxone + ocular washes v kanamycin 75mg IM + gentamicin ointment Kanamycin 75mg stat IM + tetracycline ointment	122 GON	Clinical and microbiological response to treatment of GON	3/46 completers of 61 infants receiving ceftriaxone had recurrent cultures v 3/42 completers of 61 infants receiving kanamycin + gentamicin/ tetracycline ointment (not significant)	• Between 59–79% complete for each group • Up to 59% penicillinase producing strains • Masking unknown
Heggie et al., 1985[44] USA	10% sulfacetamide sodium 4 hourly for 14 days v oral erythromycin estolate 50 mg/kg/day for 14 days	37 CTON	Persistent conjunctival infection in CTON	Persistence of conjunctival infection in 1/15 (7%) of the oral erythromycin group and (8/14) 57% of the sulfacetamide sodium group (P<0·002)	• 8 non-compliant subjects excluded • 29 analysed
Patamasucon et al., 1982[45]	1% erythromycin ointment v oral erythromycin estolate 30 mg/kg/day or erythromycin ethylsuccinate 40 mg/kg/day	53 randomised 41 analysed (19 topical)	• Giemsa stain, culture and clinical signs time to resolution, relapse rates • Nasopharyngeal cultures	• Topical v all oral erythromycin • Clinical resolution: no significant difference and	• Oral treatment group older, shorter duration and more females • Masking and randomisation

(Continued)

Table 11.3   (Continued)

Author	Intervention	No. study ON type	Outcome	Result	Comment
				time to culture negative comparable • Relapse rates: 21% topical *v* 13·6% oral (not significant) • Nasopharyngeal cultures: 8 positive post-treatment with topical *v* none oral	method unknown • Adverse effects: 2 cases of rashes with topical, 4 cases of transient diarrhoea with oral erythromycin
Stenberg and Mardh, 1991[46]	Oral erythromycin ethylsuccinate 200 mg divided 10 days (14 infants) *v* oral 25 mg roxithromycin 10 days (14 infants)		• Clinical and microbiological cure rates in CTON	• Persistent culture positive 4/14 erythromycin *v* 5/14 roxithromycin • All but 1/28 clinically cured	• Single-blind RCT • 1 neonate had watery stools for 2 days, 2 other neonates had abdominal pain during treatment

GON gonococcal opthalmia; CPC cumulative probability of cure; CTON chlamydial ophthalmia; IM intramuscular

the study by Patamasucon *et al.*[45] compared to oral erythromycin estolate or ethinylsuccinate (14% relapse rates). Stenberg and Mardh[46] found that microbiological eradication rates appear similar for oral erythromycin ethylsuccinate 200 mg compared to oral 25 mg roxithromycin both given for 10 days (29% and 36% persistence respectively).

Comment

The standard required by regulatory authorities indicates that trials should be double-blind and that clinical efficacy correlates less well with *in vitro* activity than most other infectious agents. The efficacy should be 95% cure with a lower bound of 90%. The outcome is the eradication of chlamydia or clinical response in some indications. Three follow-up visits are recommended, depending on duration, and samples should be repeated at all visits. Relapse and persistent infections are common and should be defined. Of these three studies, one was a single blind trial and in another neither the masking status nor method of

randomisation was given. For these studies, relapse or persistence rates ranged from 7% to 29% with oral erythromycin. The trial by Heggie *et al.* provides a completers-only analysis. The use of topical therapy only is also unattractive as a proportion of infants will have extraocular infection.

Implications for practice

The decision of whether an active prophylactic policy is adopted for a health region depends upon whether there is a high or low risk of chlamydia or *Neisseria gonorrhoeae* and the effectiveness of other health policies in finding and treating high-risk/infected mothers and neonates. For low-risk communities, the risk benefit of silver nitrate prophylaxis appears to be marginal with an absolute risk reduction of 8%. The majority of cases were untreated and resolved. The benefits of prophylaxis for higher risk or poorly resourced communities are less clearly established in recent research but suggest lower incidences and attack rates for chlamydial and gonococcal conjunctivitis in a high-risk population following prophylaxis.

Treatment of established conjunctivitis infection requires awareness of up-to-date region-specific guidelines regarding antibiotic susceptibility and neonatal dosing.

Implications for research

We need monitoring of the incidence and susceptibility of neonatal gonococcal and chlamydial conjunctivitis in different regions around the world, particularly with increasing STD trends. Given the varied circumstances of different areas, specific methodologies must be developed to carry out this surveillance with collaboration between many medical and scientific disciplines: epidemiology, microbiology, ophthalmology, genitourinary medicine and obstetrics. Benefits of prophylaxis in high-risk populations could be clarified. Treatment of ON requires continued monitoring of resistance patterns and investigation of efficacious agents appropriate for this indication and population.

References

1. Credé CSF. Die Verhutung der Augenentzundung der Neugeborenen [Prevention of inflammatory eye disease in the newborn]. *Archiv Gynaekol* 1881;**17**:50–3 (in German).
2. Murray CL, Lopez AD. *Global Health Statistics Volume II*. Boston, MA: Harvard University Press, 1996.
3. Schaller UC, Klauss V. Is Credé's prophylaxis for ophthalmia neonatorum still valid? *Bull World Health Organ* 2001;**79**:262–3.
4. Lund RJ, Kibel MA, Knight GJ, van der Elst C. Prophylaxis against gonococcal ophthalmia neonatorum. A prospective study. *S Afr Med J* 1987;**72**(9):620–2.
5. Bell TA, Sandstrom KI, Gravett MG *et al.* Comparison of ophthalmic silver nitrate solution and erythromycin ointment for prevention of natally acquired *Chlamydia trachomatis*. *Sex Transm Dis* 1987;**14**(4):195–200.
6. Winceslaus J, Goh BT, Dunlop EM *et al.* Diagnosis of ophthalmia neonatorum. *BMJ* (Clin Res Ed) 1987;**295**(6610):1377–9.
7. Sandstrom I. Etiology and diagnosis of neonatal conjunctivitis. *Acta Paediatr Scand* 1987;**76**(2):221–7.
8. Rapoza PA, Quinn TC, Kiessling LA, Taylor HR. Epidemiology of neonatal conjunctivitis. *Ophthalmology* 1986;**93**(4):456–61.
9. Barry WC, Teare EL, Uttley AH *et al. Chlamydia trachomatis* as a cause of neonatal conjunctivitis. *Arch Dis Child* 1986;**61**(8):797–9.
10. Pierce JM, Ward ME, Seal DV. Ophthalmia neonatorum in the 1980s: incidence, aetiology and treatment. *Br J Ophthalmol* 1982;**66**(11):728–31.
11. Schachter J, Grossman M, Holt J, Sweet R, Goodner E, Mills J. Prospective study of chlamydial infection in neonates. *Lancet* 1979;**2**(8139):377–80.
12. Buisman NJ, Abong Mwemba T, Garrigue G, Durand JP, Stilma JS, van Balen TM. Chlamydia ophthalmia neonatorum in Cameroon. *Doc Ophthalmol* 1988;**70**(2–3):257–64.
13. Iroha EO, Kesah CN, Egri-Okwaji MT, Odugbemi TO. Bacterial eye infection in neonates, a prospective study in a neonatal unit. *West Afr J Med* 1998;**17**(3):168–72.
14. Nsanze H, Dawodu A, Usmani A, Sabarinathan K, Varady E. Ophthalmia neonatorum in the United Arab Emirates. *Ann Trop Paediatr* 1996;**16**(1):27–32.
15. Gururaj AK, Ariffin WA, Vijayakumari S, Reddy TN. Changing trends in the epidemiology and management of gonococcal ophthalmia neonatorum. *Singapore Med J* 1992;**33**(3):279–81.
16. Desenclos JC, Garrity D, Scaggs M, Wroten JE. Gonococcal infection of the newborn in Florida, 1984–1989. *Sex Transm Dis* 1992;**19**(2):105–10.
17. Dannevig L, Straume B, Melby K. Ophthalmia neonatorum in northern Norway. II. Microbiology with emphasis on *Chlamydia trachomatis*. *Acta Ophthalmol (Copenh)* 1992;**70**(1):19–25.
18. Dannevig L, Straume B, Melby K. Ophthalmia neonatorum in northern Norway. I: Epidemiology and risk factors. *Acta Ophthalmol (Copenh)* 1992;**70**(1):14–18.
19. Mabey D, Hanlon P, Hanlon L, Marsh V, Forsey T. Chlamydial and gonococcal ophthalmia neonatorum in the Gambia. *Ann Trop Paediatr* 1987;**7**(3):177–80.
20. Jarvis VN, Levine R, Asbell PA. Ophthalmia neonatorum: study of a decade of experience at the Mount Sinai Hospital. *Br J Ophthalmol* 1987;**71**(4):295–300.
21. Frost E, Yvert F, Ndong JZ, Ivanoff B. Ophthalmia neonatorum in a semi-rural African community. *Trans R Soc Trop Med Hyg* 1987;**81**(3):378–80.
22. Laga M, Plummer FA, Nzanze H *et al.* Epidemiology of ophthalmia neonatorum in Kenya. *Lancet* 1986;**2**(8516):1145–9.
23. Fransen L, Nsanze H, Klauss V *et al.* Ophthalmia neonatorum in Nairobi, Kenya: the roles of *Neisseria gonorrhoeae* and *Chlamydia trachomatis*. *J Infect Dis* 1986;**153**(5):862–9.
24. World Health Organization. *Global prevalence and incidence of selected curable sexually transmitted infections, overview and estimates*. Geneva: World Health Organization, 2001.
25. Department of Health and Human Services. *Sexually Transmitted Disease Surveillance, 1999*. Atlanta: Centers for Disease Control and Prevention (CDC), September 2000.
26. Klauss V, Schwartz EC. Other conditions of the outer eye. In: Johnson GJ, Minassian DC, Weale R, eds. *The epidemiology of eye disease*. London: Chapman & Hall, 1998.
27. Centers for Disease Control and Prevention. *1998 Guidelines for treatment of sexually transmitted diseases*. *Morb Mortal Wkly Rep* 1998;**47**(No. RR–1):1–118.
28. *Canadian STD Guidelines 1998*. Laboratory Centre for Disease Control (Canada). Division of STD Prevention and Control. Health Canada Ottawa, 1998.
29. Guidelines for the management of sexually transmitted infection. World Health Organization. WHO/HIV_AIDS/2001.01 Geneva, 2001.
30. Bell TA, Grayston JT, Krohn MA, Kronmal RA. Randomized trial of silver nitrate, erythromycin and no eye prophylaxis for the prevention of conjunctivitis among newborns not at risk for gonococcal ophthalmitis. Eye prophylaxis study group. *Pediatr* 1993;**92**(6):755–60.
31. Wahlberg V. Reconsideration of Credé Prophylaxis. A study of maternity and neonatal care. *Acta Paediatr Scand* 1982;**295**(Suppl):1–73.
32. Isenberg SJ, Apt L, Yoshimori R, Leake RD, Rich R. Povidone-iodine for ophthalmia neonatorum prophylaxis. *Am J Ophthalmol* 1994;**118**(6):702–6.
33. Hammerschlag MR, Chlandler JW, Alexander ER *et al.* Erythromycin ointment for ocular prophylaxis of neonatal chlamydial infection. *JAMA* 1980;**244**(20):2291–3.
34. Brussieux J, Boisivon A, Theron HP, Faidherbe C, Machado N, Michelon B. Prevention of neonatal conjunctivitis. A comparative clinical and bacteriologic study of 2 eyedrops: silver nitrate and oxytetracycline chlorhydrate. *Ann Pediatr* 1991;**38**(9):637–41.
35. Hick JF, Block DJ, Ilstrup DM. A controlled study of silver nitrate prophylaxis and the incidence of nasolacrimal duct obstruction. *J Pediatr Ophthalmol Strabismus* 1985;**22**(3):92–3.
36. Laga M, Plummer FA, Piot P *et al.* Prophylaxis of gonococcal and chlamydial ophthalmia neonatorum. A comparison of silver nitrate and tetracycline. *N Engl J Med* 1988;**318**(11):653–7.
37. Isenberg SJ, Apt L, Wood M. A controlled trial of povidone-iodine as prophylaxis against ophthalmia neonatorum. *N Engl J Med* 1995;**332**(9):562–6.

38. Chen JY. Prophylaxis of ophthalmia neonatorum: comparison of silver nitrate, tetracycline, erythromycin and no prophylaxis. *Pediatr Infect Dis J* 1992;**11**(12):1026–30.

39. Hammerschlag MR, Cummings C, Roblin PM, Williams TH, Delke I. Efficacy of neonatal ocular prophylaxis for the prevention of chlamydial and gonococcal conjunctivitis. *N Engl J Med* 1989; **320**(12):769–72.

40. Fransen L, Nsanze H, D'Costa L, Brunham RC, Ronald AR, Pilot P. Single-dose kanamycin therapy of gonococcal ophthalmia neonatorum. *Lancet* 1984;**2**:1234–7.

41. Laga M, Naamara W, Brunham RC *et al.* Single-dose therapy of gonoccal ophthalmia neonatorum with ceftriaxone. *New Engl J Med* 1986;**315**(22):1382–5.

42. Note for Guidance on the Pharmacodynamic Section of the SPC for Anti-Bacterial Medicinal Products. Efficacy Working Party. Committee for Proprietary Medicinal Products. London 1997 Publ. No. CPMP/EWP/520/96.

43. Beam TR, Gilbert DN, Kunin CM. Guidelines for the evaluation of anti-infective drug products. *Clin Infect Dis* 1992;**15**(Suppl 1):S5–32.

44. Heggie AD, Jaffe AC, Stuart LA, Thombre PS, Sorensen RU. Topical sulfacetamide *v* oral erythromycin for neonatal chlamydial conjunctivitis. *Am J Dis Child* 1985;**138**(6):564–6.

45. Patamasucon P, Rettig PJ, Faust KL, Nelson JD. Oral v topical erythromycin therapies for chlamydial conjunctivitis. *Am J Dis Child* 1982;**136**:817–21.

46. Stenberg K, Mardh PA. Treatment of chlamydial conjunctivitis in newborns and adults with erythromycin and roxithromycin. *J Antimicrob Chemother* 1991;**28**(2):301–7.

12 Unilateral amblyopia

Cathy Williams

Background

Unilateral amblyopia has been a subject of controversy in recent years. In two recent Australian prospective, population-based surveys, amblyopia of 6/9 or worse was found in 3·06% (95% CI 2·59–3·53) of 4721 individuals aged 40 to 92 in Victoria[1] and amblyopia of 6/12 or less was present in 2.9% of 3654 adults aged over 49 years in Sydney.[2] A recent British birth cohort study found a cumulative incidence for amblyopia (defined as >0·1 LogMAR units between the acuities of the two eyes) by 37 months of age of 2·5% (95% CI 2–3%) in 3490 children.[3]

There is little evidence regarding whether or not unilateral amblyopia is disabling. Certain professions are precluded, which does represent a limitation of life choices for affected individuals.[4] The effects on an individual of losing the sight in one eye will be potentially more profound for individuals with unilateral amblyopia than for individuals with two eyes that see equally well. A recent national study estimated that the projected lifetime risk of this happening to an individual with unilateral amblyopia was at least 1·2% (95% CI 1·1–1·4) and the minimum risk of permanent visual impairment by 95 years of age was 32·9 (95% CI 29·1–36·9) per 100 000 total population.[5] Thus even if the extent to which amblyopia is disabling is unclear, there is an associated greater risk of untreatable significant visual impairment later in life, and this is worth avoiding if possible.

Question

Are there effective treatments for amblyopia?

The evidence

Data from 11 randomised studies are summarised in Table 12.1.[6–16] Many of these studies are now very old and therefore of questionable relevance. In a few small trials, some of which were of low quality, levodopa has been found to produce greater visual acuity improvement than placebo. We found no published randomised trials of treatment for amblyopia in preschool children that include a no-treatment arm.

Comment

The interventions are either time consuming (visual stimulation, red filters) or potentially hazardous (levodopa) and so are unlikely to enter conventional treatment plans unless there is compelling, direct evidence of their greater effectiveness than placebo or conventional treatment with occlusion, which was not the case in any of the studies. As the participants in the pharmacological studies were usually older children or adults who had already been refractory to occlusion alone, the extent to which these results can be generalised to all children with amblyopia is unknown.

None of these studies provide direct evidence that without treatment, visual acuity in individuals with amblyopia is static or worsens whereas treatment improves visual acuity. Whilst observational and/or uncontrolled studies have reported improvements in acuity in association with conventional occlusion, which are not seen when compliance with treatment is poor,[17,18] these studies cannot distinguish whether non-compliance *per se*, or other underlying differences in the type or quality of the visual deficits, or other patient characteristics that themselves affect the compliance, account for differences in outcome.

Question

What is the effectiveness of screening for amblyogenic factors or for amblyopia?

The evidence

A review published in 1997 by the NHS-CRD[19] highlighted the lack of high-quality data on the key issue of visual outcomes in screened versus unscreened populations. However, a recent report giving follow up data from a randomised controlled trial quoted a significantly lower prevalence of amblyopia by seven and a half years of age and better average results in children treated for amblyopia, in a group that was offered an intensive programme of repeated vision screening before three years, as compared with the control group, which was offered screening at three years only[20] (both groups were offered school-entry screening).

Table 12.1 Summary of results from randomised intervention studies for the treatment of amblyopia

Authors	Quality issues	Study population	Interventions: experimental v control	Primary outcome	Follow up	Results; experimental v control	P value
Clements 1968[6]	Randomisation method not stated. Masking not stated	Children (4–8 years) with strabismic amblyopia and eccentric fixation	Occlusion + red filter versus occlusion only	"Cured" (Snellen VA improved to 6/12 or better) or not		No differences between groups in numbers who were cured	Not given
Fletcher et al., 1969[7]	Randomisation method not stated. Masking: single blind	173 children with amblyopia	Pleoptics (retraining of fixation and stimulation of amblyopic eye) versus occlusion	VA improved or not (by 2 lines or more)	1–3 years	No differences between groups	Not given
Nyman et al., 1983[8]	Randomisation method not stated. Masking not stated	50 amblyopic children (4–6 years) with interocular acuity difference of 2 Snellen lines	5–10 visual stimulation treatments versus occlusion	No. of Snellen lines of improvement in acuity of amblyopic eye	NG	Mean (SD) improvement similar in each group: 3·11 lines (1·05) v 3·30 (1·26)	0·50
Keith et al., 1980[9]	Randomisation method not stated. Masking: single blind	67 children (5–14 years) with amblyopia, 43 of whom had had previous surgery, occlusion or both	6 brief weekly periods of occlusion plus viewing gratings versus same treatment with grey background	LogMAR improvement in amblyopic eye	1 week after last treatment	Mean improvements (based on several tests) not different between groups.	Not given
Mehdorn et al., 1981[10]	Randomisation method "according to a random sequence". Masking not stated	22 children (3–11 years) with no organic eye defects, "mental defects", nystagmus, uncooperative children/parents or inconvenient address	Visual stimulation with gratings versus visual stimulation with pictures	VA: Decimal version of VA test (SG, single E or numbers)	Mean follow up 12 weeks	No means given. Overlapping data points for the two groups on before v after plots	Not given
Gottlob et al., 1992[11]	Randomisation method not stated. Masking double blind	20 patients (12–58 years) with strabismic or anisometropic amblyopia	Crossover design: levodopa or placebo for 1 week, then nil for 1 week, then alt treatment 1 week, then nil 1 week	LogMAR improvement in amblyopic eye	Weekly, then 4 weeks after start	Mean VA in amblyopic eyes improved only after levodopa in both groups. No changes after placebo	<0·05
Leguire et al., 1993[12]	Randomisation method by pharmacy dept. Masking: double blind	20 children (5–13 years), who had failed to respond to occlusion or who presented at 9 years or older	Single doses of levodopa + occlusion (2 groups) versus placebo + occlusion	LogMAR improvement in amblyopic eye	5 hours	0·1 in combined levodopa groups v 0·0 in placebo group	Not given

(Continued)

Table 12.1 *(Continued)*

Authors	Quality issues	Study population	Interventions experimental v control	Primary outcome	Follow up	Results; experimental v control	P value
Leguire et al., 1993[13]	Randomisation method: by pharmacy dept Masking: double blind	10 amblyopic children (6–14 years) previously refractory to treatment	Levodopa tds + occlusion for 3 weeks v placebo + occlusion	LogMAR improvement in amblyopic eye	1 month after last dose	Levodopa group v placebo group had improvement by 0·27 v 0·16 at 3 weeks and 0·12 v 0·07 in placebo group	Not given
Gottlob et al., 1995[14]	Randomisation method not stated Masking: double blind	33 adults with strabismic or aniso amblyopia	Levodopa, tds for 3 weeks v placebo	LogMAR improvement in amblyopic eye	At end of treatment, then 1 and 2 months after last dose	Levodopa group improved during study, whereas placebo group did not (means not given)	<0·05
Leguire et al., 1998[15]	Randomisation method: numbers drawn from hat Masking: single blind	13 children (7–12 years), who had failed to respond to occlusion or penalisation	Occlusion + levodopa for 7 weeks v levodopa alone	Improvement as mean lines on LogMAR chart	End of treatment and 4 weeks after last dose	Greater improvement in occlusion group (2·1 lines) v non-occlusion group (0·8 lines). Maintained at 4 weeks	0·02 0·01
Procianoy et al., 1999[16]	Randomisation method: block randomised after stratification for weight Masking: double blind	78 children (7–17 years) with strabismic amblyopia (either refractory to previous treatment or >8 years on presentation	levodopa + occlusion v placebo + occlusion for 1 week	Mean Snellen (LogMAR equivalent) improvement in acuity of amblyopic eye	2 hours after last dose	Greater for levodopa group than placebo group: 0·14 v	0·023 0·06

SG, Sheridan Gardiner letter test; tds, three times daily; alt, alternative

Refractive errors, especially high hypermetropia and anisometropia, are well documented to precede clinically detectable amblyopia,[21] although the exact causal relationships involved are not clear.[22,23] Two randomised trials in the UK have examined the effectiveness of early treatment of refractive errors as a means of preventing amblyopia. In the first study, provision of full-strength spectacles to highly hypermetropic infants at six months had no overall effect on visual acuity but did produce more children who could see 6/12 or better in the subgroup who complied with the spectacles.[24] In the second trial, provision of partial strength spectacles to infants who were highly hypermetropic at nine months reduced the number of children who failed an acuity test, despite refractive correction, at four years of age.[25]

Two prospective controlled evaluations of preschool vision screening have been carried out, but using different outcomes. One study (with the groups matched for age, sex and socioeconomic status) found that vision screening of kindergarten children did reduce the prevalence of children with poor vision (uncorrected vision 20/40 or less) six to 12 months later.[26] The other study (with no matching of the groups) found no difference in the prevalence of children with amblyopia, (defined as 6/9 or worse on testing by the school nurse), between the previously screened and unscreened groups.[27] In this latter study, the prevalence of amblyopia was unexpectedly low, which may have been due to under-ascertainment of the target condition.

Comment

Several other studies have used historical comparisons to assess the effect of a screening programme, but the results are difficult to interpret without knowledge of potentially relevant changes in the population that could affect the results, such as in diagnostic criteria, treatment practices or numbers of low birth weight children or children with a family history of ocular defects. Even in the prospective studies, differences in unmatched factors (for example, family history of ocular defects) between the groups may have affected the results. The only randomised study compared screening at different times, rather than screening versus no screening. Although the results of this study support the hypothesis that early treatment is better than later treatment, further data from studies of pragmatic screening programmes versus no or minimal screening are needed.

Conclusion

Better data are needed in order to enhance the evidence base available for the management of this condition, particularly regarding the degree to which it is disabling, the effectiveness of treatment at different ages, the most appropriate screening and treatment methods to use in different age groups and the overall cost-effectiveness of widespread or targeted strategies on whole populations.

Implications for practice

At present, population screening for amblyopia does not satisfy all the National Screening Committee's (NSC) quality criteria for appraising the viability, effectiveness and appropriateness of screening. Additional problems to consider include the difficulties of obtaining adequate population coverage in the post-infancy but preschool years and the need to ensure that any vision screening offered is complementary to the existing continuum of child health surveillance measures. The existing data have led the Children's Subgroup of the NSC to recommend that pending the results of ongoing and future studies, primary orthoptic screening should be offered at school entry to all children, and this is now recommended practice.[28]

Implications for research

In order to answer the key question of whether or not treatment of amblyopia is effective, several dedicated studies to assess the results in specific populations, of relevant interventions and using all relevant outcomes, are needed. A trial based in the United Kingdom is in progress involving children aged three to five years with anisometropic amblyopia and comparing the outcomes from occlusion and spectacles versus spectacles alone versus no treatment. The results will be available in late 2003.[29]

A study in 379 Native American children aged three to five years, found that non-cycloplegic screening for refractive error was more effective as a tool to screen for amblyogenic levels of astigmatism than was visual acuity testing.[30] A randomised controlled trial nested within a birth cohort study has also found that photorefraction was more sensitive than visual acuity testing or cover testing for strabismus, when screening for amblyopia itself, in children aged up to 37 months.[3] Similar studies on different populations, using amblyopia rather than refractive error as the outcome, are needed in order to define the protocols most likely to provide any benefits in realistic screening programmes for amblyopia.

References

1. Brown SA, Weih LM, Fu CL, Dimitrov P, Taylor HR, McCarty CA. Prevalence of amblyopia and associated refractive errors in an adult population in Victoria, Australia. *Ophthalmic Epidemiol* 2000;**7**: 249–58.

2. Attebo K, Mitchell P, Cumming R, Smith W, Jolly N, Sparkes R. Prevalence and causes of amblyopia in an adult population. *Ophthalmol* 1998;**105**:154–9.

3. Williams C, Harrad RA, Harvey I, Sparrow JM, ALSPAC Study Team. Screening for Amblyopia in Preschool Children: Results of a population-based, randomized controlled trial. *Ophthalmic Epidemiol* 2001;**8**:279–95.

4. Adams GG, Karas MP. Effect of amblyopia on employment prospects. *Br J Ophthalmol* 1999;**83**:380.

5. Rahi J, Logan S, Timms C, Russell-Eggitt I, Taylor D. Risk, causes, and outcomes of visual impairment after loss of vision in the non-amblyopic eye: a population-based study. *Lancet* 2002;**360**:597–602.

6. Clements D. Treatment of eccentric fixation by the use of a red filter. *Br J Ophthalmol* 1968;**52**:929–31.

7. Fletcher M, Abbott W, Girard L *et al.* Biostatistical studies. Results of biostatistical study of the management of suppression amblyopia by intensive pleoptics versus conventional patching. *Am Orthoptic J* 1969;**19**:8–30.

8. Nyman KG, Singh G, Rydberg A, Fornander M. Controlled study comparing CAM treatment with occlusion therapy. *Br J Ophthalmol* 1983;**67**:178–80.

9. Keith C, Howell E, Mitchell D, Smith S. Clinical trial of the use of rotating grating patterns in the treatment of amblyopia. *Br J Ophthalmol* 1980;**64**:597–606.

10. Mehdorn E, Mattheus S, Schuppe A, Klein U, Kommerell G. Treatment for amblyopia with rotating gratings and subsequent occlusion. *Int Ophthalmol* 1981;**3**:161–6.

11. Gottlob I, Charlier J, Reinecke RD. Visual acuities and scotomas after one week levadopa administration in human amblyopia. *Invest Ophthalmol Vis Sci* 1992;**33**:2722–8.

12. Leguire L, Rogers G, Bremer D, Walson P, McGregor M. Levodopa/Carbidopa for childhood amblyopia. *Invest Ophthalmol Vis Sci* 1993;**34**:3090–5.

13. Leguire LE, Walson PD, Rogers GL, Bremer DL, McGregor ML. Longitudinal study of levodopa/carbidopa for childhood amblyopia. *J Pediatr Ophthalmol Strabismus* 1993;**30**:354–60.

14. Gottlob I, Wizov SS, Reinecke RD. Visual acuities and scotomas after 3 weeks' levodopa administration in adult amblyopia. *Graefe's Arch Clin Exp Ophthalmol* 1995;**233**(7):407–13.

15. Leguire L, Rogers G, Walson P, Bremer D, McGregor M. Occlusion and Levodopa–Carbidopa treatment for childhood amblyopia. *J Am Acad Paediatr Ophthalmol Strabismus* 1998;**2**:257–64.

16. Procianoy E, Fuchs F, Procianoy L, Procianoy F. The effect of increasing doses of levodopa on treatment with strabismic amblyopia. *J Am Assoc Paediatr Ophthalmol Strabismus* 1999;**3**:337–40.

17. Lithander J, Sjostrand J. Anisometropic and strabismic amblyopia in the age group 2 years and above: a prospective study of the results of treatment. *Br J Ophthalmol* 1991;**75**:111–16.

18. Cleary M. Efficacy of occlusion for strabismic amblyopia: can an optimal duration be identified? *Br J Ophthalmol* 2000;**84**:572–8.

19. Snowdon S, Stewart-Brown S. Preschool vision screening: Results of a systematic review. CRD Report 9. York: NHS Centre for Reviews and Dissemination, University of York, 1997.

20. Williams C, Northstone K, Harrad R, Sparrow J, Harvey I, ALSPAC Study Team. Amblyopia treatment outcomes after screening before 3 years *v.* at 3 years of age – follow-up from a randomised trial. *BMJ* 2002;**324**:1549–51.

21. Ingram RM. Refraction as a basis for screening children for squint and amblyopia. *Br J Ophthalmol* 1977;**61**:8–15.

22. Fielder A, Moseley M. Anisometropia and amblyopia – chicken or egg? [Editorial]. *Br J Ophthalmol* 1996;**80**:857–8.

23. Almeder L, Peck L, Howland H. Prevalence of anisometropia in volunteer laboratory and school screening populations. *Invest Ophthalmol Vis Sci* 1990;**31**:2448–55.

24. Ingram RM, Arnold PE, Dally S, Lucas J. Results of a randomised trial of treating abnormal hypermetropia from the age of 6 months. *Br J Ophthalmol* 1990;**74**:158–9.

25. Atkinson J, Braddick O, Bobier B *et al.* Two infant vision screening programmes: Prediction and Prevention of Strabismus and amblyopia from photo- and videorefractive screening. *Eye* 1996;**10**:189–98.

26. Feldman W, Milner R, Sackett B, Gilbert S. Effects of preschool screening for vision and hearing on prevalence of vision and hearing problems 6–12 months later. *Lancet* 1980;**2**:1014–16.

27. Bray L, Clarke M, Jarvis S, Francis P, Colver A. Preschool vision screening: a prospective comparative evaluation. *Eye* 1996;**10**:714–18.

28. Hall DB, Elliman D. *Health for all children, 4th edn.* Oxford: Oxford University Press, 2003.

29. The Lancet. Protocol Reviews. Protocol ref 00PRT/1 http://thelancet.com/info/info.isa?n1=authorinfo&n2=Protocol+reviews&uid=14297

30. Miller JM, Dobson V, Harvey EM, Sherrill DL. Comparison of preschool vision screening methods in a population with a high prevalence of astigmatism. *Invest Ophthalmol Vis Sci* 2001;**42**:917–24.

13 Infantile esotropia

Lorraine Cassidy, Jugnoo S Rahi

Background

Infantile esotropia is the term used to describe a large angle comitant convergent squint with an onset between three and six months of age, commonly associated with hypermetropia, cross fixation, inferior oblique overaction, dissociated vertical deviation, latent nystagmus and asymmetry of monocular OKN.[1,2] It has a prevalence of 1% and accounts for up to 54% of all esotropias in industrialised countries.[3–5]

Once refractive errors and amblyopia have been treated, the main goal of surgical treatment of infantile esotropia is to achieve some degree of binocular single vision (BSV). To obtain full, normal BSV is rare,[6–8] and subnormal or gross stereopsis is generally considered an acceptable result.[9,10] Gross stereopsis is reported to be achievable in up to 50% of cases.[11–14]

Cosmesis is also an important outcome, as squint can have psychosocial implications for the affected child and parents,[15] particularly if it remains uncorrected into adulthood.[16]

Von Noorden *et al.*[17] have proposed the following taxonomy:

- "subnormal binocular vision" being the optimal result
- "microtropia" being a desirable result
- a "residual small angle eso/exotropia" as a cosmetically acceptable result
- a large angle eso/exotropia as a cosmetically unacceptable result.

The issues

Currently two major issues in the management of infantile esotropia are the optimal timing for surgical correction[18] and the emerging use of botulinum toxin A (BTXA) as an adjunct or alternative to surgical alignment.

Over the past two decades, injection of botulinum toxin has become established as an important adjunct to surgery and as the primary treatment for some types of squints. It has recently been increasingly used in young children.[19–21]

Question

In children with infantile esotropia does early alignment (six months or under), compared with alignment at two years, result in better binocular single vision, better cosmesis and better long-term alignment?

The evidence

We found no randomised controlled trials that address this question. The Early Surgery for Congenital Esotropia Trial (ESCET) is an United States National Institute of Health funded multi-centre, randomised prospective study, which is currently underway and results are anticipated in 2004.[22,23] This trial will compare the outcome of children operated on between the ages of 11 to 18 weeks with those operated on between the ages of 28 to 32 weeks. The primary outcome is stereoacuity, and secondary outcomes are motor alignment, fusion, dissociated deviations and re-operations.

Comment

Observational clinical and laboratory studies suggest that accurate alignment before the age of two years may be more beneficial than later surgery in terms of achieving binocularity.[4,9,24] In a retrospective study of 40 children with infantile esotropia, all of whom had surgery aged 22 months or less and achieved alignment at a mean of 24 months (range 7 to 48 months), Rowe[25] reported that 22·5% achieved binocular vision and 60% achieved a small angle (<20 prism dioptres) esotropia postoperatively. Nevertheless, surgical alignment after the age of two years does not preclude the attainment of subnormal binocular vision or microtropia.[26]

It has been demonstrated that normal infants show an abrupt onset of stereopsis in the time period of three to five months of age.[27] As this would require motor alignment, it is increasingly argued that children with infantile esotropia should undergo surgery as soon as possible. However, observational data regarding the additional benefits of very early treatment in the first year of life are inconsistent.[8,22,26,28–30] In an analysis of 16 patients, Ing found that those who underwent surgery at five months or younger did not have significantly better binocularity at seven years compared with those undergoing surgery at older ages.[31] Helveston *et al.*[32] achieved measurable stereopsis in 40% of infantile esotropes who were aligned at a mean of 4·4 months. This group also demonstrated that very early alignment (age two to four months) did not increase the chance of achieving "fine" stereoacuity (i.e. 50 seconds of arc).

Question

In children with infantile esotropia does primary treatment with using botulinum toxin, compared with conventional primary surgical alignment, result in better binocular single vision, better cosmesis and better long-term alignment?

The evidence

We found no trials comparing alignment using botulinum toxin with surgery as the primary procedure.

Comment

To date, only observational clinical studies suggest that botulinum toxin may have a role as the primary approach in some children with infantile esotropia.[33] Findings of a recent trial in children with residual squint following a primary surgical procedure suggest that botulinum toxin A confers greater benefits than a second surgical procedure, as it is a more rapid and less invasive procedure but with a similar outcome.[34]

Implications for practice

The issue of when to operate remains contentious. Whether very early surgery in the first year of life confers benefit needs to be established through ongoing and future trials. The results of the ESCET trial should provide information that is currently lacking. Observational and laboratory evidence suggests a benefit of surgical alignment at age two years or under. Equally, the increasing interest in botulinum toxin as an alternative or adjunct to surgery requires investigation through trials.

Implications for research

For both questions, long-term alignment and patient-based, subjective measures of outcome should be addressed.

References

1. Von Noorden GK. A reassessment of infantile esotropia (XLIV Edward Jackson Memorial Lecture). *Am J Ophthalmol* 1988;**105**:1–102.
2. Norcia AM. Abnormal motion processing and binocularity; infantile esotropia as a model system for effects of early interruptions of binocularity. *Eye* 1996;**10**:259–65.
3. Scobee RG. Esotropia. Incidence, etiology and results of therapy. *Am J Ophthalmol* 1951;**34**:817.
4. Costenbader FD. Infantile esotropia. *Trans Am Optical Soc* 1961;**59**:397–429.
5. Nordlow W. Age distribution of onset of esotropia. *Br J Ophthalmol* 1953;**37**:359.
6. Taylor DM. How early is early surgery in the management of strabismus? *Arch Ophthalmol* 1963;**70**:752–6.
7. Parks MM. Congenital esotropia with a bifixation result. Report of a case. *Doc Ophthalmol* 1984;**58**:109–14.
8. Wright KW, Edelman PM, McVey JH, Terry AP, Liu M. High grade stereoacuity after early surgery for congenital esotropia. *Arch Ophthalmol* 1994;**112**:913.
9. Ing MR. Early surgical alignment for congenital esotropia. *J Pediatr Ophthalmol Strabismus* 1983;**20**:11–18.
10. Hiles DA, Watson BA, Biglan AW. Characteristics of infantile eotropia following early bimedial rectus recessions. *Arch Ophthalmol* 1980;**98**:697–703.
11. Mohindra I, Zwaan J, Held R, Brill S, Zwaan F. Development of acuity and stereopsis in infants with esotropia. *Ophthalmology* 1985;**92**:691.
12. Birch EE, Stager DR. Monocular acuity and stereopsis in infantile esotropia. *Invest Ophthalmol Vis Sci* 1985;**26**:1624.
13. Birch EE, Stager DR, Barry P, Everett ME. Prospective assessment of acuity and stereopsis in amblyopic infantile esotropia following early surgery. *Invest Ophthalmol Vis Sci* 1990;**31**:758–65.
14. Birch EE, Stager DR, Barry P, Everett ME. Random dot stereoacuity following surgical correction of infantile esotropia. *J Pediatr Ophthalmol Strabismus* 1995;**32**:231–5.
15. Tolchin JG, Lederman ME. Congenital (infantile) esotropia: psychiatric aspects. *J Pediatr Ophthalmol Strabismus* 1978;**15**:160–3.
16. Oltisky SE, Sudesh S, Graziano A *et al.* The negative psychosocial impact of strabismus in adults. *J AAPOS* 1999;**3**:209–11.
17. Von Noorden GK, Isaza A, Parks MM. Surgical treatment of congenital esotropia. *Trans Am Acad Ophthalmol Otolaryngol* 1972;**76**:1465–78.
18. Ing MR. The timing of surgical alignment for congenital (infantile) esotropia. *J Pediatr Ophthalmol Strabismus* 1999;**36**:61–8.
19. Robert PY, Jeaneau-Bellego E, Bertin P, Adenis JP. Value of delayed botulinum toxin injection in esotropia in the child as first line treatment. *J Fr Ophthalmol* 1998;**21**:508–14.
20. Schiavi C, Benedetti P, Scorolli L, Campos EC. Nouve indicazioni all'uso della tossina botulinica. *Atti Soc Oftalm Lonbarda* 1992;**47**:345–8.
21. Tucker MG, NcNeer KW, Spencer RF. The incidence of latent nystagmus in infantile esotropia patients treated early with bimedial botulinum toxin A. *Invest Ophthalmol Vis Sci* 1997;**38**:S112.
22. Birch E, Stager D, Wright K, Beck R. The natural history of infantile esotropia during the first six months of life. Pediatric Eye Disease Investigator Group. *J AAPOS* 1998;**2**:325–8.
23. Spiegel PH, Wright KW. Optimum timing for surgery for congenital esotropia. *Semin Ophthalmol* 1997;**12**:166–70.
24. Taylor DM. Is congenital esotropia functionally curable? *Trans Am Optical Soc* 1972;**70**:529–76.
25. Rowe FJ. Long-term postoperative stability in infantile esotropia. *Strabismus* 2000;**8**:3–13.
26. Shauly Y, Prager TC, Mazow ML. Clinical characteristics and long-term postoperative results of infantile esotropia. *Am J Ophthalmol* 1994;**117**:183–9.
27. Birch E. Stereopsis in infants and its development ratio to visual acuity. In: Simon SK, ed. *Early Visual Development Normal and Abnormal.* New York: Oxford University Press, 1993: pp. 224–36.

28. Zak TA, Morin D. Early surgery for infantile esotropia: results and influence of age upon results. *Can J Ophthalmol* 1982;**17**: 213–18.

29. Clarke WN. Very early *v.* early or late surgery for infantile esotropia. *Can J Ophthalmol* 1995;**30**:240–1.

30. Nixon RB, Helveston EM, Miller K, Archer SM, Ellis FD. Incidence of strabismus in neonates. *Am J Ophthalmol* 1985;**100**:798–801.

31. Ing MR. Outcome of surgical alignment before six months of age for congenital esotropia. *Ophthalmology* 1995;**102**:2041–5.

32. Helveston EM, Neely DF, Stidham DB, Wallace DK, Plager DA, Spru. Results of early alignment of congenital esotropia. *Ophthalmology* 1999;**106**:1716–26.

33. McNeer KW, Tucker M, Spencer RF. Management of essential infantile esotropia with botulinum toxin A: review and recommendations. *J Pediatr Ophthalmol Strabismus* 2000;**37**:63–7.

34. Tejedor J, Rodriguez JM. Early retreatment of infantile esotropia: comparison of reoperation and botulinum toxin. *Br J Ophthalmol* 1999;**83**:783–7.

14 Accommodative esotropia

Michael Clarke

Background

Definition

Accommodative esotropia is a type of convergent strabismus that is thought to arise because of inappropriate convergence due to increased accommodative effort.[1] This can occur either because excessive accommodation is required to overcome a hypermetropic refractive error, or because of inappropriate gearing between accommodation and convergence (High AC/A ratio). The diagnosis is made on the basis of the response to the correction of significant hypermetropic refractive errors or the prescription of additional plus lenses for near fixation.

Three forms are recognised:

1 Refractive – esotropia eliminated by correction of hypermetropic refractive error
2 Non-refractive – esotropia present at near only despite correction of any hypermetropic refractive error but eliminated by plus lenses at near
3 Mixed – esotropia at distance eliminated by hypermetropic correction but requires plus lenses to eliminate esotropia at near fixation.

When the deviation responds completely to correction with lenses it is termed fully accommodative. Where the deviation reduces in size but is not completely eliminated by refractive correction, it is termed partially accommodative.

Incidence/prevalence

Although accommodative esotropia is occasionally seen in infancy, the condition most commonly presents in the third or fourth year of life when a convergent strabismus is seen, particularly for near fixation. There is frequently a family history of a similar deviation. Graham estimated the prevalence per thousand of fully and partially accommodative strabismus at 6·7 and 15·3 respectively.[2]

Aetiology

The cause of fully accommodative refractive esotropia is a hypermetropic refractive error, which is usually bilateral and reasonably symmetrical. Not all significant bilateral, hypermetropic refractive errors lead to an esotropia; in some cases bilateral amblyopia occurs if accommodation is not used to overcome the error. Very asymmetrical or unilateral refractive errors usually lead to unilateral amblyopia.

Non-refractive accommodative esotropia is caused by a high ratio of accommodative convergence: accommodation (AC/A). Little is known about the constitutional factors associated with the range of AC/A ratio or about whether it changes over time.

Prognosis

Fully accommodative esotropia, by definition, responds completely to refractive correction or the use of plus lenses at near sight. Normal binocular single vision is demonstrable when this is in place. In some cases, it is possible to reduce the strength of the lenses over time until the child is able to control the strabismus without refractive correction.

Partially accommodative esotropia does not respond fully to refractive correction or plus lenses at near. Plus lenses at near are not indicated unless there is a functional benefit from their use (which is not the case in partially accommodative esotropia). Surgery is required if it is desired to reduce the angle of strabismus further. Even following surgical correction in addition to refractive correction, perfect ocular alignment and good responses to tests of stereoscopic vision are not usually achieved.

The issues

Given the relationship between hypermetropic refractive errors and accommodative esotropia, the possibility exists that early detection and prophylactic treatment of refractive error might reduce the incidence of this type of strabismus. Similarly, early treatment of fully accommodative esotropia might prevent the deterioration of this type of strabismus into a partially accommodative esotropia with a worse prognosis for binocular single vision. Surgical treatment of fully accommodative esotropia has been proposed as an alternative to refractive correction, and the possibility now exists for surgical correction of refractive error as an alternative to spectacle or contact lens correction. Finally, where surgical treatment is undertaken for partially accommodative esotropia, preoperative adaptation with prisms has been proposed as a useful manoeuvre to demonstrate the full extent of the strabismus and avoid surgical undercorrection.

Question

Does early correction of hypermetropic refractive errors lead to a reduction in the incidence of accommodative esotropia?

The evidence

This question has been examined by Ingram *et al.* in a series of papers. In the first,[3] 306 children aged one year with bilateral spherical hypermetropia of +2·00 DS dioptre sphere or more, or with anisometropia of +1·00 DS or cylinder were randomly allocated to spectacle correction or no treatment and followed until three and a half years of age. Treated children were divided into two groups – compliers and non-compliers with spectacle wear. It is not clear how this distinction was made. Although the incidence of squint at three and a half years was less in the treated group (19/129 compared to 28/136 in non-treated group) this was not statistically significant ($P = 0·28$) Compliers and non-compliers in the treatment group were not analysed separately.

In a second paper,[4] 372 children aged six months with +4D of hypermetropia in any meridian were randomised to spectacle correction or no treatment. There was no difference in the incidence of strabismus in the 285 children followed to three and a half years. Further analysis of these children[5] showed that strabismus was found more commonly in those children whose refractive error remained at or above +3·50 DS. Those children who consistently wore spectacle correction were more likely to remain significantly hypermetropic.

Comment

Despite these findings, it is widely held that early correction of refractive error is important in preventing strabismus[6] and this belief is fundamental to the use of techniques such as photoscreening in preliterate children.[7] This view is supported by the work of Atkinson *et al.*[8] This study had two phases of recruitment. In the first, every infant living in the city of Cambridge was offered an examination at the age of six to eight months. Cycloplegic photorefraction was undertaken on the 3166 infants (74% of those offered appointments) who attended. In the second phase, all children born in a two year period were offered screening at around eight months of age. Appointments were sent to 5923 and 5091 attended. Non-cycloplegic videorefraction was performed. A control group was selected

randomly from the same clinic as children meeting the refractive criteria for follow up.

Children who were hypermetropic in infancy but who did not comply with spectacle wear were 13 times more likely to develop strabismus than controls, compared to a four-fold increase in risk in children who were compliant with spectacle wear compared to controls ($P<0·05$).

The results of Atkinson *et al.* and Ingram *et al.* are contradictory with regard to the benefit of prophylactic spectacle wear on the incidence of strabismus. Atkinson *et al.* speculate that this is due to differences in the protocol for spectacle prescription and in the degree of compliance. Atkinson *et al.* do not specify their method of randomisation and seem to have excluded children who were not compliant with spectacle wear (as judged by questioning whether the child wore spectacles 50% of the time) from the analysis although this is not explicitly stated. Both studies agree that the presence of a high refractive error in infancy is predictive of the later development of strabismus and amblyopia.

Question

Is surgical treatment an alternative to refractive correction in the treatment of accommodative esotropia?

The evidence

No trials were found comparing the two approaches.

Comment

Surgical treatment of fully accommodative strabismus has been advocated in the European literature, particularly by Gobin,[9,10] but this approach has not found favour in the English-speaking world because of concern about the possibility of late overcorrection and diplopia following surgery without refractive correction.

Question

Does uncorrected fully accommodative esotropia become partially accommodative?

The evidence

No trials were found that address this issue.

Comment

There is a widespread clinical belief that neglected fully accommodative esotropia develops a non-accommodative component with a poorer sensory outcome after treatment.[1]

Question

Is preoperative prism adaptation necessary to determine the amount of surgery required to correct partially accommodative esotropia?

The evidence

The surgical treatment of acquired esotropia frequently results in undercorrection of the deviation. The Prism Adaptation Study[11] (PAS) was a randomised multi-centre clinical trial of patients with acquired esotropia who had a residual angle of 12 prism dioptres or greater with refractive correction. The PAS considered whether the preoperative use of prisms helped to determine more accurately the target angle for surgical correction, so reducing the incidence of undercorrections.

Of the 3574 patients screened, 333 were randomised. One of the exclusion criteria was the presence of a strabismus at near greater than 10 D larger than at distance. This would exclude many patients with partially accommodative esotropia.

One hundred and ninety-nine patients were randomised to preoperative treatment with prisms and 134 underwent surgery for the amount of strabismus present at recruitment. The amount of prism required to neutralise the strabismus was placed on spectacles and the patient was re-examined at weekly intervals with additional prism correction being applied until there was evidence of a fusion response (in which case the patient was designated a prism responder) or the deviation stabilised or was overcorrected without evidence of fusion (prism non-responder). Prism non-responders also underwent surgery for the amount of strabismus measured at recruitment. Prism responders were then randomised either to surgery for the entry angle or surgery based on the prism-adapted angle. Surgery was standardised and checked photographically. The primary end-point was the distance deviation measured by a masked observer six months after surgery. A successful outcome was defined as 8 D or less of esotropia or exotropia.

The overall success rate among patients who underwent prism adaptation was 83% compared to 72% among those patients who did not undergo prism adaptation ($P = 0.04$). Those patients who showed a prism response had a motor alignment success of 89% compared to 79% for prism responders operated on for their entry angle ($P = 0.23$). The observed benefits were concentrated mainly in the patients who built up to larger angles in the prism adaptation process and underwent surgery for their adapted angles.

Comment

Although prism adaptation is widely used for accommodative esotropia, the exclusion of patients with a near angle more than 10 D than the distance angle means that most cases of accommodative esotropia were excluded from the analysis and so the benefits of prism adaptation for this class of patients remains uncertain.

Question

Is surgical treatment of refractive error an alternative to conventional refractive correction in accommodative esotropia?

The evidence

Refractive surgery has been used to correct the hypermetropic refractive error of some patients with accommodative esotropia,[12] but there are no randomised trials of the outcome of this approach.

Implications for practice

There is a lack of agreement about the benefits of prophylactic refractive correction with regard to the subsequent development of accommodative esotropia. The amount of refractive error that requires prophylactic correction in this age group (to benefit both esotropia and amblyopia) will continue to be based on eminent opinion and professional consensus. There is little evidence to support surgical treatment for fully accommodative esotropia. While there is evidence that there is a marginal benefit of prism adaptation on a subclass of esotropia, the benefits of prism adaptation for accommodative esotropia are not proven. Refractive surgery, particularly for hypermetropia, remains an experimental procedure and its use in children with accommodative esotropia is ethically dubious.

Implications for research

Long-term, well-designed studies are required to provide guidance about prophylactic correction of refractive error in the paediatric age group. Such studies would help guide the use of photoscreening and other screening techniques.

References

1. Lambert SR. Accommodative esotropia. *Ophthalmol Clin North Am* 2001;**14**:425–31.
2. Graham PA. Epidemiology of strabismus. *Br J Ophthalmol* 1974;**58**:224–31.
3. Ingram R, Walker C, Wilson J, Arnold P, Lucas J, Dally S. A first attempt to prevent amblyopia and squint by spectacle correction of abnormal refractions from the age of 1 year. *Br J Ophthalmol* 1985;**69**:851–3.

4. Ingram R, Arnold P, Dally S, Lucas J. Results of a randomised trial of treating abnormal hypermetropia from the age of 6 months. *Br J Ophthalmol* 1990;**74**:158–9.
5. Ingram R, Arnold P, Dally S, Lucas J. Emmetropisation, squint and reduced visual acuity after treatment. *Br J Ophthalmol* 1991;**75**:414–16.
6. Kvarnstrom G, Jakobsson P, Lennerstrand G. Visual screening of Swedish children: an ophthalmological evaluation. *Acta Ophthalmol Scand* 2001;**79**:240–4.
7. Simons K. Photoscreening. *Ophthalmology* 2000;**107**:1619–20.
8. Atkinson J, Braddick O, Robier B *et al.* Two infant vision screening programmes: prediction and prevention of strabismus and amblyopia from photo- and videorefractive screening. *Eye* 1996;**10**:189–98.
9. Gobin M. Strabismes accommodatifs, peut-on les operer? [Should accommodative strabismus be operated on?] *J Francais d'Ophthalmol* 1992;**15**:483–91.
10. Gobin MH. Surgery for fully accommodative esotropia. *Binocular Vis Q* 2001;**16**:80–2.
11. Group PARS. Efficacy of prism adaptation in the surgical management of acquired esotropia. *Arch Ophthalmol* 1990;**108**:1248–56.
12. Stidham DB, Borissova O, Borrisov V, Prager TC. Effect of hyperopic laser in situ keratomileusis on ocular alignment and stereopsis in patients with accommodative esotropia. *Ophthalmology* 2002;**109**:1148–53.

15 Childhood exotropia

Sarah Richardson, Lawrence Gnanaraj

Background

Definition

Exotropia is a manifest divergent deviation of the visual axes; a latent divergent deviation is known as exophoria. Nearly 50% of exo deviations occur in the first year of life and there is sex preponderance towards females.[1] Exotropia is common in neonates but usually resolves by three months of age.[2]

Childhood exotropia may be primary (no systemic or ocular disease) or secondary. The secondary form may be associated with ocular abnormalities, neurological diseases and various craniofacial syndromes.

Primary childhood exotropia may be classified as constant or intermittent (Table 15.1).

Prevalence

Concomitant exo deviations occur less frequently than eso deviations with a ratio of approximately 1:3[3]; exophoria is more common than exotropia. The overall prevalence of exo deviations has been reported to be 0·4%,[4] occurring more frequently at latitudes with higher levels of sunlight.[5]

Constant exotropia and infantile exotropia

Clinical characteristics

Infantile exotropia is a large, constant, concomitant exotropia with onset within the first 12 months of life. The deviation usually alternates and is the same angle for near and distance fixation: a constant unilateral exotropia should raise suspicions of other pathology. Subjects may develop dissociated vertical deviation (DVD).[6,7] The distribution of refractive error is not significantly different from the normal population; amblyopia due to strabismus rather than anisometropia is seen in some patients (0–25%).[8]

Other types of constant exotropia are thought to develop from a decompensation of an exophoria or a basic intermittent exotropia and are therefore discussed under intermittent exotropia. It is often difficult to differentiate this type of exotropia from infantile exotropia if it presents in later life.

Table 15.1 Types of exotropia

Types	Constant exotropia	Intermittent exotropia
Subtypes	Infantile	Near Distance Basic (non-specific)* Decompensated exophoria*

*May become constant

Prevalence and aetiology

The prevalence is low, with a reported rate of 1 in 30 000.[9] The cause of primary infantile exotropia is unknown. Multiple genetic and intrauterine factors have been suggested.

Management options

The objective of surgical correction is to realign the eyes to a stable angle closer to orthotropia. Non-surgical management includes correction of refractive error and occlusion if there is associated amblyopia. Surgical correction of the squint is required in almost all patients early in life to maximise the chance of restoring binocular single vision.[9–11]

Questions

1 Does early surgery achieve a better motor and sensory outcome?
2 Is there a role for botulinum toxin injection as an alternative or adjunct to surgery?

The evidence

We found no randomised control trials relevant to management options for this condition.

Comment

The literature suggests that the chance of achieving binocular single vision will be maximised if the surgery is undertaken early in life although the functional prognosis is poor for constant exotropia present from early infancy.[12] Published reports suggest that optimal motor and sensory fusion are achieved in children whose eyes were aligned successfully before the age of two years.[9–11] It is also suggested that surgery should be planned as soon as a stable angle can be measured after the diagnosis is made.

Botulinum toxin injection into the extraocular muscles as an alternative treatment for strabismus has been in practice since 1978. Its role in the management of infantile esotropia has been reported.[13] There are no large studies published yet on its role for the treatment of infantile exotropia.

Intermittent exotropia

Intermittent exotropia is divided into near, distance, basic intermittent exotropia and decompensating exophoria. Whilst near exotropia is clearly a separate clinical entity, the latter three subgroups are similar in many respects and it is common to find them described and managed as one in the literature. Most of the principles and techniques described for the management of distance exotropia apply also to that of basic intermittent exotropia and decompensating exophoria and they are therefore not repeated in detail in these sections.

Near exotropia

Clinical characteristics

Near exotropia describes an exotropia present for only near fixation; normal binocular single vision can usually be demonstrated for distance fixation. It may also be described as a convergence weakness/insufficiency type of intermittent exotropia. It is characterised by equal vision, poor binocular convergence, normal sensory fusion and poor positive motor fusion. Symptoms of diplopia, headache and asthenopia are associated with near fixation; binocular function is thought to deteriorate rapidly after the onset.[14] Clinically it may resemble convergence palsy or convergence insufficiency.

Prevalence and aetiology

There are no data on the prevalence of this condition; it usually presents in older children or adults.[15] A low AC/A ratio has been suggested as a cause of near exotropia[15] although Plenty[16] found that this was a common finding in many normal adults and children. Presbyopia has also been suggested as a possible causative factor.

Management options

The objective of treatment is to restore binocular alignment, improve positive fusion and binocular convergence. It has been suggested that near exotropia may be associated with acquired myopia[15] and that correction of this may be sufficient to restore binocular alignment; other authorities suggest that the prevalence of refractive errors is the same in exotropia as in the non-strabismic population.[1,17]

Exercises or prisms may be used to improve positive fusion and binocular convergence.[18,19] Surgery is recommended if there is a poor response to conservative treatment or there is a large angle of deviation.[12,20] Various surgical procedures have been suggested,[12,21,22] usually involving resection of the medial rectus muscle. Complications include the risk of surgical overcorrection in the distance with diplopia; this may be successfully managed with prisms.[12]

Question

Which treatment approach is most effective in improving symptoms and restoring satisfactory alignment?

The evidence

We found no randomised controlled trials of any treatment modalities for this condition.

Comment

Observational studies report a good surgical success rate: Von Noorden[12] reported success in four out of six patients. In Kraft's series of 14 patients all had a near postoperative angle of <10 prism dioptres and no troublesome diplopia in the distance.[21]

Distance exotropia

Clinical characteristics

Normal binocular single vision is present for near fixation but a constant or intermittent exotropia occurs for distance fixation. The distance angle of deviation is at least 10 prism dioptres larger than the near deviation. The exotropia is typically noticed when the subject is daydreaming, tired or unwell and observers may also notice a tendency to close one eye in sunlight. Patients are rarely symptomatic of diplopia as suppression occurs when the deviation is manifest.[23]

Distance exotropia may be subdivided into true or simulated types. In simulated distance exotropia the deviation initially appears greater for distance, but when proximal or accommodative convergence is removed the deviation for near increases. True distance exotropia remains unchanged when tested under these conditions. If control for near fixation deteriorates it is hard to differentiate from basic intermittent exotropia.

Prevalence and aetiology

There are no data on the prevalence of this condition. The aetiology is unknown but various mechanical, anatomical and innervational factors have been suggested.[24]

Management options

The primary aim of intervention is to create binocular alignment in the distance whilst preserving/improving alignment for near fixation.

Von Noorden[12] recommends intervention if the deviation is noticed at least 50% of waking hours or if there is deterioration of control for near fixation. Intermittent exotropia is generally held to be progressive in nature although some have been observed to remain unchanged and some even to improve over years of observation.[25] Decompensation carries the risk of developing a constant manifest strabismus and a loss of binocular single vision. Surgical success is usually defined as the restoration of normal binocular single vision near and distance. Small angle deviations are thought to improve with conservative management by exercising fusion,[12,18] eliminating suppression[26] or inducing accommodation using minus lenses[27,28] but the efficacy of these treatments remains debatable.[12,29]

Questions

1. Is there an optimum age for surgical intervention?
2. Does the type of distance exotropia (i.e. whether it is true or simulated) affect the management options?
3. Does the type of surgical procedure have an effect on the outcome of surgery?
4. Is initial surgical overcorrection likely to improve the long-term outcome?

The evidence

We found no randomised controlled trials relevant to any management option for this condition.

Comment

The reported success rate of surgery varies from 95%[30] to 40%,[31] but this should be regarded cautiously as other types of intermittent exotropia are sometimes included. There is controversy regarding the optimum age for surgery: some[11,20,32] are in favour of early surgery and others[12,28,33] of late.

It has been suggested that simulated distance exotropia should be treated with a unilateral lateral rectus recession plus medial rectus resection and that true distance exotropia should undergo bilateral lateral rectus recessions[14,31,34,35] However, a study by Kushner[36] suggested that bilateral lateral rectus recessions may be effective in correcting simulated distance exotropia. A single lateral rectus recession has been suggested as an alternative for both.[37]

Surgical intervention carries the risk of long-term overcorrection and loss of binocular single vision (Hardesty *et al.* 6%,[38] Dunlap 20%[39]). However, initial surgical overcorrection may be planned, as it is thought by some authors[20,28,40] to be more likely to give satisfactory long-term alignment.

Basic (non-specific) exotropia

Clinical characteristics

In many respects basic intermittent exotropia is similar to intermittent distance exotropia. The main differences are that it becomes manifest intermittently for near as well as distance fixation and there is less than 10 prism dioptres difference between the angle of deviation at these distances. It is usually unilateral but if amblyopia is present it is generally due to anisometropia. Patients demonstrate suppression when the deviation is manifest and binocular single vision when it is controlled. However, it will often decompensate with age[15] and present as a constant exotropia. The presence of suppression then means that it may not be possible to demonstrate potential for binocular single vision pre-operatively, but it is often possible to achieve this with successful management.

Prevalence and aetiology

There are no data on the prevalence of this condition. Diminished amplitude of accommodation has been suggested as a contributory factor for decompensation.[15]

Management options

The aim of treatment is to achieve a cosmetically acceptable, stable alignment and, if possible, to restore binocular single vision.

Treatment is indicated if the deviation is noticed to be manifest frequently or there is deterioration of binocular function. Whilst the deviation is intermittent, conservative measures to improve fusional control may be attempted (as described above). However, surgery is the mainstay of treatment.

Assessment of the potential for binocular single vision preoperatively using fresnel prisms or botulinum toxin has been suggested. It is also appropriate to check for postoperative diplopia in patients who do not demonstrate potential for fusion.

> **Questions**
>
> 1 Is unilateral or bilateral surgery more effective in restoring satisfactory alignment and binocular single vision?
> 2 Does the age at surgery influence the outcome?

The evidence

We found no randomised controlled trials evaluating the effectiveness of any management option.

Comment

Unilateral lateral rectus recession and medial rectus resection on the non-fixing eye is thought to be the procedure of choice[12,15] although other evidence[36] suggests that bilateral lateral rectus recessions can be used with equal success.

If a child presents with a constant squint but a history of intermittent exotropia, early surgical correction is thought to be more likely to result to restore fusion.

Decompensated exophoria

Clinical characteristics

Decompensation of a basic exophoria can result in an intermittent exotropia of the same angle near and distance; onset may be at any age. It is usually characterised by a constant unilateral deviation and equal vision in both eyes. Unlike basic intermittent exotropia, decompensated exophoria presents with symptoms of diplopia, blurred vision and asthenopia. Normal binocular single vision is demonstrable but often with a reduced positive fusion amplitude and reduced convergence.

Prevalence and aetiology

There are no data on the prevalence of this condition. As for distance exotropia, various mechanical, anatomical and innervational factors have been suggested[24] as causative but none has been proved conclusively.

Management options

The objective of treatment is to restore satisfactory alignment and good binocular control.

As for basic and distance types of intermittent exotropia, conservative treatment may be attempted but most cases require surgical intervention.

> **Questions**
>
> 1 Is there a role for conservative treatment as an alternative or adjunct to surgery?
> 2 Is satisfactory alignment with good binocular control more likely to be achieved with unilateral or bilateral surgery?

The evidence

We found no randomised controlled trials relevant to any management options for this condition.

Comments

Conservative treatment in the form of fusion exercises and/or prisms may be of value in symptomatic patients. However, it is thought that most cases will also require surgery to achieve functional binocular alignment.

There does not seem to be any evidence to suggest that unilateral lateral rectus recession combined with medial rectus resection is better than bilateral lateral rectus recession in achieving initial or delayed satisfactory postoperative alignment. The advantage of unilateral surgery is the availability of the fellow eye if more surgery is needed. In patients with very large angle squint it may be necessary to operate on more than two muscles involving both eyes.

Implications for practice

As there are no randomised controlled trials in this area of clinical practice it has been difficult to resolve the controversies regarding indications for intervention, the most appropriate treatment option and the timing of surgery.

Implications for research

There is a clear need for randomised controlled trials to improve the evidence base for the management of these conditions. Long-term observational studies are also needed to observe the rate of progression/recovery as this is presently not known.

References

1. Gregersen E. The polymorphous exo patient. Analysis of 231 consecutive cases. *Acta Ophthalmol* 1969;**47**:579.
2. Nixon RB, Helveston EM, Miller M, Archer SM, Ellis FD. Incidence of strabismus in neonates. *Am J Ophthalmol* 1985;**100**:798–801.
3. Friedman Z, Neumann E, Hyams SW *et al.* Ophthalmic screening of 38,000 children, age 1 to 2½ years, in child welfare clinics. *J Pediatr Ophthalmol* 1980;**17**:261.
4. Graham PA. Epidemiology of strabismus. *Br J Ophthalmol* 1974;**58**:224–31.
5. Jenkins R. Demographics: Geographic variations in the prevalence and management of exotropia. *Am Orthoptic J* 1992;**42**:82.
6. Cohen RL, Moore S. Primary dissociated vertical deviation. *Am Orthoptic J* 1980;**30**:107–8.
7. Helveston EM. Dissociated vertical deviation: a clinical and laboratory study. *Trans Am Ophthalmol Soc* 1980;**78**:734–79.
8. Biglan AW, Davis JS, Cheng KP *et al.* Infantile exotropia. *J Pediatr Ophthalmol Strabismus* 1996;**33**:79.
9. Biedner B, Marcus M, David R *et al.* Congenital constant exotropia: surgical results in six patients. *Binocular Vis Eye Muscle Surg Q* 1993;**8**:137.
10. Rubin SE, Nelson LB, Wagner RS *et al.* Infantile exotropia in healthy children. *Ophthalmic Surg* 1988;**19**:792.
11. Parks MM, Mitchell PR. Concomitant exodeviations. In: Tasman W, Jaeger EA, eds. *Clinical Ophthalmology, vol. 1.* Philadelphia: Lippincott-Raven, 1996, p. 3.
12. Von Noorden GK. *Binocular vision and ocular motility: Theory and management of strabismus, 5th edn.* St Louis: Mosby, 1996, p. 351.
13. Scott AB, Magoon EH, McNeer KW *et al.* Botulinum treatment of childhood strabismus. *Ophthalmology* 1990;**97**:1434.
14. Burian HM. Exodeviations: their classification, diagnosis and treatment. *Am J Ophthalmol* 1966;**62**:1161.
15. Ansons AM, Davis H. *Diagnosis and management of ocular motility disorders, 3rd edn.* Oxford: Blackwell Science, 2001, pp. 260–83.
16. Plenty J. A new classification for intermittent exotropia. *Br Orthoptic J* 1988;**45**:19–22.
17. Schlossman A, Boruchoff SA. Correlation between physiologic and clinical aspects of exotropia. *Am J Ophthalmol* 1955;**40**:53.
18. Cooper EL, Leyman IA. The management of intermittent exotropia. A comparison of the results of surgical and non-surgical treatment. In: Moore S, Mein J, Stockbridge L, eds. *Orthoptics Past, Present and Future. Transactions of 3rd International Orthoptic Congress.* New York: Stratton Intercontinental, 1976, p. 563.
19. Sanfilippo S, Clahane AC. The immediate and long-term results of Orthoptics in exo deviations. In: *1st International Congress of Orthoptists.* St Louis: Mosby Year Book, 1968, p. 300.
20. Knapp P. Divergent deviations. In: Allen JH, ed. *Strabismic Ophthalmic Symposium II.* St Louis: Mosby Year Book, 1958, p. 364.
21. Kraft SP, Levin AV, Enzenauer RW. Unilateral surgery for exotropia with convergence weakness. *J Pediatr Ophthalmol Strabismus* 1995;**32**:183.
22. Snir M, Axer-Siegel R, Shalev B *et al.* Slanted lateral rectus recession for exotropia with convergence weakness. *Ophthalmology* 1999;**106**:992.
23. Parks M. Sensorial adaptations in strabismus. In: Duane TD, ed. *Ocular Motility and Strabismus.* Hagerstown, MD: Harper & Row, 1975, p. 67.
24. Burian HM. Pathophysiology of exodeviations. In: Manley DR, ed. *Symposium on horizontal ocular deviations.* St Louis: Mosby Year Book, 1971, p. 119.
25. von Noorden GK. Some aspects of exotropia. Presented at Wilmers Residents' Association, John Hopkins Hospital, Baltimore, April 26 1966.
26. Chutter CP. Occlusion treatment of intermittent divergent strabismus. *Am Orthop J* 1977;**27**:80.
27. Caltrider N, Jamplosky A. Overcorrecting minus lens therapy for treatment of intermittent exotropia. *Ophthalmology* 1983;**90**:1160.
28. Jampolsky A. Management of exodeviations. In: *Strabismus. Symposium of the New Orleans Academy of Ophthalmology.* St Louis: Mosby Year Book, 1962.
29. Rosenbaum AL. Exodeviations. In: *Current Concepts in Paediatric Ophthalmology & Strabismus.* Ann Arbor, MI: University of Michigan, 1993, p. 41.
30. Richard JM, Parks MM. Intermittent exotropia: surgical results in different age groups. *Ophthalmology* 1983;**90**:1172.
31. Burian HM, Spivey BE. The surgical management of exodeviations. *Am J Ophthalmol* 1965;**59**:603.
32. Pratt-Johnson JA, Barlow JM, Tillson G. Early treatment in intermittent exotropia. *Am J Ophthalmol* 1977;**84**:689–94.
33. Baker JD, Schweers M, Petranuk J. Is earlier surgery a sensory benefit in the treatment of intermittent exotropia? In: Lennerstrand G, ed. *Advances in Strabismology. Proceedings of 8th meeting of International Strabismological Association*, Maastricht, Dept 10–12, 1988. Buren, The Netherlands: Aeolus Press, 1999, p. 289.
34. von Noorden GK. Divergence excess and simulated divergence excess: diagnosis and surgical management. *Ophthalmology* 1969;**26**:719.
35. Parks MM. Concomitant exodeviations. In: Duane TD, ed. *Ocular Motility and Strabismus.* Hagerstown, MD: Harper & Row, 1975, p. 113–22.
36. Kushner BJ. Selective surgery for intermittent exotropia based on distance/near differences. *Arch Ophthalmol* 1998;**116**:324–8.
37. Olitsky SE. Early and late postoperative alignment following unilateral lateral rectus recession for intermittent exotropia. *J Paediatr Ophthalmol Strabismus* 1998;**35**:146.
38. Hardesty HH, Boynton JR, Keenan JP. Treatment of intermittent exotropia. *Arch Ophthalmol* 1978;**96**:268.
39. Dunlap EA. Overcorrections in horizontal strabismus surgery. In: *Symposium on Strabismus. Transactions of the New Orleans Academy of Ophthalmology.* St Louis: Mosby Year Book, 1971, p. 255.
40. Scott WE, Mash AJ. The postoperative results and stability of exodeviations. *Arch Ophthalmol* 1981;**99**:1814.

16 Prevention of myopia progression

Ian Flitcroft

Background

Definition

Myopia can be defined as an optical mismatch between the refractive surfaces of the eye and the position of the macula as determined by axial length whereby for distant targets and relaxed accommodation, the optical image plane is anterior to the retina. Despite the recognised linkage between myopia and axial elongation, definitions of myopia rarely include this parameter.

Aetiology

There is abundant evidence for both environmental and genetic factors in the aetiology of myopia and the debate on aetiology has polarised into nature versus nurture.[1] The apparently contradictory nature of this large evidence base suggests significant gene-environment interactions may exist.

Prognosis and clinical significance

Uncorrected refractive errors represent a major cause of loss of vision and refractive errors have been listed as one of the five priority conditions in the World Health Organization's "Vision 2020" initiative. In developed countries the vast majority of myopic people will have normal visual acuity with appropriate optical correction, but myopia has significant public health consequences from a variety of perspectives – financial, psychological, quality of life and direct and indirect risks of blindness. Direct and indirect costs of myopia in the United States population were estimated for 1990 at US$4·8 billion.[2] High levels (>10D) of myopia are associated with an impact on quality of life comparable with keratoconus.[3] Direct causes of vision loss in myopia are principally myopic macula degeneration. In Hong Kong this has been reported as the second commonest cause of low vision.[4] Myopia has been reported to be a risk factor for a range of other conditions including retinal detachment,[5] glaucoma[6] and cataract.[7,8]

Prevalence of myopia

The prevalence of myopia varies with age, geography, educational achievement, occupation and birth cohort. The most commonly cited prevalence figure for Western populations, derived from the National Health and Nutrition Examination Survey in 1972, is 25%.[9] In some Far Eastern countries the current levels are much higher, with levels in Taiwanese high school children of 84% in 16–18 year olds.[10] Myopic prevalence in children has been correlated with increasing urbanisation and within racially similar groups varies between city and country locations.[11] In contrast, some populations show very low levels of myopia with a reported prevalence of 2·9% in Melanesian school children.[12] Prevalence in specific populations has been observed to rise significantly over time. Within Inuit Eskimo populations this has been linked with the introduction of westernised patterns of living and education.[13] In Singapore there has been a rise in myopic prevalence from 26% to 43% in a little over a decade.[14] Limited studies in the West have also pointed to an increasing prevalence with higher myopic prevalence within younger cohorts in cross-sectional studies but these findings have been questioned.[15–17]

Clinical trials of myopia progression

There is wide variation in methods and criteria for defining myopia in clinical studies. Principal areas of variation include differences in the use of cycloplegia prior to refraction, differing methods of refraction and different threshold values when converting spherical/cylindrical refraction to a single parameter. Some studies even fail to record the refractive criteria used to define myopia. These variations hinder comparisons of different studies when used as part of the inclusion criteria. In relation to myopic progression the majority of studies use changes in refraction (subject to the above variations in technique). Some studies have also measured axial length, which provides a valuable additional parameter in light of the comparability issues with ocular refraction.

The evidence

Despite the vast literature on myopia progression, a recent systematic review of myopic progression[18] identified only 10 clinical trials that met their criteria. This reflects the fact that this literature includes a large number of uncontrolled or poorly controlled studies and retrospective case series. Efforts to alter the progression of myopia in humans have emphasised alteration of suspected environmental factors, particularly those related to near work.

Optical interventions

The rationale for optical treatments for the secondary or primary prevention of myopia derives from the large epidemiological literature relating myopia to near work activity. The growing animal literature on the optical regulation of eye growth in primates[19] has also led to expectations that optical manipulation will be effective in humans.

Optical undercorrection and overcorrection of myopia

Animal studies have indicated that negatively powered lenses can lead to myopic eye growth and it has been suggested that on this basis myopes should be undercorrected.[19] One randomised study showed no statistical difference between full time wear of full correction with part-time (distance only) wear of full correction.[20]

Most school age children show a progression to less hyperopic or more myopic refractions but the rate of change is greater for myopes than hyperopes.[21] This has been cited as a rationale for rendering children functionally hyperopic by overcorrection of myopic errors. A trial of overcorrection of myopia showed no significant effects of +0·75 D overcorrections as compared to full correction.[22]

A randomised trial of deliberate undercorrection, sufficient to reduce vision to 6/12, has demonstrated over 24 months that progression in the undercorrected group was −1·00 D as compared to −0·77 D in the fully corrected group.[23] Although the difference was small, it reached statistical significance.

Comment

A single trial has addressed the issue of undercorrection of myopia and indicates that undercorrection is associated with faster myopic progression than full correction. This study recruited only Malay and Chinese subjects and the differences were of small magnitude but the results suggest that human eye growth is sensitive to optical factors and that full correction of myopia is preferable to undercorrection. There is no firm evidence that overcorrection has any impact on human myopic progression.

Bifocal glasses

By reducing accommodative demand and hence increasing accommodative accuracy for near tasks it is proposed that bifocals should reduce myopic progression. There is much literature on this form of intervention but few randomised clinical trials. These are summarised in Table 16.1.

The Houston Myopia Control Study did not show any overall significant effect of bifocal over single vision glasses. This large study was undermined by the large drop-out rate (more than 40%).[24] A later reanalysis of this and previous studies from the same group suggested a benefit from bifocals for people with nearpoint esophoria.[29] A small trial with esophoric myopes showed a non-significant trend for bifocals to reduce the rate of myopic progression[25] and a larger follow-on trial from the same group showed a significantly lower rate of myopic progression with bifocal glasses.[26] Two large studies with low drop-out rates showed no significant impact of bifocals on myopic progression.[20,28] A study on United States navy academy students (young adults) showed no impact but very low progression rates in the control group and high loss to followup.[27,30]

Comment

Apart from a possible effect on a subset of children with near esophoria, there is no convincing evidence for a clinically beneficial effect of bifocals on myopic progression.

Multifocal/progressive spectacle lenses

Progressive spectacle lenses have recently been examined as an alternative to bifocals in the belief that they provide a better method of reducing accommodative demand at a range of distances (Table 16.2). A study in Hong Kong[31] showed significant changes in both myopic progression and vitreous chamber elongation. This study used alternate allocation rather than true randomisation and was unmasked. A combined atropine and progressive lens trial from Taiwan did not show a significant impact of progressive lenses alone.[32] Two randomised trials have recently reported results comparing single vision glasses with progressive/varifocal lenses. The Hong Kong

Table 16.1 **Bifocal studies**

Authors/study name	No. of subjects		Subject age range (yrs)	Trial length (yrs)	Treatment groups	Myopic progression dioptres/year (positive = increasing myopia)
	n = start	n = finish				
Grovesnor et al., Houston Myopia Control Study, 1987[24]	207	124	6–15	3	• Single vision glasses (control) • Bifocal +1 add • Bifocal +2 near add	• 0.34 • 0.36 • 0.34 No significant difference
Fulk and Cyert, 1996[25]	32	28		1·5	• Single vision glasses (control) • Bifocal +1·5 add All with near esophoria	• 0·57 • 0·35 No significant difference
Fulk et al., 2000[26]	82	75	6–12·9	2·5	• Single vision glasses (control) • Bifocal +1·5 add All with near esophoria	• 0·50 • 0·40 Significant (<0·05) adjusting for age, small but significant impact on vitreous chamber growth
Parssinen et al., 1989[20]	240	237	8·8–12·8	3	• Single vision glasses (SV) • Single vision for distance (SVD) • Bifocal add +1·75	• 0·49 (right eyes) • 0·59 • 0·56 Significant difference between SV and SVD left eye only. Other comparisons no significant difference
Shotwell, 1984[27]	235	61	17–21	4	• Tinted (sham/control) • Bifocal add +1·5 • Bifocal add +1·25 with 4 D prism	• 0·058 • 0·068 • 0·038 No significant difference (note adult subjects)
Jensen, 1991[28]	159	147	9–12	2 (3 for timolol group)	• Single vision glasses (control) • Bifocal add +2 • Timolol	• 0·57 • 0·48 • 0·59 No significant difference

Progessive Lens Myopia Control Study did not show any significant benefit of progressive lenses at 2 years.[33] The Correction of Myopia Evaluation Trial (COMET), an ongoing large multi-centre NEI sponsored trial, reported three-year results with a small but statistically significant effect of progressive lenses on reducing myopic progression.[34] The treatment effect was most apparent in the first year and also more apparent in subjects with initial poor accommodation responses.

Comment

The COMET trial has provided evidence indicating that progressive lenses can have a statistically significant effect on myopic progression but this difference could not be considered clinically significant. Future investigations and ongoing reports from the COMET study are required to understand fully the potential for progressive lenses in myopia control.

Table 16.2 Varifocal studies

Author/study name	No. of subjects		Subject age range (yrs)	Trial length (yrs)	Treatment groups	Myopic progression dioptres/year (positive = increasing myopia)
	n = start	n = finish				
Leung and Brown, 1999[31]	79	68	9–12	2	• Single vision glasses (control) • Varifocal add + 1·5 • Varifocal add + 2·0	• 0.62 • 0.38 • 0.33 Statiscally significant varifocal *v* control
Shih *et al.*, 2001[32]	227	188	6–13	1·5	• Single vision glasses • Varifocal • Varifocal + 0·5% Atropine	• 0·93 • 0·79 • 0·14 No significant difference between single vision and varifocal group without atropine
Edwards *et al.* 2002[33]	298	254	7–10·5	2	• Single vision • Varifocal add + 1·5	• 0·63 • 0·56 No Significant difference between groups at 2 years
Gwiazda *et al.*, Correction of Myopia Evaluation Trial (COMET) 2003[34]	469	N/A	6–11	3	• Single vision glasses • Varifocal add + 2·0	• 0·49 • 0·43 Significant difference (*P* = 0·004) over 3 years between groups with most of effect in first year.

Prisms with bifocals

The rationale for the use of prisms with bifocals for reading is to reduce the convergence and accommodative demands of near work. A single randomised trial has been reported on the use of prisms (included in Table 16.1).[27,30] The study randomised 232 students from a Naval Academy Preparatory School to tinted spectacles, +1·25 D with a total of 4Δ base-in or +1·5 D bifocal. After four years there was no significant differences between groups. The study had a high loss to follow-up and examined an adult population where the control group showed a very low rate of myopic progression.

Comment

The lack of clinical trials in this area means that no conclusions can be drawn about their effects.

Contact lenses: conventional and orthokeratology

A range of contact lens types has been examined for their impact on myopic progression. Orthokeratology is a technique that involves fitting flatter than normal hard contact lenses and is claimed by its proponents to reduce myopia and myopic progression, primarily by corneal flattening. A single randomised trial, the Berkeley Orthokeratology Study,[35] has examined this technique (Table 16.3). Of 80 subjects randomised, 21 were lost to follow-up. Larger reductions were observed in the orthokeratology group than the conventional lens group but these did not persist after lens wear was stopped. In a small study with poor follow up, soft hydrophilic lenses were reported to have no impact on myopic progression as compared to single vision glasses.[36]

Table 16.3   Contact lens studies

Author/study name (randomised trials)	No. of subjects		Subject age range (yrs)	Trial length (yrs)	Treatment groups	Myopic progression dioptres/year (positive = increasing myopia)
	n = start	n = finish				
Polse *et al.*, 1983 Berkeley Orthokeratology Study[35]	80	59	20–35	1·26	• Orthokeratology contact lens	−0·97 (reduction)
					• Conventional hard contact lens	−0·49 (reduction)
						Significantly difference at end of contact lens wear (*P*<0·01)
					After cessation (mean 95 days)	
					• Orthokeratology contact lens	0·19
					• Conventional hard contact lens	0·13
						No significant difference
Andreo, 1990[36]	56	11 (at 3 years)	14–19	3	• Single vision glasses	0·245
					• Hydrophillic soft contact lens	0·261
						Weight averaged across age groups
						No significant difference

Comment

The contact lens and myopia progression (CLAMP) study is currently underway. This study aims to address the design flaws of previous rigid gas permeable (RGP) studies and examine if the effects of hard contact lenses are solely corneal or whether, as suggested by previous studies, part of the effect relates to changes in axial elongation.[37] Prior to the availability of these results the evidence is at best equivocal.

Summary of optical interventions

There is a very limited number of published clinical trials on optical interventions (undercorrection, overcorrection, bifocal, varifocal glasses and contact lenses) for myopic progression. This body of evidence does not provide unequivocal evidence of a beneficial effect of any of the described interventions. Two major well-designed trials (COMET and CLAMP) are underway and should provide much greater clarity with regard to progressive addition lenses and hard contact lenses.

Pharmacological interventions

Antimuscarinic agents

Antimuscarinic eye drops, atropine in particular, have long been advocated for reducing myopic progression. The original rationale for atropine was that by reducing or abolishing accommodation associated with near work, the proposed tendency of near work to lead to myopia could be reduced or abolished. Subsequent animal studies indicated that a non-accommodative action of atropine was likely with a possible scleral and or retinal site of action and that the action may be mediated by the M1 muscarinic receptor subtype.[38]

A small number of randomised clinical trials have examined atropine or other antimuscarinic eye drops in myopia (see Table 16.4). In an identical twin study, tropicamide was found not to have a significant impact on myopic progression.[39] The three randomised studies on atropine did show a statistically significant reduction in myopic progression.[32,40,41] The atropine treatment groups all included either bifocal or varifocal glasses as an additional intervention compared to the control

Table 16.4   Topical medication

Authors/study name	No. of subjects		Subject age range (yrs)	Trial length (yrs)	Treatment groups	Myopic progression dioptres/year (positive = increasing myopia)
	n = start	n = finish				
Antimuscarinic eye drops						
Yen et al., 1989[41]	247	96	6–14	1	• Single vision + saline drops	• 0·914
					• Single vision + 1% cyclopentolate	• 0·578
					• Bifocal + 1% atropine alternate days	• 0·219
						Significant difference (*P* < 0·01)
Shih et al., 1999[40]	200	186	6–13	2	• Single vision + 0·5% cyclopentolate	• 1·06
					• Single vision + 0.1% atropine	• 0·47
					• −0·75 D undercorrection + 0·25% atropine	• 0·55
					• Bifocal + 2 D + 0·5%atropine	• 0·04
						Significant difference (*P* < 0·01) all groups *v* cyclopentolate
Shih et al., 2001[32]	227	188	6–13	1.5	• Single vision glasses	• 0·93
					• Varifocal	• 0·79
					• Varifocal + 0·5% atropine	• 0·14
						Significant difference between varifocal + atropine *v* single vision (*P* < 0·00001)
Schwartz, 1981[39]	26	25	7–13	8.5	• Monozygotic myopic twins	(Paired analysis in study, group figures given)
					• Twin 1 : bifocal + 1·25 D + 1% tropicamide	• 0·245
					• Twin 2 : single vision	• 0·275
						No significant difference
Betablocker eye drops						
Jensen, 1991[28]	159	147	9–12	3	• Single vision glasses (control)	• 0·57
					• Timolol	• 0·59
						No significant difference

groups but one study[32] included a varifocal group without atropine that did not show a significant impact compared with single vision glasses. The lack of effect in this latter study for varifocal glasses without atropine suggests that the effect of a combination of varifocal glasses and atropine is principally attributable to atropine. One of these studies also showed a very high loss to follow up.[41]

Comment

Topical atropine is the only intervention for myopic progression with consistent evidence of short-term benefit on myopic progression, though several issues remain unresolved. All these studies have been conducted by the same group on a Chinese population. In view of the racial variations in myopic prevalence, confirmation in other populations is important to ascertain whether or not these results may be generalised.

The high drop-out rates from many atropine studies reflects the poor tolerability of combined atropine/bifocal therapy. Although the risks of long-term atropine use have been questioned on theoretical grounds in relation to retinal or lens phototoxicity and premature presbyopia, no long-term safety studies have been conducted. Photochromic lenses have been advocated to address the mydriatic consequences of atropine,[42] but have not been subject to controlled trials.

Following animal studies on the effectiveness of selective M1 agent in experimental myopia,[38,43–45] two randomised trials are currently underway on pirenzepine gel, one in Singapore and the other a multi-centre trial with 10 centres in the United States, Hong Kong and Thailand. Pirenzepine has minimal mydriatic and cycloplegic effects compared to atropine and, if effective, may be better tolerated and less prone to cycloplegia-related risks.

Betablockers

The primary rationale for use of betablockers in myopia is that increased intraocular pressure (IOP) may increase or be a primary driver for axial elongation in myopia. There is some evidence for an association between IOP and myopia in humans.[46,47] A single randomised trial of timolol compared to single vision glasses and bifocal glasses showed no significant beneficial impact of timolol on myopic progression despite a reduction in IOP (Table 16.4).[28]

Implications for practice

Atropine eye drops, in combination with either bifocal or multifocal spectacles, is the only intervention shown in more than one randomised clinical trial to reduce myopic progression. However, there is insufficient evidence to support routine clinical introduction of atropine for reducing myopic progression due to the lack of clear evidence as to the risks and benefits of prolonged cycloplegia in childhood. This is in keeping with the conclusions of other reviews on myopic progression.[18]

None of the other interventions covered in this chapter may be considered appropriate for clinical introduction at this stage but several large trials currently underway may alter the status of hard contact lenses, varifocal glasses and antimuscarinic eye drops.

Implications for research

Evaluating a treatment for routine clinical use carries a high burden of proof in relation to both effectiveness and the risk/benefit relationship. Evidence of the existence of an effect requires a lower level of proof. The existing studies do provide evidence that the natural history of myopic progression can be modified by pharmacological means with atropine and possibly also by some optical interventions. This provides a justification that there is merit in further, careful clinical evaluation of the current proposed interventions of myopic progression. The major trials currently underway represent a great advance towards the style of study that is required to address these questions. Standardisation of the criteria for defining myopia and methods of measuring refraction would greatly enhance the ability to compare trials or perform meta-analysis.

The existing evidence also provides an indication that the results of experimental myopia in animal models have at least limited application to human myopia since atropine has proved effective in a range of animal models.[28,43,48] Better understanding of the basic cellular and biochemical mechanisms regulating eye growth will provide a more rational basis for framing questions for future clinical interventions. This suggests that a parallel clinical and basic science approach is warranted.

References

1. Mutti DO, Zadnik K, Adams AJ. Myopia. The nature versus nurture debate goes on. *Invest Ophthalmol Vis Sci* 1996;**37**:952–7.
2. Javitt JC, Chiang YP. The socioeconomic aspects of laser refractive surgery. *Arch Ophthalmol* 1994;**112**:1526–30.
3. Rose K, Harper R, Tromans C *et al.* Quality of life in myopia. *Br J Ophthalmol* 2000;**84**:1031–4.
4. Yap M, Cho J, Woo G. A survey of low vision patients in Hong Kong. *Clin Exp Optom* 1990;**73**:19–22.
5. The Eye Disease Case–control Study Group. Risk factors for idiopathic rhegmatogenous retinal detachment. *Am J Epidemiol* 1993;**137**:749–57.
6. Mitchell P, Hourihan F, Sandbach J, Wang JJ. The relationship between glaucoma and myopia: the Blue Mountains Eye Study. *Ophthalmology* 1999;**106**:2010–15.
7. Leske MC, Chylack LT Jr, Wu SY. The lens opacities case–control study. Risk factors for cataract. *Arch Ophthalmol* 1991;**109**:244–51.
8. Lim R, Mitchell P, Cumming RG. Refractive associations with cataract: the Blue Mountains Eye Study. *Invest Ophthalmol Vis Sci* 1999;**40**:3021–6.
9. Sperduto RD, Seigel D, Roberts J, Rowland M. Prevalence of myopia in the United States. *Arch Ophthalmol* 1983;**101**:405–7.
10. Lin LL, Shih YF, Tsai CB *et al.* Epidemiologic study of ocular refraction among schoolchildren in Taiwan in 1995. *Optom Vis Sci* 1999;**76**:275–81.

11. Zhan MZ, Saw SM, Hong RZ *et al.* Refractive errors in Singapore and Xiamen, China – a comparative study in school children aged 6 to 7 years. *Optom Vis Sci* 2000;**77**:302–8.

12. Garner LF, Kinnear RF, McKellar M, Klinger J, Hovander MS, Grosvenor T. Refraction and its components in Melanesian schoolchildren in Vanuatu. *Am J Optom Physiol Opt* 1988;**65**:182–9.

13. Johnson GJ, Matthews A, Perkins ES. Survey of ophthalmic conditions in a Labrador community. I. Refractive errors. *Br J Ophthalmol* 1979;**63**:440–8.

14. Tay MT, Au Eong KG, Ng CY, Lim MK. Myopia and educational attainment in 421,116 young Singaporean males. *Ann Acad Med Singapore* 1992;**21**:785–91.

15. Attebo K, Ivers RQ, Mitchell P. Refractive errors in an older population: the Blue Mountains Eye Study. *Ophthalmology* 1999;**106**:1066–72.

16. The Framingham Offspring Eye Study Group. Familial aggregation and prevalence of myopia in the Framingham Offspring Eye Study. *Arch Ophthalmol* 1996;**114**:326–32.

17. Mutti DO, Zadnik K. Age-related decreases in the prevalence of myopia: longitudinal change or cohort effect? *Invest Ophthalmol Vis Sci* 2000;**41**:2103–7.

18. Saw SM, Shih-Yen EC, Koh A, Tan D. Interventions to retard myopia progression in children: an evidence-based update. *Ophthalmology* 2002;**109**:415–21.

19. Hung LF, Crawford ML, Smith EL. Spectacle lenses alter eye growth and the refractive status of young monkeys. *Nat Med* 1995;**1**:761–5.

20. Parssinen O, Hemminki E, Klemetti A. Effect of spectacle use and accommodation on myopic progression: final results of a three-year randomised clinical trial among schoolchildren. *Br J Ophthalmol* 1989;**73**:547–51.

21. Mantyjarvi MI. Changes of refraction in schoolchildren. *Arch Ophthalmol* 1985;**103**:790–2.

22. Goss DA. Overcorrection as a means of slowing myopic progression. *Am J Optom Physiol Opt* 1984;**61**:85–93.

23. Chung K, Mohidin N, O'Leary DJ. Undercorrection of myopia enhances rather than inhibits myopia progression. *Vis Res* 2002;**42**:2555–9.

24. Grosvenor T, Perrigin DM, Perrigin J, Maslovitz B. Houston Myopia Control Study: a randomised clinical trial. Part II. Final report by the patient care team. *Am J Optom Physiol Opt* 1987;**64**:482–98.

25. Fulk GW, Cyert LA. Can bifocals slow myopia progression? *J Am Optom Assoc* 1996;**67**:749–54.

26. Fulk GW, Cyert LA, Parker DE. A randomised trial of the effect of single-vision *v.* bifocal lenses on myopia progression in children with esophoria. *Optom Vis Sci* 2000;**77**:395–401.

27. Shotwell AJ. Plus lenses, prisms, and bifocal effects on myopia progression in military students. *Am J Optom Physiol Opt* 1981;**58**:349–54.

28. Jensen H. Myopia progression in young school children. A prospective study of myopia progression and the effect of a trial with bifocal lenses and beta blocker eye drops. *Acta Ophthalmol Suppl* 1991;(Suppl 200):1–79.

29. Goss DA, Grosvenor T. Rates of childhood myopia progression with bifocals as a function of nearpoint phoria: consistency of three studies. *Optom Vis Sci* 1990;**67**:637–40.

30. Shotwell AJ. Plus lens, prism, and bifocal effects on myopia progression in military students. Part II. *Am J Optom Physiol Opt* 1984;**61**:112–17.

31. Leung JT, Brown B. Progression of myopia in Hong Kong Chinese schoolchildren is slowed by wearing progressive lenses. *Optom Vis Sci* 1999;**76**:346–54.

32. Shih YF, Hsiao CK, Chen CJ, Chang CW, Hung PT, Lin LL. An intervention trial on efficacy of atropine and multi-focal glasses in controlling myopic progression. *Acta Ophthalmol Scand* 2001;**79**:233–6.

33. Edwards MH, Li RW, Lam CS, Lew JK, Yu BS. The Hong Kong progressive lens myopia control study: study design and main findings. *Invest Ophthalmol Vis Sci* 2002;**43**:2852–8.

34. Gwiazda J, Hyman L, Hussein M *et al.* A randomized clinical trial of progressive addition lenses versus single vision lenses on the progression of myopia in children. *Invest Ophthalmol Vis Sci* 2003;**44**:1492–500.

35. Polse KA, Brand RJ, Vastine DW, Schwalbe JS. Corneal change accompanying orthokeratology. Plastic or elastic? Results of a randomised controlled clinical trial. *Arch Ophthalmol* 1983;**101**:1873–8.

36. Andreo LK. Long-term effects of hydrophilic contact lenses on myopia. *Ann Ophthalmol* 1990;**22**:224–7, 229.

37. Walline JJ, Mutti DO, Jones LA *et al.* The contact lens and myopia progression (CLAMP) study: design and baseline data. *Optom Vis Sci* 2001;**78**:223–33.

38. Stone RA, Lin T, Laties AM. Muscarinic antagonist effects on experimental chick myopia. *Exp Eye Res* 1991;**52**:755–8.

39. Schwartz JT. Results of a monozygotic cotwin control study on a treatment for myopia. *Prog Clin Biol Res* 1981;**69**(Pt C):249–58.

40. Shih YF, Chen CH, Chou AC, Ho TC, Lin LL, Hung PT. Effects of different concentrations of atropine on controlling myopia in myopic children. *J Ocul Pharmacol Ther* 1999;**15**:85–90.

41. Yen MY, Liu JH, Kao SC, Shiao CH. Comparison of the effect of atropine and cyclopentolate on myopia. *Ann Ophthalmol* 1989;**21**:180–2, 187.

42. Romano PE. There's no longer any need for randomised control groups; it's time to regularly offer atropine and bifocals for school myopia; comments on evidence-based medicine. *Binocul Vis Strabismus Q* 2001;**16**:12.

43. Tigges M, Iuvone PM, Fernandes A *et al.* Effects of muscarinic cholinergic receptor antagonists on postnatal eye growth of rhesus monkeys. *Optom Vis Sci* 1999;**76**:397–407.

44. Cottriall CL, McBrien NA. The M1 muscarinic antagonist pirenzepine reduces myopia and eye enlargement in the tree shrew. *Invest Ophthalmol Vis Sci* 1996;**37**:1368–79.

45. Leech EM, Cottriall CL, McBrien NA. Pirenzepine prevents form deprivation myopia in a dose dependent manner. *Ophthalmic Physiol Opt* 1995;**15**:351–6.

46. Pruett RC. Progressive myopia and intraocular pressure: what is the linkage? A literature review. *Acta Ophthalmol Suppl* 1988;**185**:117–27.

47. Quinn GE, Berlin JA, Young TL, Ziylan S, Stone RA. Association of intraocular pressure and myopia in children. *Ophthalmology* 1995;**102**:180–5.

48. McBrien NA, Moghaddam HO, Reeder AP. Atropine reduces experimental myopia and eye enlargement via a nonaccommodative mechanism. *Invest Ophthalmol Vis Sci* 1993;**34**:205–15.

Section IV

Adnexal

Michael J Wearne, Editor

Adnexal: mission statement

This section highlights the evidence available for the management of certain diseases of the ocular adnexae. Entropion and ectropion represent eyelid malpositions that are commonly seen in ophthalmology clinics, but the optimal approach for correction remains controversial. Thyroid eye disease is complicated ophthalimic condition that is relatively rare, and, therefore, lends itself to an evidence-based approach to establish best practice. Endoscopic lacrimal surgery for epiphora has advanced considerably over recent years and careful viewing of the results of controlled trials allows comparison to be made with more traditional surgical techniques. An evidence-based approach for all these conditions furthers our goal and responsibility to provide better care for our patients.

17 Entropion and ectropion

Kostas G Boboridis, Michael J Wearne

Background

Entropion

Entropion is an eyelid malposition characterised by the inward turning of the lid margin, lashes and sometimes the external skin against the globe. Depending on the aetiology, acquired entropion can be classified as involutional, spastic or cicatricial. An involutional entropion is one of the commonest lower lid malpositions in the elderly population and is the most frequently corrected in clinical practice.[1] There are no published prevalence data, but it is usually encountered in people older than 60 years, with an equal sex distribution.[2] It is mainly caused by senile vertical lid laxity in the form of attenuation or dehiscence of the lower lid retractors and horizontal laxity in the form of canthal tendon elongation.[3,4] The pathophysiological changes in eyelids with entropion are similar to those seen in ectropion. However, in entropion, hypertrophy of the orbicularis and Riolan muscles, septal atrophy and tarsal thinning allow overriding of the preseptal over the pretarsal muscle, resulting in inward rolling of the lid margin.[2,5,6] Spastic entropion is considered an early form of involutional entropion with the same causative factors and cicatricial entropion is often due to scarring and contracture of the posterior lid lamella.

Patients may complain of a chronic foreign body sensation, redness, tearing and discharge. Constant rubbing of the eyelid margin against the ocular surface can cause a chronic conjunctivitis or corneal abrasions. Secondary corneal thinning, corneal ulceration and perforation may occur in untreated cases.[7,8] Non-surgical temporary treatments include topical symptomatic support with antibiotic or lubricating ointments, taping the lid to the cheek or chemical denervation of the orbicularis muscle with botulinum toxin injections.[9,10] Surgical correction is considered the only long-term treatment and over the years more than 80 procedures have been described addressing one or more of the causative factors.[11] Horizontal lid laxity has been corrected by stabilising the preseptal orbicularis muscle to the lateral orbital rim with or without tightening of the lateral canthal tendon.[12,13] Vertical lid laxity has been reduced by tightening the lower lid retractors, indirectly with the Wies procedure or directly with the Jones retractor plication procedure.[11,14–16] Procedures such as Quickert procedure or Jones retractor plication with a lateral canthal sling, address both vertical and horizontal lid laxity.[17–19] The same principles apply in the management of spastic entropion.

Interventions used to correct a cicatricial entropion include tarsal fracture or posterior lid lamella lengthening with a mucous membrane graft combined with everting sutures.[20,21]

Ectropion

Ectropion refers to an eyelid malposition in which the lid is everted from its normal apposition to the globe. Acquired ectropion is classified as involutional, mechanical, cicatricial or paralytic. Although prevalence data do not exist, involutional ectropion is undoubtedly the commonest type seen in clinical practice. This tends to occur in older people due to horizontal eyelid and canthal ligament laxity, and attenuation of the lower lid retractors. Another aetiological factor may be a larger than normal tarsal plate mechanically overcoming the normal or decreased tone of the preseptal/pretarsal orbicularis muscle.[22] Mechanical eversion of the lower lids can result from ill-fitting spectacles or lesions weighing down the eyelid. Cicatricial ectropion tends to be due to skin shortage or scarring of the anterior lamella of the eyelid, and paralytic ectropion is secondary to a facial nerve weakness.

Patients with a lower lid ectropion may experience ocular discomfort, recurrent conjunctivitis, epiphora and lagophthalmos (incomplete closure of the eyelids). Although topical therapies may help in mild cases, the eyelid malposition usually requires surgical correction. Many different procedures have been described to treat lower lid ectropion. Pentagonal wedge resections[23] have been widely used to correct involutional ectropion for many years. The popularity of this procedure has declined recently as it may exacerbate medial and lateral canthal ligament laxity. A tarsal strip procedure has the advantage of shortening the lid laterally, followed by reattachment to the lateral orbital rim.[24–26] Reinserting the lower eyelid retractors, either in isolation, or in conjunction with horizontal lid tightening, is another technique preferred by some ophthalmologists.[27,28]

Medial involutional ectropion can also be corrected by a number of different procedures. Excision of a diamond of tarso-conjunctival tissue with inverting sutures,[29] the "lazy-T" repair with a full thickness lid resection,[30] plication of a lax medial canthal tendon[31] or a medial tarsal strip procedure[32] are all techniques in current use.

Interventions used for a cicatricial ectropion include a Z-plasty,[33] or placement of a full thickness skin graft or flap.[34] Correction of a paralytic ectropion may involve lid tightening but with additional medial canthoplasty. Autogenous fascia or synthetic devices can also be used in severe cases to create a supportive "sling" for the lid.[35]

Questions

What is the effect of the various interventions for involutional entropion?

What is the optimum technique for the surgical correction of involutional lower eyelid ectropion?

The evidence

We found one Cochrane review of interventions for involutional lower lid entropion that did not contain any trials.[36] We did not find any randomised controlled trials where one intervention for either involutional entropion or ectropion has been compared to another method of treatment.

Comment

There are no available data from randomised trials to provide evidence for the most effective intervention for the correction of involutional entropion or ectropion. The large number of suggested surgical procedures for both eyelid malpositions, often addressing similar pathophysiological factors, may be interpreted as suggesting that the understanding of the disease process has been limited.

The current information available relating to the treatment of entropion and ectropion comes from non-randomised studies. These vary significantly on key issues including methodology and follow up, such that the apparent success rate of each procedure is open to misinterpretation.[37] Current clinical practice is probably formulated by surgeons' understanding of the pathophysiological causative changes associated with involutional eyelid changes, along with results from personnel experience or uncontrolled retrospective case series studies.

Implications for practice

There are many non-randomised case series and retrospective studies that have reported on the number of

overcorrections and recurrences associated with different techniques. The studies suggest that for entropion the recurrence rate is higher when vertical lid laxity is corrected in isolation[15] as compared to a combined technique that involves additional horizontal lid shortening.[17,18,38] Other non-trial evidence suggests that inferior retractor plication may have a further beneficial role in achieving a satisfactory long-term outcome.[39–41]

Interpretation of these data should be considered with caution since these results have not been verified by randomised controlled trials.

Implications for research

There is a clear need for sufficiently large, high-quality randomised trials to establish the effectiveness of interventions for entropion and ectropion.

References

1. Levine RM, El-Toukhy E, Schaefer JA. Entropion. In: Levine RM, ed. *Smith's Ophthalmic Plastic and Reconstructive Surgery, 2nd edn.* St. Louis, MO: Mosby, 1998, pp. 271–89.
2. Dalgleish R, Smith JL. Mechanics and histology of senile entropion. *Br J Ophthalmol* 1966;**50**(2):79–91.
3. Collin JRO. Entropion and trichiasis. In: Collin JRO (ed). *A Manual of Systematic Eyelid Surgery, 2nd edn.* London: Churchill Livingstone, 1989: pp. 7–26.
4. Benger RS, Musch DC. A comparative study of eyelid parameters in involutional entropion. *Ophthal Plast Reconstr Surg* 1989;**5**(4): 281–7.
5. Bashour M, Harvey J. Causes of involutional ectropion and entropion – age-related tarsal changes are the key. *Ophthal Plast Reconstr Surg* 2000;**16**(2):131–41.
6. Sisler HA, Labay GR, Finlay JR. Senile ectropion and entropion: a comparative histopathological study. *Ann Ophthalmol* 1976;**8**(3): 319–22.
7. Musch DC, Sugar A, Meyer RF. Demographic and predisposing factors in corneal ulceration. *Arch Ophthalmol* 1983;**101**(10):1545–8.
8. Tse DT. *Oculoplastic Surgery.* Pennsylvania: JB Lippincott Company, 1992.
9. Clarke JR, Spalton DJ. Treatment of senile entropion with botulinum toxin. *Br J Ophthalmol* 1988;**72**(5):361–2.
10. Neetens A, Rubbens MC, Smet H. Botulinum A-toxin treatment of spasmodic entropion of the lower eyelid. *Bull Soc Belge d'Ophthalmol* 1987;**224**:105–9.
11. Jones LT, Reeh MJ, Wobig JL. Senile entropion. A new concept for correction. *Am J Ophthalmol* 1972;**74**(2):327–9.
12. Olver JM, Barnes JA. Effective small-incision surgery for involutional lower eyelid entropion. *Ophthalmology* 2000;**107**(11):1982–8.
13. Wheeler JM. Spastic entropion correction by orbicularis transplantation. *Trans Am Ophthalmol Soc* 1938;**36**:157–62.
14. Jones LT, Reeh MJ, Tsujimura JK. Senile entropion. *Am J Ophthalmol* 1963;**55**:463–9.
15. Wies FA. Surgical treatment of entropion. *J Int Coll Surg* 1954;**21**:758–60.
16. Wies FA. Spastic entropion. *Trans Am Acad Ophthalmol Otolaryngol* 1955;**59**:503–6.
17. Collin JR, Rathbun JE. Involutional entropion. A review with evaluation of a procedure. *Arch Ophthalmol* 1978;**96**(6):1058–64.
18. Carroll RP, Allen SE. Combined procedure for repair of involutional entropion. *Ophthal Plast Reconstr Surg* 1991;**7**(2):123–7.

19. Lance SE, Wilkins RB. Involutional entropion: A retrospective analysis of the Wies procedure alone or combined with a horizontal shortening procedure. *Ophthal Plast Reconstr Surg* 1991;**7**(4):273–7.

20. Baylis HI, Silkiss RZ. A structurally oriented approach to the repair of cicatricial entropion. *Ophthal Plast Reconstr Surg* 1987;**3**(1):17–20.

21. Elder MJ, Dart JK, Collin R. Inferior retractor plication surgery for lower lid entropion with trichiasis in ocular cicatricial pemphigoid. *Br J Ophthalmol* 1995;**79**(11):1003–6.

22. Bashour M, Harvey J. Causes of involutional ectropion and entropion – age-related tarsal changes are the key. *Ophthal Plast Reconstr Surg* 2000;**16**(2):131–41.

23. Smith B, Cherubini TD. *Oculoplastic Surgery: a compendium of principles and techniques*. St. Louis, MO: CV Mosby, 1970.

24. Tenzel RR, Buffam FV, Miller GR. The use of the "lateral canthal sling" in ectropion repair. *Can J Ophthalmol* 1977;**12**:199–202.

25. Anderson RL, Gordy DD. The tarsal strip procedure. *Arch Ophthalmol* 1979;**97**:323–4.

26. Weber PJ, Popp JC, Wulc AE. Refinements of the tarsal strip procedure. *Ophthalmic Surg* 1991;**22**:687–91.

27. Putterman AM. Ectropion of the lower eyelid secondary to Muller's muscle-capsulopalpebral fascia detachment. *Am J Ophthalmol* 1978;**85**:814–17.

28. Tse DT, Kronish JW, Buus D. Surgical correction of lower eyelid ectropion by reinsertion of the retractors. *Arch Ophthalmol* 1991;**109**:427–31.

29. Tse DT. Surgical correction of punctal malposition. *Am J Ophthalmol* 1985;**100**:339–40.

30. Smith B. The 'lazy-T' correction of ectropion of the lower punctum. *Arch Ophthalmol* 1976;**94**:1149–50.

31. Edelstein JP, Dryden RM. Medial palpebral tendon repair for medial ectropion of the lower eyelid. *Ophthal Plast Reconstr Surg* 1990;**6**:28–37.

32. Jordan DR, Anderson RL, Thiese SM. The medial tarsal strip. *Arch Ophthalmol* 1990;**108**:120–4.

33. Putterman AM. Combined Z-plasty and horizontal shortening procedure for ectropion. *Am J Ophthalmol* 1980;**89**:525–30.

34. Hurwitz JJ, Lichter M, Rodgers J. Cicatricial ectropion due to essential skin shrinkage: treatment with rotational upper-lid pedicle flaps. *Can J Ophthalmol* 1983;**18**:269–73.

35. Arion HG. Dynamic closure of the lids in paralysis of the orbicularis muscle. *Int Surg* 1972;**57**:48–50.

36. Boboridis K, Bunce C. Interventions for involutional lower lid entropion (Cochrane Review). In: Cochrane Library. Issue 4. Oxford: Update Software, 2002.

37. Glatt HJ. Follow-up methods and the apparent success of entropion surgery. *Ophthal Plast Reconstr Surg* 1999;**15**(6):396–400.

38. Danks JJ, Rose GE. Involutional lower lid entropion: to shorten or not to shorten? *Ophthalmology* 1998;**105**(11):2065–7.

39. Dryden RM, Leibsohn J, Wobig J. Senile entropion. Pathogenesis and treatment. *Arch Ophthalmol* 1978;**96**(10):1883–5.

40. Van den Bosch WA, Rosman M, Stijnen T. Involutional lower eyelid entropion: Results of a combined approach. *Ophthalmic Surg Lasers* 1998;**29**(7):581–6.

41. Boboridis K, Bunce C, Rose GE. A comparative study of two procedures for repair of involutional lower lid entropion. *Ophthalmology* 2000;**107**(5):959–61.

18 Thyroid eye disease

Michael J Wearne, Silvia Wengrowicz

Background

Thyroid eye disease (also known as dysthyroid eye disease, thyroid orbitopathy or thyroid ophthalmopathy) is a disease of the orbit that predominantly affects the extraocular muscles.[1] It is the most common cause of unilateral or bilateral proptosis in adults, due to enlarged eye muscles and an increase in orbital fat. The term thyroid eye disease can be misleading. Although it is often related to Graves' disease and thyroid autoimmunity, it can also occur in people who have normal thyroid gland function.

Thyroid eye disease most often affects young to middle aged adults, and is more common in females. It is considered to be an autoimmune inflammatory condition[2,3] but the precise pathogenesis remains unclear. There is no laboratory test for thyroid eye disease, and the diagnosis is usually made clinically or radiologically. The classical signs are unilateral or bilateral proptosis, restricted eye movements, upper or lower eyelid retraction, eyelid and conjunctival oedema and, rarely, visual failure secondary to a compressive optic neuropathy.[4]

The natural history of thyroid eye disease is poorly documented in the literature, but it is often stated that there is an acute phase of disease with active orbital inflammation prior to an inactive fibrotic stage. A proportion of patients improve spontaneously, a factor that needs to be considered when assessing the effectiveness of any treatment.[5] Recognised risk factors that may influence ocular prognosis include cigarette smoking,[6] radioiodine treatment of thyrotoxicosis[7] and uncontrolled thyroid dysfunction.[8]

Patients with thyroid eye disease are selected for treatment based on the activity and severity of the condition.[9,10] In the absence of a treatment based on knowledge of the precise pathogenesis, a variety of therapeutic approaches have been proposed, chiefly various systemic immunosuppressive agents. Steroid therapy has been commonly used to manage thyroid eye disease for several decades, but many areas of controversy exist. Glucocorticoids have often been administered systemically in the initial stages of active orbital disease.[11] Studies have tried to assess the benefit and side effects of intravenous pulsed high-dose steroids, followed by oral treatment[12] or oral administration alone.[13] There are, however, no clear guidelines regarding the best route, optimum dose or duration of treatment, the role of uncontrolled risk factors or the effectiveness of steroids when combined with other immunosuppressive therapies.

Alternative methods exist that attempt to suppress active thyroid eye disease and reports of using orbital radiotherapy date back to 1936.[14] The success rate associated with this treatment modality is also controversial, and the role of orbital radiotherapy in limiting the secondary effects of ocular inflammation remains poorly defined.[15] This chapter concentrates on assessing what evidence exists for the use of steroid therapy and orbital radiotherapy in the clinical management of thyroid eye disease.

Question

What is the effectiveness of glucocorticoid therapy in reducing activity and severity of thyroid eye disease in patients when other risk factors have been controlled?

The evidence

A search of the Cochrane controlled trials register (CENTRAL) identified no randomised controlled trials for thyroid eye disease comparing steroids with a placebo group. Six published studies were found as prospective randomised controlled trials, but all looked at steroids versus, or in combination with, radiotherapy,[16,17] immunosuppressive drugs,[18,19] somatostatin analogues[20] or intravenous immunoglobulins.[21] Initial oral doses equivalent to 60–100 mg/day prednisone and tapered down for several months led to favourable responses within several weeks in about 60% of cases (range 40–100%). Ocular improvements include less soft tissue swelling, enhanced motility and an increase in optic nerve function, but benefit for proptosis is less evident. Combination therapies appear to be more effective in these trials.

Low dose oral prednisone (0·4–0·5 mg/kg/day for one month and tapering in three months) was shown in a randomised controlled study to be effective for preventing worsening ophthalmopathy after radioiodine treatment for hyperthyroidism.[22] The eye changes after radioiodine are usually mild and transient, but it is worth considering oral steroids in high-risk cases.

Only one prospective, single-blind randomised study was found providing comparative data of high-dose intravenous and oral glucocorticoid treatment in association with orbital radiotherapy.[23] The intravenous route seems to be more effective and better tolerated than the oral route.

Other routes of administration have been tried in an attempt to increase the efficacy and decrease the side effects of steroids. Local retrobulbar glucocorticoids were shown to be less effective than the systemic route in a randomised controlled study.[24]

Question

What evidence exists that orbital radiotherapy has a beneficial role in the treatment of active thyroid eye disease?

The evidence

A Cochrane systematic review on the role of radiotherapy in thyroid eye disease is currently underway. This review will include randomised controlled trials in which orbital radiotherapy was compared to sham orbital radiotherapy or to no intervention.[25] The primary outcomes used were to evaluate changes in standardised indices of clinical activity before and after intervention, and to assess the time from treatment to the end of the active phase of the disease. Only one trial[26] was deemed to meet the inclusion criteria for the review. The study was a double-blind, randomised trial in which consecutive patients referred to the study centre were assessed using predefined criteria for inclusion. Allocation concealment of those patients enrolled appears to have been adequate. The radiotherapist providing the treatment was not masked, but was not involved in the pre- or post-treatment outcome measurements. The recipients of care and the persons responsible for outcome assessments were both unaware of the assigned therapy. There were no apparent systematic differences in care provided apart from the treatment being evaluated, nor were there differences in outcome assessments for the two groups.

Sixty patients judged to have moderate thyroid eye disease, who had been euthyroid for at least three months, were enrolled. Thirty were assigned retrobulbar radiotherapy using a dose of 20 Gy in ten fractions over 12 days, and 30 to receive sham irradiation. All patients were examined one day before and four, 12 and 24 weeks after treatment by the same ophthalmologist.

The qualitative treatment outcome was successful in 18 of 30 (60%) irradiated patients versus nine of 29 (31%) sham irradiated patients at 24 weeks (relative risk (RR) 1·9, 95% confidence interval (CI) 1·0–3·6, P = 0·04). This difference was chiefly due to a motility improvement in the radiotherapy group (14/17 = 82%) compared to the sham irradiated patients (4/15 = 27%) (RR = 3·1, CI 1·3–7·4, P = 0·004). Other clinical outcome measures, such as eyelid swelling and proptosis, were not significantly different between the two groups. Apart from the exclusion of one patient from the analysis at 12 weeks because of recurrence of hyperthyroidism, the study quality was considered to be at low risk of bias.

A double-blind trial of prednisone versus radiotherapy in patients with moderately severe eye disease confirmed findings from uncontrolled studies that these two treatment modalities are equally effective.[17]

Discussion

Thyroid eye disease provides many challenges for researchers assessing the impact of various treatment modalities. It remains relatively uncommon, the natural history is not well documented and large variations can occur in disease duration and activity. Clinical evaluation, in a reproducible manner, can be difficult, with no existing standard objective or subjective technique.

Despite being established therapies for thyroid eye disease, the role and effectiveness of steroids and retrobulbar irradiation is unclear. The literature is littered with conclusions and statements from mainly uncontrolled open clinical trials. The complexities involved in studying patients with thyroid eye disease make an evidence-based approach essential. There are no formal randomised controlled trials comparing steroids with a placebo. The paper by Mourits *et al.*[26] is the only double-blind, randomised clinical trial assessing the success associated with retrobulbar irradiation identified from an extensive search. The methodology and study design suggest that the risk of bias is low and therefore their conclusions that radiotherapy improves, but does not cure, motility impairment in patients with moderate Graves' orbitopathy, are likely to be valid.

Implications for practice

The intravenous administration of glucocorticoids seems to be more effective and better tolerated than the oral route in the treatment of severe thyroid eye disease, although there is only one published randomised study comparing oral and intravenous glucocorticoid treatment associated with orbital radiotherapy.[23] One patient with transient non-infectious hepatitis was described in this study and in another report there was a case of fatal liver damage.[27] There is a need to carefully monitor patients' liver status before and during treatments and to establish new intravenous steroid schedules in severe thyroid eye disease to prevent liver toxicity or exacerbation of previous asymptomatic autoimmune chronic hepatitis.

Implications for research

Many issues in the treatment of moderately severe thyroid eye disease remain unclear. The impact of steroid therapy, including the optimum dose and route, is not clearly established. Similarly little is known regarding the best radiation dose, most appropriate timing for the treatment and the success of using irradiation in combination with other modalities. In an era of evidence-based medicine the use of steroids and orbital irradiation for thyroid eye disease require further evaluation, using prospective randomised trials, in order that best practice can be further established.

References

1. Perros P, Kendall-Taylor P. Pathogenesis of thyroid-associated ophthalmopathy. *Trends Endocrinol Metab* 1993;**4**:270–5.
2. Kriss JP, Konishi J, Herman M. Studies on the pathogenesis of Graves' ophthalmopathy (with some related observations regarding therapy). *Recent Prog Horm Res* 1975;**31**:533–66.
3. Yamada M, Li AW, Wall JR. Thyroid-associated ophthalmopathy: clinical features, pathogenesis and management. *Crit Rev Clin Lab Sci* 2000;**37**:523–49.
4. Burch HB, Wartofsky L. Graves' ophthalmopathy: current concepts regarding pathogenesis and management. *Endocrine Rev* 1993;**14**: 747–93.
5. Perros P, Crombie AL, Kendall-Taylor P. Natural history of thyroid associated ophthalmopathy. *Clin Endocrinol* 1995;**42**:45–50.
6. Solberg Y, Rosner M, Belkin M. The association between cigarette smoking and ocular diseases. *Surv Ophthalmol* 1998;**42**:535–47.
7. Marcocci C, Bartalena L, Bogazzi F, Bruno-Bozzio G, Pinchera A. Relationship between Graves' ophthalmopathy and type of treatment of Graves' hyperthyroidism. *Thyroid* 1992;**2**:171–8.
8. Prummel MF, Wiersinga WM, Mourits MP, Koorneef L, Berghout A, Van der Gaag R. Amelioration of eye changes of Graves' ophthalmopathy by achieving euthyroidism. *Acta Endocrinol (Copenh)* 1989;**121**(Suppl 2):185–9.
9. Bahn RS, Gorman CA. Choice of therapy and criteria for assessing treatment outcome in thyroid-associated ophthalmopathy. *Endocrinol Metab Clin North Am* 1987;**16**:391–407.
10. Ad hoc committee. Classification of eye changes of Graves' disease. *Thyroid* 1992;**2**:235–6.
11. Wiersinga WM. Immunosuppression in endocrine ophthalmopathy: Why and when? In: Kahaly G, eds. *Endocrine ophthalmopathy. Molecular, Immunological and Clinical Aspects, Vol 25*. Basel: Krager, 1993, pp. 120–30.
12. Kendall-Taylor P, Crombie AL, Stephenson AM, Hardwick M, Hall K. Intravenous methylprednisolone in the treatment of Graves' ophthalmopathy. *BMJ* 1988;**297**:1574–8.
13. Krassas GE, Heufelder AE. Immunosuppressive therapy in patients with thyroid eye disease: an overview of current concepts. *Eur J Endocrinol* 2001;**144**:311–18.
14. Thomas HM, Woods AC. Progressive exophthalmos following thyroidectomy. *Bull Hopkins Hosp* 1936;**59**:99–113.
15. Bartalena L, Pinchera A, Marcocci C. Management of Graves' ophthalmopathy: reality and perspectives. *Endocrinol Rev* 2000;**21**:168–99.
16. Bartalena L, Marcocci C, Chiovato L *et al.* Orbital cobalt irradiation combined with systemic corticosteroids for Graves' ophthalmopathy: comparison with systemic corticosteroids alone. *J Clin Endocrinol Metab* 1983;**56**:1139–44.
17. Prummel M, Mourits M, Blank L, Berghout A, Koornneef L, Wiersinga W. Randomised double-blind trial of prednisone versus radiotherapy in Graves' ophthalmopathy. *Lancet* 1993;**342**:949–54.
18. Kahaly G, Schrezenmeir J, Krause U, Schweikert B, Meuer S, Muller W. Cyclosporin and prednisone *v.* prednisone in treatment of Graves' ophthalmopathy: a controlled, randomised and prospective study. *Eur J Clin Invest* 1986;**16**:415–22.
19. Prummel M, Mourits M, Berghout A *et al.* Prednisone and cyclosporine in the treatment of severe Graves' ophthalmopathy. *N Engl J Med* 1989;**321**:1353–9.
20. Kung AWC, Michon J, Tai KS, Chan FL. The effect of somatostatin versus corticosteroid in the treatment of Graves' ophthalmopathy. *Thyroid* 1996;**6**:381–4.
21. Kahaly G, Pitz S, Müller-Forell W, Hommel G. Randomized trial of intravenous immunoglobulins versus prednisolone in Graves' ophthalmopathy. *Clin Exp Immunol* 1996;**106**:197–202.
22. Bartalena L, Marcocci C, Bogazzi F *et al.* Relation between therapy for hyperthyroidism and the course of Graves' ophthalmopathy. *N Engl J Med* 1998;**338**:73–8.
23. Marcocci C, Bartalena L, Tanda ML *et al.* Comparison of the effectiveness and tolerability of intravenous or oral glucocorticoids associated with orbital radiotherapy: results of a prospective, single-blind, randomized study. *J Clin Endocrinol Metab* 2001;**86**: 3562–7.
24. Marcocci C, Bartalena L, Panucucci M *et al.* Orbital cobalt irradiation combined with retrobulbar or systemic corticosteroids for Graves' ophthalmopathy: a comparative study. *Clin Endocrinol* 1987;**27**: 33–42.
25. Wearne MJ, Henshaw K. Radiotherapy for thyroid eye disease [protocol]. In: Cochrane Collaboration. *Cochrane Library*. Issue 2. Oxford: Update Software, 2002.
26. Mourits MP, van Kempen-Harteveld ML, Garcia MB, Koppeschaar HPF, Tick L, Terwee CB. Radiotherapy for Graves' orbitopathy: randomised placebo-controlled study. *Lancet* 2000;**355**:1505–9.
27. Weissel M, Hauff W. Fatal liver failure after high dose glucocorticoid pulse therapy in a patient with severe thyroid eye disease. *Thyroid* 2000;**10**:521.

19 Lacrimal obstruction

Vinidh Paleri, Andrew K Robson, Michael Bearn

Background

Obstruction of the nasolacrimal duct commonly presents as epiphora and is diagnosed by the presence of obstruction evident on lacrimal syringing. The cause of duct obstruction is often unknown but may occur secondary to bacterial infection and rarely to tumours. It is four to five times more common in females because the duct in women is more angulated and shorter in diameter.[1] The prevalence of obstruction in asymptomatic individuals increases with age, ranging from 9–10% at 40 years to 35–40% at 90 years.[2] There is a racial predominance in whites and Asians, with blacks being less commonly affected.[3]

External dacryocystorhinostomy is the traditional procedure for the management of nasolacrimal duct obstruction. This technique was described in 1904 by Toti[4] and various modifications of the procedure have since been developed.[5,6,7] The procedure involves making an external incision on the skin over the lacrimal sac and removing the bone underlying the sac that separates it from the nose. The sac is then opened to create a drainage site into the nose. This procedure has reported success rates of 85–95%.[6–8] The disadvantages of the external approach include scarring, haemorrhage and wound infection.

The endonasal approach was first introduced in 1893 by Caldwell,[9] before the introduction of the external approach. However, wide acceptance of this procedure was hampered by difficulties in visualising the operating site. The advent of the rigid Hopkins rod telescope (which provides an excellent wide-angled view inside the nose) and developments in endoscopic nasal and paranasal sinus surgery, rekindled the interest in the endonasal approach to the lacrimal sac. The procedure involves identifying the bone underlying the lacrimal sac from within the nose, removing it and opening the sac to create a drainage port into the nose. Success rates of 68–85% have been reported.[10–14] The advantage of the endonasal technique is the absence of an external wound that may be prone to infection, less bleeding, limited tissue injury and reduced postoperative stay. Various techniques have been used to create the functioning conduit from the lacrimal sac into the nasal cavity in the endonasal technique. These include bone drills and various lasers to vaporise bone. Massaro *et al.*[15] first described the use of the Argon blue green laser for

endonasal dacryocystorhinostomy. Potassium titanyl phosphate (KTP), carbon dioxide, holmium: YAG (yttrium–aluminium–garnet), neodymium: YAG, and the combined carbon dioxide neodymium: YAG (CO_2–Nd: YAG) are other lasers that have been used.[10–14]

Scarring at the operative site due to fibrous tissue commonly causes surgical failures. Thus, reducing the scarring process by suppressing fibroblast proliferation can logically lead to a reduction in failure rates. Mitomycin C and 5-fluorouracil are two antimetabolites that are used in glaucoma surgery for this purpose. Mitomycin C is an alkylating antibiotic isolated from *Streptomyces caespitosus* and 5-fluorouracil is a pyrimidine analogue, both capable of suppressing fibroblast proliferation.

Question

In patients with primary acquired nasolacrimal duct obstruction free of concurrent nasal disease needing dacryocystorhinostomy, is one surgical approach (external versus endonasal) superior to the other in terms of:

● success rates as determined by duct patency and symptomatic relief after at least six months of follow up
● postoperative complications
● operative time for the procedure and duration of hospital stay
● cost-effectiveness
● patient preference for or satisfaction with either approach?

The evidence

A Cochrane systematic review is underway,[16] which includes trials of external dacryocystorhinostomy using any of the standard described techniques and endonasal surgery performed using the laser or the mechanical drill to open the lacrimal sac into the nose, with or without use of antimetabolites at the operated site. The review excludes trials of people with congenital or secondary nasolacrimal sac obstruction and trials when the follow up period was of less than six months. Two RCTs were identified that satisfied the inclusion criteria.[17,18]

Table 19.1 Outcome results from Hartikainen *et al.* (1998)[17] and Hartikainen *et al.* (1998)[18]

Outcome measures	External	Endonasal laser	Endonasal drill
No. of procedures	32	32	32
Patency rates after primary procedure (%)	91	63	75
Patency rates after revision procedure (%)	97	94[19]	97
Symptom relief (%)	84	59	59
Epistaxis	1	0	2
Procedure time (mins)	78 (SD ±13)	23 (SD ±6)	38 (SD ±13)

Both trials were conducted at the same institution and from the data provided in both papers, the same group undergoing external dacryocystorhinostomy (using the technique of Dupuy–Dutemps) were compared to two variations of the endonasal procedure (CO_2–Nd:YAG laser and mechanical drill).

Both trials included patients with primary acquired nasolacrimal duct obstruction, symptomatic for longer than one year, where the site of obstruction was confirmed to be distal to the lacrimal sac after syringing and/or dacryocystography. The primary outcome measure was patency of the nasolacrimal system on syringing one year postoperatively. Other outcomes studied included complications and the time of operation. Questionnaires pertaining to the presence of tearing and appearance of the scar (for the external approach) were used to assess patient satisfaction.

The duct patency rates following primary surgery as ascertained by syringing were 91% for the external group, 63% and 75% for the endonasal laser and drill groups, respectively. However, after revision surgery for those patients who failed the primary surgery, the success rates were comparable (Table 19.1). The external approach thus has a relative benefit of 1·4 (95% CI 1·08–1·93) over the endonasal laser procedure and 1·2 (95% CI 0·96–1·51) over the endonasal drill approach. It is also evident from Table 19.1 that the endonasal approaches take approximately half the time compared to the external approach. The complication rates among the various approaches are not significantly different, despite limited middle turbinate resections in 31% of patients undergoing endonasal drill approach.

Comment

The results indicate that primary success rates in terms of patency and symptomatic relief are better for the external approach. The difference in success rates after the primary procedure between the external and the endonasal laser approaches are significant.[18] The endonasal approaches certainly take less time compared to the external approach

but the issues of hospital stay, cost-effectiveness and patient satisfaction have not so far been addressed.

Question

In patients with primary acquired nasolacrimal duct obstruction free of concurrent nasal disease needing dacryocystorhinostomy, does the use of topical antimetabolites during the procedure through the external or endonasal approach lead to better success rates following the surgery?

The evidence

Seven published trials[20–26] were identified that satisfied inclusion criteria (Table 19.2). The paper by Zilelioğlu[25] was excluded from analysis as concurrent nasal pathology needing surgery was present in four patients. All other papers analysed the effect of antimetabolites on the external procedure except Bakri,[26] who studied the success rates of endonasal laser dacryocystorhinostomy with and without 5-fluorouracil.

From the description of the operation provided, it would appear that the technique of Dupuy–Dutemps has been used by all the studies where external dacryocystorhinostomy has been performed. The trials used mitomycin C in varying concentrations: 0·2 mg/ml,[20,21,23,24] 0·5 mg/ml[21,22] and 1 mg/ml.[22] Two trials used 5-fluorouracil at concentrations of 0·5 mg/ml,[26] 2·5 mg/ml[22] and 5 mg/ml.[22] The contact duration of the antimetabolite at the surgical site also varied: two minutes,[24] five minutes[21] and 30 minutes.[20,23] Yalaz *et al.*[22] do not mention the contact duration and the cases in this study treated with 5-fluorouracil have been excluded from the meta-analysis. We have not attempted to differentiate studies based on the contact duration as there is evidence to show that one minute's exposure is as effective as five minutes' exposure.[27] Two studies from the same centre[20,23] used silicone tube intubation of all eyes for six months. The others[21,22,24] have not followed this practice.

Table 19.2   Quality assessments of trials using antimetabolites

Parameters	Liao et al.[20]	You and Fang[21]	Yalaz et al.[22]	Kao et al.[23]	Gonzalvo Ibanez et al.[24]	Zilelioğlu et al.[25]	Bakri (personal communication)
Allocation concealment	A	B	B	A	B	B	A
Method of allocation	A	B	B	A	B	B	A
Exclusions	B	A	A	B	B	C	B
Follow up	A	A	A	A	A	A	A
Complications	A	A	B	A	A	B	A

A, adequate; B, unclear; C, in adeaquate

Study	Mitomycin C n/N	Control n/N	RR (95% CI fixed)	Weight %	RR (95% CI fixed)
Gonzalvo Ibanez et al., 2000[24]	9/9	5/8		6·5	1·60 (0·94, 2·74)
Kao et al., 1997[23]	7/7	7/8		8·0	1·14 (0·88, 1·49)
Liao et al., 2000[20]	42/44	31/44		38·1	1·35 (1·11, 1·66)
Yalaz et al., 1999[22]	19/20	18/20		22·1	1·06 (0·88, 1·26)
You and Fang 2001[21]	30/32	16/18		25·2	1·05 (0·88, 1·27)
Total (95% CI)	107/112	77/98		100·0	1·21 (1·09,1·35)

Test for heterogeneity chi-square = 6·86 df = 4 P = 0·14

Test for overall effect Z = 8·45 P = 0·0006

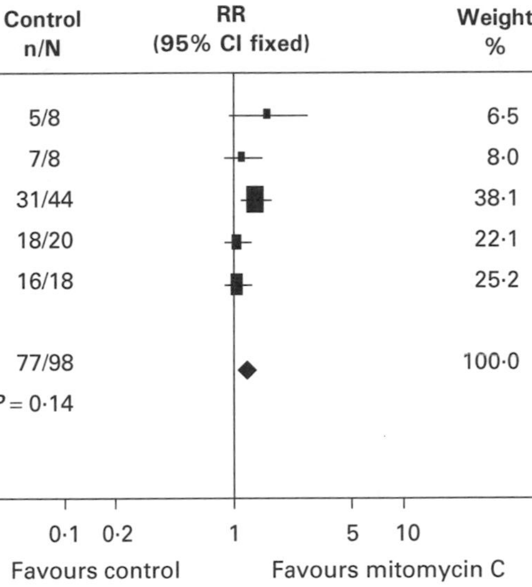

0·1 0·2   1   5 10

Favours control   Favours mitomycin C

Figure 19.1   Meta-analysis of trials studying the effect of mitomycin C on external dacryocystorhinostomy

All the included studies mention outcome in terms of symptom free rates, with three trials[20,21,24] noting the patency rates of the nasolacrimal system as confirmed by irrigation. Pooling the results of the included studies,[17–21,24] 97% of eyes patent to irrigation are asymptomatic. The symptom relief rates have been used for meta-analysis. Minimum follow-up of six months has been achieved in all the included studies, ranging from six months to 42 months. The relative benefit provided by use of mitomycin C during external dacryocystorhinostomy in each of the studies is shown in Figure 19.1. The 95% confidence intervals of the cumulative relative benefit do not contain unity (1·09 to 1·35), therefore indicating a significant increase in symptom control rates when mitomycin C is used.

Bakri's study[26], which randomised 167 patients undergoing endonasal laser dacryocystorhinostomy to a control or 5-fluorouracil group found no significant difference in symptom control rates between the groups. It is interesting that Yalaz et al.,[22] who also used 5-fluorouracil for the external procedure, found no benefit although Yalaz et al.[22] accept that their study group was quite small.

Comment

The evidence presented suggests that use of mitomycin C during external dacryocystorhinostomy will provide a relative benefit (symptom relief) of 21% (95% CI 9–35%). There appears to be no increased risk of complications with the use of mitomycin C. No randomised controlled trials have studied the effect of mitomycin C on success rates with the endonasal approach, but we believe that a similar benefit will be evident as the same site is being subjected to the antimetabolite exposure, albeit transnasally. A wide range of concentrations has been used for the purpose and the ideal strength remains to be determined.

Implications for practice and research

The best current evidence suggests that a primary external dacryocystorhinostomy is more successful, in terms of duct patency and symptomatic improvement, compared to the endonasal approach. The endonasal techniques do have the advantage of tending to be quicker and avoiding an external scar. The issues of hospital stay and cost-effectiveness have not been adequately addressed.

Meta-analysis data provide evidence in favour of the peroperative use of mitomycin C in external dacryo-cystorhinostomy. More information is required regarding the optimum dose and contact time.

References

1. Hurwitz JJ, Rutherford S. Computerised survey of lacrimal surgery patients. *Ophthalmology* 1986;**83**:14.
2. Dalgleish R. Idiopathic acquired lacrimal drainage obstruction. *Br J Ophthalmol* 1967;**51**:463.
3. Santos Fernandez J. De la disposition anatomica del canal nasoen el Negro, que explicasumenor predisposicion a las afeccicions da las dias lagrimales. *Arch Oftal Hisp Am* 1903;**3**:193.
4. Toti A. Nuovo metodo conservatore di cura radicale delle suppurazioni croniche del sacco lacrimale (Dacriocistorinostomia). *Clin Mod Firenze* 1904;**10**:385–7.
5. Dupuy–Dutemps B. Procede plastique de dacryocystorhinostomie et ses resultants. *Annales d'Oculistique* 1921;**158**: 241–61.
6. Rosen M, Sharir M, Moverman DC, Rosner M. Dacryocystorhinostomy with silicone tubes: evaluation of 253 cases. *Ophthalmic Surg* 1989;**20**:115–19.
7. Becker BB. Dacryocystorhinostomy without flaps. *Ophthalmic Surg* 1988;**19**:419–27.
8. Tarbet KJ, Custer PL. External dacryocystorhinostomy: surgical success, patient satisfaction and economic cost. *Ophthalmology* 1995;**102**: 1065–70.
9. Caldwell GW. Two new operations for obstruction of the nasal duct. *New York Med J* 1893;**57**:581–2.
10. Reifler DM. Results of endoscopic KTP laser assisted dacryocystorhinostomy. *Ophthal Plast Reconstr Surg* 1993;**9**: 231–6.
11. Woog JJ, Metson R, Puliafito CA. Holmium: YAG endonasal laser dacryocystorhinostomy. *Am J Ophthalmol* 1993;**116**:1–10.
12. Kong YT, Kim TI, Kong BW. A report of 131 cases of endoscopic laser lacrimal surgery. *Ophthalmology* 1994;**101**:1793–800.
13. Seppa H, Grenman R, Hartikainen J. Endonasal CO_2–Nd: YAG laser dacryocystorhinostomy. *Acta Ophthalmologica* 1994;**72**:703–6.
14. Boush GA, Lemke BN, Dortzbach RK. Results of endonasal laser assisted dacryocystorhinostomy *Ophthalmology* 1994;**101**:955–9.
15. Massaro BM, Gonnering RS, Harris GJ. Endonasal laser dacryocystorhinostomy. A new approach to nasolacrimal duct obstruction. *Arch Ophthalmol* 1990;**108**:1172–6.
16. Paleri V, Robson A, Bearn M. Endonasal versus external dacryocystorhinostomy for nasolacrimal duct obstruction (Protocol for a Cochrane Review). In: *Cochrane Library*. Issue 4. Oxford: Update Software, 2002.
17. Hartikainen J, Antila J, Varpula M, Puukka P, Seppa H, Grenman R. Prospective randomized comparison of endonasal endoscopic dacryocystorhinostomy and external dacryocystorhinostomy. *Laryngoscope* 1998;**108**:1861–6.
18. Hartikainen J, Grenman R, Puukka P, Seppa H. Prospective randomized comparison of external dacryocystorhinostomy and endonasal laser dacryocystorhinostomy. *Ophthalmology* 1998;**105**:1106–13.
19. Hartikainen J, Grenman R, Puukka P, Seppa H. External dacryocystorhinostomy versus endonasal laser dacryocystorhinostomy (comment). *Ophthalmology* 1999;**106**:647–9.
20. Liao SL, Kao SC, Tseng JH, Chen MS, Hou PK. Results of intraoperative mitomycin C application in dacryocystorhinostomy. *Br J Ophthalmol* 2000;**84**:903–6.
21. You YA, Fang CT. Intraoperative mitomycin C in dacryo-cystorhinostomy. *Ophthal Plast Reconstr Surg* 2001;**17**:115–19.
22. Yalaz M, Firinciogullari E, Zeren H. Use of mitomycin C and 5-fluorouracil in external dacryocystorhinostomy. *Orbit* 1999;**18**: 239–45.
23. Kao SCS, Liao CL, Tseng JHS, Chen MS, Hou PK. Dacryo-cystorhinostomy with intraoperative mitomycin C. *Ophthalmology* 1997;**104**:86–91.
24. Gonzalvo Ibanez FJ, Fuertes Fernandez I, Fernandez Tirado FJ, Hernandez Delgado G, Rabinal Arbues F, Honrubia Lopez FM. External dacryocystorhinostomy with mitomycin C. Clinical and anatomical evaluation with helical computed tomography. *Arch Soc Esp Oftalmol* 2000;**75**:611–18.
25. Zilelioğlu G, Uğurbaş SH, Anadolu Y, Akner M, Aktürk T. Adjunctive use of mitomycin C on endoscopic lacrimal surgery *Br J Ophthalmol* 1998;**82**:63–6.
26. Bakri K, Jones NS, Downes R, Sadig SA. Intraoperative fluorouracil in endonasal laser dacryocystorhinostomy. *Arch Otolarynglol Mead Neck Surg* 2003;**129**:233–5.
27. Jampel HD. Effect of brief exposure to mitomycin C on viability and proliferation of cultured human Tenon's capsule fibroblasts. *Ophthalmology* 1992;**99**:1471–6.

Section V

Cornea and external disease

Linda Ficker, Editor

Cornea: mission statement

The common causes of corneal blindness worldwide are trachoma, herpes simplex and contact lens associated bacterial keratitis. These topics are included in this section. Common causes of presentation to emergency departments include trauma and recurrent erosions, the latter being difficult to manage, and a topic of this section.

Corneal transplants have a relatively small role to play in the management of corneal disease, but are very valuable where other means of visual rehabilitation such as contact lens fitting is not adequate or appropriate. The problem of transplant rejection, particularly in high risk transplants remains unresolved and clinical trials have attempted to address these issues. This topic warrants inclusion in a future edition of evidence-based medicine.

20 Trachoma

Denise Mabey

Background

Definition

Active trachoma is chronic inflammation of the conjunctiva caused by infection with *Chlamydia trachomatis*. The World Health Organization classification for active trachoma defines mild trachoma (grade TF) and severe trachoma (grade TI). Scarring trachoma is caused by repeated active infection by *C. trachomatis* in which the upper eyelid is shortened and distorted (entropion) and the lashes abrade the eye (trichiasis). Blindness results from corneal opacification, which is related to the degree of entropion/trichiasis.

Incidence/prevalence

Trachoma is the world's leading cause of preventable blindness and is second only to cataract as an overall cause of blindness.[1] Globally, active trachoma affects an estimated 150 million people, most of them children. About 5·5 million people are blind or at risk of blindness as a consequence of trachoma. Trachoma is a disease of poverty regardless of geographical region. Scarring trachoma is prevalent in large regions of Africa, the Middle East, south-west Asia, the Indian subcontinent, and Aboriginal communities in Australia, and there are also small foci in Central and South America.[1] In areas where trachoma is constantly present at high prevalence, active disease is found in more than 50% of preschool children and may have a prevalence of 60–90%.[2] The prevalence of active trachoma decreases with increasing age, with less than 5% of adults showing signs of active disease.[2] Although similar rates of active disease are observed in male and female children, the later sequelae of trichiasis, entropion and corneal opacification are more common in women than men and as many as 75% of women and 50% of men over the age of 45 years who had trachoma as children may show signs of scarring disease.[3]

Aetiology/risk factors

Active trachoma is associated with young age and with situations in which there is close contact between people. Discharge from the eyes and nose may be a source of further re-infection.[4] Sharing a bedroom with someone who has active trachoma is a risk factor for infection.[5] Facial contact with flies is held to be associated with active trachoma, but studies reporting this relationship employed weak methods.[6]

Prognosis

Corneal damage from trachoma is caused by multiple processes. Scarring may cause an inadequate tear film and a dry eye may be more susceptible to damage from inturned lashes, leading to corneal opacification. The prevalence of scarring and consequent blindness increases with age and, therefore, is most commonly seen in older adults.[7]

Treatement options

The WHO-led campaign for elimination of blinding trachoma uses the SAFE strategy of Surgery, Antibiotics, Facial cleanliness and Environmental improvement.

Question

What are the effects of public health interventions in reducing active trachoma?

The evidence

Two systematic reviews[6,8] and one additional RCT[9] were identified. The first systematic review[6] identified one RCT and one pilot study for an RCT, the second systematic review[9] identified the same RCT and pilot study as the first review plus two subsequent RCTs (see comment below).

Promotion of face washing

Both reviews identified one RCT[10] that compared promotion of face washing plus 30 days of daily topical tetracycline (ointment) versus 30 days of daily topical tetracycline alone in 1417 Tanzanian children aged one to seven years. The trial found that promotion of face washing plus topical tetracycline increased the likelihood of children having a clean face on at least two of three follow up visits, although the result was not significant (odds ratio for having a clean face with face washing plus topical tetracycline versus topical tetracycline alone 1·6, 95% CI 0·94–2·74). The RCT also found that promotion of face washing plus topical tetracycline versus topical tetracycline alone significantly reduced the risk of severe trachoma after one year (OR for severe trachoma 0·62, 95% CI 0·40–0·97), but found that this reduction was not significant for all grades of trachoma combined (OR for mild and severe trachoma 0·81, 95% CI 0·42–1·59). The RCT found that when all participants from intervention and control villages were pooled, children who had a sustained clean face were significantly less likely to have active trachoma than those who had ever had a dirty face (OR 0·58, 95% CI 0·47–0·72). The additional RCT[9] recruited 1143 children in 36 communities in Australia and compared three groups: daily face washing (performed by a teacher); daily face washing (performed by a teacher) plus daily topical tetracycline (as drops for one week each month); and no intervention. Trachoma was defined as the presence of at least one follicle or some papillae on the upper tarsal plate (this study pre-dated the present World Health Organization definition of trachoma). Losses to follow up were treated as being trachoma positive. The RCT found no significant difference between face washing alone versus no intervention in the number of children with trachoma after three months (191/246 (78%) with face washing alone versus 160/211 (76%) with no intervention; relative risk 1·0; CI not provided). It also found that face washing plus tetracycline drops versus no intervention significantly reduced the number of children with trachoma after three months (215/312 (69%) with face washing plus topical tetracycline versus 160/211 (78%) with no intervention; RR 0·9; CI not provided).

Fly control using insecticide

The reviews identified one pilot study for an RCT (414 children younger than 10 years) that compared spraying of deltamethrin for three months versus no intervention in two pairs of villages.[11] One pair received the intervention or none in the wet season and one pair received the intervention or none in the dry season. There were a total of 191 children under 10 years of age in the control villages and 223 children in the intervention villages. The pilot study found that spraying of deltamethrin significantly reduced the number of new cases of trachoma (World Health Organization classification) after three months (RR 0·25, 95% CI 0·09–0·64).

Comment

Cluster randomisation used in the RCTs and the pilot study limits the power to detect differences between

groups, and makes interpretation of the results for individual children difficult.[9–11] The RCT comparing promotion of face washing plus topical tetracycline versus topical tetracycline alone was too small to rule out a clinically important effect.[10] The two subsequent RCTs identified by the second systematic review compared antibiotics versus health education plus face washing, and it was not possible to extract data relating to the health education and face washing interventions separately.[8] The additional RCT pre-dates the simplified World Health Organization classification of trachoma, limiting the applicability of the results.[9]

Question
What are the effects of antibiotics in reducing active trachoma?

The evidence

There has been a Cochrane review that identified 12 antibiotic treatment trials for active trachoma.[12] The comparisons were of any antibiotic treatment against placebo/no treatment and of oral antibiotic treatment against topical antibiotic treatment. A further RCT, not included in the review, has compared topical plus oral treatment with the oral antibiotic azithromycin[13] and found no significant difference between treatments.

Antibiotic treatment versus placebo or no treatment

The Cochrane review of antibiotics for trachoma considered topical treatment, oral treatment or any combination compared with placebo/no treatment.[12] The results of the trials that compare an oral antibiotic to placebo/no treatment and the trials that compare a topical antibiotic to placebo/no treatment show high degrees of heterogeneity in their outcomes. A synthesis of the results to give a summary statistic was therefore not performed but point estimates of relative risk were given. For the outcome of active trachoma, the trials did not show a significant effect of antibiotics but suggested a lowering of risk at three and 12 months after treatment. This was similarly the case for the outcome of laboratory evidence of trachoma.

Oral versus topical antibiotics

The Cochrane review of antibiotics for trachoma cites the results of four trials that compared an oral with a topical treatment for active trachoma.[12] The results showed highly significant degrees of heterogeneity for both the outcome measures of active trachoma and the laboratory evidence of infection. Point estimates of relative risk were given but no summary statistic was calculated because of the heterogeneity. Three of the trials were small and low powered. The fourth trial compared mass treatment in which people were treated irrespective of disease status and were randomly allocated by village (cluster randomisation). The results suggest that oral treatment is neither more nor less effective than topical treatment for the outcomes of active trachoma at three and 12 months. Azithromycin was significantly better than topical treatment at reducing laboratory evidence of infection with heterogeneity showing a *P* value of 0·036.

Comment

No harms were reported but adverse reactions to systemic antibiotics were not recorded in the trial protocols.

Question

What are the effects of surgical treatments for scarring trachoma (entropion and trichiasis)?

The evidence

Three RCTs were identified, two of which compared surgical interventions versus each other for entropion/trichiasis[14,15] and the third compared village-based versus health centre-based tarsal rotation surgery for major trichiasis.[16]

Surgical technique

The two RCTs that compared surgical interventions versus each other defined operative success as no lashes in contact with the globe in primary position of gaze and complete lid closure with gentle voluntary effort. The first RCT[14] compared five surgical techniques in Omani villagers. Analysis was not by intention to treat and the power of the trial was low. The second RCT of 200 eyelids in Oman compared bilamellar tarsal rotation versus tarsal advance and rotation.[15] It found that tarsal rotation significantly increased operative success after 25 months (relative risk (RR) for failure, tarsal advance and rotation *v* tarsal rotation 3·1, 95% CI 1·9–5·2).

Location of surgery

One RCT compared village-based versus health centre-based tarsal rotation surgery for major trichiasis.[16] It found that attendance rates were not significantly different between interventions (57/86 (66%) *v* 32/72 (44%); RR 1·5, 95% CI not provided). The RCT also found that there was no significant difference between interventions in operative success rate (defined as no evidence of trichiasis) after three months.

Harms

Adverse outcomes of interventions were corneal exposure, ulceration, phthisis bulbi and severe recurrent trichiasis.[14] In the two RCTs that compared different surgical techniques versus each other, major trichiasis and defective closure after surgical procedures for scarring trachoma were more common after eversion splinting, tarsal advance, and tarsal grooving than after bilamellar tarsal rotation and tarsal advance and rotation.[14,15] Cryoablation of the eyelashes can cause necrosis of the lid margin, corneal ulcers, and in the RCT in which cryoablation was used it was the only procedure associated with onset of phthisis bulbi (two cases out of 57).

Implications for practice

Face washing is beneficial for intense trachoma if used in conjunction with topical antibiotics. Fly spraying reduces the incidence of active trachoma. No conclusions can be drawn on the effectiveness of antibiotic treatment for active trachoma, although there is a suggestion of a reduction in the point prevalence of the relative risk for those treated with antibiotics. The bilamellar tarsal rotation procedure is the surgical procedure least associated with recurrence.

Implications for research

The WHO Global Elimination of Blinding Trachoma programme has endorsed the donation of azithromycin for the treatment of trachoma in selected countries. This provides the setting for determining whether antibiotics are an effective treatment and whether they have a place in the surgical treatment of entropion/trichiasis.

References

1. Thylefors B, Negrel AD, Pararajasegaram R *et al.* Global data on blindness. *Bull World Health Organ* 1995;**73**:115–21.
2. West SK, Munoz B, Turner VM, Mmbaga BB, Taylor HR. The epidemiology of trachoma in central Tanzania. *Int J Epidemiol* 1991;**20**:1088–92.
3. Courtright P, Sheppard J, Schachter J, Said ME, Dawson CR. Trachoma and blindness in the Nile Delta: current patterns and projections for the future in the rural Egyptian population. *Br J Ophthalmol* 1989;**73**:536–40.

4. Bobo L, Munoz B, Viscidi R, Quinn T, Mkocha H, West S. Diagnosis of *Chlamydia trachomatis* eye infection in Tanzania by polymerase chain reaction/enzyme immunoassay. *Lancet* 1991;**338**:847–50.

5. Bailey R, Osmond C, Mabey DC, Whittle HC, Ward ME. Analysis of the household pattern of trachoma in a Gambian village using a Monte Carlo simulation procedure. *Int J Epidemiol* 1989;**18**:944–51.

6. Emerson PM, Cairncross S, Bailey RL, Mabey DC. Review of the evidence base for the "F" and "E" components of the SAFE strategy for trachoma control. *Trop Med Int Health* 2000;**5**:515–27.

7. Munoz B, West SK. The forgotten cause of blindness. *Epidemiol Rev* 1997;**19**:205–17.

8. Pruss A, Mariotti SP. Preventing trachoma through environmental sanitation: a review of the evidence base. *Bull World Health Organ* 2000;**78**:258–66.

9. Peach H, Piper S, Devanesen D *et al.* Trial of antibiotic drops for the prevention of trachoma in school-age Aboriginal children. *Annu Rep Menzies Sch Health Res* 1986:74–6.

10. West S, Munoz B, Lynch M *et al.* Impact of face washing on trachoma in Kongwa, Tanzania. *Lancet* 1995;**345**:155–8.

11. Emerson PM, Lindsay SW, Walraven GE *et al.* Effect of fly control on trachoma and diarrhoea. *Lancet* 1999;**353**:1401–3.

12. Mabey D, Fraser-Hurt N. Antibiotics for trachoma (Cochrane Review). In : The Cochrane Collaboration: *Cochrane Library.* Issue 1. Oxford: Update Software, 2002.

13. Bailey RL, Arullendran P, Whittle HC, Mabey DC. Randomised controlled trial of single-dose azithromycin in treatment of trachoma. *Lancet* 1993;**342**:453–6.

14. Reacher MH, Huber MJ, Canagaratnam R, Alghassany A. A trial of surgery for trichiasis of the upper lid from trachoma. *Br J Ophthalmol* 1990;**74**:109–13.

15. Reacher MH, Munoz B, Alghassany A *et al.* A controlled trial of surgery for trachomatous trichiasis of the upper lid. *Arch Ophthalmol* 1992;**110**:667–74.

16. Bowman RJ, Soma OS, Alexander N *et al.* Should trichiasis surgery be offered in the village? A community randomised trial of village *v.* health centre-based surgery. *Trop Med Int Health* 2000;**5**:528–33.

21 Corneal abrasion and recurrent erosion

David F Anderson

Background

Definitions

Corneal abrasion comprises a defect in the corneal epithelial surface with or without breach of Bowman's layer and implies that no substantial loss of stromal tissue has occurred. If, subsequently, microtrauma, insufficient to separate a healthy epithelium from the basement membrane, results in a corneal epithelial defect, the diagnosis of recurrent corneal erosion (RCE) is made.

Incidence

The incidence of hospital presentation of traumatic corneal abrasion (TCA) has been recorded in 11–12·9% of new presentations to eye accident and emergency units.[1] Some 36% of patients at initial hospital presentation with RCE had a history of trauma and epithelial microcysts, 23% were patients with anterior basement membrane dystrophy alone and 7% had anterior basement membrane dystrophy and a history of trauma.[2]

Aetiology

Recurrent corneal erosion syndrome arises when abnormal adhesion between basal corneal epithelial cells and their basement membrane allows microtrauma at the ocular surface to cause detachment of the regenerating epithelial sheets. Corneal abrasion and RCE are associated with superficial corneal trauma, anterior basement membrane dystrophy (ABMD) or a combination of both.[2] Traumatic cases may lead to RCE in otherwise normal eyes or in those with an underlying defect of the epithelial basement membrane or its deposition.[2]

Natural history

Studies have measured healing times in one of two ways: either the time to closure of the epithelial defect in days or the rate of healing over a defined period of time (usually 24 hours). Those studies that measured time to defect closure for the largest defects (those larger than 4/mm²) from TCA reported a maximal healing time of 4·2 ± 0·5 days (mean ± SD) independent of treatment employed. Patients presenting with RCE were more likely to have suffered trauma than ABMD or ABMD and a history of trauma[2] and lesions of the lower half of the cornea were more frequent than those in the upper half ($P < 0.0001$).[2] In the three studies evaluated[2,4,5] all patients received treatment or patient numbers were too small to determine the recurrence rate without treatment.

Question

Does padding the eye make a difference to the rate of healing of the epithelial defect in TCA?

The evidence

Padding the eye is based upon the assumption that preventing upper eyelid excursion over regenerating corneal epithelium during blinking allows the formation of adhesion complexes to proceed in the absence of shearing forces and accelerates epithelial healing.

Five prospective RCTs investigated the time to closure of the epithelial defect, or rate of healing of an epithelial defect, over a 24-hour period secondary to a TCA[1,3,6–8] (Table 21.1).

Kaiser *et al.*[3] randomised the largest series of 223 patients (22 exclusions) with TCA secondary to direct corneal trauma (n = 120) or removal of superficial corneal foreign body (n = 81, 40% of total) to receive antibiotic ointment and cycloplegia with (Group I) or without (Group II) pressure pad. Follow up was daily. There was no statistical difference on presentation between the two groups in patient age and gender, time to presentation or abrasion size. In both aetiology groups of TCA larger abrasions (larger than 4/mm² in area) took longer to heal than smaller abrasions, but those patients who were not padded demonstrated significantly faster healing ($P < 0.05$). Thirteen per cent of patients in the padded group had removed their pad by 24-hour follow up, and all patients on the no pad group completed treatment (analysis performed on an

Table 21.1 Trial outcomes and characteristics

Authors	No. randomised	Intervention/ groups	Antibiotic/ cycoplegia	Inclusion criteria	Exclusion criteria	Principal outcome measure	Results	Significance
Öhman and Fagerholm, 1998[5]	56	• I PTK + manual debridement • II Manual debridement	Yes/No	RCE >3/12 of symptoms	Corneal dystrophy	• RCE recurrence rate • Visual acuity • Refraction	• Lower recurrence in group I • No significant difference • No significant difference	$P<0\cdot005$ $P=$ not stated $P=$ not stated
Kirkpatrick et al., 1993[8]	44	• I Pad • II No pad	Yes/Yes	1st episode of TCA	Foreign body	• Closure of epithelial defect • Pain	• Faster in group II • No significant difference	$P=0\cdot04$ $P=$ not stated
Kaiser et al., 1995[3]	223	• I Pad • II No pad	Yes/Yes	TCA Foreign body	Corneal dystrophy	• Rate of healing • Pain at 24 hours	• Faster in group II for foreign body and TCA • Less pain in group II	$P<0\cdot05$ $P<0\cdot01$
Patterson et al., 1996[9]	50	• I Pad • II No pad	Yes/No	TCA	–	• Pain at 24 hours	• Pre- and post-treatment scores lower in group I	$P=$ not stated
Acheson et al., 1987[7]	28	• I Pad • II BCL	Yes/Yes	TCA >4/mm²	–	• Pain at 24 hours • Closure of defect	• Less in group II • Faster in group II	$P<0\cdot05$ $P<0\cdot05$
Campanile et al., 1997[7]	74	• I Pad • II No pad	Yes/Yes	TCA Foreign body	–	• Closure of defect	• Faster in group II at 24 hours	$P=0\cdot02$
Arbour et al., 1997[6]	48	• I Pad • II No pad	Yes/Yes	TCA RCE >1/mm²	Foreign body	• Closure of defect • Pain • Insomnia	• No difference • No difference • No difference	$P=$ not stated $P=$ not stated $P=$ not stated
Hope-Ross et al. 1994[4]	30	• I Lubricants • II Oral tetracycline	NA	RCE	–	• Recurrence • Healing rate • Symptoms	• Lowest in groups II and III • Fastest in groups II and III • Lowest in groups II and III	$P=0\cdot04$ $P=0\cdot0003$ $P=0\cdot001$ $P=0\cdot001$ $P=0\cdot005$

(Continued)

Table 21.1 *(Continued)*

Authors	No. randomised	Intervention/ groups	Antibiotic/ cycoplegia	Inclusion criteria	Exclusion criteria	Principal outcome measure	Results	Significance
		• III Oral tetracycline + topical prednisolone						
Jayamanne et al., 1997[10]	40	• I Diclofenac 0·1% • II Placebo	Yes/No	TCA	RCE Corneal dystrophy Previous corneal disease	• Pain	• Lowest in group I	*P*<0·002
Szucs et al., 2000[11]	49	• I Diclofenac 0·1% • II Placebo	Yes/Yes	TCA	Pain <30% of visual analogue scale	• Pain 2 hours after treatment	• Lowest in group I	*P*=0·002

PTK, phototherapeutic keratectomy; RCE, recurrent corneal enosion; TCA, traumatic corneal abrasion

intention to treat basis), exhibiting better compliance with the treatment.

To measure precisely the rate of closure of the epithelial defect following corneal erosion, Arbour et al.[6] studied the digitised images of slit lamp photographs of healing erosions taken daily and analysed using image analysis software. Two groups of patients were compared: group I underwent double eye patching (n = 25), whilst group II were not patched (n = 22). All patients were treated with topical cycloplegia and antibiotic and were prescribed oral analgesia. To avoid pathology arising at the level of Bowman's layer, cases of foreign body removal were specifically excluded. No statistically significant difference was found between groups for the rate of closure of epithelial defect measured either by reduction in total area with time, or reduction over time of the radius of the largest circle included in the defect (linear speed of re-epithelialisation). The trial had 92% power to detect a 6-hour delay of epithelial closure between the two groups and 95% power to detect a 12-hour delay. The authors concluded that patching a corneal erosion did not significantly accelerate re-epithelialisation.

Campanile et al.[7] compared the rate of healing of TCA in patients who were padded compared with those who were not. Of 74 patients who met the inclusion criteria, 64 were evaluated. The abrasion was measured at the slit lamp and transposed to a calibrated grid sheet from which the area was calculated. All patients were treated with topical antibiotic and cycloplegia. There was no statistical difference in the mean size of the abrasion before treatment but at 24-hour follow up the defects were significantly smaller ($P = 0.028$) in the non-patched group. All epithelial defects were completely closed by 72 hours.

Forty-four patients with a first episode of TCA were randomised by Kirkpatrick et al.[8] into two groups treated by chloramphenicol ointment and cycloplegia with (group I) or without (group II) a double eye pad and bandage. Closure of the epithelial defect was significantly faster in group II ($P = 0.04$). By the end of the 24-hour follow up period, however, 49% of eye bandages were no longer in place, 29% were reported as having fallen off whilst the patient was asleep and 20% had been removed due to discomfort. The number of patients failing to attend follow up was similar between groups although follow up varied from two to seven months.

The effectiveness of a bandage soft contact lens (BCL) in the primary treatment of TCA of large surface area (>4/mm^2) was investigated by Acheson et al. in 1987.[1] Patients with abrasions from all causes were randomised to two treatment groups: occlusive pad and bandage (group I) or standard size BCL (group II). Both groups were treated with topical antibiotic and cycloplegics. Time to epithelial healing was measured by daily follow up and was significantly faster in

group II ($P < 0.05$). All epithelial defects had closed by four days.

Comment

These studies concluded that padding the eye either made no difference to the rate of healing or that treatment with topical antibiotic and cycloplegia alone or BCL led to statistically faster healing of the defect. Potential sources of bias in these studies included compliance, size of defect and use of topical medication. Compliance tended to be higher in the no-pad groups and the number of non-compliant patients, i.e. those who removed the pad early, were particularly high in Kirkpatrick et al.'s study.[8] Although in the BCL treatment arm of Acheson et al.'s study[1] only one patient failed to re-attend for six days, the loss to follow up of a patient with a TCA and a BCL in situ might be of particular concern in view of the risk of infectious keratitis.

Those studies that examined larger defects[3,6,7] reported that these defects took longer to heal but found no delay in healing rate in those patients who were not padded. Although padding the eye would have resulted in those patients being unable to instil topical medication that might have had an effect on healing rate, all patients in the studies reported were treated with topical antibiotic and cycloplegia at presentation and seen 24 hours later.

Evidence suggests that padding may decrease corneal oxygenation and tear clearance rate, increase the epithelial exposure time to infective and toxic products and increase corneal temperature, all of which would favour bacterial growth. Padding the eye also precludes binocular vision, which may lead to secondary morbidity.

Question

Which treatment modalities are the most effective in reducing the pain and discomfort of TCA?

The evidence

Symptoms of TCA were assessed by seven RCTs examining the effects of pad compared with no pad (n = 4),[3,6,8,9] pad compared with BCL (n = 1)[1] and treatment with topical diclofenac 0·1% compared with placebo (n = 2).[10,11]

In Kaiser et al.'s study of 223 patients (22 exclusions) with TCA secondary to direct corneal trauma or removal of superficial corneal foreign body, patients in the no-pad treatment arms reported significantly less pain at 24 hours ($P < 0.01$) as well as a greater difference in pain score at 24-hour follow up compared with presentation ($P < 0.05$) for both aetiologies.[3] Patients were questioned about their level of pain, which was then assessed on a scale of 0 to 10.

Although patients were allowed oral analgesia, the use of these was not monitored by the investigators.

The use of prescribed oral analgesia was recorded by Arbour et al.[6] and pain was measured using a visual analogue scale (VAS; uncalibrated 100 mm line) in their study of 48 patients with symptoms from TCA or RCE randomised to undergo pad or no pad following topical antibiotic and cycloplegia. This study also recorded insomnia quantified as a difference between the number of hours actually versus usually slept. No statistical difference between groups was noted for mean or maximal pain score, hours of insomnia or use of prescribed analgesia.

Pain measured at 24-hour follow up compared with pain at presentation was selected as the main outcome measure in 33 patients randomised by Patterson et al.[9] to treatment with topical antibiotic with (group I) or without (group II) a pressure pad. The change in mean pain score at 24-hour follow up was not significantly different between the padded and non-padded groups although absolute pain scores measured on a VAS were higher pre- and post-treatment in the non-padded group, suggesting possible selection bias. Patient selection was not consecutive and with the sample size and difference in starting pain scores the power of the study to detect a real difference between groups may have been limited.

Kirkpatrick et al.'s[8] study of the outcomes of patients treated for TCA by chloramphenicol ointment and cycloplegia with or without a double eye pad and bandage showed no statistically significant difference between the two groups for difference in pain scores. The pain score was a secondary outcome measure of the trial and was measured using a VAS. As before, the relatively high rate of non-compliance with treatment in the padded group may well have masked any true treatment effect.

Acheson et al.[1] investigated the pain experienced by patients with TCA of large surface area (>4/mm^2). Patients were treated with topical antibiotic and cycloplegics and randomised to receive an occlusive pad and bandage (group I) or standard size BCL (group II). Pain as assessed by VAS was recorded as a percentage of that experienced at presentation and was significantly less at follow up in group II ($P<0.05$).

Jayamanne et al.[10] explored the effectiveness of topical diclofenac 0·1% compared with placebo on pain arising from TCA. Forty patients were randomised to receive topical diclofenac 0·1% (n = 20) (group I) or normal saline (placebo) (n = 20) four times daily (group II). No specific instructions regarding the use of oral analgesics were given, no cycloplegics or eye pads were used and all patients were followed up on a daily basis until re-epithelialisation was complete. Pain was assessed in three ways: using a VAS comprising an uncalibrated 100 mm-long horizontal line, using a categorical quantitative pain scale, for example, mild, moderate, severe and using a categorical qualitative pain scale, for example, foreign body-like, headache-like. At time of presentation there was no statistically significant difference in pain, but by day one the VAS and categorical pain scores were significantly lower in group I ($P<0.002$, $P <0.02$, respectively) using distribution-free analysis (Wilcoxon rank sum test).

The safety and efficacy of diclofenac sodium 0·1% in the treatment of TCA was also assessed by Szucs et al.[11] Forty-nine patients were treated with topical antibiotic and cycloplegia and topical diclofenac 0·1% four times daily (group I) or control four times daily (Group II) for 24 to 36 hours, and no eye pad was used. Pain was measured by VAS comprising a calibrated 100 mm-long horizontal line, but the size of the abrasion was not measured. The primary outcome measure was improvement of pain two hours after first treatment, which was assessed by structured telephone call promoting the patient to mark the VAS in their possession and record any rescue oral analgesia they had been prescribed. The two-hour pain score was significantly better in group I, 3·1 (95% CI 2·3–4·0, $P= 0.002$) compared with group II, 1·0 (95% CI 0·1–2·0, $P= 0.002$). Twenty per cent (95% CI 4–36%) of patients in group I took oral analgesia compared with 42% (95% CI 22–62%) of controls, although this difference did not achieve statistical significance.

Comment

The use of an eye pad did not significantly reduce pain or insomnia due to TCA,[3,6,8,9] in fact in the largest study, patients reported greater pain when padded.[3] The use of a BCL for large TCA[1] was associated with significantly less pain compared with using an eye pad. Treatment with topical diclofenac 0·1% led to significantly less pain reported when compared with placebo.[10,11]

Question
Does excimer laser treatment influence the rate of recurrence of RCE?

The evidence

Öhman et al.[5] randomised 56 patients with RCE to undergo excimer laser phototherapeutic keratectomy (PTK) ablation following manual epithelial debridement (group I) or epithelial debridement alone (group II). A Summit ExciMed was used to perform a 6·5 mm central maximal diameter ablation of 5 μm unless the debridement area was large or eccentric when additional zones were treated. Patients were followed up for 12 months. Trauma was an associated condition in 46% of cases of both groups. The

Table 21.2 Performance and quality of trials

Author/s	Performance bias: masked?	Attrition bias: follow up	CI quoted	Placebo controlled	Intention to treat analysis
Öhman and Fargerholm, 1998[5]	Non-masked	Not stated	No	No	No
Kirkpatrick et al., 1993[8]	Non-masked	16% did not complete, similar between groups	No	No	No
Kaiser et al., 1995[3]	Non-masked	13% of padded patients removed pad	Standard deviation	No	No
Patterson et al., 1996[9]	Non-masked Non-consecutive	34% did not complete, similar between groups	No	No	No
Acheson et al., 1987[1]	Non-masked	7% in BCL and 21% in pad group did not complete	Standard deviation and standard error of mean	No	Yes
Campanile et al., 1997[7]	Masked	9·4% removed pad, 9·0% DNC in no pad group	No	No	No
Arbour et al., 1997[6]	Non-masked	2% (1 patient) did not complete: group not stated	Mean + standard deviation 95% power to detect 12-hr difference	No	No
Hope-Ross et al., 1997[4]	Non-masked	3·3% (1 patient) discontinued tetracycline	No	No	Yes
Jayamanne et al., 1997[10]	Masked	All completed	No	Yes	N/A
Szucs et al., 2000[11]	Masked	All completed	Yes	Yes	N/A

BCL, bandage soft contact lens; RCE, recurrent corneal erosion; TCA, traumatic corneal abrasion; DNC, did not complete

RCE recurrence rate was significantly lower in group I (P <0·005). There was no statistical difference between groups for any other outcome measure. No patients treated by PTK who experienced RCE (7%) required retreatment.

Comment

Five studies investigated the rate of healing and seven outcomes of different treatments on the pain experienced by patients with TCA and RCE. Only one study of padding compared with no pad was single-masked (investigator), indicating that performance bias might have been an influencing factor in comparing outcomes within the populations studied (Table 21.2). Of the three studies examining the effects of pharmacological intervention, two of topical diclofenac 0·1% and one of oral tetracycline, only the topical diclofenac 0·1% studies were double-masked.

No study showed that padding the eye following a TCA arising from primary trauma or from removal of a corneal foreign body accelerated healing or reduced pain. Three RCTs found that healing was significantly faster in the no-pad group and three that pain at follow up was significantly lower in the no-pad group. This evidence would suggest that the primary management of TCA should not include padding the eye in addition to topical antibiotics and cycloplegics. Interestingly, when the effect of upper lid excursion was eliminated by the use of a BCL, both pain and healing at 24 hours was significantly faster and compliance with wearing the lens better than wearing a pad. Those RCTs that examined the effect of topical diclofenac 0·1% both concluded that the pain associated with TCA was significantly lower both two hours[11] and 24 and 48 hours after presentation.[10] Only one study recorded the use of rescue oral analgesia,[9] which might have been a significant factor in pain modulation in the other trials.

Accurate measurement of healing rate (by grid drawing[7] or computer image analysis software[6]) is important since in all studies the maximal time to closure of the defect was five days, with the majority closed by 48 hours. The natural history of TCA is of particular relevance to healthcare economists when more expensive treatments such as fitting a BCL are advocated.

Implications for practice

No trial suggested that application of a pressure pad, or pad and bandage, quickened epithelial healing or reduced the pain or discomfort of TCA. Treatment by topical cycloplegia and antibiotic alone led to healing rates that were at least as fast or significantly faster and levels of pain at follow up that were equivalent or significantly lower than additional padding. Use of a BCL was associated with significantly less pain and faster epithelial healing from large ($>4/mm^2$) abrasions compared to padding, whilst patients treated with topical diclofenac 0·1% reported significantly less pain both two and 24 hours after TCA.

A significantly lower recurrence rate for RCE was observed in patients treated by excimer laser in addition to manual epithelial debridement, with more than 90% of patients recurrence-free for 12 months following treatment. The use of oral tetracycline for three months was also associated with a lower recurrence rate of RCE and faster epithelial closure. This effect was observed whether or not patients were treated with topical prednisolone 0·5% for seven days.

Implications for research

Further work is clearly needed to determine the true natural history of RCE and to determine if treatments other that excimer laser may reduce recurrence rates below that obtained with topical lubricant treatment alone. Specifically, a trial comparing BCL and topical medication to topical medication alone is needed in TCA.

References

1. Acheson JF, Joseph J, Spalton DJ. Use of soft contact lenses in an eye casualty department for the primary treatment of traumatic corneal abrasions. *Br J Ophthalmol* 1987;**71**:285–9.
2. Hykin PG, Foss AE, Pavesio C, Dart JKG. The natural history and management of recurrent corneal erosion: A prospective randomised trial. *Eye* 1994;**8**:35–40.
3. Kaiser PK, the corneal abrasion patching study group. A comparison of pressure patching versus no patching for corneal abrasions due to trauma or foreign body removal. *Ophthalmology* 1995;**102**:1936–42.
4. Hope-Ross MW, Chell PB, Kervick GN, McDonnell PJ, Jones HS. Oral tetracycline in the treatment of recurrent corneal erosions. *Eye* 1994;**8**:384–8.
5. Öhman L, Fagerholm P. The influence of excimer laser ablation on recurrent corneal erosions: A prospective randomized study. *Cornea* 1998;**17**:349–52.
6. Arbour JD, Brunette I, Boisjoly HM, Shi ZH, Dumas J, Guertin MC. Should we patch corneal erosions? *Arch Ophthalmol* 1997;**115**:313–17.
7. Campanile TM, St Clair DA, Benaim M. The evaluation of eye patching in the treatment of traumatic corneal epithelial defects. *J Emerg Med* 1997;**15**:769–74.
8. Kirkpatrick JNP, Hoh HB, Cook SD. No eye pad for corneal abrasion. *Eye* 1993;**7**:468–71.
9. Patterson J, Fetzer D, Krall J, Wright E, Heller M. Eye patch treatment for the pain of corneal abrasion. *Southern Med J* 1996;**89**:227–9.
10. Jayamanne DGR, Fitt AWD, Andrews RM, Mitchell KW, Griffiths PG. The effectiveness of topical diclofenac in relieving discomfort following traumatic corneal abrasions. *Eye* 1997;**11**:79–83.
11. Szucs PA, Nashed AH, Allegra JR, Eskin B. Safety and efficacy of diclofenac ophthalmic solution in the treatment of corneal abrasions. *Ann Emerg Med* 2000;**35**:131–7.

22 Herpes simplex keratitis

Alonso Rodriguez

Background

Herpetic keratitis is an important public health issue with deep social and economic repercussions. In the United States alone, herpes simplex virus (HSV) eye disease affects approximately 400 000 to 500 000 people, with an estimated 48 000 episodes of active HSV eye disease annually.[1,2]

HSV has been identified as the single most frequent cause of corneal opacities in developed countries.[3] Each episode can bring inflammation, structural damage and corneal scarring that eventually leads to opacities of the cornea and blindness. It is a leading cause for corneal grafting.[4] The survival rate for corneal grafts performed for HSV keratitis ranges from 14% to 61%.[5,6]

Treatment options

Over the past three decades, much has been written about the treatment and prophylaxis of herpes simplex virus ocular infection. Unfortunately, much of this has been based on clinical impression or uncontrolled, potentially biased trials. Even if the conclusions from these reports are valid, they cannot be accepted as proven evidence unless confirmed by randomised controlled trials that provide solid scientific backing to the conclusions derived.

> ## Question
>
> In patients with dendritic, epithelial herpetic keratitis, which antivirals have been shown to be the most effective?

The evidence

The earliest trials comparing different antiviral agents showed that trifluorothymidine (F_3T, trifluridine) was more effective than idoxuridine (IDU) in the treatment of dendritic and amoeboid (geographic) ulcers ($P<0.005$).[7] Other authors showed that F_3T was more effective than traditional debridement, but that debridement combined with F_3T was not superior to F_3T alone,[8] and that topical adenine arabinoside

(Ara-A, vidarabine) was equally effective in treating dendritic herpetic ulcers when compared to topical F_3T.[9]

At the end of the 1970s, a new drug, aciclovir (ACV), was introduced for the treatment of herpetic disease. This drug, in theory, would be more selective against infected cells and therefore less toxic to the corneal epithelium.[10] The first controlled trials proved that topical ACV was an effective antiviral agent for treating ulcerative herpetic keratitis, and that it was at least as active as Ara-A, IDU, or F_3T[11–25] (Tables 22.1 and 22.2). A recent systematic review of controlled clinical trials concluded that currently available and investigational antiviral agents (excluding IDU) are all effective and nearly equivalent.[29] One study,[23] however, also found a significantly lower rate of superficial punctuate epitheliopathy with ACV when compared to IDU ($P = 0.0096$). Others have shown that ACV produces a significantly more rapid healing rate when combined with minimal debridement than ACV alone ($P <0.025$),[30] although this has not been corroborated by others.[31]

A double-blind RCT of 60 patients showed topical ACV to be superior to IDU in healing times and rates in dendritic corneal ulceration[26,27] (Tables 22.1 and 22.2). A later trial also demonstrated that oral ACV (400 mg five times a day) is as effective as locally applied aciclovir (3% ophthalmic ointment five times a day) in the management of herpes simplex dendritic corneal ulceration, and thus oral medication appears to be an acceptable alternative for patients unable or unwilling to use local treatment for their disease.[32] In many countries, however, the higher cost of oral medication remains an important issue in selecting the antiviral of choice.

The search continues for newer, more effective antiviral agents that are better tolerated. Recently, ganciclovir has been introduced for the treatment of herpes simplex keratitis. Ganciclovir is an antiviral agent, structurally related to aciclovir, with an antiviral broad spectrum of activity, which includes cytomegalovirus, Epstein-Barr virus, adenovirus, herpes zoster and herpes simplex. A recent report of two RCTs comparing ACV ointment with ganciclovir gel for the treatment of dendritic and geographic ulceration[32] showed ganciclovir gel 0·05% and 0·15% to have equal efficacy to topical ACV in the treatment of

Table 22.1 Comparison of combined healing rate for herpes simplex epithelial keratitis in reported results

Report	Sample size (n)	No. of patients with geographic ulcers	% Combined healing rate					P
			Aciclovir 3% ointment	Adenine arabinoside 3% ointment	Idoxuridine 0·5% ointment	Trifluoro-thymidine 2% ointment	Ganciclovir gel	
McGill et al.[11]	57	0	100	97	–	–	–	>0·05
Pavan-Langston et al.[12]	41	5	95	90	–	–	–	>0·05
Yeakley et al.[13]	40	1	100	95	–	–	–	ns
Laibson et al.[14]	73	5	97	92	–	–	–	ns
Denis et al.[15]	23	NA	93	78	–	–	–	0·33
Jackson et al.[16]	66	7	97	88	–	–	–	>0·05
Genée and Maith[17]	28		78	57	–	–	–	ns
Coster et al.[18]	60	6	100	–	100 (1% ointment)	–	–	>0·05
Colin et al.[19]	52	NA	92	–	88	–	–	0·5
La Lau et al.[20,21]	59	0	87	–	–	82	–	ns
Høvding[22]	50	0	92	–	–	96	–	ns
McCulley et al.[23]	64	12	83·3	–	85·3	–	–	ns
Young et al.[24,25]	93	8	94	84				NA
Collum et al.[26,27]	60	0	100		76	–	–	<0·01
Colin et al.[28] Trial 1	67	6	72	–	–	–	0·05% gel: 81 0·15% gel: 85	0·66
Colin et al.[32] Trial 2	37	1	71	–	–	–	0·15% gel: 83	0·44

ns, not statistically significant; NA, value not available from data in the report

ulcerative herpes simplex keratitis (Tables 22.1 and 22.2). Additionally, they found local tolerance to be significantly superior with ganciclovir, with fewer complaints of discomfort (stinging, burning) or blurred vision after application (trial 1: $P = 0·05$, trial 2: $P = 0·045$). Another report also failed to find any statistically significant difference in rate of healing of herpes simplex dendritic keratitis, treated with either ACV 3% ointment, or ganciclovir 0·15% gel.[33] Other antivirals will probably find their place in the current treatment arsenal. Valaciclovir, a pro-drug of aciclovir, appears promising although long-term studies of efficacy are still lacking.

Comment

Aciclovir has become the standard treatment for herpetic ulcerative keratitis throughout the world. Topically, it has been proven to be at least as effective as Ara-A or F_3T, as well as being better tolerated. In cases where the patient is not able to use topical preparations, oral ACV is an equivalent option. New drugs such as ganciclovir have been shown to be as efficient as ACV although few randomised trials comparing their results are available.

Question

Is there evidence supporting the use of aciclovir, or any other antiviral, in treating the geographic form of epithelial herpetic ulceration?

The evidence

There is less written in the literature about the treatment of geographic or amoeboid ulcers when compared to the more common dendritic ulceration, and few trials have studied this form of keratitis as a separate entity. Treatment of geographic ulcers has been more difficult, perhaps because of the frequent association of steroid use prior to the start of antivirals, and thus success in the treatment of these lesions would seem a more sensitive therapeutic test to differentiate the effect of different antivirals that prove to be highly active in treating less challenging dendritic ulcers. In several reports, results in treating geographic ulcers were extracted from larger series treating dendritic ulcers, and included small numbers of patients from which a statistically significant conclusion could not be determined.

Table 22.2 Comparison of time to heal (days) for herpes simplex epithelial keratitis in reported results

Report	Sample size (n)	No. of patients with geographic ulcers	Aciclovir 3% ointment	Adenine arabinoside 3% ointment	Idoxuridine 0·5% ointment	Trifluoro-thymidine 2% ointment	Ganciclovir gel	P
				Time to heal (days)				
McGill et al.[11]	57	0	4.5	6.2	–	–	–	>0·05
Pavan-Langston et al.[12]	41	5	3·8	5·2	–	–	–	>0·05
Yeakley et al.[13]	40	1	4·42	4·45	–	–	–	ns
Laibson et al.[14]	73	5	3·9	5·0	–	–	–	ns
Denis et al.[15]	23	NA	7·4	5·9	–	–	–	ns (Students t = 1·85)
Jackson et al.[16]	66	7	6·26	7·07	–	–	–	>0·05
Genée and Maith[17]	28	NA	6·5	8·0	–	–	–	ns
Coster et al.[18]	60	6	NA	–	NA (1% ointment)	–	–	>0·05
Colin et al.[19]	52	NA	7·5	–	9·0	–	–	<0·05
La Lau et al.[20,21]	59	0	6·3	–	–	7·0	–	ns
Høvding[22]	50	0	6·7	–	–	5·9	–	ns
McCulley et al.[23]	64	12	5·9	–	7·2	–	–	ns
Young et al.[24,25]	93	8	6·7	9·2	–	–	–	<0·01
Collum et al.[26,27]	60	0	4·4	–	9·2	–	–	<0·01
Colin et al.[28] Trial 1	67	6	10	–	–	–	0·05% gel: 7 0·15% gel: 7	0·31
Colin et al.[28] Trial 2	37	1	7	–	–	–	0·15% gel: 6	0·056

ns, not statistically significant; NA, value not available from data in the report

A RCT that included 30 patients found topical F_3T to be more effective than Ara-A in dealing with amoeboid ulcers (logrank $P = 0·05$).[34] A more recent trial treated 51 patients in a dual-centre, double-blind comparison of topical ACV and Ara-A in geographic ulcers[35] and found both drugs to be effective and of equal potency in the management of geographic herpetic ulcerations.

Comment

Since few trials have addressed the treatment of geographic ulcers independently, more trials are warranted in order to establish if ACV, or any other antiviral agent, is preferable for treating these patients.

Question

In patients with stromal herpetic keratitis, what evidence is there for combining corticosteroids with antivirals for treatment, and does the use of steroids carry a higher rate of recurrence?

The evidence

It is believed that stromal keratitis, particularly the disciform variety, is largely an immunological condition.[36] With this presumption, antiviral treatment should be more effective if combined with steroids. An early trial showed that aciclovir combined with steroids is more effective than ACV alone, and that ACV without concomitant use of steroids does not provide effective control of disciform keratitis.[37] This randomised trial of 40 patients, however, included patients who were using topical steroids prior to randomisation, and thus was potentially biased by selecting patients with steroid dependent keratitis. The same authors performed a similar trial, but in 30 patients who never had used steroids in the past.[38] Even in these patients, a combination of aciclovir and steroids proved to be superior to ACV alone in the treatment of disciform keratitis. Using the Mantel Cox test, patients receiving ACV and steroids were shown to heal significantly more quickly than those receiving ACV alone, suggesting that it is necessary to use corticosteroids to promote healing in disciform keratitis.

Additionally, this study found no significant statistical differences in recurrence rates when comparing patients who had and had not received steroids.

The effect of topical steroids has been recently addressed by a multi-centre RCT, the Herpetic Eye Disease Study (HEDS). A randomised, double masked, placebo controlled clinical trial was designed, in which patients with active herpes simplex stromal keratitis who had not received any corticosteroids for at least 10 days before enrolment were treated with topical F_3T and either topical prednisolone or placebo over 10 weeks.[39] The planned sample size was 178 patients. However, enrolment was stopped at 106 patients, after the primary objective, determination of the time to treatment failure, was satisfied, and a statistically significant difference in the primary outcome between the treatment groups had been established. The median time to treatment failure was 98 days for the steroid group (95% CI, 81 to > 120 days) and 17 days for the placebo group (95% CI, 14–27 days). This difference proved to be highly significant in favour of the steroid group ($P < 0.001$). The time from randomisation to resolution of active herpes keratitis was also significantly shorter for the steroid group (steroid group: median, 26 days; 95% CI, 14–49 days; placebo group: median, 72 days; 95% CI, 44–123 days, $P < 0.001$). Additionally, there was no statistically significant difference in recurrence rates between the two treatment groups ($P = 0.9$).

Other RCTs have addressed the results of using different antivirals. A trial involving 30 patients, all with dilute betamethasone, reported that there is no significant difference either in the time to heal or rate of healing between ACV and Ara-A when combined with corticosteroids in treatment of disciform keratitis. However, they found a significantly lower rate of superficial punctuate keratopathy with ACV ($P = 0.02$), suggesting ACV is a more appropriate drug because of its low toxicity.[40]

A randomised trial of 39 patients published in 1990 compared topical and systemic aciclovir in the management of herpetic disciform keratitis, in patients receiving topical prednisolone 0.05%.[41] No statistically significant difference was demonstrated in resolution times for the clinical signs studied, or in time required for complete healing. Additionally, no difference was found in recurrence rates over a three-year follow-up. The authors concluded that oral ACV treatment is an effective alternative to ophthalmic ointment in the management of herpetic disciform keratitis.

The benefits of using oral ACV in herpes simplex stromal keratitis have recently been studied by the HEDS. In a randomised, double masked, placebo controlled trial of 104 patients, either oral ACV (400 mg five times daily) or placebo was used, along with a standard regimen of topical prednisolone and F_3T to treat patients with active HSV stromal keratitis, without concomitant epithelial keratitis,

treated with steroids.[42] Sample size was chosen so that a 5%, one-tailed test would have an 80% chance of detecting a doubling of the median time to treatment failure. This study found no statistically significant difference overall in time to treatment failure between the aciclovir treated group and the placebo treated group ($P = 0.46$). Oral ACV did not significantly delay the time to treatment failure, decrease the proportion of patients who failed treatment, increase the proportion of patients whose keratitis resolved, decrease the time to resolution, or increase best corrected visual acuity. Thus, oral ACV given in addition to standard treatment (topical antiviral and steroid) provided additional benefits of such a small magnitude that no statistical and clinical significance could be determined.

Comment

It can be concluded that the treatment of stromal herpetic keratitis should involve an antiviral agent as well as a steroid, and the usefulness of ACV, either topical or oral, has already been determined. Studies have proven the importance of steroids in promoting healing, and their safety in terms of recurrences. Combining topical plus oral antivirals, however, does not provide an additional level of protection.

Question

What evidence is there for the use of prophylactic aciclovir to prevent recurrent herpes simplex keratitis?

The evidence

In 1967, a randomised controlled trial that studied the effect of IDU or placebo and their ability to prevent dendritic keratitis recurrence in patients receiving steroids, established the importance of topical antivirals in reducing the rate of recurrence of HSV epithelial keratitis during corticosteroid treatment of HSV disciform keratitis.[43] In 1978, a similar trial demonstrated the importance of topical antivirals (F_3T) in reducing the rate of recurrence of HSV epithelial keratitis during steroid treatment of HSV keratouveitis.[44] A recent study of the risk factors for HSV epithelial keratitis recurrence during treatment of stromal keratitis or iridocyclitis[45] recruited 260 patients who were all receiving topical F_3T for active stromal keratitis and/or iridocyclitis without epithelial keratitis. Patients were examined for HSV epithelial keratitis during 16 weeks and were enrolled in one of three parallel trials. One trial compared the effects of a 10-week course of topical placebo with a tapering dosage of topical steroids. Another compared a 10-week course of oral ACV with oral placebo in patients receiving topical prednisolone phosphate (and F_3T) for stromal keratitis, and the third trial compared oral ACV with oral placebo in patients receiving topical prednisolone phosphate for iridocyclitis. In all these trials, patients were also receiving topical F_3T. Overall, epithelial keratitis developed in 4·6% of the patients, and no statistically significant differences in the occurrence of HSV epithelial keratitis between any of the groups were found. Thus, adding oral ACV to a standard topical antiviral treatment with F_3T did not provide additional benefits, nor did steroids provide additional risks when under antiviral treatment.

The Herpetic Eye Disease Study (HEDS) has recently addressed the subject of efficacy of oral ACV prophylaxis in preventing stromal keratitis or iritis in patients with HSV epithelial keratitis treated with a topical antiviral agent.[46] This prospective, randomised, double masked, placebo-controlled study enrolled patients with active epithelial keratitis who were treated with topical F_3T or Ara-A and were randomised to a three-week course of oral ACV, 400 mg five times a day or placebo, and were followed up for one year. Although the sample size needed was calculated at 502 patients, recruitment was stopped at 287, because of lack of evidence of benefit in the group that had been treated with oral ACV. The cumulative probability of developing stromal keratitis or iritis for the 12 month follow-up period (after stopping topical or oral antivirals) was 12% in the ACV group and 11% in the placebo group; the comparison of Kaplan–Meier curves by the log-rank test showed no statistically significant difference ($P = 0·92$). There was no evidence of a beneficial effect of the treatment in any group based on whether epithelial keratitis, stromal keratitis, or iritis had occurred in the past or based on the duration of symptoms of epithelial keratitis at the time of trial enrolment. However, the development of stromal keratitis or iritis was more common in patients with a history of HSV eye disease before the episode of epithelial keratitis ($P = 0·01$).

Another problem ophthalmologists face when treating herpes keratitis is recurrences in patients who will be receiving topical steroids for prolonged periods, such as in steroid dependent stromal keratitis or in patients who have had a penetrating keratoplasty (PK). A recent RCT reported for the first time the effect of postoperative oral ACV on the survival of corneal grafts.[4,47] This compared the risk of recurrence in 14 eyes that underwent PK and received postoperative aciclovir (800–1000 mg/day for 12–15 months) with nine eyes that underwent PK but did not receive ACV. Both groups received topical prednisolone 1% four times daily after surgery, tapered over three months. With a follow up of 16·5 months, they showed that postoperative oral ACV significantly reduces the risk of HSK recurrence following PK (rate of recurrence: 0% in the ACV group, and 44% in the control group, $P < 0·05$ by x^2).

Comment

The evidence shows that adding oral antivirals to a standard treatment that includes topical antivirals does not provide additional protection from HSV recurrences, whether epithelial or stromal. Nevertheless, recurrences are more frequent in patients with a history of prior herpetic episodes, and it seems logical to target prophylaxis at these high risk groups. In patients who have undergone corneal grafts, aciclovir prophylaxis has proven to be important in preventing recurrences. Since few randomised controlled studies have tackled this issue, it is still to be determined how long this prophylactic treatment needs to be in order to provide long lasting protection.

Implications for practice

Aciclovir has an established role in the treatment of HSV keratitis, whether in its topical or oral form. Its efficacy has been proven against "first generation" drugs (IDU, Ara-A, F_3T). Newer drugs surely will continue to be developed, such as ganciclovir, and these will need to be compared with ACV not only in terms of their clinical effectiveness in dendritic, disciform, and other types of keratitis, but also for their tolerance and toxicity. In stromal keratitis, the combination of an antiviral agent such as aciclovir with a topical steroid has been shown to be both safe and effective.

Implications for research

In spite of these results, there are many issues that still need to be addressed with regard to HSV keratitis treatment and prophylaxis. Most trials have focused on epithelial dendritic keratitis and stromal disciform keratitis. There are few reports that have been directed at studying the treatment of geographic corneal ulcers, and no randomised trial has been performed to study the effect of oral antivirals on necrotising stromal keratitis, although data extracted from broader trials appear to be promising.[41] Another issue that must be studied more carefully is that of drug induced toxicity, particularly when one is about to give prophylactic treatment for extended periods. Few trials have provided substantial evidence about drug related toxicity with the use of various topical antivirals. Some ancillary information has been gathered from larger series that have studied other variables, but to date, no randomised trial has focused entirely on toxicity.

The dosage and duration of treatment required for prophylactic antiviral medication has so far been determined empirically. Although recent reports back the need for prophylactic medication, no trial has addressed the optimal dosage, frequency and duration of treatment. Future trials will probably help define the optimal protocols for prophylactic treatment.

References

1. National Institutes of Health. Workshop on the treatment and prevention of herpes simplex virus infections. *J Infect Dis* 1973;**127**: 117–19.

2. Liesang TJ, Melton LJ, Daly PJ, Ilstrup DM. Epidemiology of ocular herpes simplex: incidence in Rochester, Minn, 1950 through 1982. *Arch Ophthalmol* 1989;**107**:1155–9.

3. Dawson CR, Togni B. Herpes simplex eye infections: clinical manifestations, pathogenesis and management. *Surv Ophthalmol* 1976; **21**:121–35.

4. Foster CS, Barney NP. Systemic acyclovir and penetrating keratoplasty for herpes simplex keratitis. *Doc Ophthalmol* 1992; **80**:363–9.

5. Langston RHS, Pavan-Langston D, Dohlman CH. Penetrating keratoplasty for herpetic keratitis – prognosis and therapeutic determinants. *Trans Am Acad Ophthalmol Otol* 1975;**79**:577.

6. Foster CS, Duncan J. Penetrating keratoplasty for herpes simplex keratitis. *Am J Ophthalmol* 1981;**92**:336.

7. Wellings PC, Awdry PN, Bors FH, Jones BR, Brown DC, Kaufman HE. Clinical evaluation of trifluorothymidine in the treatment of herpes simplex corneal ulcers. *Am J Ophthalmol* 1972;**73**:932–42.

8. Parlato CJ, Cohen EJ, Sakauye CM, Dreizen NG, Galentine PG, Laibson PR. Role of debridement and trifluridine (trifluorothymidine) in herpes simplex dendritic keratitis. *Arch Ophthalmol* 1985;**103**: 673–5.

9. Coster DJ, McKinnon JR, McGill JI, Jones BR, Fraunfelder FT. Clinical evaluation of adenine arabinoside and trifluorothymidine in the treatment of corneal ulcers caused by herpes simplex virus. *J Infect Dis* 1976;**133**(Suppl):A173–7.

10. Jones BR, Coster DJ, Fison PN, Thompson GM, Cobo LM, Falcon MG. Efficacy of acycloguanosine (Wellcome 248u) against herpes simplex corneal ulcers. *Lancet* 1979;**1**:243–4.

11. McGill J, Tormey P, Walker CB. Comparative trial of acyclovir and adenine arabinoside in the treatment of herpes simplex corneal ulcers. *Br J Ophthalmol* 1981;**65**:610–13.

12. Pavan Langston D, Lass J, Hettinger M, Udell I. Acyclovir and vidarabine in the treatment of ulcerative herpes simplex keratitis. *Am J Ophthalmol* 1981;**92**:829–35.

13. Yeakley WR, Laibson PR, Michelson MA, Arentsen JJ. A double-controlled evaluation of acyclovir and vidarabine for the treatment of herpes simplex epithelial keratitis. *Trans Am Ophthalmol Soc* 1981;**79**:168–9.

14. Laibson PR, Pavan Langston D, Yeakley WR, Lass J. Acyclovir and vidarabine for the treatment of herpes simplex keratitis. *Am J Med* 1982;**73**:281–5.

15. Denis J, Thenault Giono S, Ray Cohen ML, Tournoux A, Pouliquen Y. Traitement de l'herpes oculaire en double insu: vira A et acyclovir. *Bull Soc Ophtalmol Fr* 1983;**83**:25–9.

16. Jackson WB, Breslin CW, Lorenzetti DW, Michaud R, Dube I. Treatment of herpes simplex keratitis: comparison of acyclovir and vidarabine. *Can J Ophthalmol* 1984;**19**:107–11.

17. Genée E, Maith J. Wirksamkeitsvergleich von acyclovir und vidarabine bei oberflächlichen herpeskeratitiden. *Klin Monatsblatter Augenheilkunde* 1987;**191**:30–3.

18. Coster DJ, Wilhelmus KR, Michaud R, Jones BR. A comparison of acyclovir and idoxuridine as treatment for ulcerative herpetic keratitis. *Br J Ophthalmol* 1980;**64**:763–5.

19. Colin J, Tournoux A, Chastel C, Renard G. Keratite herpetique superficielle. Traitement comparatif en double insu par acyclovir et idoxuridine. *Nouv Presse Med* 1981;**10**:2969–70.

20. La Lau C, Oosterhuis JA, Versteeg J *et al*. Multicenter trial of acyclovir and trifluorothymidine in herpetic keratitis. *Am J Med* 1982;**73**:305–6.

21. La Lau C, Oosterhuis JA, Versteeg J *et al*. Acyclovir and trifluorothymidine in herpetic keratitis: A multicentre trial. *Br J Ophthalmol* 1982;**66**:506–8.

22. Høvding G. A comparison between acyclovir and trifluorothymidine ophthalmic ointment in the treatment of epithelial dendritic keratitis. A double blind, randomised parallel group trial. *Acta Ophthalmol* 1989;**67**:51–4.

23. McCulley JP, Binder PS, Kaufman HE, O'Day DM, Poirier RH. A double-blind, multicenter clinical trial of acyclovir v idoxuridine for treatment of epithelial herpes simplex keratitis. *Ophthalmol* 1982;**89**:1195–200.

24. Young BJ, Patterson A, Ravenscroft T. A randomised double blind clinical trial of acyclovir (Zovirax) and adenine arabinoside in herpes simplex corneal ulceration. *Br J Ophthalmol* 1982;**66**: 361–3.

25. Young BJ, Patterson A, Ravenscroft T. Double-blind clinical trial of acyclovir and adenine arabinoside in herpetic corneal ulceration. *Am J Med* 1982;**73**:311–12.

26. Collum LM, Benedict-Smith A, Hillary IB. Randomised double-blind trial of acyclovir and idoxuridine in dendritic corneal ulceration. *Br J Ophthalmol* 1980;**64**:766–9.

27. Collum LM, Logan P, Hillary IB, Ravenscroft T. Acyclovir in herpes keratitis. *Am J Med* 1982;**73**:290–3.

28. Colin J, Hoh HB, Easty DL *et al*. Ganciclovir ophthalmic gel (Virgan;0·15%) in the treatment of herpes simplex keratitis. *Cornea* 1997;**16**:393–9.

29. Wilhelmus KR. Interventions for herpes simplex virus epithelial keratitis. In: Cochrane Collaboration. *Cochrane Library*. Issue 4. Oxford: Update Software, 2002.

30. Wilhelmus KR, Coster DJ, Jones BR. Acyclovir and debridement in the treatment of ulcerative herpetic keratitis. *Am J Ophthalmol* 1981;**91**:323–7.

31. Jensen KB, Nissen SH, Jessen F. Acyclovir in the treatment of herpetic keratitis. *Acta Ophthalmol* 1982;**60**:557–63.

32. Collum LM, McGettrick P, Akhtar J, Lavin J, Rees PJ. Oral acyclovir (Zovirax) in herpes simplex dendritic corneal ulceration. *Br J Ophthalmol* 1986;**70**:435–8.

33. Hoh HB, Hurley C, Claoue C *et al*. Randomised trial of ganciclovir and acyclovir in the treatment of herpes simplex dendritic keratitis: a multicentre study. *Br J Ophthalmol* 1996;**80**:140–3.

34. Coster DJ, Jones BR, McGill JI. Treatment of amoeboid herpetic ulcers with adenine arabinoside or trifluorothymidine. *Br J Ophthalmol* 1979;**63**:418–21.

35. Collum LM, Logan P, McAuliffe Curtin D, Hung SO, Patterson A, Rees PJ. Randomised double-blind trial of acyclovir (Zovirax) and adenine arabinoside in herpes simplex amoeboid corneal ulceration. *Br J Ophthalmol* 1985;**69**:847–50.

36. Pepose JS. Herpes simplex keratitis: role of viral infection versus immune response. *Surv Ophthal* 1991;**35**:345–52.

37. Collum LM, Logan P, Ravenscroft T. Acyclovir (Zovirax) in herpetic disciform keratitis. *Br J Ophthalmol* 1983;**67**:115–18.

38. Collum LM, Power WJ, Collum A. The current management of herpetic eye disease. *Doc Ophthalmol* 1992;**80**:201–5.

39. Wilhelmus KR, Gee L, Hauck WW *et al*. Herpetic Eye Disease Study. A controlled trial of topical corticosteroids for herpes simplex stromal keratitis. *Ophthalmol* 1994;**101**:1883–95.

40. Collum LM, Grant DM. A double blind comparative trial of acyclovir and adenine arabinoside in combination with dilute betamethasone in the management of herpetic disciform keratitis. *Curr Eye Res* 1987;**6**:221–4.

41. Porter SM, Patterson A, Kho P. A comparison of local and systemic acyclovir in the management of herpetic disciform keratitis. *Br J Ophthalmol* 1990;**74**:283–5.

42. Barron BA, Gee L, Hauck WW *et al*. Herpetic Eye Disease Study. A controlled trial of oral acyclovir for herpes simplex stromal keratitis. *Ophthalmol* 1994;**101**:1871–82.

43. Patterson A, Jones BR. The management of ocular herpes. *Trans Ophthalmol Soc UK* 1967;**87**:59–84.

44. Sundmacher R. Tryfluorothymidinprophylaxe bei der Steroidtherapie herpetischer keratouveitiden. *Klin Monatsblatter Augenheilkunde* 1978;**173**:516–19.

45. Wilhelmus KR, Dawson CR, Barron BA *et al.* Risk factors for herpes simplex virus epithelial keratitis recurring during treatment of stromal keratitis or iridocyclitis. Herpetic Eye Disease Study Group. *Br J Ophthalmol* 1996;**80**:969–72.
46. Herpetic Eye Disease Study Group. A controlled trial of oral acyclovir for the prevention of stromal keratitis or iritis in patients with herpes simplex virus epithelial keratitis. The Epithelial Keratitis Trial. *Arch Ophthalmol* 1997;**115**:703–12.
47. Barney NP, Foster CS. A prospective randomized trial of oral acyclovir after penetrating keratoplasty for herpes simplex keratitis. *Cornea* 1994;**13**:232–6.

23 Suppurative keratitis

Stephanie L Watson

Background

Definition

Suppurative keratitis (SK) is a severe infection of the cornea characterised by focal polymorphonuclear leucocytic infiltration, typically with surrounding inflammatory cells, oedema and an overlying epithelial defect.[1] It is usually caused by bacteria or fungi, and rarely by amoebic or viral infection.

Incidence

The incidence of SK is not accurately known.[1] Incidence rates for bacterial keratitis (BK), and microbial keratitis (MK), include ulcerative keratitis as well as SK. In the developing world, MK is responsible for at least 1·5 million new cases of unilateral blindness every year.[2] It is a rare cause of blindness in the developed world but has significant associated morbidity.[3,4] Worldwide the estimated incidence of BK is approximately 2 per 100 000 population.[1] The pattern of SK depends on geographic, environmental and climatic factors.[4,5] In the UK, bacteria account for over 90% of SK in cool northern climates[6,7] and 60% in hot southern climates.[8,9] In tropical climates, fungi are responsible for up to 50% of cases and are usually filamentous.[10–15]

Aetiology

Suppurative keratitis occurs when the ocular defence mechanisms are disrupted.[4] This may be caused by contact lens wear, corneal trauma or surgery, post-herpetic corneal disease, corneal anaesthesia, exposure, keratoconjunctivitis sicca, or ocular surface disease.[1,16–18] Contact lens wear is the greatest risk factor for bacterial and amoebic keratitis in developed countries.[16,19] Contact lens wearers are exposed to increased numbers of microbes, via bacterial biofilms on contact lens cases,[20,21] and have reduced resistance to infection, due to corneal hypoxia and trauma.[22,23] In developing countries, corneal trauma, particularly agricultural injury, is the commonest risk factor.[24,25] In Africa, fungal keratitis has been associated with HIV infection.[26]

Prognosis

Suppurative keratitis may result in corneal scarring and opacity leading to severe visual disability.[4,17,27] Progression of SK can cause corneal perforation, scleritis, endophthalmitis, panophthalmitis, loss of the eye and even potentially fatal cavernous sinus thrombosis.[28,29] This is typically rapid in untreated *Psuedomonas* keratitis[30] and slower with fungal keratitis.[31] Prompt diagnosis and treatment can improve the prognosis.[16]

Question

In patients with bacterial SK what is the best topical antibiotic therapy?

The evidence

Nine papers report eight randomised controlled clinical trials[18,27,32–37] that investigated antibiotic therapy in bacterial keratitis. A further trial[38] examined whether hyaluronate improves the efficacy of fortified antibiotics by prolonging drug contact time via increased viscosity.[39] The details of each trial are summarised in Table 23.1. Four trials[18,27,33,34] were of sufficient quality. Two trials[32,37] were not double-masked. Four trials[32,35,37,38] were not large enough, particularly for subgroup analysis. Patients with BK are a diverse group, therefore subgroup analysis is usually required. Significance levels were not provided by all studies. There were no placebo controlled trials.

The inclusion criterion for the trials was patients with BK. Two studies[27,33] randomised patients with clinical BK but only analysed a subset of patients who were culture positive.[40] One study[38] excluded 10 patients with significant amounts of the same bacteria in both eyes. Four studies[32,35,37,38] included moderate ulcers to remove the bias associated with having different sized ulcers. Two studies[18,27] only included those with a best-corrected visual acuity of 20/200 or better in the involved eye. Exclusion criteria were microbiological evidence of fungal keratitis, patients with only one eye, pregnant women, patients with diabetes and allergy to study medications. One study also excluded an unknown number of patients who stopped taking the study medication. They did not state which medication was stopped or the reason for discontinuation.

Results

One small and four large RCTs of sufficient quality found that there was little difference in efficacy between fluoroquinolone monotherapy and combination fortified antibiotic therapy in achieving healing (cure) or resolution of BK. One study reported significantly greater toxicity[34] and two studies[27,33] found significantly more discomfort with fortified antibiotics. In clinically identified cases of BK positive culture rates were around 50%; staphylococci were most commonly isolated. Fluoroquinolone (ciprofloxacin or ofloxacin) monotherapy can replace fortified antibiotic therapy in the management of moderate bacterial keratitis. Trials should continue to determine the most frequent organisms and their sensitivities.

Comment

The inclusion criteria for some trials was clinically suspected BK, while other trials required microbiological confirmation of BK but this has only moderate sensitivity, such that cases may be excluded. Clinical criteria may allow more cases of BK to be included, however, all non-bacterial cases may not be excluded. Corneal swabs and conjunctival scrapings are less reliable than corneal scrapes. Most of the trials used different study medications or a different concentration of the same medication preventing direct comparison of the results. Further, the single centre studies may only be applicable to patients in a similar setting, as SK varies with geographic location and climate. The main outcome measure was epithelial healing; this may not reflect the rate of bacterial killing. Several studies also included clinical features in their outcome measures. One study identified possible confounders, such as a greater number of cases with *Pseudomonas* in the fortified antibiotic group than the ciprofloxacin group, but did not adjust for them.

Question

In patients with bacterial SK what is the role of topical steroids when used with topical antibiotic therapy?

The evidence

We found one prospective, randomised, controlled clinical trial of 40 patients in which topical antibiotics alone

(n = 19) were compared to topical antibiotics and steroids (n = 21).[41] This RCT was unmasked (patients and investigators) and small. Patients with central or paracentral bacterial corneal ulcers severe enough to warrant hospital admission were included. All patients had a corneal scrape for microscopy and culture. Patients with fungal isolates, perforated ulcers or descemetocoeles, underlying viral keratitis, atopic ulcers, no light perception vision, or aged less than 13 years were excluded. Prior to analysis of the healing rate six out of 21 in the steroid group and eight out of 19 in the non-steroid group were excluded due to a persistent epithelial defect, uncontrolled infection or the requirement for other therapy.

Results

There was no statistical difference in the final VAs for the two groups, though both had a statistically significant improvement in VA ($P < 0.001$ for the steroids group and $P < 0.01$ for the non-steroid group, paired analysis by t test). The mean healing rate was not significantly different, 0.36 mm^2/day for the steroid group and 0.30 mm^2/day for non-steroid group (Student's t test, no P values given). There were eight complications in the steroid group and 10 in the non-steroid group (no P values given).

Comment

The single RCT conducted was not of sufficient quality to confirm or exclude important clinical effects of steroid drops in bacterial keratitis. The results may not be applicable to patients at other centres, as the inclusion criterion was BK "severe enough to warrant hospital admission" and this will vary between different centres. The trial was too small to confirm or exclude important clinical effects of steroid drops in bacterial keratitis. Important sources of error in this trial were selection bias, observer bias, measurement bias and confounding in the analysis of healing rates. Limited evidence suggested that topical steroids added to topical antibiotic regimens for BK might not delay healing nor increase complications. Further RCTs should be conducted to investigate topical steroid therapy in BK.

A single RCT found significantly faster healing when hyaluronate was added to topical antibiotics. This trial was too small and not of sufficient quality to allow hyaluronate to be recommended for clinical use in MK. Hyaluronate cannot be routinely recommended for use in MK until further RCTs are conducted.

Table 23.1 Clinical trials of antibiotic therapy in bacterial keratitis

Clinical trial	Location	Population	Inclusion criteria	Interventions	Primary outcome	Secondary outcome	Secondary outcome	Secondary outcome	Secondary outcome	Microbiology	Side effects
Reddy, 1988[32]	SD Eye Hospital, Hyperabad, India	82	Clinical	Group 1: framycetin 0·5% n = NI Group 2: chloramphenicol 0·4% n = NI Group 3: gentamicin 0·3% n = NI, Group 4: neomycin 1700 units, gramicidin 0·0025%, polymixin B sulphate 5000 units n = NI	Good to very good clinical response: framycetin 91% gentamicin 77% chloramphenicol 56% neomycin 61% (no P values given). A response occurred earlier in framycetin group					Most frequent isolates: Staphylococcus, Pneumococcus, Streptococcus, Psuedomonas. More isolates sensitive to framycetin	None reported
Gandolfi et al, 1992[38]	Istituto di Oftamologia, Parma, Italy	26	Conjunctival scrapings	Tobramycin 1·5% in saline* n = 13 Tobramycin 1·5% in sodium Hyaluronate n = 13	Time to healing: saline 5·9 ± 1·5 days v hyaluronate 3·5 ± 0·9 days (P<0·001)					Most frequent isolates: S. aureus S. epidermidis P. aeruginosa	None reported
O'Brien et al, 1995[27]	28 centres in the USA	248	Clinical	Ofloxacin 0·3% (2 bottles) n = 73 Fortified cefazolin 10·0% and Tobramycin 1·5% n = 67	Portion healed: ofloxacin 7 days: 37% 28 days: 89% v fortified therapy 7 days: 38% 28 days: 86% (P=0·70)	Resolution of infiltrate at day 28: ofloxacin 83% v fortified therapy 82% (P=0·49)	Biomicroscopic findings (6 signs graded): no significant difference between the 2 groups (P=0·41)	Patient symptoms: burning and stinging was less in the ofloxacin group (P<0·001)		Positive cultures in 140/248 (56%) Most frequent isolates: Staphylococcus sp, S. aureus	Treatment discontinued due to lack of efficacy by 3 patients (2 ofloxacin) and due to side effects by 6 patients (5 fortified therapy)

(Continued)

Table 23.1 (Continued)

Clinical trial	Location	Population	Inclusion criteria	Interventions	Primary outcome	Secondary outcome	Secondary outcome	Secondary outcome	Microbiology	Side effects
Hyndiuk et al., 1996[33]	28 centres in the USA, Europe, and India	324	Clinical	Ciprofloxacin 0·3% (2 bottles) n = 160 (82 analysed), Fortified cefazolin 5·0% and tobramycin 1·33% n = 164 (94 analysed)	Overall clinical efficacy (physician judgement): ciprofloxacin 91·5% v fortified therapy 86·2% (P=0·34).	Resolution of clinical signs and symptoms (P>0·08) and the time to cure (P=0·55) were similar	Treatment failures: ciprofloxacin 8·5% v fortified therapy 13·8%		Most frequent isolates: S. epidermidis, P. aeruginosa, S. aureus Coagulase negative staphylococcus	Ciprofloxacin group reported less discomfort (P=0·01)
The ofloxacin study group, 1997[34]	Moorfields Eye Hospital, London and Manchester Royal Eye Hospital, UK	122	Clinical	Ofloxacin 0·3% and saline (placebo) n = 59 Fortified cefuroxime 5·0% and gentamcin 1·5% n = 59	Proportion cured at 14 days: ofloxacin 62·1% v fortified therapy 67·9% ratio, 1·09; 95% CI, 0·83–1·43; P=0·52	Proportion cured at 7 days: ofloxacin 52·5% versus fortified therapy 57·6% [ratio, 1·10; (95% CI, 0·79–1·52); P=0·58]			Positive cultures in 49/122 (40%) Most frequent isolates: S. aureus P. aeruginosa coagulase negative staphylococcus	Toxicity; Ofloxacin 10·2% v fortified therapy 50·8% (ratio, 5·00; 95% CI, 2·25–11·11; P<0·0001)
Panda et al, 1999[35] Khokkar 2000[36]	Dr R Prasad Centre for Ophthalmic Services, New Delhi, India	30	Microbiological	Ofloxacin 0·3% and saline (placebo) n = 15 Fortified cefazolin 10% and tobramycin 1·5% n = 15	Ulcer resolution: ofloxacin 93% v fortified therapy 87% (no P values given)	Time to healing: ofloxacin 15·0 ± 3·86 days v fortified therapy 15·46 ± 3·86 days (P=0·46)	Time to symptom relief: ofloxacin 7·8 ± 1·54 days v fortified therapy 8·33 ± 1·54 days (P=0·05)	Subjective improvement in VA: BCVA of ≥ 20/200 in all except for one eye	Most frequent isolates: Staphylococcus aureus, Coagulase negative Staphylococci	None reported
Kosrirukvongs and Buranapongs, 2000[37]	Siriraj Hospital, Bangkok, Thailand	41	Clinical	Ciprofloxacin 0·3% n = 17 Fortified cefazolin 5% and	Treatment efficacy (signs and symptoms graded):	Time to healing: ciprofloxacin 15·6 ± 8·6 days	VA improvement in success cases: ciprofloxacin		Gram stain and/or positive cultures in 21/41 (51·2%),	White crystalline precipitate noted in

(Continued)

Table 23.1 (Continued)

Clinical trial	Location	Population	Inclusion criteria	Interventions	Primary Outcome	Secondary outcome	Secondary outcome	Secondary outcome	Microbiology	Side effects
				gentamicin 1·4% n = 24	ciprofloxacin 70·6% v fortified therapy 62.5% (P=0·839)	v fortified therapy 14·6 ± 5·8 days (P=0·726)	66·7% v fortified therapy 62·5% (P=0·516)		Most frequent isolates: P. aeruginosa, S. aureus, S. pneumoniae	17·6% of ciprofloxacin group.
Venkatesh Prajna et al., 2001[18]	Aravind Eye Hospital, Madurai, India	217	Microbiological	Ofloxacin 0·3% n = 112 Ciprofloxacin 0·3% n = 105	Time to healing: Ofloxacin 13.7 days v ciprofloxacin 14·4 days (P=0·80).	Proportion healed: Ofloxacin 85% v Ciprofloxacin 77% (P=0·32)	Biomicroscopic findings: similar in the 2 groups		Most common isolates: S. pneumoniae P. aeruginosa	Burning and stinging most frequent. No treatment was discontinued due to side effects. White crystalline precipitate in 20% of ciprofloxacin group

NI, not indicated
*the saline contained preservatives.

Table 23.2 Clinical trials of antifungals in fungal keratits

Clinical trial	Study population (n)	Location	Inclusion and exclusion criteria	Interventions	Outcome measure 1	Outcome measure 2	Microbiology	Side effects
Rahman et al., 1997[24]	60	Aravind Eye Hospital, Madurai, India	Patients with suppurative keratitis who had fungal elements identified on microscopy and confirmed on culture. Excluded patients with only one eye or diabetes, children under 1 year, perforated corneas, polymicrobial infections, and those unwilling to participate or unable to attend for follow up. Also excluded 12 patients with severe ulcers, as they would have a poor prognosis with natamycin therapy, and two patients lost to follow up	Three concentrations of topical chlorhexidine gluconate (0·05%, 0·1% and 0·2% in aqueous solution) v natamycin 5%	Favourable response at day 5; Natamycin v chlorhexidine concentrations: 0·05% RE 1·17 ($P > 0·1$) 0·1% RE 1·43 ($P > 0·1$) 0·2% RE 2·00 ($P = 0·051$). Patients with no prior antifungal treatment 0·2% RE 2·20 ($P = 0·043$)	Cure at day 21; Natamycin versus Chlorhexidine concentrations: 0·2% RE 1·67 ($P > 0·1$). 0·05%, 0·1% less efficacous than 0·2%		None reported.
Rao et al., 1997[42]	8	Medical Research Foundation, Sankara Nethralaya, Chennai, India	Patients with fungal keratitis. Exclusion criteria not stated	Topical natamycin 5% v topical fluconazole 0·2% and oral fluconazole 100 mg bd	Natamycin 3/4 healed; average time 19·7 days; one deteriorated requiring a PK v		Filamentous fungi in all cases	

Table 23.2 (Continued)

Clinical trial	Study population (n)	Location	Inclusion and exclusion criteria	Interventions	Outcome measure 1	Outcome measure 2	Microbiology	Side effects
					Fluconazole 0/4 healed; average time 8 days. (On switching to natamycin, 2 resolved and 2 required PK)			
Rahman et al., 1998[31]	71	Chittagong Eye Institute and Training Complex, Bangladesh	Patients with suppurative keratitis who had fungal elements identified on microscopy and confirmed on culture. Excluded patients with only one eye or diabetes, children under 1 year, perforated corneas, polymicrobial infections, and those unwilling to participate or unable to attend for follow up	Topical chlorhexidine gluconate 0·02% v natamycin 2·5%	Favourable response at day 5; chlorhexidine group 31/35 (88·6% efficacy) 2 ulcers healed v natamycin group 18/35 (51·4% efficacy; RE 1·7; 95% CI 1·24–2·63; $P<0·001$; for severe ulcers the RE was 7·33)	Cure at 21 days; Non-severe ulcers: chlorhexidine group 66·7% healed v natamycin group 36% healed (RE 1·85; CI 1·01–3·39; $P=0·04$). Severe ulcers: None healed (3 healed by day 60 in chlorhexidine group)	Aspergillus (22) Fusarium (22)	Temporary punctate epithelial keratopathy in one chlorhexidine patient, who may have received topical treatment more frequently than prescribed

* RE = relative efficacy

Evidence-based Ophthalmology

Question

In patients with fungal SK what is the best topical antifungal therapy?

The evidence

We found three prospective, randomised controlled clinical trials on the treatment of fungal keratitis in developing countries[24,31,42] (Table 23.2). One trial enrolled only eight participants and was discontinued after interim analysis revealed an extremely poor clinical response to fluconazole.[42] It was not stated whether this trial was masked. Of the two remaining trials, one was masked and in the other the clinical staff could not be masked due to the different appearance of the medications. One trial was too small, particularly for subgroup analysis, and did not adequately control for confounders.[24] The two trials used different concentrations of natamycin, preventing a direct comparison of the results. These trials were conducted in tropical settings in the developing world such that their results are not transferable to other clinical settings.

Results

The two large RCTs supported the use of chlorhexidine for the treatment of filamentous fungal keratitis when specific antifungal therapy is not available.[24,31] One small RCT suggested that topical and oral fluconazole might not be the agent of choice for treatment of fungal keratitis in India, possibly due to the predominance of filamentous fungi.[42]

Comment

Available RCTs are not of sufficient quality to determine the most appropriate antifungal therapy for use in developing countries where the availability of antifungals is limited. RCTs are needed to establish the most appropriate antifungal therapy in a variety of clinical settings. Until the results of such trials are available therapy should be based on microbiological findings[25] and local epidemiological data of fungal type and sensitivity. Limited evidence suggests that chlorhexidine may be used instead of natamycin in tropical settings where the availability of antifungals is limited.

Implications for practice

Patients with SK are a diverse group with different risk factors and infecting organisms. Antibiotic monotherapy can replace combination therapy in bacterial SK.

Implications for research

Further RCTs are needed to address the role of steroids in BK and to determine the best antifungal therapy in a variety of settings. The quality of future clinical studies would be improved by a faster and more reliable method for diagnosis of SK, such as polymerase chain reaction. Larger studies, particularly multi-centre trials, would allow valid subgroup analysis and ensure that study results are more widely applicable. At the same time, trials should continue to gather local data for monitoring and the selection of the appropriate therapy.

References

1. Wilhelmus KR. Bacterial keratitis. In: Pepose JS, Holland GN, Wilhelmus KR, eds. *Ocular Infection and Immunity.* St Louis: Mosby, 1996, pp. 973–81.
2. Whitcher JP, Srinivasan M, Upadhyay MP. Prevention of corneal ulceration in the developing world. *Int Ophthalmol Clin* 2002;**42**:71–7.
3. Dart JKG, Seal DV. The pathogenesis and therapy of *Pseudomonas aeruginosa* keratitis. *Eye* 1988;**2**(Suppl):S46–55.
4. Schaefer F, Bruttin O, Zografos L, Guex-Crosier Y. Bacterial keratitis: a prospective clinical and microbiological study. *Br J Ophthalmol* 2001;**85**:842–7.
5. Houang E, Lam D, Fan D, Seal D. Microbial keratitis in Hong Kong: relationship to climate, environment and contact-lens disinfection. *Trans Royal Soc Trop Med Hygiene* 2001;**95**:361–7.
6. Asbell P, Stenson S. Ulcerative keratitis. Survey of 30 years' laboratory experience. *Arch Ophthalmol* 1982;**100**:77–80.
7. Coster DJ. Inflammatory disease of the outer eye. *Trans Ophthalmol Soc UK* 1979;**99**:463–80.
8. Liesegang TJ, Forster RK. Spectrum of microbial keratitis in South Florida. *Am J Ophthalmol* 1980;**90**:38–47.
9. Katz NNK, Wadud SA, Ayazuddin M. Corneal ulcer disease in Bangladesh. *Ann Ophthalmol* 1983;**15**:834–6.
10. Rahman MM. Management of fungal corneal ulcer. *Trans Ophthalmol Soc Bangladesh* 1981;**9**:12–19.
11. Williams G, Billson F, Husain R, Howlader SA, Islam N, McClellan K. Microbiological diagnosis of suppurative keratitis in Bangladesh. *Br J Ophthalmol* 1987;**71**:315–21.
12. Dunlop AAS, Wright ED, Howlander SA *et al.* Suppurative corneal infection in Bangladesh: a study of 142 cases examining the microbiological diagnosis, clinical and epidemiology features of bacterial and fungal keratitis. *Aust NZ J Ophthalmol* 1994;**22**:105–10.
13. Willams G, McClellan K, Bilson F. Suppurative keratitis in rural Bangladesh; the value of gram stain in planning management. *Int Ophthalmol* 1991;**15**:131–5.
14. Hagan M, Wright E, Newman M, Dolin P, Johnson G. Causes of suppurative keratitis in Ghana. *Br J Ophthalmol* 1995;**79**:1024–8.
15. Yee RW, Kosrirukvongs P, Meenakshi S, Tabbara KF. Fungal keratitis. In: Tabbara KF, Hyndiuk RA, eds. *Infections of the Eye, 2nd edn.* Little, Brown and Company, 1995.
16. Dart JKG, Stapleton F, Minassian D. Contact lenses and other risk factors in microbial keratitis. *Lancet* 1991;**338**:650–3.
17. Diamond JP, White L, Leeming JP, Bing Hoh H, Easty DL. Topical 0·3% ciprofloxacin, norfloxacin and ofloxacin in treatment of bacterial keratitis: a new method for comparative evaluation of ocular drug penetration. *Br J Ophthalmol* 1995;**79**:606–609.
18. Venkatesh Prajna N, George C, Selvaraj S, Lu KL, McDonnell PJ, Srinivasan M. Bacteriologic and clinical efficacy of ofloxacin 0·3% versus ciprofloxacin 0·3% ophthalmic solutions in the treatment of patients with culture-positive bacterial keratitis. *Cornea* 2001;**20**:175–8.

19. Duguid IGM, Dart JK, Morlet N *et al.* Outcome of Acanthamoeba keratitis treated with polyhexamethyl biguanide and propamidine. *Ophthalmology* 1997;**104**:1587–92.
20. Elder MJ, Stapleton F, Evans E, Dart JKG. Biofilm-related infections in ophthalmology. *Eye* 1995;**9**:102–9.
21. Stapleton F, Dart J. Psuedomonas keratitis associated with biofilm formation on a disposable soft contact lens. *Br J Ophthalmol* 1995;**79**:864–5.
22. Dart JKG. Contact lens and prosthesis infections. In: Jaeger E, Tasman W, eds. *Duane's Foundations of Clinical Ophthalmology Vol 2.* Philadelphia: Lippincott-Raven, 1996.
23. Liesegang TJ. Contact lens-related microbial keratitis: Part I: Epidemiology. *Cornea* 1997;**16**:125–31.
24. Rahman MR, Minassian D, Srinivasan M, Martin MJ, Johnson GJ. Trial of chlorhexidine gluconate for fungal corneal ulcers. *Ophthalmic Epidemiol* 1997;**4**:141–9.
25. O'Day DM. Fungal keratitis. In: Pepose JS, Holland GN, Wilhelmus KR, eds. *Ocular Infection and Immunity.* St Louis: Mosby, 1996, p. 1048.
26. Mselle J. Fungal keratitis as an indicator of HIV infection in Africa. *Trop Doct* 1999;**29**:133–5.
27. O'Brien TP, Maguire MG, Fink NE, Alfonso E, McDonnell P and the Bacterial Keratitis Study Research Group. Efficacy of ofloxacin *v* cefazolin and tobramycin in the therapy for bacterial keratitis. *Arch Ophthalmol* 1995;**113**:1257–65.
28. Brenner M. Bacterial corneal ulcer, endophthalmitis, and embolic phenomena. *Ann Ophthalmol* 1984;**16**:334–40.
29. Liesegang TJ. Bacterial keratitis. *Infect Dis Clin North Am* 1992;**6**:815–29.
30. Van Bijsterveld OP, Jager GV. Infectious diseases of the conjunctiva and cornea. *Curr Opin Ophthalmol* 1996;**7**:65–70.
31. Rahman MR, Johnson GJ, Husain R, Howlader SA, Minassian DC. Randomised trial of 0·2% chlorhexidine gluconate and 2·5% natamycin for fungal keratitis in Bangladesh. *Br J Ophthalmol* 1998;**82**:919–25.
32. Reddy PR. Topical antibiotics in the management of corneal ulcer. *Ind J Ophthalmol* 1988;**36**:95–7.
33. Hyndiuk RA, Eiferman RA, Caldwell DR *et al.*, the Ciprofloxacin Bacterial Keratitis Study Group. Comparison of Ciprofloxacin ophthalmic solution 0·3% to fortified tobramycin-cefazolin in treating bacterial corneal ulcers. *Ophthalmology* 1996;**103**:1854–63.
34. The Ofloxacin Study Group. Ofloxacin monotherapy for the primary treatment of microbial keratitis. A double-masked, randomised, controlled trial with conventional dual therapy. *Ophthalmology* 1997;**104**:1902–9.
35. Panda A, Ahuja R, Srinivas S. Comparison of topical 0·3% ofloxacin with fortified tobramycin plus cefazolin in the treatment of bacterial keratitis. *Eye* 1999;**13**:744–7.
36. Khokhar S, Sindhu N, Mirdha BR. Comparison of topical 0·3% ofloxacin to fortified tobramycin-cefazolin in the therapy of bacterial keratitis. *Infection* 2000;**28**:149–52.
37. Kosrirukvongs P, Buranapongs W. Topical ciprofloxacin for bacterial corneal ulcer. *J Med Assoc Thail* 2000;**83**:776–82.
38. Gandolfi SA, Massari A, Orsoni JG. Low-molecular-weight sodium hyaluronate in the treatment of bacterial corneal ulcers. *Graefe's Arch Clin Exp Ophthalmol* 1992;**230**:20–3.
39. Adler CA, Maurice DM, Paterson ME. The effect of viscosity of the vehicle on the penetration of fluorescein into the human eye. *Exp Eye Res* 1971;**11**:34–42.
40. Baker RS, Flowers CW Jr, Casey R, Fong DS, Wilson MR. Efficacy of ofloxacin versus cefazolin and tobramycin in the therapy for bacterial keratitis. *Arch Ophthalmol* 1996;**114**:632–3.
41. Carmichael TR, Gelfand Y, Welsh NH. Topical steroids in the treatment of central and paracentral ulcers. *Br J Ophthalmol* 1990;**74**:528–31.
42. Rao SK, Madhavan HN, Rao G. Fluconaxole in filamentous fungal keratitis. *Cornea* 1997;**16**:700.

Section VI

Uveitis

Carlos Pavesio, Editor

Uveitis: mission statement

Even though the incidence of uveitis is much lower than many other blinding conditions, it still represents an important cause of visual loss in individuals of working age and, in some parts of the world, is responsible for blindness on a very large scale. Some causes of uveitis can be clearly identified, especially the infectious ones in which case specific therapy can be instituted and cure can usually be achieved. This is not always as easy as it may seem, as can be seen in the chapter on Toxoplasmosis and Onchocerciasis.

The majority of cases have no specific diagnosis and are considered idiopathic, being driven by an immune-mediated mechanism. These are treated with anti-inflammatory and immunosuppressive agents in an attempt to control the progressive damage caused by the uncontrolled inflammation. Not much is known about many of these conditions and very little evidence exists to support the use of most of the agents currently used. The chapter entitled Idiopathic sight-threatening uveitis demonstrates this very clearly.

Anterior uveitis represents the most common form of intraocular inflammation seen in practice, but it is interesting to note that very few studies have dealt with this subject properly. On the other hand CMV retinitis, a much more recent problem, has had a large number of very good RCTs to demonstrate the efficacy of antiviral therapy in controlling progression of this blinding condition in HIV-infected patients. This certainly reflects the difference between the two conditons in terms of their impact as a cause of visual loss, but may also reflect the huge financial drive behind the RCTs in CMV retinitis.

Overall, the chapter dealing with the conditions mentioned above highlight the need for properly designed trials, which is the only way to answer the many questions we are still asking in our daily practice.

24 Ocular toxoplasmosis

Carlos Pavesio

Background

Toxoplasmic retinochoroiditis is the most frequent form of posterior uveitis, accounting for 20–60% of the cases.[1-3] It is caused by the protozoan, *Toxoplasma gondii*, and can be acquired congenitally, most frequently during late stages of pregnancy, or during postnatal life, due to exposure to contaminated water, food, direct exposure to cats' faeces, or inhalation of spores. Ocular toxoplasmosis is commonly attributed to congenital infection, but the role of acquired infection appears to be more important than previously thought. Lesions seen in the retina may actually be more frequently the result of a remote acquired infection rather than a late manifestation of a congenital transmission.[4] The evidence available suggests that at least two-thirds of ocular toxoplasmosis is caused by postnatal infection.[5]

Primary ocular disease occurs more frequently during acute systemic infection, but may also occur during the course of the chronic phase of systemic disease.[6,7] Case reports show that new lesions can appear for the first time as early as two months after onset of infection,[8] or as late as five years.[9] Recurrences are typical of both the congenital form and of the chronic phase of postnatally acquired disease.[10,11] The risk of recurrence of lesions in cohorts of prenatally infected children and case series of patients with postnatal disease appear to be similar (8–40%), but are based on small numbers.[5]

Many theories have been proposed to explain the typical recurrences, but it seems that active invasion of retinal cells by organisms released by a ruptured retinal cyst is the most likely explanation.

Severe morbidity and visual loss is frequently associated with congenital infection. More than 82% of congenitally infected individuals not treated as infants develop retinal lesions by adolescence, many with loss of vision. Information regarding visual loss in postnatal infection is limited.

Ability to control or eradicate the disease will depend on the use of treatment that can destroy the intracellular, cystic form, of the parasite. Also, limitation of retinal damage may be achieved by more effective control of the infection after initial clinical presentation of an active focus of retinitis.

Several different anti-toxoplasma drug therapy regimes can be used to treat this condition, with most of the information derived from uncontrolled series or reports. The real impact of treatment on the natural history of active disease, or on the risk of recurrences is currently unknown.

Questions

1 What is the evidence that current medical therapy is effective in controlling active disease?
2 What is the evidence that recurrences can be reduced or eliminated by the use of currently available drugs?

The evidence

We found six randomised controlled trials and one systematic review on the medical treatment of ocular toxoplasmosis. Three studies compared some form of intervention with controls.[12-14] In two of them the controls received placebo,[12,13] and in the third one, a study on prophylactic therapy,[14] only patients with inactive disease were included and treatment was compared with no treatment, without a placebo.

The study by Perkins *et al.*,[12] used Daraprim as therapy for four weeks in 113 patients presenting with active uveitis, regardless of having a typical retinal lesion or not. The outcome was defined as improved or not improved inflammation, and this finding was correlated with treatment given and toxoplasma serologic reaction. The cases were analysed also on the basis of the anatomic distribution of the uveitis (anterior, posterior, or pan-uveitis). For the patients who were serologically negative for toxoplasma there was no difference between the Daraprim and the placebo group. The toxoplasma positive patients treated with placebo showed a similar response to the toxoplasma negative patients (50% improvement). The toxoplasma positive patients treated with Daraprim showed 76% improvement, which was found to be significant. More details about this study can be found in the systematic review recently published.[15]

At the time this paper was written there was a feeling that ocular toxoplasmosis could not be diagnosed on clinical grounds and the patients included did not necessarily have the typical retinal lesion, which today is considered diagnostic in the immunocompetent individual. The presence of positive serology in the absence of a retinal lesion does not establish a causal relationship, but only represents exposure of this patient to toxoplasma. Analysis of the data by anatomic distribution of the uveitis is confronted with the problem of small numbers, and does not achieve significance. No clear information is provided about the use of cortisone. Even though the proportion of patients receiving this drug did not differ significantly between the toxoplasma positive and negative, treated and untreated groups, the information on its use in posterior or pan-uveitis is not provided, and it is possible that the improvement seen was more related to the use of cortisone than to Daraprim. There is no information about visual impairment or recurrence rate.

The study by Acers[13] was designed to compare the use of pyrimethamine, trisulfapyridines and prednisolone with placebo combined with prednisolone. Only 20 patients matching the criteria of a focus of retinitis, a positive serology and exclusion of other causes were included. No mention is made of the method of randomisation and no distinction as to severity of the inflammatory process, anatomical site, duration, and frequency of recurrences. More details about this study can be found in the recent systematic review.[15] All patients showed improvement by three weeks and almost complete clearing after eight weeks. Only patients with macular lesions ended up with poor visual acuity. Two relapses, one in each group, were reported over two years. According to this study steroid therapy is as efficacious as specific antimicrobial therapy with pyrimethamine. No final details on numbers followed up or long-term visual acuity were provided.

The study by Silveira *et al.*[11] had the objective of determining the effect of long-term intermittent therapy with trimethoprim/sulfamethoxazole on recurrences of toxoplasmic retinochoroiditis. Sixty-one patients received the drug therapy and 63 were controls, without placebo. The regime involved the use of one tablet of the combination drug every three days for up to 20 consecutive months. All patients had inactive disease at inclusion, and a new focus of necrotising retinitis defined a recurrence (end-point). Randomisation was done using a computer-generated list (1:1 ratio). Medications were administered in a non-masked fashion and the examining ophthalmologist was also not masked. Recurrences were found in 6·6% of patients in the treatment group and in 23·8% of the patients in the control group, which was statistically significant. There were no qualitative differences in recurrent lesions between groups. There was no statistical difference for the average time for recurrence between groups. No information on vision is available. The non-masking may have introduced bias during examination, and the data, as recognised by the authors, only support the protective effect of active therapy. No data on follow up, after the discontinuation of therapy, are available and no conclusions can be drawn for long lasting effects of this approach.

A recent prospective, randomised multi-center study[6] has compared the efficacy, safety and tolerability of two treatment regimens: one combining pyrimethamine and sulfadiazine, and the other combining pyrimethamine and azythromycin, both given for a period of four weeks. Both groups received folinic acid and oral prednisone from day three. The presence of an active focus of toxoplasmic retinitis, within the major temporal vascular arcades, was essential for inclusion in the study. The assignment to one of the treatments was done by a randomisation protocol. A total of 46 patients entered the study, with 24 receiving the regimen with azythromycin and 22 receiving the sulfadiazine. On clinical examination no differences were found between the groups in terms of time needed for resolution of inflammation, in the decrease in size of retinal lesions, and improvement of visual acuity of more than 0·5 logMAR units. There was also no difference in the recurrence rate for those patients followed up for one year. Adverse effects were more frequent, but not statistically significant, in the sulfadiazine group.

The study shows similar efficacy between the two regimens used, with reduced frequency of adverse effects in the azythromycin group. Due to the unmasked nature of the study, bias by the ophthalmologist cannot be excluded when comparing response to therapy between the two groups. Also, the number of patients was too small to detect real differences between the two groups, especially when considering the long follow up and recurrence data.

Two studies compared the use of oral therapy with pyrimethamine and sulfadiazine against sub-conjunctival clindamycin, without a control group.[16,17] Both studies used systemic steroids, but in one of them this was only started after 48 hours of specific therapy.[17] No randomisation method is reported in these studies.

The inclusion criteria included a typical clinical and angiographic lesion suggestive of toxoplasmosis, exclusion of other causes and a positive serology. All lesions were inducing reduction in vision either because of location or intense vitritis.

The patients were followed up for 20–24 months in one study and up to 19 months in the other. Both studies showed that no significant differences between the groups could be found in terms of subjective improvement, visual acuity recovery, and healing of the retinal lesion. Poor visual outcome was associated with macular lesions. Recurrences occurred in both groups with a higher frequency in the pyrimethamine/sulfadiazine group, but without reaching significance.

The conclusion was that sub-conjunctival clindamycin is as effective as systemic therapy with pyrimethamine and sulfadiazine, with the advantage of avoiding systemic side effects, but was unable to prevent recurrences. Both studies involve a small number of patients and no clear randomisation method is described. This does not exclude the possibility that the improvement was actually due to the systemic steroid therapy used in both groups. The follow up period is not long enough to allow proper conclusions about recurrences.

The final study by Mets *et al.*,[18] had the purpose of determining the natural history of treated and untreated congenital toxoplasmosis and the impact on vision. Children were included if they had confirmed infection and were less than 2·5 months in age. Untreated children during the first year of life were historical controls. Children were randomised to treatments A or C (both groups received pyrimethamine and sulfadiazine, the difference being that group A received the pyrimethamine daily for two months followed by three days a week for one year, while group C had the daily treatment prolonged for six months, before reducing to three days a week for the rest of the year). The randomisation was stratified for severity, prior maternal treatment, and certainty of diagnosis at birth, and was based on a random number table, with treatment assigned in blocks of varying size. All patients were evaluated prospectively up to 15 years of age.

The most common eye manifestation was chorioretinal scars, most commonly in the peripheral retina. The severity of eye disease was worse in the historical control group (less severe systemic or neurologic disease), and no statistical difference could be found between the two treatment groups.

Development of active lesions following discontinuation of therapy was seen in 13% of treated patients during 189 patient-years of follow up, and in 44% of the controls during 160 patient-years of follow up. Treatment did not prevent new lesions appearing and the recurrence rate between the two treatment groups was not significant (7% for group A and 4% for group C).

Owing to ethical implications, there were no concomitant untreated controls. No direct comparisons can be made between the treated patients and the historical controls because the difference in severity of disease presentation and different ages would induce bias. The historical patients were comparable to only 20% of the treated patients who had no or mild clinical involvement at birth.

This study, even though including groups not directly comparable, showed a trend towards reduction of reactivation of ocular disease for those children with congenital toxoplasmosis who were offered prolonged therapy in the postnatal period. No differences could be found between the lower and higher dosage regime.

Summary

In spite of the fact that the aetiological agent for toxoplasmosis was identified at the beginning of the twentieth century and that the drugs currently being used have been in use for several decades, few randomised clinical trials looking into their true efficacy in controlling active disease or preventing recurrences could be found. This is certainly related to the difficulty in performing such studies, which is related to the self-limiting character of this infection, its different clinical presentations, and also factors related to host and parasite. The most frequently used drugs (pyrimethamine, sulfadiazine, other sulfonamides and clindamycin) were tested in these studies, and in one study a new alternative regimen (pyrimethamine combined with azythromycin) was tested.

No clear evidence that the therapeutic regimens had a beneficial effect on the outcome of active lesions could be found. Reduction in the size of the lesions and improvement in vision was certainly shown in the study by Bosch-Driessen and colleagues,[6] but this study had no control group. The study by Silveira and colleagues[11] shows a protective prophylactic effect of the drug therapy used, but no follow-up data, after discontinuation of therapy, are available to show long-term protection. The other studies comparing different forms of therapy could not show any significant difference and the improvement demonstrated may have been simply the effect of systemic steroid therapy used. The study by Bosch-Driessen *et al.*[6] shows similar efficacy with less toxicity with the use of azythromycin, and this finding has affected the treatment policy of their group. The only study looking into therapy in congenital disease also shows a trend towards reduction in recurrences, but longer follow-up is needed to confirm this observation. It did not allow for comparisons with the control group since this was a historical control showing different severity of disease and including children of different age groups.

Implications for research

The available data do not allow a conclusive answer to the questions proposed and properly designed studies are clearly necessary.

Implications for practice

Current practice in the management of toxoplasmic retinitis involves the use of courses of anti-toxoplasmic drugs in cases where lesions are threatening critical structures such as the macula and optic nerve, and also in cases of large lesions causing significant vitritis. The combination of pyrimethamine/sulfadiazine and corticosteroids seems to be the most frequently used,[19] but discontinuation of therapy occurs in about 25% of the cases because of bone marrow suppression or allergic reactions. The few clinical trials discussed in this review do not show a significant advantage of one regimen over the other in terms of efficacy during the acute disease or for long-term protection against new relapses. The prolonged use of intermittent therapy was shown to reduce attacks during therapy, but it does not represent a practical solution for most cases since there is no evidence that it can reduce the long-term risk of attacks after discontinuation of therapy. It may be an interesting alternative, as pointed out by the authors, for the management of those individuals with macular lesions in whom a new attack may result in severe visual loss, but long-term toxicity of this regimen needs to be assessed. The introduction of azythromycin as a first line agent, in combination with pyrimethamine, seems to be an interesting alternative. The study by Bosch-Driessen et al.[6] has shown similar efficacy with less toxicity of this combination in comparison to the classic regimen. Even though numbers were small this seems to be the best contribution to practical management found in the studies analysed in this review.

References

1. Miettenen. Incidence of uveitis in Northern Finland. *Acta Ophthalmol* 1993;**77**:371–7.
2. Wakefield D, Dunlop I, McCluskey PJ *et al.* Uveitis: aetiology and disease associations in an Australian population. *Aust NZ J Ophthalmol* 1986;**14**:181–7.
3. Secchi A, Tagnan S, Salmaso M *et al.* Uveitis in Italy: 10 years of experience in a referral center. In: Ohno S, Aoki K, Usui M, Uchio E, eds. *Uveitis today.* Amsterdam: Elsevier Science, 1998, pp. 232–8.
4. Holland GN. Reconsidering the pathogenesis of ocular toxoplasmosis. *Am J Ophthalmol* 1999;**128**:502–5.
5. Gilbert R, Stanford M. Is ocular toxoplasmosis caused by prenatal or postnatal infection? *Br J Ophthalmol* 2000;**84**:224–6.
6. Bosch-Driessen LH, Verbraak FD, Suttorp-Schulten MSA *et al.* A prospective, randomized trial of pyrimethamine and azythormycin *v* pryrimethamine and sulfadiazine for the treatment of ocular toxoplasmosis. *Am J Ophthalmol* 2002;**134**:34–40.
7. Bosch-Driessen LE, Berendschot TT, Ongkosuwito JV, Rothova A. Ocular toxoplasmosis: clinical features and prognosis of 154 patients. *Ophthalmology* 2002;**109**(5):869–78.
8. Couvreur J, Thulliez P. Acquired toxoplasmosis of ocular or neurologic site: 49 cases. *Presse Med* 1996;**25**:438–42.
9. Leblanc A, Bamberger J, Guillien F *et al.* Acquired toxoplasmic chorioretinitis with a late onset. *Arch Fr Pediatr* 1985;**42**:37–9.
10. Bosch-Driessen EH, Rothova A. Recurrent ocular disease in postnatally acquired toxoplasmosis. *Am J Ophthalmol* 1999;**128**:421–5.
11. Silveira C, Belfort R Jr, Muccioli C *et al.* A follow-up study of *Toxoplasma gondii* infection in southern Brazil. *Am J Ophthalmol* 2001;**131**:351–4.
12. Perkins ES, Smith CH, Schofield PB. Treatment of uveitis with pyrimethamine (Daraprim). *Br J Ophthalmol* 1956;**40**:577–86.
13. Acers T. Toxoplasmic retinochoroiditis: a double blind therapeutic study. *Arch Ophthalmol* 1964;**71**:92–6.
14. Silveira C, Belfort Jr R, Muccioli C *et al.* The effect of long-term intermittent trimethoprim/sulfamethoxazole treatment on recurrences of toxoplasmic retinochoroiditis. *Am J Ophthalmol* 2002;**134**: 41–6.
15. Gilbert RE, See SE, Jones LV, Stanford MS. Antibiotics versus control for toxoplasma retinochoroiditis (Cochrane Review). In: Cochrane Collaboration: *Cochrane Library.* Issue 4. Oxford: Update Software, 2002.
16. Colin J, Harie JC. Chorioretinites presumes toxoplasmiques: etude comparative des traitments par pyrimethamine et sulfadiazine ou clindamycine. *J Fr Ophthalmol* 1989;**3**:161–5.
17. Jeddi A, Azaiez A, Bouguila H *et al.* Interet de la clindamycine dans le traitement de la toxoplasmose oculaire. *J Fr Ophthalmol* 1997;**20**: 418–22.
18. Mets MA, Holfels E, Boyer KM *et al.* Eye manifestations of congenital toxoplasmosis. *Am J Ophthalmol* 1996;**122**:309–24.
19. Engstrom Jr RE, Holland GN, Nussenblatt RB, Jabs DA. Current practices in the management of ocular toxoplasmosis. *Am J Ophthalmol* 1991;**111**:601–10.

25 Onchocerciasis

Henry Ejere

Background

Onchocerciasis (river blindness) is a filarial infestation caused by the nematode, *Onchocerca volvulus*. Onchocerciasis is endemic in 34 countries: 26 in the African region, six in the region of the Americas and two in the Eastern Mediterranean.[1] Recent estimates indicate that about 18 million people are infected globally, of whom 99% are in Africa and a further 120 million people (the majority from Africa) are believed to be at risk of developing the disease.[2] Onchocerciasis causes severe skin disease but the main public health importance of the disease is blindness. About 270 000 people are estimated to be irreversibly blind and a further 500 000 severely visually disabled.[3]

Onchocerciasis is transmitted from person to person by black flies that breed in fast flowing rivers. The infective worms enter the human body through the bite of the black fly and develop into mature adult worms (macrofilariae). Macrofilariae mate and adult female worms produce millions of microfilariae, which migrate throughout the skin and to the eye. Microfilariae may be visualised in the cornea or anterior chamber by the slit lamp. Onchocercal eye disease generally develops after a long exposure to onchocercal infection, although eye lesions may occur rapidly when the intensity of infection is high. The main pathological changes seen in the eye appear to be related to the local death of the microfilariae. Dead microfilariae precipitate a severe inflammatory reaction, which leads to characteristic lesions affecting the anterior segment of the eye – punctate keratitis, sclerosing keratitis and iridocyclitis. The pathogenesis of posterior segment lesions – chorioretinitis and optic neuritis is less clear. An autoimmune theory has been described based on the observed structural similarity between an *Onchocerca volvulus* antigen (Ov39) and a human retinal antigen (hr44).[4] According to this theory, chorioretinal pathology initiated by the presence of local microfilariae may progress even in the absence of the organism.[5] The main pathways to blindness due to onchocerciasis are sclerosing keratitis, chorioretinitis and optic nerve disease.

Ivermectin (marketed as Mectizan) is currently used as the drug of choice in the control of onchocerciasis. The microfilaricidal properties of ivermectin in people with onchocerciasis have been reported[6] and some studies show that 150 micrograms/kg body weight of ivermectin is optimal.[7] It is believed that sustained annual delivery of ivermectin could prevent a substantial proportion of onchocercal eye disease and blindness in endemic communities.[8] The World Health Organization (WHO) has defined a new global strategy for controlling onchocerciasis that is based on yearly administration of single doses of ivermectin to affected populations. In 1987, Merck, the manufacturer of ivermectin, pledged to provide, at no cost, all the drugs necessary to overcome onchocerciasis as a public health problem. The African Programme for Onchocerciasis Control (APOC) and the Onchocerciasis Elimination Programme for the Americas (OEPA) currently promote mass treatment with ivermectin in hyper- and meso-endemic communities. Since 1987 more than 65 million doses of ivermectin have been donated for distribution.[2]

Question

What are the effects of ivermectin on visual loss and eye lesions in people with onchocerciasis?

The evidence

A systematic review of randomised controlled trials of ivermectin for onchocercal eye disease is published in the *Cochrane Library*.[9] The review included all randomised controlled trials with at least one year follow-up comparing ivermectin against placebo in people with onchocercal eye disease or at risk of developing eye disease. Participants are normally resident in onchocercal endemic communities. Treatment was defined according to the recommended dose of 150 micrograms/kg ivermectin tablets given annually or semi-annually. The outcomes used were incidence of visual loss (unilateral or bilateral) including visual field loss, proportion of people with or progression in punctate keratitis, sclerosing keratitis, iridocyclitis, chorioretinitis, or optic nerve disease. Adverse effects outcomes were also included as reported in the trials. Parasitological outcomes such as microfilarial counts in the cornea and anterior chamber were considered.

Five randomised controlled trials were included in the review.[8,10–13] Outcomes from some of the original trials

Table 25.1 Effect of ivermectin on visual acuity loss (new cases)

Study	Ivermectin n/N (%)	Placebo n/N (%)	Odds ratio	95% CI
Abiose *et al.*, 1993[8]	–	–	–	–
Dadzie *et al.*, 1989[10]	–	–	–	–
Newland *et al.*, 1988[11]	0/52	0/48	–	–
Taylor *et al.*, 1989[12]	0/8	0/9	–	–
Whitworth *et al.*, 1991[13]	7/296 (2·4)	7/272 (2·6)	0·92	0·32–2·65

Table 25.2 Effect of ivermectin on visual field loss (new cases)

Study	Ivermectin n/N (%)	Placebo n/N (%)	Odds ratio	95% CI
Abiose *et al.*, 1993[8]	34/314 (10·8)	58/322 (18)	0·56	0·36–0·87
Dadzie *et al.*, 1989[10]	–	–	–	–
Newland *et al.*, 1988[11]	0/52	0/48	–	–
Taylor *et al.*, 1989[12]	0/8	1/9	0·15	0·00–7·67
Whitworth *et al.*, 1991[13]	–	–	–	–

were reported separately in other papers.[14–17] Only original trials are primarily referenced in the review. Allocation concealment was adequate in all trials. Recipients and providers of care were masked in all trials, as were outcome assessors. Information on follow-up was obtained from the authors of one trial.[13] Follow-up rates were unclear in other trials. Results were analysed in two trials on the basis of an intention to treat principle.[11,12] The five trials randomised a total of 10 198 participants. One of the trials[8] initially randomised 8136 people who were five years old and above but later excluded 5091 individuals from analysis, who were either below the age of 15 years or were found to have optic nerve disease at baseline. Three trials were dose-finding studies and compared three different doses of ivermectin against placebo.[10–12] Only data for participants in the 150 micrograms ivermectin and placebo groups were extracted from these trials.

Two of the studies were undertaken in the Bassa County of Liberia,[11,12] one study was undertaken in northern Nigeria,[8] one study in northern Ghana[10] and one in southern Sierra-Leone.[13] All the studies recruited participants normally resident in endemic onchocercal communities. In all trials ivermectin at a dose of 150 micrograms per kilogram of body weight (micrograms/kg) was compared with placebo. Ivermectin was given as a single dose annually in all the studies except one, in which ivermectin was given six monthly.[13] Duration of treatment ranged from one to three years. Assessment of outcome measures was by ocular examination undertaken by

specialist doctors or specially trained eye nurses and included visual acuity or visual field assessment, slit lamp examination, and skin snip tests. Outcomes were defined, measured, and reported differently in the trials making a statistical pooling of results inappropriate. A narrative summary therefore follows.

Effect of ivermectin on visual loss (visual acuity and visual field)

All five trials obtained baseline data on visual acuity but only one trial explicitly reported figures of incidence of visual loss.[13] This trial found no statistically significant difference between ivermectin and placebo in the incidence of visual acuity loss from any cause (odds ratio 0·92, 95% CI 0·32–2·65). In other trials, visual acuity loss was either not observed or not explicitly reported (Table 25.1). In one trial,[8] a statistically significant reduction in the odds of visual field loss between ivermectin and placebo groups was reported (odds ratio 0·56, 95% CI 0·36–0·87). There was no statistically significant difference in visual field loss between the treatment groups in another trial (Table 25.2).[12]

Effect on anterior segment lesions

One trial[13] reported a beneficial effect of ivermectin on punctate keratitis compared to placebo (odds ratio 0·28, 95% CI 0·18–0·43). Data on punctate keratitis were incomplete for three trials,[10–12] therefore a summary

Table 25.3   Effect of ivermectin on punctate keratitis (proportion of people with PK)

Study	Ivermectin n/N (%)	Placebo n/N (%)	Odds ratio	95% CI
Abiose *et al.*, 1993[8]	–	–	–	–
Dadzie *et al.*, 1989[10]	–	–	–	–
Newland *et al.*, 1988[11]	–	–	–	–
Taylor *et al.*, 1989[12]	–	–	–	–
Whitworth *et al.*, 1991[13]	27/288 (9·4)	75/263 (28·5)	0·28	0·18–0·43

Table 25.4   Effect of ivermectin on sclerosing keratitis (proportion of people with SK or progression in pre-existing SK)

Study	Ivermectin n/N (%)	Placebo n/N (%)	Odds ratio	95% CI
Abiose *et al.*, 1993[8]	–	–	–	–
Dadzie *et al.*, 1989[10]	–	–	–	–
Newland *et al.*, 1988[11]	–	–	–	–
Taylor *et al.*, 1989[12]	0/8	2/9 (22·2)	0·13	0·01–2·35
Whitworth *et al.*, 1991[13]	82/293 (28·3)	93/267 (34·8)	0·74	0·52–1·06

Table 25.5   Effect of ivermectin on iridocyclitis

Study	Ivermectin n/N (%)	Placebo n/N (%)	Odds ratio	95% CI
Abiose *et al.*, 1993[8]	–	–	–	–
Dadzie *et al.*, 1989[10]	2/42 (4·8)	0/38	6·88	0·42–112·42
Newland *et al.*, 1988[11]	–	–	–	–
Taylor *et al.*, 1989[12]	–	–	–	–
Whitworth *et al.*, 1991[13]	39/291 (13·4)	57/263 (21·7)	0·56	0·36–0·87

Table 25.6   Effect of ivermectin on corneal or anterior chamber microfilariae (proportion of people with MF count > 1)

Study	Ivermectin n/N (%)	Placebo n/N (%)	Odds ratio	95% CI
Abiose *et al.*, 1993[8]	–	–	–	–
Dadzie *et al.*, 1989[10]	–	–	–	–
Newland *et al.*, 1988[11]	–	–	–	–
Taylor *et al.*, 1989[12]	–	–	–	–
Whitworth *et al.*, 1991[13] (Corneal MF count > 1)	17/285 (6)	61/263 (23·2%)	0·24	0·15–0·39
Whitworth *et al.*, 1991[13] (AC MF count > 1)	10/285 (3·5)	91/263 (34·6)	0·13	0·08–0·2

statistic could not be calculated (Table 25.3). Two trials reported a reduction in the odds of sclerosing keratitis in the ivermectin group compared to placebo but this was not statistically significant (Table 25.4). A statistically significant beneficial effect of ivermectin on iridocyclitis was reported in one trial[13] (odds ratio 0·56, 95% CI 0·36–0·87). However, in another trial[10] a potentially harmful effect of

ivermectin on iridocyclitis was reported, but this was not statistically significant (odds ratio 6·88, 95% CI 0·42–112·42) (Table 25.5). One trial[13] reported a beneficial effect of ivermectin on corneal and anterior chamber microfilarial count (Table 25.6). Data were incomplete in three trials,[10–12] therefore a summary statistic could not be calculated.

Table 25.7 Effect of ivermectin on chorioretinitis including retinal pigment epithelial atrophy (new cases or progression)

Study	Ivermectin n/N (%)	Placebo n/N (%)	Odds ratio	95% CI
Abiose *et al.*, 1993[8]	–	–	–	–
Dadzie *et al.*, 1989[10]	0/42	0/38	–	–
Newland *et al.*, 1988[11]	0/52	7/48 (14·6)	0·11	0·02–0·50
Taylor *et al.*, 1989[12]	0/8	0/9	–	–
Whitworth *et al.*, 1991[13]	28/278 (10·1)	15/250 (6)	1·72	0·92–3·21

Table 25.8 Effect of ivermectin on optic nerve disease (new cases or proportion with optic nerve disease)

Study	Ivermectin n/N (%)	Placebo n/N (%)	Odds ratio	95% CI
Abiose *et al.*, 1993[8]	45/1750 (2·6)	71/1772 (4·0)	0·64	0·44–0·92
Dadzie *et al.*, 1989[10]	0/42	0/38	–	–
Newland *et al.*, 1988[11]	0/52	0/48	–	–
Taylor *et al.*, 1989[12]	0/8	0/9	–	–
Whitworth *et al.*, 1991[13]	22/281 (7·8)	14/251 (5·6)	1·43	0·73–2·81

Effect of ivermectin on posterior segment lesions

One trial[11] reported a beneficial effect of ivermectin on chorioretinitis (odds ratio 0·11, 95% CI 0·02–0·50) but another trial[13] reported a potential harmful effect of ivermectin on chorioretinitis, but this was not statistically significant (odds ratio 1·72, 95% CI 0·92–3·21). No events were observed in the ivermectin or placebo group in two trials (Table 25.7).[10,12] One trial[9] reported a beneficial effect of ivermectin in reducing the incidence of optic nerve disease compared to placebo (odds ratio 0·64, 95% CI 0·44–0·93). However, another trial[13] reported an opposite effect with ivermectin more likely to produce a harmful effect on optic nerve disease compared to placebo, though this was not statistically significant (odds ratio 1·43, 95% CI 0·73–2·81). Three trials[10–12] did not observe any retinal or optic nerve changes in either the ivermectin or placebo group (Table 25.8).

Adverse reactions associated with ivermectin treatment

One trial[13] did not find any statistically significant difference between ivermectin and placebo in adverse reactions of any kind (odds ratio 1·40, 95% CI 0·88–2·24). These reactions were either mild, moderate, or severe and included cutaneous reactions, musculoskeletal reactions, fever, swelling of the face, joints and limbs, headaches and dizziness, lymphadenopthy, eye reactions and nodule pain.

One trial[10] reported a higher risk of severe symptomatic postural hypotension in the ivermectin group compared to placebo (odds ratio 7·44, 95% CI 1·23–45·05).

Summary

The effect of ivermectin in preventing visual loss is an outcome of importance to people at risk of blindness from onchocerciasis. An interesting phenomenon is the fact that although all trials collected baseline information on visual acuity, only one trial explicitly reported figures on incidence of visual loss. It is uncertain whether the paucity of reporting of visual outcomes in most trials is related to a lack of beneficial effect of treatment. Length of follow up is an important factor when considering effect on vision. Most of the trials included in the review had follow-up ranging from one to three years. Perhaps a longer period of follow up would be necessary to observe any appreciable difference in visual outcomes between the treatment groups. However, one trial[8] reported a beneficial effect of ivermectin on visual field loss within a three-year period. One trial[13] consistently indicated a beneficial effect of ivermectin on anterior segment lesions including effect on cornea and anterior chamber microfilariae, except for sclerosing keratitis where the effect was not statistically significant (Tables 25.3–25.6). This is not surprising as sclerosing keratitis represents a long-standing disease with subsequent scarring of the cornea. Any observed benefit would most likely have been due to chance. The effect of ivermectin on posterior segment lesions (chorioretinitis and optic nerve disease) is inconsistent between trials. One trial[13] indicates a potential increase in the risks of chorioretinitis and optic atrophy even though these findings were not statistically significant. However, another trial[8] reported a statistically significant beneficial effect of ivermectin in reducing the incidence of optic nerve disease. However, this trial initially randomised children younger than 15 years but excluded them from analysis on the basis of a low prevalence of optic nerve disease, which incidentally was the main outcome of interest. An intention to treat analysis was not presented and since children formed a large proportion of the initially randomised population, it is not clear to what extent their exclusion from analysis could have affected the observed effect size. The observed result was unlikely to have been invalidated if the decision to exclude children from analysis had been taken *a priori* and well documented in the study protocol or protocol amendment. On the other hand, a *post hoc* decision taken after observation of a low event rate in children can introduce bias and calls for a cautious interpretation of the results. One trial[10] reports a statistically significant risk of postural hypotension with ivermectin treatment. While ivermectin has been associated with postural hypotension in field studies,[18,19] the finding in this trial may have been exaggerated by the trial's small sample size.

Implications for practice and policy

Ivermectin may reduce the incidence of visual field loss but data from currently available trials are insufficient to conclude that ivermectin has a beneficial effect in preventing visual acuity loss in onchocercal eye disease. Some of the trials demonstrate that ivermectin may be effective in reducing anterior segment lesions, but its effectiveness in reducing posterior segment lesions, particularly chorioretinitis, is inconclusive. A potential benefit of ivermectin on optic nerve disease cannot be excluded but this has to be cautiously interpreted against the background of the uncertainty created by the exclusion of children from the trial that reported this benefit.[8]

Implications for research

Blindness and visual impairment are important public health concerns in onchocerciasis. It is therefore important that visual outcomes are evaluated more thoroughly in future trials of ivermectin, given ethical considerations. The duration of these trials should be sufficiently long to be able to detect meaningful changes in visual acuity. The search for alternative drugs or drug combination for onchocerciasis is underway.[20,21] Although details of these studies are not yet available, it seems likely that these drugs or drug combinations could represent the comparison treatment in future trials of ivermectin for onchocerciasis.

References

1. Johnson G, Minassian DC, Weale R, eds. *The Epidemiology of Eye Disease*. London: Chapman & Hall, 1998.
2. World Health Organization. *Onchocerciasis (River blindness)*. Fact sheet No. 95 Revised 2000. Geneva: WHO.
3. Rolland A. Results of 2 eye examinations carried out with an interval of 6 years in 2 Upper Volta villages where onchocerciasis is endemic. *Bull World Health Organ* 1974;**51**(3):257–61.
4. Cooper PJ, Guderian RH, Proano R, Taylor DW. Absence of cellular responses to a putative autoantigen in onchocercal chorioretinopathy. Cellular autoimmunity in onchocercal chorioretinopathy. *Invest Ophthalmol Vis Sci* 1996;**37**(9):1717–19.
5. Cooper PJ, Guderian RH, Proano R, Taylor DW. The pathogenesis of chorioretinal disease in onchocerciasis. *Parasitol Today* 1997;**13**:94–8.
6. Aziz MA, Diallo S, Diop IM, Lariviere M, Porta M. Efficacy and tolerance of ivermectin in human onchocerciasis. *Lancet* 1982;**2**(8291):171–3.
7. White A, Newland HS, Taylor HR *et al.* Controlled trial and dose finding study of ivermectin for treatment of onchocerciasis. *J Infect Dis* 1987;**156**(3):463–70.
8. Abiose A, Jones BR, Cousens SN *et al.* Reduction in incidence of optic nerve disease with annual ivermectin to control onchocerciasis. *Lancet* 1993;**341**(8838):130–4.
9. Ejere H, Schwartz E, Wormald R. Ivermectin for onchocercal eye disease (river blindness) (Cochrane Review). In: Cochrane collaboration: *Cochrane Library*. Issue 3. Oxford: Update Software, 2001.
10. Dadzie KY, Awadzi K, Bird AC, Schulz-Key H. Ophthalmological results from a placebo controlled comparative 3-dose ivermectin study in the treatment of onchocerciasis. *Trop Med Parasitol* 1989;**40**:355–60.
11. Newland HS, White AT, Greene BM *et al.* Effect of single-dose ivermectin therapy on human onchocerca volvulus infection with onchocercal ocular involvement. *Br J Ophthalmol* 1988;**72**:561–9.
12. Taylor HR, Semba RD, Newland HS *et al.* Ivermectin treatment of patients with severe ocular onchocerciasis. *Am J Trop Med Hyg* 1989;**40**(5):494–500.
13. Whitworth JAG, Gilbert CE, Mabey DM, Maude GH, Morgan D, Taylor DW. Effects of repeated doses of ivermectin on ocular onchocerciasis: community-based trial in Sierra Leone. *Lancet* 1991;**338**:1100–3.
14. Cousens SN, Cassels-Brown A, Murdoch I *et al.* Impact of annual dosing with ivermectin on progression of onchocercal visual field loss. *Bull World Health Organ* 1997;**75**(3):229–36.
15. White A, Newland HS, Taylor HR *et al.* Controlled trial and dose finding study of ivermectin for treatment of onchocerciasis. *J Infect Dis* 1987;**156**(3):463–70.
16. Whitworth JAG, Morgan D, Maude GH, Downham MD, Taylor DW. A community trial of ivermectin for onchocerciasis in Sierra Leone: adverse reactions after the first five treatment rounds. *Trans R Soc Trop Med Hyg* 1991;**85**:501–5.
17. Whitworth JAG, Morgan D, Maude GH, Luty AJF, Taylor DW. A community trial of ivermectin for onchocerciasis in Sierra Leone: clinical and parasitological responses to four doses given at six-monthly intervals. *Trans R Soc Trop Med Hyg* 1992;**86**:277–80.
18. Chijioke CP, Okonkwo PO. Adverse events following mass ivermectin therapy for onchocerciasis. *Trans R Soc Trop Med Hyg* 1992;**86**(3):284–6.
19. De-Sole G, Remme J, Awadzi K *et al.* Adverse reactions after large-scale treatment of onchocerciasis with ivermectin: combined results from eight community trials. *Bull World Health Organ* 1989;**67**(6):707–19.
20. Taylor M. Filarial nematodes: a bug's life? *Filarial Update* 2000;**2**(1):10–11.
21. Hoerauf, A, Mand, S, Adjei, O, Fleischer, B, Buttner DW. Depletion of wolbachia endobacteria in *Onchocerca volvulus* by doxycycline and microfilaridermia after ivermectin treatment. *Lancet* 2001;**357**(9266):1415–16.

26 Idiopathic (autoimmune) sight-threatening uveitis

Philip I Murray

Background

Uveitis, a term correctly used to describe inflammation of the uveal tract (iris, ciliary body, choroid) alone, actually comprises a large group of diverse diseases affecting not only the uvea but also the retina, optic nerve and vitreous. Uveitis usually occurs in people of working age and is a major cause of severe visual impairment.

Although the number of people blind from uveitis is unknown, it has been estimated that uveitis accounts for 10% of severe visual handicap in the USA.[1] Another study found 35% visual impairment or blindness, mainly due to posterior uveitis.[2] The prevalence of uveitis in western countries is reported to be 38 per 100 000[3] with an annual incidence of 14 to 17·5 per 100 000[3–5] and a maximum occurrence in the 20–50 years age group. As uveitis is rarely included in surveys of the causes of blindness these values are probably an underestimate. The most important cause both of blindness and visual impairment is cystoid macular oedema.[2] This can have serious economic consequences with many days off work or job losses, may interfere with or prevent driving and, in the younger age group, interfere significantly with education.

The International Uveitis Study Group classification[6] separates uveitis by anatomical localisation of the disease, according to the major visible signs: anterior, posterior, pan and intermediate. The course of the disease can be described as acute, chronic (greater than three months' duration) and recurrent. In the majority of cases of endogenous uveitis, the aetiology is unknown. Some cases are a manifestation of a systemic disease such as sarcoidosis or Behçet's disease, whilst others are only associated with various conditions, such as the HLA-B27-related group of diseases. Although one can attach a label to a number of uveitis syndromes, such as Fuchs' heterochromic cyclitis or Vogt-Koyanagi-Harada disease, the actual cause underlying these conditions is unknown. In a prospective study of 865 patients, a definitive association with a systemic disease was determined for 220 (26%) patients and a relationship with a subclinical disorder could be presumed in 201 (23%) cases.[7]

Little is known about either the aetiology or the pathogenesis of this group of diseases, but they are thought to be autoimmune in nature. Treatment is often very long term, is directed towards dampening the resulting immune and inflammatory cascade and aims to reduce tissue damage. Although present treatment is successful in some cases, it is restricted by the required long-term use and the significant side effects of the drugs.

Question

In patients with sight-threatening idiopathic uveitis, what is the evidence that medical therapy is effective in:

- preventing loss of vision
- improving vision
- controlling inflammation
- preventing relapses of inflammation?

The evidence

The bibliographic databases searched were: *Cochrane Library*, MEDLINE (PubMed), EMBASE (Ovid), Science Citation Index (Web of Science) and NHS Economic Evaluation.

Box 26.1 Criteria for inclusion/exclusion of studies and trials

- Inclusion Criteria

Population:	Patients with sight-threatening uveitis
Intervention:	Systemic medical therapy compared to another systemic therapy or placebo
Outcomes:	Visual acuity, control of inflammation, relapse rate, side-effects of therapy
Study design:	Randomised controlled trials (RCTs)

- Exclusion criteria

  Non-randomised studies
  Animal studies
  Anterior uveitis
  Presumed infectious uveitis
  Traumatic uveitis
  Postoperative uveitis
  Non-medical therapy (surgery, laser, radiation, cryotherapy)

One reviewer, using explicit predetermined criteria, made the inclusion and exclusion decisions. These decisions were made independently of the inspection of trial results. Trials and studies were only included if they met the criteria shown in Box 26.1.

A total of 16 RCTs were identified that fulfilled the criteria. Of these, one had been retracted by the journal and another could not be translated into English. A Cochrane review on pharmacotherapy for Behçet's disease was also identified. This review included 10 trials on Behçet's involving 679 patients, but not all the trials included patients with eye involvement. This left 15 papers for analysis. Two other papers, a meta-analysis on the treatment of Adamantiades-Behçet disease with systemic intereferon alfa,[8] and guidelines for the use of immunosuppressive drugs in patients with ocular inflammatory disorders[9] were excluded from the analysis of clinical effectiveness, but their presence was noted as essential background to the review.

Table 26.1 summarises the 14 RCTs, including the authors' conclusions. It can be seen that the majority of studies were on a heterogeneous group of uveitis conditions. Although five studies looked at Behçet's disease, other studies also included some of these patients. The inclusion criteria for all the studies differ widely; in only one study was a power calculation performed to determine the appropriate sample size, and in only three studies was the method of randomisation stated. No statistical analyses were undertaken in three studies, and in another two the statistical tests used were not mentioned. Overall, there was a wide variation in study design, outcome measures were often poorly defined, and in many studies the authors came to conclusions that could not be derived from the data presented.

Comment

Many studies failed to adequately answer the questions posed above. One possible reason for this was that a number of studies did not propose a clear-cut question or hypothesis. Where a question was identified, there was often insufficient evidence presented to answer it. Nevertheless, the Cochrane review confirmed the conclusions of two RCTs that showed the protective effects of ciclosporin and azathioprine for eye involvement in Behçet's disease.

Implications for practice

A total of 15 papers were identified dealing with the medical therapy of sight-threatening idiopathic uveitis. Overall, the quality of evidence for the effectiveness of therapies is poor.

Implications for research

Basic questions need to be identified that could be answered in the form of well-designed, multi-centre studies with clear outcome measures using homogeneous groups of patients.

References

1. National Institutes of Health. *Interim report of the National Advisory Eye Council support for visual research.* Washington, DC: US Department of Health, Education and Welfare, 1976.
2. Rothova A, Suttorp-van Schulten MSA, Treffers WF, Kijlstra A. Causes and frequency of blindness in patients with intraocular inflammatory disease. *Br J Ophthalmol* 1996;**80**:332–6.
3. Vadot E, Barth E, Billet P. Epidemiology of uveitis – preliminary results of a prospective study in Savoy. In: Saari KM, ed. *Uveitis update.* Amsterdam: Elsevier, 1984, pp. 13–16.
4. Darrell RW, Wagener HP, Kurland LT. Epidemiology of uveitis. *Arch Ophthalmol* 1962;**68**:502–15.
5. Tran VT, Auer C, Guex-Crosier Y, Pittet N, Herbort CP. Epidemiology of uveitis in Switzerland. *Ocul Immunol Inflamm* 1994;**2**:169–76.
6. Bloch-Michel E, Nussenblatt RB. International uveitis study group recommendations for the evaluation of intraocular inflammatory disease. *Am J Ophthalmol* 1987;**103**:234–6.
7. Rothova A, Buitenhuis HJ, Meenken C *et al.* Uveitis and systemic disease. *Br J Ophthalmol* 1992;**76**:137–41.
8. Zouboulis CC, Orfanos CE. Treatment of Adamantiades-Behçet disease with systemic interferon alfa. *Arch Dermatol* 1998;**134**:101–6.
9. Jabs DA, Rosenbaum JT, Foster CS *et al.* Guidelines for the use of immunosuppressive drugs in patients with ocular inflammatory disorders: recommendations of an expert panel. *Am J Ophthalmol* 2000;**130**:492–513.
10. James DG, Carstairs LS, Trowell J, Sharma OP. Treatment of sarcoidosis. Report of a controlled therapeutic trial. *Lancet* 1967;**2**:526–8.
11. Schlaegel TF Jr, Weber JC. Double-blind therapeutic trial of isoniazid in 344 patients with uveitis. *Br J Ophthalmol* 1969;**53**:425–7.
12. Abdalla MI, Bahgat N E-D. Long-lasting remission of Behçet's disease after chlorambucil therapy. *Br J Ophthalmol* 1973;**57**:706–11.
13. Aktulga E, Altac M, Muftuoglu A *et al.* A double blind study of colchicine in Behçet's disease. *Haematologica* 1980;**65**:399–402.
14. BenEzra D, Cohen E, Chajek T *et al.* Evaluation of conventional therapy versus cyclosporine A in Behçet's syndrome. *Transplant Proc* 1988;**20**(3 Suppl 4):136–43.
15. Masuda K, Nakajima A, Urayama A, Nakae K, Kogure M, Inaba G. Double-masked trial of cyclosporin versus colchicines and long-term open study of cyclosporin in Behçet's disease. *Lancet* 1989;**1**:1093–6.
16. Yazici H, Pazarli H, Barnes CG *et al.* A controlled trial of azathioprine in Behçet's syndrome. *N Engl J Med* 1990;**322**:281–5.
17. de Vries J, Baarsma S, Zaal MJW *et al.* Cyclosporin in the treatment of severe chronic idiopathic uveitis. *Br J Ophthalmol* 1990;**74**:344–9.
18. Nussenblatt RB, Palestine AG, Chan CC, Stevens G Jr, Mellow SD, Green SB. Randomized, double-masked study of cyclosporine compared to prednisolone in the treatment of endogenous uveitis. *Am J Ophthalmol* 1991;**112**:138–46.
19. de Smet MD, Rubin BI, Whitcup SM, Lopez JS, Austin HA, Nussenblatt RB. Combined use of cyclosporine and ketoconazole in the treatment of endogenous uveitis. *Am J Ophthalmol* 1992;**113**:687–90.
20. Farber MD, Lam S, Tessler HH, Jennings TJ, Cross A, Rusin MM. Reduction of macular oedema by acetazolamide in patients with chronic iridocyclitis: a randomised prospective crossover study. *Br J Ophthalmol* 1994;**78**:4–7.
21. Whitcup SM, Csaky KG, Podgor MJ, Chew EY, Perry CH, Nussenblatt RB. A randomized, masked, cross-over trial of acetazolamide for cystoid macular edema in patients with uveitis. *Ophthalmology* 1996;**103**:1054–63.
22. Nussenblatt RB, Gery I, Weiner HL *et al.* Treatment of uveitis by oral administration of retinal antigens: results of a phase I/II randomized masked trial. *Am J Ophthalmol* 1997;**123**:583–92.

Table 26.1 Summary of 14 relevant RCTs

Paper	Inclusion criteria	Exclusion criteria	Power calculation?	How randomised?	No. of patients	Treatment protocol	Outcome measures	Follow up	Results	Statistical analysis	Authors' conclusions
James et al., 1967[10]	Histologically confirmed sarcoidosis with multi-system involvement	Received either trial drug or active treatment in previous 6 months	No	Not stated	84 (24 with ocular involvement)	Prednisolone or oxyphenbutazone v placebo	Not stated	6 months	Not given	Test not stated	Not given
Schlaegel and Weber, 1969[11]	All uveitis patients including those with a possible diagnosis of tuberculosis	None	No	Not stated	344	Isoniazid v placebo	An "improvement"	4 weeks	38 patients improved on isoniazid, 38 patients improved on placebo	Chi-square	Infectious tuberculosis is rarely a cause of endogenous uveitis
Abdalla and Bahgat, 1973[12]	Behçet's disease	Not stated	No	Not stated	14	Chlorambucil plus steroid v steroid	An "improvement" in signs of uveitis	40 months	Remission in all 4 patients with posterior uveitis in the chlorambucil group	Not done	Chlorambucil is beneficial
Aktulga et al., 1980[13]	Behçet's disease	Not stated	No	Not stated	35	Colchicine v placebo	An "improvement"	Not stated	3/8 placebo and 3/7 colchicine patients improved	Test not stated	No effect
Ben Ezra et al., 1988[14]	Behçet's disease	Any abnormal laboratory test	No	Selecting a sealed envelope at "random"	40	Ciclosporin v conventional treatment (17/20 steroid)	Visual acuity and "control" of inflammation	?24 months	Improvement in visual acuity on ciclosporin	Not done	Encouraging beneficial effect
Masuda et al., 1989[15]	Behçet's disease with acuity < 20/40 and = 2 episodes of ocular	Not stated	No	Not stated	96	Ciclosporin v colchicine	Frequency of ocular attacks, visual acuity, ocular signs	16 weeks	Significant reduction in frequency and severity of ocular	Chi-square	Ciclosporin more beneficial than colchicine

(Continued)

Table 26.1 (Continued)

Paper	Inclusion criteria	Exclusion criteria	Power calculation?	How randomised?	No. of patients	Treatment protocol	Outcome measures	Follow up	Results	Statistical analysis	Authors' conclusions
	inflammation during previous 16 weeks								attacks in ciclosporin group		
Yazici et al, 1990[16]	Behçet's disease – group 1: <40 years, duration of disease = 24 months and no uveitis; group 2: patients with uveitis	Irreversible, bilateral eye disease; unable to asess fundi; live more than 1 day's journey away; on immunosuppressives within the previous 3 months	No	Not stated	Group 1:25; group 2: 48	Azathioprine v placebo; systemic steroids allowed for exacerbations	Withdrawals due to eye disease; development of new eye disease; hyopyon uveitis; corticosteroid treatment; visual acuity	24 months	Azathioprine resulted in a statistically lower rate of withdrawal and higher rate of absence of eye disease, less hypoyon uveitis and less second eye involvement	Life tables; Fisher's exact test; t test	Azathioprine effective in controlling the progression of eye disease
de Vries et al, 1990[17]	Active idiopathic posterior, pan or intermediate uveitis; insufficient response to steroids; best corrected acuity of 0.5 or less in the better eye (except for patients with Behçet's disease). Also included patients with sarcoidosis and birdshot	Under 18 years; presumed infectious uveitis; end-stage disease with irreversible retinal damage; corneal or lens opacities limiting fundal view; contraindication to study medication; anticipated intra-ocular surgery during the study	No	Not stated	27	Ciclosporin and steroid v placebo and steroid	Visual acuity; inflammatory activity	12 months	Mean acuity and inflammatory activity same for both groups; initially patients fared better when on ciclosporin 10 mg/kg/day	Kaplan–Meier survival curves, Wilcoxon rank sum test	Ciclosporin has a place between corticosteroids and cytostatic agents in the treatment of severe, chronic idiopathic uveitis
Nussenblatt et al, 1991[18]	Intermediate posterior non-infectious uveitis =	Anticipated intra-ocular surgery during first 6 months	No	Not stated	56	Course A: ciclosporin v prednisolone. If failed at	Improvement in visual acuity of 15 letters or	12 months	Acuity or vitreal haze improved in 13/28	Test not stated	Systemic steroids should be considered

(Continued)

Table 26.1 (Continued)

Paper	Inclusion criteria	Exclusion criteria	Power calculation?	How randomised?	No. of patients	Treatment protocol	Outcome measures	Follow up	Results	Statistical analysis	Authors' conclusions
	10 years; active bilateral disease with acuity of = 20/40 in both eyes. Included patients with sarcoidosis, VKH and birdshot	of the study; on immunosuppressives for at least one month before entering the study; IDDM or uncontrolled hypertension; pregnancy				three months then assigned to Course B: swapped to prednisolone v ciclosporin. If failed at three months then assigned to Course C: ciclosporine and prednisolone	more in at least one eye; or improvement of at least two increments on the vitreal haze scoring scheme		(46%) in each group. Macular oedema resolved in 7/15 in ciclosporin group and in 10/16 in prednisolone group, which was not significant		the preferred treatment in the vast majority of patients, but ciclosporin is a logical possible alternative to steroids in those patients who are unable to continue steroid therapy
de Smet et al., 1992[19]	Endogenous uveitis (4 Behçet, 1 sarcoidosis, 5 intermediate) controlled with ciclosporin and prednisone	Not stated	No	Not stated	10	Cyclosporin and prednisone and ketoconazole v cyclosporin and prednisone and placebo	Number of flare ups	3 months	4/4 patients on ketaconozoled did not have a flare-up, while 4/6 on placebo had flare-ups	Not done	Addition of ketaconazole seemed to be effective in maintaining remission; further studies are needed
Farber et al., 1994[20]	Chronic idiopathic iridocyclitis; = 18 years old; cystoid macular oedema documented by fluorescein angiography; visual acuity of 20/40 to 20/200	History of liver or kidney disease; cardiovascular disease; chronic obstructive pulmonary disease; IDDM; abnormal electrolytes; hypersensitivity to sulfonamides; pregnancy;	No	Not stated	30	Acetazolamide v placebo, then washout period; then placebo v acetazolamide (crossover trial)	Visual acuity; vitreous fluorophotometry	28 days	No difference between the two groups. Mean acuity improved by 12% at 14 days and 14% at 28 days in the acetazolamide	Chi square; Fisher's exact test; Student's paired t-test	Acetazolamide appears to improve visual acuity, particularly in patients <55 years

(Continued)

Table 26.1 *(Continued)*

Paper	Inclusion criteria	Exclusion criteria	Power calculation?	How randomised?	No. of patients	Treatment protocol	Outcome measures	Follow up	Results	Statistical analysis	Authors' conclusions
		systemic or perocular steroid in the previous month							group as compared to 4% and 2% in the placebo group. Patients <55 years did better		
Whitcup et al., 1996[21]	Intermediate, posterior or panuveitis with visual acuity = 20/40 in at least one eye with cystoid macular oedema documented on fluorescein angiography; at least 8 years old; weight at least 35 kg; systemic therapy allowed	Patients receiving a carbonic anhydrase inhibitor; hypersensitivity to sulphonamides or acetazolamide or fluorescein; marked renal or hepatic dysfunction; abnormal electrolytes; hazy media due to cataract or vitreous opacity that would obscure fluorescein angiography; macular hole; choroidal neovascularisation	Yes	Generated from a random number chart in blocks of 6	40	Acetazolamide v placebo, then washout period; then placebo v acetazolamide (crossover trial)	Amount of cystoid macular oedema on fluorescein angiography; a 3 line (15 letter) or greater difference in visual acuity	28 days	Statistically significant decrease in macular oedema in the acetazolamide group. No period difference in the effect on visual acuity	Followed the approach of Senn (regressing the outcome variable on a treatment indicator adjusts for period effects). Subgroup analyses using regression models and Z tests	Although the overall treatment effect of aceatzolamide is small, there may be a role for this medication. Should expect only a short-term therapeutic benefit. Would recommend acetazolamide for chronic cystoid macular oedema in uveitis if other medications are ineffective

(Continued)

Table 26.1 *(Continued)*

Paper	Inclusion criteria	Exclusion criteria	Power calculation?	How randomised?	No. of patients	Treatment protocol	Outcome measures	Follow up	Results	Statistical analysis	Authors' conclusions
Nussenblatt et al, 1997[22]	Non-pregnant patients with intermediate and posterior uveitis; systemic therapy with one or more immunosuppressive agents; well-or moderately-controlled uveitis; cell-mediated immune response to retinal S antigen; included patients with Behçet's disease, sarcoidosis, VKH, birdshot, multifocal choroiditis, serpiginous choroidopathy	Infectious causes of uveitis; significant cardiac, haematological, hepatic or renal disease; other medical illnesses	No	Generated from a random number chart in blocks of 12	45	Four therapy groups; placebo; retinal mixture; retinal mixture and retinal S antigen; retinal S antigen	Primary end-point: a loss in either eye in the best corrected visual acuity of 10 letters or more; an increase in either eye in two grades of vitreous activity	12 months	Time to development of primary end-point was not statistically significantly different for any of the four treatment groups; group on retinal S antigen alone appeared to be tapered off their immunosuppressive medication more successfully than patients on placebo	Life-table analyses; Breslow generalised Wilcoxon statistic; Cox proportional hazards model	Suggest a trend and possible therapeutic effect in the use of retinal S antigen for the treatment of uveitis

VKH, Vogt-Koyanagi-Harada disease; IDDM, insulin dependent diabetes mellitus

27 Cytomegalovirus retinitis in patients with AIDS

Adnan Tufail

Background

Definition

Cytomegalovirus retinitis (CMV-R) is a necrotising retinitis caused by a double-stranded DNA virus that affects immunosuppressed or congenitally infected individuals.

Aetiology

Sight-threatening CMV disease only occurs in immuno-suppressed individuals. Following primary infection, CMV is disseminated by the blood stream to various organs. In immunosuppressed hosts, retinal infection can occur at the time of primary infection or after reactivation of latent CMV. Whether latent CMV exists in retinal cells remains to be clarified. It is assumed, however, that in patients with chronic infection the virus reaches the eye to cause CMV-R by haematogenous spread after reactivation elsewhere in the body.[1]

Infection with CMV is very common among the general population, but in most cases it does not cause clinically apparent disease. Cytomegalovirus is, however, a well-known cause of serious, even life-threatening, disease in immunosuppressed individuals, and in congenitally infected newborns.

All current specific treatments for CMV-R suppress CMV replication but do not eliminate the virus from the eye. Retinitis therefore eventually reactivates with lesion enlargement. Reactivation may be due to a number of factors, including inadequate drug delivery, resistant CMV strains and increasing immunosuppression.

Epidemiology in patients with AIDS

Cytomegalovirus retinitis is the most common ocular infection in patients with AIDS in the United States.[2–5] The reported prevalence of AIDS-related CMV-R, before the use of highly active antiretroviral therapy (HAART), varied from 4% of ambulatory patients (primarily intravenous drug abusers)[6] to 34% of eyes in an autopsy series of male homosexuals.[7] Cytomegalovirus retinitis is uncommon among African patients with AIDS, possibly due to death from other opportunistic infections before CMV disease can occur.[8]

With the introduction of HAART in the 1990s, there has been a fall in the incidence of CMV-R in the United States, and there is also a reducing proportion of Caucasian homosexual males of the total new presentations of CMV-R. In a study by Palella and associates they found that the incidence of cytomegalovirus retinitis declined from about 17 per 100 person-years to less than 4 per 100 person-years by mid 1997.[9]

Cytomegalovirus retinitis is reported less commonly among HIV-infected children than among HIV-infected adults.[10] Cytomegalovirus retinitis in HIV-infected children generally does not develop for several years after birth, which reflects its association with declining immune function. Although CMV-R has been reported in HIV-infected infants,[11–14] its occurrence at birth is not diagnostic of AIDS, since it may be a manifestation of congenital cytomegalic inclusion disease.

Prognosis

CMV-R results in relentless progression of disease resulting in expanding areas of retinal necrosis, unless treated by anti-CMV drugs or controlled by immune reconstitution. In the pre-HAART era, prognosis for retention of useful vision in patients with CMV-R was reasonable on treatment with anticytomegalovirus therapies. At six months after the start of intravenous (IV) ganciclovir (GCV) or foscarnet therapy, at least 88% of patients retained 6/12 or better vision in the better eye.[3] With the advent of HAART, maintenance anti-CMV medications may be stopped in individuals who develop immune reconstitution and, providing immune recovery is adequately maintained, the retinitis remains inactive. However, despite stable retinitis, vision may still be affected by immune-recovery uveitis. (Three of 14 patients lost more than three lines of vision in a study by Whitcup *et al*.[15])

The evidence

The types of studies included here are all randomised clinical controlled trials where anti-CMV-R treatments in AIDS patients were compared with respect to preventing progression of disease and all randomised controlled clinical trials where chronic maintenance therapy for CMV-R was discontinued after initiation of HAART.

There are no randomised controlled trials investigating the efficacy of intravitreal ganciclovir and foscarnet. No randomised controlled clinical trials have been published regarding discontinuation of CMV-R therapy after initiation of HAART. However, prospective non-randomised intervention trials have been published.[15] Detailed summaries of the randomised controlled trials are given in table 27.1, with general comments on individual drugs below.

Intravenous ganciclovir

Intravenous GCV has been shown in a small randomised trial[16] (n = 25, with 14 excluded) to be statistically significantly better in increasing time to progression of retinitis versus deferred therapy (42 *v* 16 days, *P* = 0·07). This study was carried out at a time when no other treatment was available and so suffers from the limitations of the study design and of a non-standard definition of progression. This study also introduced the now established treatment schedule of giving an initial high "induction" dose therapy for two to three weeks followed by a lower dose "maintenance" therapy to control clinically inactive retinitis. The efficacy of ganciclovir has been supported in other trials.[3]

Problems associated with intravenous therapy include those related to the drug itself, such as neutropenia, and those related to the mode of delivery, i.e. catheter-related sepsis.[17]

Oral ganciclovir

The studies evaluating the efficacy of oral GCV for therapy were carried out comparing it to IV GCV for maintenance only. Although the studies did not show any statistical difference in time to progression compared to IV

therapy (oral to IV, 50 *v* 63 days (*P* = 0·15),[17] 68 *v* 98 days (*P* = 0·63)[18] and 53 versus 66 days (*P* > 0·05),[19] there was a trend in all the studies for a longer mean time to progression in the IV group. This difference is more marked if medians and not mean times to progression are evaluated[18,19] and reaches statistical significance in one trial when clinical and not photographic end-points are evaluated.[19] Higher doses of oral GCV than the conventional 3 g/day may be more comparable in effect to IV GCV for maintenance therapy.[20] Oral GCV is therefore used only as a maintenance therapy for controlled disease and has the advantage over IV GCV of avoiding the need of a central line and its associated risk of sepsis (NNH = 11).[17]

Ganciclovir implant

Ganciclovir may be delivered by means of a sustained release device implanted surgically through the pars plana. This allows high constant levels of drug to be delivered to the treated eye but not to the rest of the body and therefore may not protect against CMV disease elsewhere. The GCV implant is significantly better at delaying median time to retinitis progression compared to both placebo (implant versus placebo, 226 *v* 15 days)[21] and IV GCV (implant versus IV, 221 *v* 71 days).[22] No difference was found in time to progression between two different implant release rates of GCV.[22] There is a higher rate of extraocular CMV disease and second eye involvement with CMV-R in patients on implant alone.[22] A trial to evaluate the combination of a GCV implant with oral GCV was underpowered and no clear conclusions can be drawn to see if oral GCV helps prevent the extraocular CMV disease associated with the use of implant alone.[23]

Prodrug valganciclovir

Valganciclovir is an orally administered prodrug that is hydrolysed to GCV. An oral dose of 900 mg achieves similar GCV blood levels as 5 mg/kg of IV GCV. In a study comparing oral valganciclovir to IV ganciclovir for untreated CMV-R no statistically significant difference was found in the median time to progression of the two treatments (oral versus IV 160 *v* 125 days).[24] The frequency of adverse events were similar between the two groups except that diarrhoea was more common in the oral group (NNH = 11) and catheter-related events were more common in the IV group (NNH = 20).[24]

Foscarnet

Intravenous foscarnet has been shown in a randomised trial[25] to be statistically significantly better in increasing time to progression of retinitis versus deferred therapy

Table 27.1 Trials of single systemic agents either in placebo controlled studies or in studies comparing different systemic routes of administration

Study name and reference	Study design, quality (all studies are RCTs unless otherwise stated)	Entry criteria/CD4 count (all studies on patients with AIDS and CMV-R)	Intervention	Outcome time to progression: primary outcome measure unless otherwise stated. (As measured by fundus photographic reading centre)	Side effects	(1) Systemic CMV treated/untreated (2) Quality of life assessment (measured using HIV-modified Medical Outcome Survey questionnaire)
Randomised prospective trial of ganciclovir maintenance therapy for cytomegalovirus retinitis[16]	25 patients randomised to immediate (n = 3) or deferred maintenance (n = 8) Note: 14 patients excluded from the analysis	**Exclusion:** hypersensitivity to GCV, on respirator, stage 3 or 4 coma	All patients received IV GCV induction 2·5 mg/kg tds. Then randomised to (1) maintenance 5 mg/kg 5 days/week or, (2) deferral of treatment to progression	Note: definition of progression different from other studies.* Median time to progression 42 days immediate treatment and 16 days deferred treatment (P = 0.07)	ANC significant change (P = 0.01) from onset of induction to nadir 1794 (± 531) cells/l to 1376 (± 473) cells/l	(1) Median survival 4·5 (± 1·3) months for immediate and 6 (± 1·1) months for deferred treatment (P = 0·9) (2) Not performed
A randomised controlled trial of foscarnet in the treatment of cytomegalovirus retinitis in patients with AIDS[25]	24 patients randomised to deferred treatment (n = 11) or FOS (n = 13)	**Entry:** untreated CMV-R outside zone 1, age = 18 to 60. **Exclusion:** low ANC, platelets, or Karnofsky score. High serum creatinine, systemic aciclovir use	FOS: 60 mg/kg tds induction for 21 days then 90 mg/kg/day adjusted for renal function or deferred untill progression	Median time to progression FOS 13·3 weeks v 3·2 weeks deferred group (P<0.001)	Electrolyte abnormalities with FOS v delayed therapy: creatinine >176·8, NNH = 4·3; magnesium <0·49, NNH 1·6; ANC <0·5 × 10⁹/l	(1) No mortality data (2) Not performed
IV v oral ganciclovir: European/ Australian comparative study of efficacy and safety in the prevention of cytomegalovirus retinitis recurrence in patients with AIDS[17]	Multi-centre RCT, 159 patients randomised 2:1 oral (n = 112): IV ganciclovir (n = 47)	**Entry:** age > 18, no progression after 2–3 weeks of IV GCV induction. **Exclusion:** >3 previous IV inductions of any drug to treat CMV, non-ocular CMV requiring treatment, low Karnofsky, ANC, platelet count, or CC, "significant" GI symptoms	All patients received 2–3 weeks induction of IV GCV (5 mg/kg bd) then randomised to either (1) oral GCV maintenance (500 mg × 6/day) or (2) IV GCV(5 mg/ kg od)	Time to progression oral median 41days (31–45), mean 50·8 (3·3); IV median 60 days (42–83), mean 63 (5·1). No statistical comparison of medians only means P = 0·15	No significant difference in adverse events. Except more infections at IV sites with IV group NNH = 11·1	(1) Only one event of systemic CMV in oral group (2) Not performed

(Continued)

Table 27.1 (*Continued*)

Study name and reference	Study design, quality (all studies are RCTs unless otherwise stated)	Entry criteria/CD4 count (all studies on patients with AIDS and CMV-R)	Intervention	Outcome time to progression: primary outcome measure unless otherwise stated. (As measured by fundus photographic reading centre)	Side effects	(1) Systemic CMV treated/untreated (2) Quality of life assessment (measured using HIV-modified Medical Outcome Survey questionnaire)
Oral ganciclovir as maintenance treatment for cytomegalovirus retinitis in patients with AIDS[18]	161 patients, of which 123 randomised to either oral GCV (n = 63), IV GCV (n = 60). 38 patients withdrawn before randomisation	**Entry:** CMV-R diagnosed within one month before entry. Age >13 years. **Exclusion:** Signs and symptoms of "serious GI disease", low ANC, platelet count, or creatinine	All patients induced with IV GCV 5 mg/kg bd for 14 days and then od for 7 days. If retinitis was stabilised then patient randomised to either (1) IV GCV 5 mg/kg od or (2) oral GCV 500 mg 6 times/day (= 3000 mg/day)	The median time to progression was 105 days (mean 96 days) for IV GCV and 48 days (68 days mean) for the oral group. IV progression oral:IV 1·08, based on means and not median data. $P = 0.63$, RR progression oral:IV 1·08, based on means and not median data	Neutropenia ($P = 0.17$), anaemia ($P = 0.02$, NNH = 5,99), and IV-catheter-related adverse events ($P = 0.006$, NNH = 2·78) were reported more frequently in the IV GCV group	(1) Median survival was 11 months in both groups (13 months mean) (2) Not performed
Oral ganciclovir for cytomegalovirus retinitis in patients with AIDS: results of two randomised studies[19]	220 patients randomised to maintenance therapy of either IV (n = 70), an oral GCV divided into either 6 daily (n = 74) or 3 daily (n = 76) doses. 20 week follow up	**Entry:** CMV-R that has responded to IV induction therapy, and not >4 months IV GCV **Exclusion:** Signs and symptoms of "serious GI disease"	All patients randomised to receive either IV GCV 5 mg/kg/d, oral GCV 500 mg 6 times daily or 1000 mg 3 times daily	Mean time to progression; (1) (photographic) was 66 days for IV GCV and 53 and 54 days for the oral GCV (500 mg ×6/day, and 1000mg ×3/day respectively) $P > 0.05$ (2) (clinical) (99:75:77 days IV:500mg:1000mg oral $P = 0.023$)	No significant differences in neutropenia but more catheter-related sepsis in the IV group	(1) No significant differences in mortality (2) Not performed
MSL–109 adjuvant therapy for CMV retinitis in patients with AIDS: the Monoclonal Antibody	209 patients randomised to MSL-109 (n = 104) and placebo (n = 105) and stratified on the	**Entry:** active CMV-R **Exclusion:** non-ocular CMV requiring treatment, low Karnofsky score	Previous treatment with GCV, FOS, or GCV-implant was permitted. The patients were then randomised to	No effect on retinitis progression (median time to progression MSL-109: placebo was 67:65 days)	No significant difference in any laboratory measures of toxicity	Mortality rate in the MSL-109 group was 0·68/person-year, and in the placebo group, 0·31/person-year ($P = 0.01$)

(*Continued*)

Table 27.1 (Continued)

Study name and reference	Study design, quality (all studies are RCTs unless otherwise stated)	Entry criteria/CD4 count (all studies on patients with AIDS and CMV-R)	Intervention	Outcome time to progression: primary outcome measure unless otherwise stated. (As measured by fundus photographic reading centre)	Side effects	(1) Systemic CMV treated/untreated (2) Quality of life assessment (measured using HIV-modified Medical Outcome Survey questionnaire)
Cytomegalovirus Retinitis Trial[41]	basis of whether newly diagnosed or relapsed retinitis was present		receive additional MSL-109 or placebo 60 mg IV infusion every 2 weeks			(2) "No substantial difference"
Parenteral cidofovir for cytomegalovirus retinitis in patients with AIDS: the HPMPC peripheral cytomegalovirus retinitis trial[28,29]	Multi-centre RCT unmasked, Stage 1: patients randomised (n = 29) 1:1 to deferred treatment: low dose CDV Stage 2: patients randomised (n = 35) 1:1:1 deferred: low dose: high dose CDV	**Entry:** untreated zone 2/3 CMV-R, CMV-R < 25% retinal area **Exclusion:** non-ocular CMV requiring treatment, cardiac disease, allergy to probenecid, nephrotoxic drug use, renal or cardiac disease. Low Karnofsky score, ANC, platelet count, or Hb. High creatinine, proteinuria >1+.	Either (1) deferred treatment until CMV-R progresses Or (2) IV CDV with 4 g of oral probenecid CDV 5 mg/kg once a week for 2 weeks induction followed by either low dose 3 mg/kg or high dose 5 mg/kg maintenance every 2 weeks	Median time to progression was 64 days (low dose CDV group) and 21 days (deferral group) ($P = 0.052$). The median time to progression was not reached in the high dose group but was 20 days in the deferral group ($P = 0.009$)	Rates (per person-year) of (1) 2+ proteinuria, 2.6 deferred, 2.8 low dose ($P > 0.2$) and 6.8 high dose ($P = 0.135$), (2) Neutropenia, and creatinine, no significant change, (3) ocular hypotony, 0.7 deferred, 0.1 low ($P = 0.25$), and 0.3 high ($P = 0.99$).	(1) Mortality rates were similar among all 3 groups, low dose: deferral = 0.34:0.37 per person-years ($P > 0.2$) and deferral:high-dose 0.24:0.60 per person-years. (2) Not performed

(Continued)

Table 27.1 *(Continued)*

Study name and reference	Study design, quality (all studies are RCTs unless otherwise stated)	Entry criteria/CD4 count (all studies on patients with AIDS and CMV-R)	Intervention	Outcome time to progression: primary outcome measure unless otherwise stated. (As measured by fundus photographic reading centre)	Side effects	(1) Systemic CMV treated/untreated (2) Quality of life assessment (measured using HIV-modified Medical Outcome Survey questionnaire)
Intravenous cidofovir for periphera cytomegalovirus retinitis in patients with AIDS. A randomised, controlled trial[30]	48 patients randomised to deferred treatment ($n=23$) or immediate treatment ($n=25$)	**Entry:** Previously untreated zone 2/3 CMV-R, CMV-R <25% retinal area, age 13–60. **Exclusion:** non-ocular CMV requiring treatment, allergy to probenecid, low Karnofsky score, ANC, or platelet count. High serum creatinine, or proteinuria >1+	Either (1) deferred treatment until CMV-R progresses or (2) IV CDV with 4 g of oral probenecid CDV 5 mg/kg once a week for 2 weeks induction followed by 5 mg/kg maintenance every 2 weeks	Median time to progression was 22 days (95% CI, 10–27 days) in the deferral group and 120 days (95% CI, 40–134 days) ($P=0.001$)	Any reaction to probenecid NNH =1·8. Proteinuria (5/41 of patients, 12%), neutropenia (6/41 of patients, 15%), elevated creatinine (2/41 of patients, 5%)	(1) Median survival 10·5% in the deferred and 13·5 months in the immediate treatment groups ($P=0.15$). (2) Not performed

*progression defined as a lesion increasing by 2 disc diameters in size, new lesion, crossed a major vessel, or entered a new sector.

Abbreviations: AZT, zidovudine; AIDS , based on the surveillance case definition adopted by the Centers for Disease Control in 1997; ANC, absolute neutrophil count; AAT, alanine aminotransferase; bd, twice a day; CC, creatinine clearance; CDV, cidofovir; CI, confidence interval; CMV-R, cytomegalovirus retinitis; FOS, foscarnet; GI, gastrointestinal; GCV, ganciclovir; HAART, highly active antiretroviral therapy; IV, intravenous; NNT, numbers needed to treat; NNH, numbers needed to harm; od, once a day; RCT, randomised controlled trial; RD, retinal detachment; RR, relative risk; tds, three times a day; VA, visual acuity.

Table 27.2 Comparative trials between different systemic therapies or doses

Study name and reference	Study design, quality (all studies RCTs unless otherwise stated)	Entry criteria/CD4 count (all studies on patients with AIDS and CMV-R)	Intervention	Outcome time to progression: primary outcome measure unless otherwise stated. (As measured by fundus photographic reading centre)	Side effects	(1) Systemic CMV treated/untreated (2) Quality of life assessment (measured using HIV-modified Medical Outcome Survey questionnaire)
Foscarnet-Ganciclovir Cytomegalovirus Retinitis Trial[26,27,34–38]	234 patients randomised to GCV (n = 127) or FOS (n = 107). Stratified randomisation: strata 1 = zone 1 or lesion >25% of retina (randomised to GCV or FOS 1:1), strata 2 = zone 2/3 and <25% of retinal involvement. Patients given 3 options: immediate treatment (GCV:FOS 1:1); deferred treatment until progression then GCV or FOS 1:1; or random assignment.	**Entry:** previously untreated CMV-R, age > 13. **Exclusion:** low ANC, high serum creatinine. AZT contraindicated during GCV induction	FOS: 60 mg/kg tds induction for 14 days then 90 mg/kg/day adjusted for renal function GCV: 5mg/kg bd induction for 14 days then 5 mg/kg/day adjusted for renal function. Treatment switched if poor control	Median time to progression GCV 56 days and 59 days FOS (P=0·685)	No significant difference in catheter infections, opportunistic infections or retinal detachment. Significant differences in ANC (FOS v GCV 0·72 v 1·3 /person-year), serum creatinine >260 mol/l (FOS v GCV 0·30 v 0·12/person-year), and number of treatment switches (FOS v GCV 36% v 11%)	(1) Mortality higher in GCV treated group. 51% v 34%, NNH=5·8 for an excess death on GCV relative to FOS. Median survival 8·5 months GCV v 12·6 months FOS (2) Not performed
Combination foscarnet and ganciclovir therapy v monotherapy for the treatment of relapsed cytomegalovirus retinitis in patients with AIDS[39]	279 patients randomised to FOS (n=89), GCV (n=94) or FOS and GCV (n=96). Note once progression of retinitis occurred a specific protocol given to decide the subsequent drugs and doses[39]	**Entry:** active CMV-R despite at least 28 days treatment with either FOS or GCV in the last 28 days. **Exclusion:** Low Karnofsky score, ANC, platelet count, or high serum creatinine. "Significant" GI symptoms	Initial therapy one of 3 options: (1) FOS 90 mg/kg bd for 14 days induction then 120 mg/kg day maintenance; (2) GCV 5 mg/kg bd induction for 14 days then 10 mg/kg/day maintenance; (3) combination therapy,	Median times to retinitis progression were as follows: FOS, 1·3 months; GCV 2 months; and combination therapy group 4·3 months (P<0·001) Rates of visual field loss: FOS, 28° per month; GCV 18° per month; and	Morbidity rates showed no significant difference between the 3 groups for the following measures, Hb, ANC, platelet count, creatinine, and opportunistic infection rate.	(1) Median survival times, FOS 8·4; GCV 9·2; and FOS+GCV 8·6 months (P=0·89). Prior therapy with GCV v FOS before enrolment on trial adjusted RR for mortality 1·44 (95% CI 1

(Continued)

Table 27.2 *(Continued)*

Study name and reference	Study design, quality (all studies RCTs unless otherwise stated)	Entry criteria/CD4 count (all studies on patients with AIDS and CMV-R)	Intervention	Outcome time to progression: primary outcome measure unless otherwise stated. (As measured by fundus photographic reading centre)	Side effects	(1) Systemic CMV treated/untreated (2) Quality of life assessment (measured using HIV-modified Medical Outcome Survey questionnaire)
			induce with drug not on at study start (at doses as above) and continue with maintenance therapy doses of current drug for 14 days then IV FOS 90 mg/kg/day and GCV 5 mg/kg/day	combination therapy group 16° per month (P<0·04).		2·09, P=0·05) (2) The mean adjusted treatment impact scores (FOS, −4; GCV −1; FOS+GCV −9·8 (P=0·03)). The mean adjusted changes in quality-of-life scores (FOS, −7; GCV −3·6; FOS+GCV −7·4 (P=0·21))
Cytomegalovirus retinitis in AIDS patients: a comparative study of IV and oral ganciclovir as maintenance therapy[40]	Randomised to either oral GCV or IV GCV	Entry: CMV-R diagnosed within one month before entry. Age >13 years Exclusion: Signs and symptoms of "serious GI disease". Low ANC, platelet count, or, creatinine clearance	All patients induced with IV GCV 5 mg/kg bd for 14 days and then 5 mg/kg od for 7 days. If retinitis was stabilised then the patient was randomised to either (1) IV GCV 5 mg/kg od or (2) oral GCV 3000 mg/day	The mean time to progression was 61 days for IV GCV and 51 days for the oral group P=0·15	IV-catheter-related adverse events (NNH = 18) were reported more frequently in the IV GCV group	(1) Median survival was 11 months in both groups (13 months mean) (2) Not performed
Randomised, controlled study of the safety and efficacy of IV cidofovir for the treatment of relapsing	150 patients randomised to CDV low dose or CDV high dose.	Entry: persistently active CMV-R not responding to FOS or GCV. Age 13–60 years, males or non-pregnant females.	IV CDV with 4 g of oral probenecid. CDV 5mg/kg once a week for 2 weeks induction followed by either low dose 3 mg/kg or high dose 5 mg/kg	The median times to progression (1) high dose group, not reached in the (less than 50% progressed, 95% CI 115- upper limit not	Nephrotoxicity 5 mg:3 mg, 25:11%, proteinuria 47%:31%, decreased intraocular pressure 9:12%	(1) Median survival 5·9 months in the high dose and 4·9 months in the low dose group (P=0·17) (2) Not performed

(Continued)

Table 27.2 *(Continued)*

Study name and reference	Study design, quality (all studies RCTs unless otherwise stated)	Entry criteria/CD4 count (all studies on patients with AIDS and CMV-R)	Intervention	Outcome time to progression: primary outcome measure unless otherwise stated. (As measured by fundus photographic reading centre)	Side effects	(1) Systemic CMV treated/untreated (2) Quality of life assessment (measured using HIV-modified Medical Outcome Survey questionnaire)
cytomegalovirus retinitis in patients with AIDS[31]		Exclusion: Unrepaired retinal detachment, allergy to probenecid, nephrotoxic drug use, renal or cardiac disease, low Karnofsky score, ANC, or platelet count, or high serum creatinine	maintenance every 2 weeks	reached), (2) low dose group 49 days (95% CI, 35–52 days) $P=0.0006$. RR of progression 3 mg: 5 mg group 1·91(95% CI, 0·7–5·3)		
High dose oral ganciclovir treatment for cytomegalovirus retinitis[20]	281 patients randomised to 3 ($n=74$), 4·5 ($n=63$) or 6 g/day ($n=67$) oral , or IV GCV ($n=57$). 16 patients withdrew after randomisation but before treatment	Entry: stable CMV-R after at least 4 weeks of IV GCV, age>13, Exclusion: > 2 episodes of CMV-R progression. Low Karnofsky, ANC, platelet count, or creatinine clearance	Oral GCV either 3, 4·5, or 6 mg/kg/day or IV GCV 5 mg/kg/day. If progressed by reading centre criteria-induced IV GCV 5 mg/kg bd. Patients withdrawn at second progression. No patient on HAART	Median days to progression 3, 4, 5, 6 g/day oral v 5mg/kg/day IV are 42 (32–52), 50(33–84), 57(44–73) and 70 (43–88) respectively. ($P=0.052$) for 3 g v IV logrank	Sepsis more common in IV group ($n=12/57$)	(1) Incidence of extraocular CMV disease "less than 3%" in all groups. Median survival 335,378,368, and 33 days for 3, 4·5, 6 mg/kg/day and IV groups respectively (2) Not performed
A controlled trial of valganciclovir as induction therapy for cytomegalovirus retinitis[24]	160 patients randomised to oral valganciclovir ($n=80$) or IV GCV ($n=80$)	Entry: previously untreated CMV-R outside 1500 microns from fovea (first 43 patients enrolled only). Exclusion: systemic anti-CMV therapy for > 3weeks or within last 3 months. Low Karnofsky score, ANC, platelet count, or creatinine clearance. Severe uncontrolled diarrhoea	Intravenous therapy GCV 5 mg/kg/day for 3 weeks (induction) followed by 5 mg/kg (maintenance) or oral valganciclovir 900 mg/twice a day for 3 weeks (induction) followed by 900 mg/day (maintenance)	Median time to progression IV:oral 125 days (95% CI 74 to undetermined): oral 160 days (95% CI 99 to undetermined). Relative risk oral:IV 0·90 (95% CI 0·58 – 1·38). Progression in first 4 weeks IV:oral 7/70:7/71 (difference 0·1%)	Adverse events oral v IV: diarrhoea (19 v 10%, NNH 11, $P=0.11$), catheter-related events 4 v 9% (no P value given). Frequency and severity of other adverse events similar between the 2 groups, neutropenia 13:14%	(1) One death in each group (2) Not performed

For abbreviations see Table 27.1.

Table 27.3 Local therapy trials

Study name and reference	Study design, quality (all studies RCTs unless otherwise stated)	Entry criteria/CD4 count (all studies on patients with AIDS and CMV-R)	Intervention	Outcome time to progression: primary outcome measure unless otherwise stated. (As measured by fundus photographic reading centre)	Side effects	(1) Systemic CMV treated/untreated (2) Quality of life assessment (measured using HIV-modified Medical Outcome Survey questionnaire)
Treatment of cytomegalovirus retinitis with an intraocular sustained-release ganciclovir implant. A randomised controlled clinical trial[21]	30 eyes of 24 patients randomised to deferred treatment (n = 16) or immediate treatment (n = 14). If unilateral disease randomised 1:1, if the contralateral eye developed CMV-R later patient given choice of treatment. If bilateral CMV-R then one eye randomised to immediate and the other to deferred	Entry: previously untreated CMV-R outside zone 1 but posterior to globe equator, age > 18 and < 60 Exclusion: low Karnofsky score, or platelet count, and the ability to undergo local eye surgery	1 microgram/h release rate ganciclovir implant, surgically placed through a pars plana wound, immediately or deferred until progression. The original trial design had an arm with implant 2 microgram/h release rate that was dropped after enrolling 2 patients for logistical reasons	Median time to progression 15 days (range 14–39) deferred treatment group and 226 days for immediate treatment (range–only 5 eyes progressed during the follow up period), of which 4/5 were reimplanted which resulted in decreased CMV-R activity in ¾.	Secondary endpoints, time to develop: (1) visceral CMV disease (95% CI, 248 to undetermined, 8/26 study patients.) (2) CMV-R in fellow eye (median 203 days, 95% CI undetermined, 14/21 study patients). Ocular morbidity (implant group: RD in 7/51 procedures, transient drop in VA in "most patients"	(1) Time to death, median 295 days (CI not given) in implant group, separate data for deferred group not given. (2) Not performed
Treatment of cytomegalovirus retinitis with a sustained-release ganciclovir implant[22]	Multi-centre, randomised, unmasked trial of 188 patients randomised to 3 groups IV GCV (n = 56), low dose implant (n = 62), and high dose implant (n = 55)	Entry: AIDS and previously untreated CMV-R, age > 18, HIV infection and CMV-R, vision better than 20/200 Exclusion: Karnofsky score < 60, platelet count < 25 × 10⁹/1, and ANC < 500 cells/mm³	Either 1 microgram/h or 2 microgram/h release rate GCV implant, surgically placed through a pars plana wound, immediately or given IV GCV 5 mg/kg bd induction followed by IV 5 mg/kg/day	Median times to progression: (1) 1 microgram/h group 221 days (95% CI, range 181 to unknown, (2) 2 microgram/h group 191 days (95% CI, range 51–96), (3) IV GCV group 71 days (95% CI, range 51–96). Not significant between implant groups (P = 0·63)	Secondary endpoints, 25-percentile time to develop visceral CMV disease 87 days implant, 119 days IV GCV (P = 0·28). Time to develop CMV-R in contralateral eye IV: implant 0·5 (95% CI, 0·2–1·4)	(1) Time to death, median 295 days (CI not given) in implant group, separate data for deferred group not given (2) Not performed

(Continued)

Table 27.3 (Continued)

Study name and reference	Study design, quality (all studies RCTs unless otherwise stated)	Entry criteria/CD4 count (all studies on patients with AIDS and CMV-R)	Intervention	Outcome time to progression: primary outcome measure unless otherwise stated. (As measured by fundus photographic reading centre)	Side effects	(1) Systemic CMV treated/untreated (2) Quality of life assessment (measured using HIV-modified Medical Outcome Survey questionnaire)
The ganciclovir implant plus oral ganciclovir v parenteral cidofovir for the treatment of cytomegalovirus retinitis in patients with acquired immunodeficiency syndrome[23]	61 patients stratified into two groups: (1) newly diagnosed CMV-R; (2) relapsed CMV-R and randomised to either oral and implant GCV (n=31) or IV cidofovir (n=30)	**Exclusion:** Low Karnofsky score, ANC, or platelet count. High serum creatinine, or proteinuria >2+ Note: trial unable to reach full recruitment due to the advent of HAART	Either (1) Oral GCV 1 g tds and GCV implant (n=31) or (2) IV cidofovir, 5 mg/kg once a week followed by 5 mg/kg every other week Note: study underpowered, interpret results with caution	Retinitis progression in GCV group 0·67 per person-year and 0·71 in the CDV group (P=0·72). Loss of VA of 15 letters or more in GCV group 0·78/person-year and 0·47 in the CDV group (P=0·28)	Significant increase in vitreous haemorrhage in GCV group (P=0·014), uveitis more common in the CDV group (P=0·066). No significant difference between the 2 groups in extraocular CMV disease rate	(1) No mortality data (2) No significant difference in general health and vision scores, but both the mental health and energy suggested significant benefit for cidofovir (P=0·01 mental health, P=0·07 energy)
Randomised controlled trial of IV fomiversen for treatment of newly diagnosed peripheral CMV-R in patients with AIDS[42]	29 patients randomised to either immediate treatment (n=18), or deferred treatment (n=10). One immediate treatment patient did not return for follow up after the initial dose	**Entry:** stable peripheral (750μm outside zone (1) CMV-R, age >18, male or non-pregnant female **Exclusion:** Karnofsky score <70, external ocular infection, presence of non-CMV-R, retinal detachment (treated or untreated)	Intravitreous inject on of 165 micrograms fomiversen 0·05 ml. Injections given at day 1, 8, and 15 for induction then alternate weeks maintenance. Note: initial dose of 330 micrograms stopped after 10 patients, as 2 reported peripheral vision loss	Median time to progression 71 days (95% CI 28 days – not determined) for immediate treatment and 13 days (95% CI 9–15 days) for deferred treatment. Difference remained significant after adjusting for the baseline HAART use	No retinal detachment among treated eyes. Ocular adverse events >4 events reported: AC inflammation 0·48/patient-year, increased IOP 0·24/patient-year. NNH not calculable	(1) Not reported (2) Not performed

(Continued)

Table 27.3 *(Continued)*

Study name and reference	Study design, quality (all studies RCTs unless otherwise stated)	Entry criteria/CD4 count (all studies on patients with AIDS and CMV-R)	Intervention	Outcome. time to progression: primary outcome measure unless otherwise stated. As measured by fundus photographic reading centre	Side effects	(1) Systemic CMV treated/untreated (2) Quality of life assessment (measured using HIV-modified Medical Outcome Survey questionnaire)
Randomised dose-comparison studies of IV fomiversen of CMV-R that has reactivated or is persistently active despite other therapies in patients with AIDS[11]	Two multi-centre (USA/Brazilian studies; EuroCanadian study) RCT unmasked, 61 patients randomised in total to either regimen A (n = 61 patients, 67 eyes), or regimen B (n = 32 patients, 39 eyes)	**Entry:** previously treated (with either GCV, FOS, or CDV) CMV-R involving zone 1 or >25% retinal area, age >18, male or non-pregnant female **Exclusion:** Karnofsky score <70, external ocular infection, presence of non-CMV-R, retinal detachment (treated or untreated)	Two regimens of intravitreous fomiversen 330 micrograms/ injection. Regimen A: 3-weekly injections at induction followed by alternate week treatment. Regimen B: injections at day 1 and 15 at induction followed by treatment every 4 weeks	USA/Brazilian study median time to progression 106 days regimen A and 267 days regimen B ($P=0.218$); EuroCanadian study median time to progression not determinable (only 4 patients progressed) regimen A and 403 days regimen B ($P=0.218$)	Main ocular adverse events reported (regimen A/B), anterior uveitis 0·85/0·26/patient-year (pt-yr), vitritis 0·5/0·20 per pt-yr, increased IOP 0·24/0·36 per pt-yr, retinal oedema 0·32/0·15 per pt-yr, vitreous haemorrhage 0·18/0·05 per pt-yr, ocular pain 0·46/0·31 per pt-yr	(1) Not reported (2) Not performed

(13.3 *v* 3·2 weeks, *P* = 0·004). Foscarnet use in this study was associated with renal (NNH = 4·3) and electrolyte abnormalities (NNH = 1·6). No statistically significant difference was found in a study comparing the efficacy of foscarnet to IV GCV (median time to progression foscarnet:GCV 59:56 days, *P* = 0·69).[26] However, mortality was higher in the GCV treated group, with median survival for GCV:foscarnet being 8·5:12·6 months.[27]

Cidofovir

Intravenous cidofovir has been shown in two randomised trials[28,29] to be statistically significantly better at increasing median time to progression of previously untreated retinitis versus deferred therapy (64 days *v* 21 days, *P* = 0·05[28] and 120 *v* 22 days, *P* = 0·001[30]). In patients who have persistently active CMV-R not responding to foscarnet or GCV cidofovir, high dose (5 mg/kg) was more effective than low dose cidofovir (3 mg/kg)[31] but was associated with more side effects such as nephrotoxicity. The major dose-limiting effect of cidofovir is nephrotoxicity, but the drug may also cause ocular hypotony and uveitis. Concomitant administration of probenecid reduces nephrotoxicity.

Fomiversen

Fomiversen is an antisense oligonucleotide which has anti-CMV activity and is delivered by intravitreous injection. Fomiversen (at 165 micrograms/injection) has been shown in a randomised trial to be statistically significantly better at increasing median time to progression of previously untreated retinitis versus deferred therapy (71 days *v* 13 days, *P* = 0·0001). In patients who have persistently active CMV-R not responding to other therapies, fomiversen 330 micrograms/injection had a similar effect at delaying progression both at intense and less intense treatment frequencies. Ocular side effects included anterior uveitis, raised ocular pressure and a retinal pigment epitheliopathy.

Answering the questions posed

In HIV-infected people with CMV-R does anti-CMV therapy reduce the risk of loss of vision?

The evidence

As the majority of trials involve the proxy measure of "progression of retinitis" rather than change in vision as the study end-point, specific comments regarding a particular therapy with respect to vision loss cannot be made in the majority of trials. There is an assumption that slowing progression of retinitis will prevent vision loss. However, some trials do address this issue (foscarnet-ganciclovir CMV-R trial).[32] This trial showed that retinal detachment was a major cause of visual loss with a risk of 18·9% at 6 months (95% CI 14–23·8%) and 39% at one year,[32] not just progression of retinopathy. It should be noted that certain interventions might themselves affect vision, by the complications of the surgical procedure itself (for example, ganciclovir implants or intravitreal injections) or by precipitating uveitis (for example, cidofovir).

In HIV-infected people with CMV-R what is the most effective anti-CMV therapy for primary treatment and re-treatment?

The evidence

Primary treatment

Foscarnet, ganciclovir (given as implant, prodrug or IV form), cidofovir and fomiversen are all significantly better than placebo at controlling progression of retinitis. MSL-109 adjuvant therapy has no effect on progression compared to placebo. Foscarnet and IV ganciclovir are equally effective. Valganciclovir is as effective as IV ganciclovir at delaying progression of retinitis. The ganciclovir implant is significantly better than IV ganciclovir at delaying progression of retinitis. Comparisons between other drugs cannot be made using times to progression alone, as the effect of different background antiretroviral treatment cannot be controlled for. There are no randomised controlled trials investigating the efficacy of intravitreal ganciclovir and foscarnet, and no comment has been made regarding these therapies.

Maintenance therapy

Foscarnet, ganciclovir (given as implant, oral, prodrug or IV form), cidofovir, and fomiversen are all significantly better than placebo at controlling retinitis progression. Comparisons between other drugs cannot be made using times to progression alone, as the effect of different background antiretroviral treatment cannot be controlled for, except when a specific trial addressed this issue. Trials designed to compare maintenance therapies showed that oral versus IV ganciclovir comparison in three trials showed no significant difference in time to progression. There was a trend, however, in all the trials of a longer time to progression in the IV group, and in one study there was a significant difference in the clinical but not the photographic mean time to progression.[19] In the oral versus IV studies, the mean and not the more usual median time to progression was used for analysis and this may mask real difference in efficacy between the groups. In the setting of patients receiving HAART, the ganciclovir implant plus oral drug and IV cidofovir have similar efficacy at controlling CMV-R progression (although this study was underpowered).

In HIV-infected people with CMV-R does the use of highly active anti-retroviral combination therapy reduce the risk of loss of vision?

The evidence

No randomised controlled trails are available. However non-randomised interventional studies suggest that anti-CMV medications may be stopped in patients with stable CMV-R and elevated CD4+ T-lymphocyte counts.[15]

Summary

Currently there is no antiviral regimen that can completely prevent progression of disease unless a certain level of immune reconstitution has been achieved. Available treatments that are significantly better than placebo at controlling retinitis at induction are ganciclovir (IV, oral, prodrug and implant forms), IV foscarnet, IV cidofovir and intravitreal fomiversen. Maintenance therapies shown to be efficacious compared to placebo include ganciclovir (oral, IV and implant), IV foscarnet, IV cidofovir and intravitreal fomiversen. Comparative studies between drugs are limited; comparisons between times to progression from different studies should be viewed with great caution due to variation in both the study populations and the antiretroviral therapy in different studies. Comparative studies have shown similar efficacy in delaying progression of retinitis for IV ganciclovir and foscarnet, IV ganciclovir and oral valganciclovir for induction of treatment, and oral and IV ganciclovir for maintenance of stable retinitis. The ganciclovir implant is more effective at delaying progression than IV ganciclovir, and a combination of foscarnet and ganciclovir is more effective than each drug alone in treating relapsed retinitis.

Implications for research

Currently, information is lacking on comparative studies between different combinations of systemic treatments and local treatments. Future studies should utilise measures of quality of life outcomes, as well as time to loss of vision and progression in their analyses. Studies are required to better understand when anti-CMV therapy may be stopped after commencement of HAART and why, after a good response to HAART, some patients develop immune reconstitution uveitis or develop reactivation of CMV-R.

Implications for practice

Given the relative lack of comparative studies choice of treatment currently needs to take into account the side effect profile, the therapeutic regimen, quality of life, the presence or absence of extraocular CMV disease (as local therapy to the eye is not effective at treating systemic disease) and previous treatment (resistance may develop). Relatively few studies have made use of quality of life data (as treatment regimens themselves may affect this) or visual acuity outcome. Most studies use the proxy measurement of effect, "progression".

In the available studies there are no randomised trials looking at the effect of HAART on control of CMV-R although non-randomised interventional studies and "expert-opinion" groups have suggested that anti-CMV therapy may be stopped once CD4+ T-cell count is above $150 \text{ cells} \times 10^6/l$ for six months.[33] Occasional cases of new CMV-R have been reported in case series on patients that fulfil these parameters (one in 60 patients in a series by Song *et al.*[43]).

References

1. Holland GN, Tufail A, Jordan MC. Cytomegalovirus disease. In: Pepose JS, Holland GN, Wilhelmus KR, eds. *Ocular Infection and Immunity.* St. Louis: Mosby-Year Book Inc, 1995, pp. 1088–129.
2. Holland GN, Pepose JS, Pettit TH, Yee RD, Foos RY. Acquired immune deficiency syndrome. Ocular manifestations. *Ophthalmology* 1983;**90**:859–73.
3. Studies of Ocular Complications of AIDS (SOCA) Research Group in collaboration with the AIDS Clinical Trials Group (ACTG). Forscarnet-ganciclovir cytomegalovirus retinitis trial: IV. Visual outcomes. *Ophthalmology* 1994;**7**:1250–61.
4. Jabs DA, Green WR, Fox R, Polk BF, Bartlett JG. Ocular manifestations of the aquired immune deficiency syndrome. *Ophthalmology* 1989;**96**:1092–9.
5. Schuman JS, Orellana J, Friedman AH, Teich SA. Aquired immunodeficiency syndrome (AIDS). *Surv Ophthalmol* 1987;**31**:384–410.
6. Rosenberg PR, Uliss AE, Friedland GH, Harris CA, Small CB, Klein RS. Acquired immunodeficiency syndrome. Ophthalmic manifestations in ambulatory patients. *Ophthalmology* 1983;**90**:874–8.
7. Pepose JS, Holland GN, Nestor MS, Cochran AJ, Foos RY. Acquired immune deficiency syndrome. Pathogenic mechanisms of ocular disease. *Ophthalmology* 1985;**92**:472–84.
8. Kestelyn P. Ocular problems in AIDS. *Int Ophthalmol* 1990;**14**:165–72.
9. Palella FJ, Delaney KM, Moorman AC *et al.* Declining morbidity and mortality among patients with advanced human immunodeficiency virus infection. *N Engl J Med* 1998;**338**:853–60.
10. Dennehy PJ, Warman R, Flynn JT, Scott GB, Mastrucci MT. Ocular manifestations in pediatric patients with acquired immunodeficiency syndrome. *Arch Ophthalmol* 1989;**107**:978–82.
11. Randomized dose-comparison studies of intravitreous fomivirsen for treatment of cytomegalovirus retinitis that has reactivated or is persistently active despite other therapies in patients with AIDS. *Am J Ophthalmol* 2002;**133**:475–83.
12. Jonckheer T, de Selys A, Pierre C *et al.* [Retinitis in an infant infected with HIV] Retinite chez un nourrisson infecte par le VIH. *Arch Fr Pediatr* 1990;**47**:585–6.

13. Levin AV, Zeichner S, Duker JS, Starr SE, Augsburger JJ, Kronwith S. Cytomegalovirus retinitis in an infant with acquired immunodeficiency syndrome. *Pediatrics* 1989;**84**:683–7.
14. Salvador F, Blanco R, Colin A, Galan A, Gil-Gibernau JJ. Cytomegalovirus retinitis in pediatric acquired immunodeficiency syndrome: report of two cases. *J Pediatr Ophthalmol Strabismus* 1993;**30**:159–62.
15. Whitcup SM, Fortin E, Lindblad AS *et al*. Discontinuation of anticytomegalovirus therapy in patients with HIV infection and cytomegalovirus retinitis. *JAMA* 1999;**282**:1633–7.
16. Jacobson MA, O'Donnell JJ, Brodie HR, Wofsy C, Mills J. Randomized prospective trial of ganciclovir maintenance therapy for cytomegalovirus retinitis. *J Med Virol* 1988;**25**:339–49.
17. The Oral Ganciclovir European and Australian Cooperative Study Group. Intravenous versus oral ganciclovir: European/Australian comparative study of efficacy and safety in the prevention of cytomegalovirus retinitis recurrence in patients with AIDS. *AIDS* 1995;**9**:471–7.
18. Drew WL, Ives D, Lalezari JP *et al*. Oral ganciclovir as maintenance treatment for cytomegalovirus retinitis in patients with AIDS. Syntex Cooperative Oral Ganciclovir Study Group. *N Engl J Med* 1995;**333**:615–20.
19. Squires KE. Oral ganciclovir for cytomegalovirus retinitis in patients with AIDS: results of two randomized studies. *AIDS* 1996;**10**(Suppl 4):S13–S18.
20. Lalezari JP, Friedberg DN, Bissett J *et al*. High dose oral ganciclovir treatment for cytomegalovirus retinitis. *J Clin Virol* 2002;**24**:67–77.
21. Martin DF, Parks DJ, Mellow SD *et al*. Treatment of cytomegalovirus retinitis with an intraocular sustained-release ganciclovir implant. A randomized controlled clinical trial. *Arch Ophthalmol* 1994;**112**:1531–9.
22. Musch DC, Martin DF, Gordon JF, Davis MD, Kuppermann BD. Treatment of cytomegalovirus retinitis with a sustained-release ganciclovir implant. The Ganciclovir Implant Study Group. *N Engl J Med* 1997;**337**:83–90.
23. The ganciclovir implant plus oral ganciclovir versus parenteral cidofovir for the treatment of cytomegalovirus retinitis in patients with acquired immunodeficiency syndrome: The Ganciclovir Cidofovir Cytomegalovirus Retinitis Trial. *Am J Ophthalmol* 2001;**131**:457–67.
24. Martin DF, Sierra-Madero J, Walmsley S *et al*. A controlled trial of valganciclovir as induction therapy for cytomegalovirus retinitis. *N Engl J Med* 2002;**346**:1119–26.
25. Palestine AG, Polis MA, De Smet MD *et al*. A randomized, controlled trial of foscarnet in the treatment of cytomegalovirus retinitis in patients with AIDS. *Ann Intern Med* 1991;**115**:665–73.
26. Foscarnet-Ganciclovir Cytomegalovirus Retinitis Trial. 4. Visual outcomes. Studies of Ocular Complications of AIDS Research Group in collaboration with the AIDS Clinical Trials Group. *Ophthalmology* 1994;**101**:1250–61.
27. Mortality in patients with the acquired immunodeficiency syndrome treated with either foscarnet or ganciclovir for cytomegalovirus retinitis. Studies of Ocular Complications of AIDS Research Group, in collaboration with the AIDS Clinical Trials Group. *N Engl J Med* 1992;**326**:213–20.
28. Parenteral cidofovir for cytomegalovirus retinitis in patients with AIDS: the HPMPC peripheral cytomegalovirus retinitis trial. A randomized, controlled trial. Studies of Ocular complications of AIDS Research Group in Collaboration with the AIDS Clinical Trials Group. *Ann Intern Med* 1997;**126**:264–74.
29. Long-term follow-up of patients with AIDS treated with parenteral cidofovir for cytomegalovirus retinitis: the HPMPC Peripheral Cytomegalovirus Retinitis Trial. The Studies of Ocular Complications of AIDS Research Group in collaboration with the AIDS Clinical Trials Group. *AIDS* 2000;**14**:1571–81.
30. Lalezari JP, Stagg RJ, Kuppermann BD *et al*. Intravenous cidofovir for peripheral cytomegalovirus retinitis in patients with AIDS. A randomized, controlled trial. *Ann Intern Med* 1997;**126**:257–63.
31. Lalezari JP, Holland GN, Kramer F *et al*. Randomized, controlled study of the safety and efficacy of intravenous cidofovir for the treatment of relapsing cytomegalovirus retinitis in patients with AIDS. *J Acquir Immune Defic Syndr Hum Retrovirol* 1998;**17**:339–44.
32. Studies of Ocular Complications of AIDS (SOCA) Research Group in collaboration with the AIDS Clinical Trials Group (ACTG). Rhegmatogenous retinal detachment in patients with cytomegalovirus retinitis: the Foscarnet-Ganciclovir Cytomegalovirus Retinitis Trial. *Am J Ophthalmol* 1997;**124**:61–70.
33. Jabs DA. Discontinuing anticytomegalovirus therapy in patients with cytomegalovirus retinitis and AIDS. *Br J Ophthalmol* 2001;**85**:381–2.
34. Studies of ocular complications of AIDS Foscarnet-Ganciclovir Cytomegalovirus Retinitis Trial: 1. Rationale, design, and methods. AIDS Clinical Trials Group (ACTG). *Control Clin Trials* 1992;**13**:22–39.
35. Morbidity and toxic effects associated with ganciclovir or foscarnet therapy in a randomized cytomegalovirus retinitis trial. Studies of ocular complications of AIDS Research Group, in collaboration with the AIDS Clinical Trials Group. *Arch Intern Med* 1995;**155**:65–74.
36. Foscarnet-Ganciclovir Cytomegalovirus Retinitis Trial: 5. Clinical features of cytomegalovirus retinitis at diagnosis. Studies of ocular complications of AIDS Research Group in collaboration with the AIDS Clinical Trials Group. *Am J Ophthalmol* 1997;**124**:141–57.
37. Rhegmatogenous retinal detachment in patients with cytomegalovirus retinitis: the Foscarnet-Ganciclovir Cytomegalovirus Retinitis Trial. The Studies of Ocular Complications of AIDS (SOCA) Research Group in Collaboration with the AIDS Clinical Trials Group (ACTG). *Am J Ophthalmol* 1997;**124**:61–70.
38. Holbrook JT, Davis MD, Hubbard LD, Martin BK, Holland GN, Jabs DA *et al*. Risk factors for advancement of cytomegalovirus retinitis in patients with acquired immunodeficiency syndrome. Studies of Ocular Complications of AIDS Research Group. *Arch Ophthalmol* 2000;**118**:1196–204.
39. Combination foscarnet and ganciclovir therapy *v* monotherapy for the treatment of relapsed cytomegalovirus retinitis in patients with AIDS. The Cytomegalovirus Retreatment Trial. The Studies of Ocular Complications of AIDS Research Group in Collaboration with the AIDS Clinical Trials Group. *Arch Ophthalmol* 1996;**114**:23–33.
40. Danner SA, Matheron S. Cytomegalovirus retinitis in AIDS patients: a comparative study of intravenous and oral ganciclovir as maintenance therapy. *AIDS* 1996;**10**(Suppl 4):S7–11.
41. MSL-109 adjuvant therapy for cytomegalovirus retinitis in patients with acquired immunodeficiency syndrome: the Monoclonal Antibody Cytomegalovirus Retinitis Trial. The Studies of Ocular Complications of AIDS Research Group. AIDS Clinical Trials Group. *Arch Ophthalmol* 1997;**115**:1528–36.
42. A randomized controlled clinical trial of intravitreous fomivirsen for treatment of newly diagnosed peripheral cytomegalovirus retinitis in patients with AIDS. *Am J Ophthalmol* 2002;**133**:467–74.
43. Song MK, Schrier RD, Smith IL, Plummer DJ, Freeman WR. Paradoxical activity of CMV retinitis in patients receiving highly active antiretroviral therapy. *Retina* 2002;**22**:262–7.

28 Anterior uveitis

Nicholas P Jones

Background

Anterior uveitis (AU) is inflammation of the anterior uvea, that is the iris, ciliary body, or both. No population-based study has established the incidence of uveitis. Most studies emanate from sub-specialist tertiary referral centres and are subject to patient selection and referral bias. Nevertheless, there is some level of agreement that in the West (from where all such studies emanate) the annual incidence of uveitis is about 15 to 20 cases per 100 000 population. McCannel[1] makes a direct contemporaneous comparison between uveitis presenting to generalists and specialists. The higher proportion of AU (about 90%) in these generalist studies is striking and almost certainly more representative of uveitis in the general population.

From these figures, one would expect an average general ophthalmologist serving a population of 90,000 in the United Kingdom to encounter a new episode of uveitis about once every three weeks, the vast majority being AU, as this is quite a common disease. A small minority of cases of AU have infective causes and require specific treatment (such as herpetic uveitis). However, the majority, despite perhaps being associated with HLA-B27 or a systemic inflammatory diseases, are idiopathic.

Untreated recurrent AU frequently led to blindness. Duke-Elder, writing in 1966,[2] found that "eventually the iris becomes widely scarred, atrophic and completely bound down to the lens by annular fibrous synechiae, the pupil becomes occluded by a connective tissue membrane, and cataract, glaucoma or phthisis results". Prior to the introduction of topical corticosteroids for uveitis in the late 1940s, treatment was confined to mydriasis and cycloplegia with heat, rest and fresh air, in some cases supplemented by sub-conjunctival mercury or iodine; oral gold, arsenic, or salicylates; fever therapy induced by repeated intramuscular cow's milk; irradiation, paracentesis, or iridectomy. Frequently unsuccessful, Duke-Elder concluded that "when all ameliorative measures have failed and the eye is shrinking or hard and painful, relief may be gained by a retrobulbar injection of alcohol … or the final expedient of evisceration or excision". The introduction of topical steroid treatment for anterior uveitis was immediately perceived as a huge success; controlled studies were not performed, but the results compared with previous experience were strikingly improved.[3,4]

Idiopathic AU is currently treated on the basis of clinical appearance. The ophthalmologist will wish to remove inflammation as quickly as possible, to provide adequate analgesia, to minimise complications largely caused by progressive scarring subsequent on the release of fibrinogen into the aqueous humour, and to restore the patient to normal vision while sparing any undesirable consequences of treatment. How is this best achieved?

Question

There is such a paucity of high-quality evidence on the management of AU that only a small number of questions can be approached. Some important questions for which there are no evidence-based answers appear in the final summary. Those that have some supporting evidence are:

1　Do topical steroids modify the course of AU?
2　Are some topical steroids better than others?
3　Are some steroids more likely to induce glaucoma?
4　Are topical or systemic non-steroidal anti-inflammatory drugs effective?
5　Are there any other effective treatments?
6　Is there any treatment available that inhibits recurrences of AU?

Question

Do topical steroids modify the course of AU?

The evidence

No controlled trials were performed when topical steroids were first introduced to treat uveitis. Their use rapidly became widespread in the early 1950s and their efficacy unquestioned. In 1979 Dunne and Travers[5] published the results of the first trial, a randomised double-masked placebo-controlled comparison of topical treatment with betamethasone or clobetasone. In addition, all patients received the same dose of cycloplegic. The test population (60, reducing to 48 after exclusions) was too small to allow analysis of the comparison between steroids to reach statistical significance. Treatment failures (all on placebo) were excluded from the analysis. However, topical betamethasone was found to be significantly better than placebo.

Young *et al.*[6] compared topical prednisolone with a topical non-steroidal anti-inflammatory drug (NSAID) and placebo in 92 patients. Cycloplegia was used. There were multiple observers, and the treatment was adjusted according to perceived clinical need, but not according to a protocol. At the 21-day stage (defined as the end-point) cases were described as cured or not cured (the term "cured" was not defined). On this basis there was no significant difference between treatments, but at seven days only prednisolone showed an effect, and at 14 days, only prednisolone and NSAID.

Comment

The Dunne and Travers study was notable for being the first in this area to use a controlled structure and appropriate statistical analysis. However, it used an empirical and subjective scoring system for measurement of efficacy and did not use a single observer. The use of symptoms to measure efficacy is of dubious validity when cycloplegics are used (even when used in an identical fashion for all patients).

In the Young study the assessment criteria were of dubious value and the sample size was again almost certainly too small.

The evidence, albeit sparse, is that topical steroids are effective in treating AU.

Question

Are some topical steroids better than others?

The evidence

Dunne and Travers[5] compared betamethasone and clobetasone but their sample size was too small. Dunne *et al.*[7] compared prednisolone with betamethasone (and a NSAID) in a three-arm randomised double-masked trial, again using cycloplegia in all patients. While betamethasone was consistently better than prednisolone, the comparison did not reach statistical significance, probably because the test population was too small.

Topical loteprednol has been compared with prednisolone acetate[8] in a randomised double-masked trial. Symptom evaluation, including pain level, was part of the assessment of efficacy, but variable doses of cycloplegia were permitted. Nevertheless, prednisolone acetate was found to be statistically better than loteprednol in its anti-inflammatory effect.

Comment

The evidence supports a difference in efficacy between certain topical steroids. Unfortunately comparisons have not been made between the most commonly used steroids.

Question

Are some steroids more likely to induce glaucoma?

The evidence

The loteprednol etabonate US uveitis study group[8] compared that drug with prednisolone acetate, in a randomised double-masked study on 175 patients. Loteprednol was felt to have a less marked effect in intraocular pressure, but the difference was not statistically significant.

Comment

No statistically significant evidence from controlled trials has been published to support the contention that different steroids are more or less likely to induce glaucoma.

Question

Are topical or systemic non-steroidal anti-inflammatory drugs (NSAIDS) effective?

The evidence

Dunne *et al.*[7] compared the topical NSAID tolmetin with prednisolone and betamethasone, in a randomised double-masked trial. This three-way comparison was too complex for a population of 71 (decreasing to 60 after exclusions) to answer the question satisfactorily. Tolmetin was the least effective of the three methods of treatment, but none of the comparisons was clinically significant. It was claimed that tolmetin was an effective treatment, but the study was not placebo-controlled.

Young *et al.*[6] compared topical tolmetin with prednisolone in a placebo-controlled trial. Tolmetin was reported to be less effective than prednisolone but more effective than placebo. No comparison reached statistical significance, possibly because of an inadequate sample size.

Sand and Krogh[9] compared topical dexamethasone with topical indometacin in 49 patients (falling to 43 after exclusions). It appears that the patients were recruited from 10 different centres, with multiple observers, and the use of cycloplegia was uncontrolled. The measures of disease activity were crude and subjective. Dexamethasone was found to be significantly better. The study concluded that indometacin was a useful alternative to a topical steroid, but this study was not placebo-controlled.

Hunter *et al.*[10] compared oral oxyphenbutazone (with topical placebo) with topical hydrocortisone (with oral placebo) in a randomised double-masked trial sponsored by its manufacturer. A single observer was used. An effect for oxyphenbutazone was reported, but the trial was not placebo-controlled and there was no statistical analysis. The choice of hydrocortisone as a steroid comparator was interesting, as this is probably the weakest of the available steroids and was not generally used to treat uveitis. There is inadequate evidence from this study for a therapeutic effect from oral oxyphenbutazone.

Comment

There is no evidence that topical or oral NSAIDs are effective in endogenous AU.

Question

Are there any other effective treatments?

The evidence

Van Rooij *et al.*[11] examined the effect of oral vitamins C and E on AU, in patients who were otherwise treated identically with topical steroid and cycloplegia. The rationale for the study was that both vitamins are known scavengers of free radicals. The study is the only one to use an objective measure of activity, in the laser cell/flare meter, and was randomised and double-masked. The study size was 145, reducing to 130 after exclusions. The vitamins did not have a significant effect on inflammation.

Comment

There is no evidence of any effective treatment for AU, other than steroids.

Question

Is there any treatment available that inhibits recurrences of AU?

The evidence

We found two studies that have addressed this issue. Palestine and Nussenblatt[12] observed the effect of oral

bromocriptine on a group of 14 patients. The study was randomised and double-masked. No effect was demonstrated over one year.

Comment

There is no evidence that any treatment can prevent recurrences of AU.

Implications for practice

Evidence of the management of AU is limited both in quantity and quality. We found only nine controlled trials that have addressed any aspect of management. The little evidence that exists does support the efficacy of topical steroids, and this treatment is well-established. Hard evidence on the efficacy of other modes of treatment requires further research.

Implications for research

One trial was excluded from review because of poor quality. Others referred to have relatively low statistical power and in several cases, poor study design. The use of topical steroids in AU is so well-established that placebo-controlled trials will be considered unethical. Nevertheless, many questions remain unanswered. What is the best mydriatic/cycloplegic regime for AU? Can cyclopentolate provoke inflammation? When, if ever, are sub-conjunctival steroids necessary? What is the true relationship between the commonly used steroids in terms of efficacy? What are the true relative risks of induced glaucoma for the different steroids, and is there simply an inverse relationship between efficacy and glaucoma induction? Are all the topical steroids cataractogenic? In what circumstances, if ever, should intracameral fibrinolysis be used? Are systemic steroids ever justified? Can we prevent recurrences of AU?

We do have the ability to answer these questions with carefully designed trials of adequate statistical power, using objective methods of assessment and controlled observation. Such studies are long overdue.

References

1. McCannel CA, Holland GN, Helm CJ *et al.* Causes of uveitis in the general practice of ophthalmology. *Am J Ophthalmol* 1996;**121**:35–46.
2. Duke-Elder S. The treatment of uveitis. In: Duke-Elder S. *System of Ophthalmology Vol IX: Diseases of the Uveal Tract*. London: Henry Kimpton, 1966, pp.167–78.
3. Duke-Elder S. The clinical value of cortisone and ACTH in ocular disease. *Br J Ophthalmol* 1951;**35**:637–71.
4. Duke-Elder S, Duthie OM, Foster J *et al.* A series of cases treated locally by cortisone. *Br J Ophthalmol* 1951;**35**:672–94.

5. Dunne JA, Travers JP. Double-blind clinical trial of topical steroids in anterior uveitis. *Br J Ophthalmol* 1979;**63**:762–7.

6. Young BJ, Cunningham WF, Akingbehin T. Double-masked controlled clinical trial of 5% tolmetin versus 0·5% prednisolone versus 0·9% saline in acute endogenous nongranulomatous anterior uveitis. *Br J Ophthalmol* 1982;**66**:389–91.

7. Dunne JA, Jacobs N, Morrison A, Gilbert DJ. Efficacy in anterior uveitis of two known steroids and topical tolmetin. *Br J Ophthalmol* 1985;**69**:120–5.

8. The Loteprednol etabonate US Uveitis Study Group. Controlled evaluation of loteprednol etabonate and prednisolone acetate in the treatment of acute anterior uveitis. *Am J Ophthalmol* 1999;**127**:537–44.

9. Sand BB, Krogh E. Topical indometacin, a prostaglandin inhibitor, in acute anterior uveitis. A controlled clinical trial of non-steroid versus steroid anti-inflammatory treatment. *Acta Ophthalmol* 1991;**69**:145–8.

10. Hunter PJL, Fowler PD, Wilkinson P. Treatment of anterior uveitis. Comparison of oral oxyphenbutazone and topical steroids. *Br J Ophthalmol* 1973;**57**:892–6.

11. van Rooij J, Schwartzenberg SG, Mulder PG, Baarsma SG. Oral vitamins C and E as additional treatment in patients with acute anterior uveitis: a randomised double masked study in 145 patients. *Br J Ophthalmol* 1999;**83**:1277–82.

12. Palestine AG, Nussenblatt RB. The effect of bromocriptine on anterior uveitis. *Am J Ophthalmol* 1988;**106**:488–9.

Section VII

Glaucoma

Richard Wormald, Editor

Glaucoma: mission statement

Glaucoma as a subspecialty holds the largest number of trials in ophthalmology, but unfortunately most of them are of limited relevance to clinical practice since they are largely comparative studies of the effect of medications or other interventions on intraocular pressure. The question, "Are interventions for lowering IOP effective in preventing progression of disease?" has been much less frequently dealt with. The former studies have been omitted from this section as they add a huge, and uninformative excess to the content of the section which needs to be brief and succinct to adhere to the overall requirements of the book.

Space limitations mean the section deals with issues relevant only to the treatment of disease. Organisation of care, and case detection methods are of course very important, but are not covered here. Management of secondary disease is also not included but there are very few trials dealing with this.

Until quite recently, the evidence base for the effectiveness of therapy has been thin, but recent National Eye Institute funded studies have changed this.

Modification of wound healing in glaucoma surgery has been the subject of numerous RCTs and hence a separate chapter focusing on these has been included.

29 Primary open angle glaucoma and ocular hypertension

Richard Wormald, Rajiv Shah

Background

Definition

Glaucoma is a group of diseases characterised by progressive optic neuropathy. It is usually bilateral but asymmetric and may occur within a wide range of intraocular pressures (IOP). All forms of glaucoma show optic nerve cupping with pallor, associated with peripheral visual field loss.

Primary open angle glaucoma occurs in people with an open drainage angle and no secondary identifiable cause. Normal tension glaucoma occurs in people with intraocular pressures consistently below 21 mmHg, which is now accepted as part of a continuous distribution of IOP as a risk factor for the disease.

Secondary forms of open angle glaucoma include pseudoexfoliation, pigment dispersion glaucoma and steroid induced glaucoma. Only pigment dispersion glaucoma has been the subject of specific intervention studies on the role of peripheral iridotomy in preventing raised IOP and optic nerve damage. The Early Manifest Glaucoma Trial included people with pseudoexfoliation.[1]

Ocular hypertension (DHT) is defined by intraocular pressure raised in one or both eyes two standard deviations above the population mean, which is normally taken as 21 mmHg but which varies somewhat between different populations. Visual function and optic nerve structure are normal. Raised intraocular pressure is an important risk factor for glaucoma.

Incidence/prevalence

Open angle glaucoma occurs in 1–2% of white people aged over 40 years, rising to 5% at 70 years. Primary open angle glaucoma accounts for two thirds of those affected, and normal tension glaucoma (NTG) for about a quarter.[1,2] In people with black African ethnic origin, glaucoma is more prevalent, presents at a younger age with higher intraocular pressures, is more difficult to control, and is the main irreversible cause of blindness in black populations in the USA and Caribbean.[2,4] Glaucoma-related blindness is responsible for 8% of new blind registrations in the UK.[5]

Incidence of primary open angle glaucoma in the largely white European population of Melbourne, Australia is estimated to be 0·5% (95% CI 0·3–0·7%) in five years in people over forty years of age for definite disease and 1·1% (95% CI 0·8–1·4%) for probable and definite disease.[6] In the largely black population of Barbados over 40 years, the overall four-year incidence was found to be 2·2% (95% CI 1·7–2·8%).[4]

The prevalence of ocular hypertension is variable in different studies. It was estimated at 2·1% in northern Italy[7] and 6·5% in Crete.[8] Other studies have found anything from 0.3%.[10] to 10%[9]

Aetiology/risk factors

The major risk factor for developing primary open angle glaucoma is raised intraocular pressure. In the ocular hypertension treatment trial control group, 10% of people with OHT developed glaucoma in five years (disc and/or field progression).[11] Lesser risk factors include increasing age, ethnic origin, family history, myopia and, in some studies, diabetes. The relationship between systemic blood pressure and intraocular pressure may be an important determinant of blood flow to the optic nerve head and, as a consequence, may represent a risk factor for glaucoma.[12] Systemic hypotension, vasospasm (including Raynaud's disease and migraine) and a history of major blood loss have been reported as risk factors for normal tension glaucoma in hospital based studies.

The aetiology of primary open angle glaucoma remains unknown but is thought to have major genetic determinants that may be numerous and interact with environmental risk factors.

Prognosis

Advanced visual field loss is found in about 20% of people with primary open angle glaucoma at diagnosis,[13] and is an important risk factor for glaucoma-related blindness.[14] Blindness results from gross loss of visual field and loss of central vision. Once early field defects have appeared, and where the intraocular pressure is greater than 30 mmHg, untreated people may lose the remainder of the visual field in three years or less.[15] As the disease progresses, people with glaucoma have difficulty moving from a bright to a darker room and judging steps and kerbs. Progression of visual field loss is often slower in normal tension glaucoma. In the Collaborative Normal-tension Glaucoma Study 40% of patients in the control arm showed no progression in five years.

Treatment

The intention of treatment is to prevent progression of visual field loss while minimising the adverse effects of treatment. Chronic glaucoma cannot be cured. Relevant outcomes of treatment are prevention of further visual field loss and preservation of optic nerve structure and function. Intraocular pressure is a surrogate outcome.

Question

What are the effects of topical medical treatments for established primary open angle glaucoma?

The evidence

We found one systematic review (16 placebo controlled RCTs, 86 comparative RCTs, 5000 people).[16] These trials included many studies that involved patients with both open angle glaucoma, "secondary" open angle conditions and ocular hypertension. These are not clearly differentiated in the review. Only trials comparing intervention with placebo were summarised. For intraocular pressure, the review found that medical treatment versus placebo significantly reduced mean intraocular pressure after a minimum of three months (16 placebo controlled RCTs; mean reduction in intraocular pressure 4·9 mmHg, 95% CI 2·5–7·3). For visual field loss, the review found no significant difference with medical treatment versus placebo after long-term follow up (three RCTs, 302 people; pooled odds ratio (OR) for any worsening of visual field loss 0·75, 95% CI 0·42–1·35). These trials were on people with ocular hypertension and the outcome was the prevention of onset of glaucoma as defined by the development of visual field loss. An update of this review has not yet been published, but a Cochrane review is in process.

Since this review there have been numerous additional trials comparing the relative effectiveness of reducing intraocular pressure but few have examined the effects of lowering intraocular pressure on conversion to glaucoma or on progression of established disease.

The Ocular Hypertension Treatment Study (OHTS)[11] was powered to detect a 40% reduction in risk of conversion to glaucoma over five years. The intervention was a 20% reduction in IOP by topical medications. These were predominantly topical betablockers initially, with an increasing proportion of prostaglandin analogues being introduced during the course of the study. The trial found a greater than 50% reduction in relative risk of conversion from 10·9% to 4·4% for visual field and/or optic disc progression (number needed to treat (NNT) 15). If only field progression is taken as the end-point, then the reduction was 4·6% to 2·2%; still a greater than 50% reduction in risk but a smaller absolute reduction (NNT 42).

The most recent trial compared betaxol to placebo in 356 ocular hypertensives stratified by baseline pattern electroretinogram (PERG) findings and age.[17] Although a delay in progression was identified in the treatment arm after follow up ranging from two to six years, it did not reach statistical significance due mainly to a lower conversion rate in controls than expected.

Systemic adverse effects of topical treatments are uncommon but may be serious, including exacerbation of chronic obstructive airways disease after use of topical betablockers. Non-selective topical betablockers can also cause systemic hypotension and reduction in resting heart rate.[18] These side effects were not reported in OHTS as being more frequent in the intervention arm but a population-based cohort study has identified an adjusted hazard ratio of developing obstructive airways disease requiring treatment in the first year after starting topical betablockers as 2·29 (95% CI 1·71–3·07), number needed to harm (NNH) 43 (95% CI 34–60).[19]

Comment

Rossetti's systematic review did not clearly define the medical treatments involved. Since the review, there have been numerous additional studies comparing the relative effectiveness of topical agents in lowering intraocular pressure but only one has been properly powered to address the question of prevention of glaucoma in ocular hypertension. Trials comparing the various topical agents are usually sponsored by the pharmaceutical industry.

Question

What are the effects of laser trabeculoplasty for established primary open angle glaucoma?

The evidence

We found no systematic review, but found four RCTs. The Early Manifest Glaucoma Trial (EMGT) compared the effects of 360 degree laser trabeculoplasty and topical betaxolol to no treatment in people with early manifest glaucoma identified in population-based screening in southern Sweden.[1] The aim of the trial was to determine whether lowering IOP in early glaucoma reduced the risk of progression. A total of 255 people were randomised to treatment or none. Follow up was for five years. Persons showing signs of progression confirmed by masked observers based on consistent changes in the visual field and/or optic disc came out of the trial and were treated appropriately. Forty-five per cent of treated persons and 62% of controls progressed. This highly significant difference gives an approximate NNT of six.

The Glaucoma Laser Trial (GLT) (203 people) found that combined treatment (initial laser trabeculoplasty followed by medical treatment) versus medical treatment alone significantly reduced intraocular pressure (1·2 mmHg greater reduction in intraocular pressure with combined treatment; $P < 0.001$), significantly (statistically not clinically) improved visual field (0·6 dB greater improvement with combined treatment; $P = 0.001$) and significantly reduced deterioration in optic disc appearance ($P < 0.005$) after a mean of seven years.[20]

Other trials have compared laser trabeculoplasty to trabeculectomy. Adverse effects of laser trabeculoplasty are mild and include a transient rise in intraocular pressure (>5 mmHg in 91/271 participants) and formation of peripheral anterior synechiae (in 93/271 participants).[1] The EMGT found a significant increase in the risk of nuclear lens opacity in the treatment group. This has also been reported in an observational study in Barbados with cataract being more common in people being treated for glaucoma compared to those untreated.[21] The cause is not known though it is thought more likely to be due to topical medication, perhaps betablockers rather than trabeculoplasty.

Comment

Participants in the EMGT were not masked to their treatment but observers of the primary outcomes were. The GLT was a multi-centre trial with multiple observers and it is not clear whether these observers were masked to the intervention.

Use of laser trabeculoplasty is variable in practice and often reserved for older patients and those with pigmented trabecular meshworks in whom the treatment is thought to be more effective. A concern is that the duration of effect is hard to predict and intraocular pressure may rise rapidly when the effect wears off.

Question

What are the effects of surgical trabeculectomy on established primary open angle glaucoma?

The evidence

There are no published systematic reviews but there are two RCTs comparing trabeculectomy to medical treatment, comparing surgery to medicine or laser and one comparing different sequences of surgery and laser in advanced glaucoma.

The Jay trial (116 people) compared trabeculectomy (followed by medical treatment when indicated) versus medical treatment (followed by trabeculectomy when medical treatment failed).[22] It found no significant difference between treatments in visual acuity ($P = 0.44$) but found that trabeculectomy versus medical treatment significantly reduced visual field loss ($P = 0.03$) after a mean of 4·6 years.

The Moorfields Laser Medicine Surgery Trial (186 people) compared medical treatment (pilocarpine +/− timolol +/− a sympathomimetic), laser trabeculoplasty and surgical trabeculectomy.[23] It found that surgical trabeculectomy versus both other treatments significantly reduced intraocular pressures ($P = 0.0001$), but found no significant difference between any of the treatments in visual acuity (results presented graphically) after five years. Visual field loss was least in the surgical group.

The Collaborative Initial Glaucoma Treatment Study (CIGTS)[24] was a large multi-centre trial in the USA comparing initial treatment of primary open angle glaucoma with either medical treatment or trabeculectomy with or without 5-fluorouracil. Six hundred and seven patients were randomised and followed up for at least four years. The main outcome measure was progression of visual field loss but other outcomes such as visual acuity and need for cataract surgery were considered. Importantly, a parallel study examined vision-related quality of life at baseline (initial diagnosis) and after four to five years' follow up. No difference was found in visual field loss. In fact, very little field progression occurred in either group. IOP was consistently lower in the surgical group and vision initially worse though similar by the end of follow up. This was because cataract surgery had dealt with the acuity loss, which was three times more common in the surgical group. Vision-related quality of life provided important information on the impact of glaucoma diagnosis at baseline but was not very different after four to five years. The surgical group was more likely to complain of ocular discomfort.[25]

The Advanced Glaucoma Intervention Study (AGIS) (776 eyes with advanced glaucoma; 451 black people, 325 white people) compared surgical trabeculectomy versus laser trabeculoplasty as initial treatments.[26] Initial surgical trabeculectomy was followed by laser trabeculoplasty and repeat surgical trabeculectomy as required; initial laser trabeculoplasty was followed by surgical trabeculectomy as required. The RCT found that in black people initial laser trabeculoplasty versus surgical trabeculectomy significantly improved vision (both visual acuity and visual field; $P < 0.01$), although in white people there was no significant difference between treatments in vision (results presented graphically) after seven years. The RCT also found that in both black and white people surgical trabeculectomy was more effective than laser trabeculoplasty in reducing intraocular pressure (significance not reported and results presented graphically).

Surgical trabeculectomy is associated with a reduction in central vision. In one study, 83% of participants lost two lines of Snellen visual acuity.[27] One RCT in people with normal tension glaucoma has found that treatment including trabeculectomy versus no treatment significantly increased cataract formation after eight years.[28] Other serious complications may occur during or after surgery, including massive choroidal haemorrhage or bacterial endophthalmitis but are too rare to be detected in trials. It is also reported that patients with advanced visual field loss may lose their residual central island of visual field following surgery (the so-called "snuff out" effect) though this is also not reported in RCTs.

Comment

Trabeculectomy is often modified with antimetabolic agents to increase the probability of success. This is dealt with in Chapter 31.

The AGIS study has reported numerous additional analyses, including the relationship between the reduction of IOP and risk of progression of visual field loss, which shows a strong indication that lowering pressure reduces the risk of progression. These results are, however, from non-randomised comparisons.

Question

What are the effects of lowering intraocular pressure in people with normal tension glaucoma?

The evidence

A Cochrane systematic review on interventions for normal tension glaucoma is in press.[28] A total of 11 trials were identified, three of which were excluded. Of the remaining eight, all examined medical interventions only apart from one, the Collaborative Normal-tension Glaucoma Study (CNTGS), which allowed medical and surgical interventions to reduce IOP by 30% in the intervention arm (61 eyes). There was no placebo in the control group (79 eyes).[29] Progression of visual field loss was defined in terms of deepening of an existing scotoma, a new or expanded field defect coming close to central vision or a fresh scotoma

in a previously normal part of the visual field. Optic disc changes were photographed and independently assessed by two ophthalmologists. The RCT found that treatment significantly reduced progression of visual field loss after 8 years (7/61 (12%) eyes with treatment *v* 28/79 (35%) eyes with no treatment; RR 0.32, 95% CI 0.15–0.70, NNT 5, 95% CI 3–9).

The RCT found that treatment (drugs +/– trabeculectomy) versus no treatment significantly increased cataract formation after eight years (23/61 (38%) with treatment versus 11/79 (14%) with no treatment; RR 2.71, 95% CI 1.4–5.1, NNH 4, 95% CI 2–10).[24] Subgroup analysis found that the excess risk of cataract formation was confined to those people treated surgically ($P = 0.0001$).

A companion paper[30] suggests that the favourable effect of intraocular pressure lowering treatment versus no treatment is evident only when the cataract inducing effect of trabeculectomy is removed.

Two additional trials[28] looked at the effect of a calcium channel blocker, brovincamine, on progression of visual field loss in normal tension glaucoma (see below) but this was not an intervention for lowering IOP.

The remaining trials in the review did not look at visual function as a primary outcome and measured either IOP or ocular blood flow as a primary outcome.

Comment

The CNIGS remains the only trial to examine the effect of lowering IOP on visual function in people with normal tension glaucoma and the effect could only be demonstrated after controlling for the effects of cataract. This trial and one other were the only ones in the review considered to be of good quality.

Question

What is the effectiveness of non-pressure lowering treatments in normal tension glaucoma?

The evidence

The two trials identified in the Cochrane review[28] were both on the calcium channel blocker, brovincamine. Sawada *et al.* randomised 28 people to 20 mg brovincamine three times daily or placebo.[31] The average follow up was 40 months. None of the 14 treated patients showed progression compared to two who progressed in the control arm. This was reported as being statistically significant ($P = 0.0123$).

Koseki *et al.* randomised 52 people to the same treatment or placebo and followed them up for two years.[32] A significant difference in mean deviation was observed between the two groups at the end of follow up but there was no difference in corrected pattern standard deviation or total deviation in the visual field analysis. The treatment seems to have been well tolerated, with only four people in the intervention arm withdrawing because of side effects.

Comment

The reviewers commented that these studies were of poor quality in terms of what could be understood from the reports. Other calcium channel blockers have been used in NTG but side effects are common. Another trial in the review suggested that prostaglandin analogues are better than betablockers in improving the calculated ocular perfusion pressure.[33] Changes in blood flow were measured in two trials looking at betaxolol[34] and dorzolamide.[35]

Question

What is the effectiveness of non-penetrating surgery for primary open angle glaucoma?

There are two types of procedure, deep sclerectomy with or without a collagen implant and viscocanalostomy in which Schlemm's canal is identified in the deep sclerectomy and opened using injected viscoelastic material.

One review found no randomised controlled trials and proposed that they should be undertaken.[36] Since then, three trials have been published: one on deep sclerectomy[37] and two on viscocanalostomy.[38,39]

Chiselita randomised the first eye of 17 patients either to standard trabeculectomy or non-penetrating deep sclerectomy (without collagen implant).[37] The other eye had the opposite treatment within six weeks. Follow up was for 18 months. Patients with trabeculectomy fared better in term of IOP control and "success". There were fewer complications in the non-penetrating surgery eyes.

Jonescu-Cuypers *et al.* randomised 10 patients each to viscocanalostomy or trabeculectomy.[38] Success was defined as IOP between 7 mmHg and 20 mmHg six to eight months after surgery. Half of the trabeculectomy procedures and none on the viscocanalostomy procedures reached this target.

O'Brart *et al.* randomised 50 eyes of 48 patients either to trabeculectomy with antimetabolites (5-fluorouracil or mitomycin) or viscocanalostomy.[39] Follow up was for at least 12 months. All the trabeculectomy group were successful compared to 64% of the viscocanalostomy group. There was no difference in visual outcomes but there were fewer complications such as bleb leakage and shallow anterior chamber in the non-penetrating group.

Comment

There are numerous uncontrolled case series discussing modifications of the procedure and different types of implant but the quality of evidence remains poor. Despite the fact that non-penetrating surgery seems safer, the technique has a learning curve and at present the increase in safety does not appear to outweigh the relative lack of effectiveness of primary open angle glaucoma.

Conclusion

The evidence base for treatment has clearly improved since the emergence of recent trials, most of which have been sponsored by the USA's National Eye Institute. However, surgical aspects of glaucoma management clearly require more evidence. Medical treatments need to be assessed on standardised end-points that are not surrogate. While there are numerous trials comparing the pressure lowering effect of different drops, this does not tell us which medication better preserves visual function.

One aspect not dealt with in this chapter is tube implant surgery for difficult cases. Trials in these situations, which are so much less frequent, are very hard to organise but some are ongoing.

Another enormous and very important issue, not dealt with here, is the detection of glaucoma, the pros and cons of screening and different methods for case finding; another issue is the organisation of care in terms of the most cost-effective and safe means of monitoring at-risk suspects and, in the future, people carrying genetic risk factors for the disease.

Implications for practice

Evidence suggests that a lower IOP is achieved surgically more reliably than by using topical medicine or laser trabeculoplasty but it is more likely to have adverse effects. Modern topical therapy seems to be equally successful in preventing visual field loss according to the CIGTS. A strong message emerging from both OHTS and EMGT is that every patient is different and that interventions need to be tailored to meet individual patients' needs, taking into account the risks and benefits of the treatment options and the longer term prognosis of the condition.

There is evidence from observational studies that an important risk factor for failure of surgical treatment is prolonged exposure to topical treatments, which suggests that a decision to operate, if it is going to be made, is better made sooner than later.

It is a good idea, therefore, when the diagnosis is made and confirmed, that an appropriate long-term plan is made for the patient's life-time management, based on the best available evidence.

Implications for research

Since we now have good evidence that sight loss from chronic glaucoma is indeed preventable, there is a much more urgent need to find efficient and expedient ways of identifying people who need treatment and then, the means to deliver it. This is especially an issue for populations of black African origin such as African Americans, African Caribbeans and Africans, probably particularly West Africans. Epidemiological research in West Africa would surely provide vital clues into the genetic and environmental determinants of the disease, but funding such research is difficult.

There is an urgent need to organise glaucoma research in order to achieve common standards of relevant clinical outcomes and to encourage collaboration. When this is achieved, it might be possible to add glaucoma to the list of preventable causes of blindness targeted by the WHO's global prevention of blindness programme – Vision 2020, the right to sight.[40]

Acknowledgements

This chapter is based on already published in *Clinical Evidence* (Wormald R, Shah R, Primary open angle glaucoma and ocular hypertension. *Clinical Evidence* (June issue 7). London: BMJ Publishing Group, 2002) by the same authors. Major changes have been made for this edition. The original chapter was, however, written by Professor Colm O'Brien and Mr Jeremy Diamond, whose contribution is gratefully acknowledged.

References

1. Heijl A, Leske MC, Bengtsson B *et al.* Reduction of intraocular pressure and glaucoma progression: results of the Early Manifest Glaucoma Trial. *Arch Ophthalmol* 2002;**120**:1268–79.
2. Sommer A, Tielsch JM, Katz J *et al.* Relationship between intraocular pressure and primary open angle glaucoma among white and black Americans. *Arch Ophthalmol* 1991;**109**:1090–5.
3. Coffey M, Reidy A, Wormald R *et al.* The prevalence of glaucoma in the west of Ireland. *Br J Ophthalmol* 1993;**77**:17–21.
4. Leske MC, Connell AM, Wu SY *et al.* Incidence of open-angle glaucoma: the Barbados Eye Studies. The Barbados Eye Studies Group. *Arch Ophthalmol* 2001;**119**:89–95.
5. Government Statistical Service. *Causes of blindness and partial sight amongst adults.* London: HMSO, 1988.
6. Mukesh BN, McCarty CA, Rait JL, Taylor HR. Five year incidence of open-angle glaucoma: the visual impairment project. *Ophthalmology* 2002;**109**:1047–51.
7. Bonomi L, Marchini G, Marraffa M, Morbio R. The relationship between intraocular pressure and glaucoma in a defined population. Data from the Egna-Neumarkt Glaucoma study. *Ophthalmology* 2001; **215**:34–8.
8. Kozobolis VP, Detorakis ET, Tsilimbaris M *et al.* Crete, Greece Glaucoma study. *J Glaucoma* 2000;**9**:143–9.
9. Dandona L, Dandona R, Srinivas M *et al.* Open angle glaucoma in southern India: The Andhra Pradesh eye disease study. *Ophthalmology* 2000;**107**:1702–9.
10. Hollows FC, Graham PA. Intra-ocular pressure, glaucoma, and glaucoma suspects in a defined population. *Br J Ophthalmol* 1966;**50**:570–86.
11. Kass MA, Heuer DK, Higginbotham EJ *et al.* The Ocular Hypertension Treatment Study: a randomized controlled trial determines that topical ocular hypotensive medication delays or prevents the onset of Primary Open Angle Glaucoma. *Arch Ophthalmol* 2002;**120**:711–13.
12. Tielsch JM, Katz J, Quigley HA *et al.* Diabetes, intraocular pressure, and primary open-angle glaucoma in the Baltimore Eye Survey. *Ophthalmology* 1995;**102**:48–53.
13. Sheldrick JH, Ng C, Austin DJ *et al.* An analysis of referral routes and diagnostic accuracy in cases of suspected glaucoma. *Ophthalmic Epidemiol* 1994;**1**:31–8.
14. Fraser S, Bunce C, Wormald R *et al.* Deprivation and late presentation of glaucoma: case-control study. *BMJ* 2001;**322**:639–43.
15. Jay JL, Murdoch JR. The rates of visual field loss in untreated primary open angle glaucoma. *Br J Ophthalmol* 1993;**77**:176–8.
16. Rossetti L, Marchetti I, Orzalesi N *et al.* Randomised clinical trials on medical treatment of glaucoma: are they appropriate to guide clinical practice? *Arch Ophthalmol* 1993;**111**:96–103.
17. Kamal D, Garway-Heath D, Ruben S *et al.* Results of the betaxolol versus placebo treatment trial in ocular hypertension. *Graefe's Arch Clin Exp Ophthalmol* 2003;**241**:196–203.
18. Diamond JP. Systemic adverse effects of topical ophthalmic agents: implications for older patients. *Drugs Aging* 1997;**11**:352–60.
19. Kirwan JF, Nightingale JA, Bunce CB, Wormald R. Beta blockers for glaucoma and excess risk of airways obstruction: population based cohort study. *BMJ* 2002;**325**:1396–7.
20. Glaucoma Laser Trial Group. The glaucoma laser trial (GLT) and glaucoma laser trial follow-up study: results. *Am J Ophthalmol* 1995;**120**:718–31.
21. Leske MC, Wu SY, Nemesure B, Hennis A and the Barbados Eye Study Group. Risk factors for incident nuclear opacities. *Ophthalmology* 2002;**109**:1303–8.
22. Jay JL, Allan D. The benefit of early trabeculectomy versus conventional management in primary open angle glaucoma relative to severity of disease. *Eye* 1989;**3**:528–35.
23. Migdal C, Gregory W, Hitchings R *et al.* Long-term functional outcome after early surgery compared with laser and medicine in open angle glaucoma. *Ophthalmology* 1994;**101**:1651–7.
24. Lichter PR, Musch DC, Gillespie BW and the CIGTS study group. Interim clinical outcomes in the Collaborative Intitial Glaucoma Treatment Study comparing initial treatment randomized to medication or surgery. *Ophthalmology* 2001;**108**:1943–53.
25. Janz NK, Wren PA, Lichter PR *et al.* The Collaborative Initial Glaucoma Treatment Study: interim quality of life findings after initial medical or surgical treatment of glaucoma. *Ophthalmol* 2001;**108**:1954–65.
26. The Advanced Glaucoma Intervention Study (AGIS). 4. Comparison of treatment outcomes within race. Seven year results. *Ophthalmology* 1998;**105**:1146–64.
27. Costas UP, Smith M, Spaeth GL *et al.* Loss of vision after trabeculectomy. *Ophthalmology* 1993;**100**:599–612.
28. Sycha T, Vass C, Findl O *et al.* Interventions for normal tension glaucoma (Cochrane review). In: Cochrane Collaboration: *Cochrane Library.* Issue 2. Oxford: Update Softwate, 2003.
29. Collaborative Normal-tension Glaucoma Study Group. Comparison of glaucomatous progression between untreated patients with normal-tension glaucoma and patients with therapeutically reduced intraocular pressure. *Am J Ophthalmol* 1998;**126**:487–97.
30. Collaborative Normal-tension Glaucoma Study Group. The effectiveness of intraocular pressure reduction in the treatment of normal-tension glaucoma. *Am J Ophthalmol* 1998;**126**:498–505.
31. Sawada A, Kitazawa Y, Yamamoto T *et al.* Prevention of visual field defect progression with brovincamine in eyes with normal tension glaucoma. *Ophthalmology* 1996;**103**:283–8.
32. Koseki N, Araie M, Yamagami J *et al.* Effects of oral brovincamine on visual field damage in patients with normal tension glaucoma. *J Glaucoma* 1999;**8**:117–23.

33. Drance SM, Crichton A, Mills RP. Comparison of the effect of latanoprost 0·005% and timolol 0·5% on the calculated ocular perfusion pressure in patients with normal tension glaucoma. *Am J Ophthalmol* 1998;**125**:585–92.
34. Harris A, Spaeth GL, Sergott RC *et al.* Retrobulbar haemodynamic effects of betaxolol and timolol in normal tension glaucoma. *Am J Ophthalmol* 1995;**120**:168–75.
35. Harris A, Arend O, Kageman L *et al.* Dorzolamide, visual function and ocular haemodynamics in normal tension glaucoma. *J Ocul Pharmacol Ther* 1999;**15**:189–97.
36. Netland PA. Non-penetrating glaucoma surgery. *Ophthalmology* 2001;**108**:416–21.
37. Chiselita D. Non-penetrating deep sclerectomy versus trabeculectomy in primary open angle glaucoma surgery. *Eye* 2001;**15**:131–2.
38. Jonescu-Cuypers C, Jacobi P, Konen W, Krieglstein G. Primary viscocanalostomy versus trabeculectomy in white patients with open-angle glaucoma: A randomized clinical trial. *Ophthalmology* 2001;**108**:254–8.
39. O'Brart DP, Rowlands E, Islam N, Noury AM. A randomised prospective study comparing trabeculectomy augmented with antimetabolites with viscocanalostomy technique for the management of open angle glaucoma uncontrolled by medical therapy. *Br J Ophthalmol* 2002;**11**:90–6.
40. Frick KD, Foster A. The magnitude and cost of global blindness: an increasing problem that can be alleviated. *Am J Ophthalmol* 2003;**135**:471–6.

30 Acute and chronic angle closure glaucoma

Richard Wormald, Rajiv Shah

Background

Definition

Acute angle closure glaucoma is a rapid and severe rise in intraocular pressure assumed to be caused by physical obstruction of the anterior chamber drainage angle. If left untreated, the eye is severely damaged in a matter of hours. The patient usually suffers severe ocular pain with or without additional referred pain over the brow often associated with nausea and vomiting. Lids may be swollen, conjunctiva and episclera deeply injected, cornea oedematous, anterior chamber shallow with an occluded angle, the pupil semidilated, sometimes distorted and fixed, changes appear in the anterior lens cortex termed "glaukomflecken" and the optic nerve becomes pale and irreversibly damaged as in ischaemic optic neuropathy after a prolonged attack. It usually occurs unilaterally but can rarely occur bilaterally simultaneously.

Patients are at risk of acute angle closure if they have a narrow anterior chamber drainage angle and shallow anterior chamber. Angle closure may cause subacute or intermittent elevation of intraocular pressure (IOP) or chronic elevation of IOP with or without optic nerve damage. Modern nomenclature requires the presence of optic nerve damage for the term glaucoma to apply.[1]

Pathogenesis

Primary acute angle closure occurs by two mechanisms: with relative pupil block and accumulation of aqueous behind the pupil pushing the peripheral iris forward thereby obstructing the drainage angle or by angle crowding and occlusion of the drainage angle by thick iris folds without pupil block.

Chronic angle closure may be simply primary open angle glaucoma with a coincident narrow angle or the morphology of the angle may be causing chronic elevation of IOP. Plateau iris syndrome is one example. The presence of synaechial closure is evidence that the peripheral iris is occluding the angle but the presence of pupil block is harder to determine. Some undertake a diagnostic iridotomy to determine whether this is the case. Modern imaging devices

for the anterior segment such as the ultrasound biomicroscope make the differential diagnosis easier.

Epidemiology

The crude incidence of acute angle closure was reported in Hong Kong as 10·4 per 100 000 per year in persons over 30 years of age.[2] In Singapore, the annual incidence of acute glaucoma presenting to hospital was 12·2 per 100 000, which was twice that of the Malays and Indians at 6·0 and 6·3 per 100 000, respectively.[3] In their cross-sectional study of people over 40 in Northern Italy, Bonomi *et al.*[4] describe how acute angle closure actually occurs in a group of people at risk with narrow drainage angles, including people suffering subacute and chronic disease. The overall prevalence of narrow angle glaucoma was found to be 0·6%. Five people had previous acute attacks resolved with treatment, three had persistent chronic glaucoma after acute attacks, three had intermittent or subacute attacks and 15 had chronic angle closure. In the Chinese population of Singapore, the overall prevalence of glaucoma was 3·2% in people aged 40–79 of which 31% was angle closure glaucoma.[5] In Mongolia, angle closure glaucoma was more prevalent than open angle disease and 6·4% of people over 40 had gonioscopically occludable angles.[6]

Part of the difficulty in describing the epidemiology of angle closure is the terminology, which is used inconsistently. An international consensus group has developed rational guidelines to resolve this issue.[1] Another problem is that gonioscopy is not routinely performed in cross-sectional studies although the use of the Van Herrick method for assessing the peripheral anterior chamber depth has been shown to be sufficiently sensitive in cross-sectional studies.[7]

Like open angle glaucoma, angle closure risk is different in different ethnic groups and seems to be most prevalent in mongoloid races. South Indians may be more prone to angle closure than northerners. In the Andhra Pradesh Eye Disease Study 2·12% of people over 30 years were found to have either angle closure glaucoma or occludable angles.[8]

Risk factors for acute angle closure reported in the above epidemiological studies include increasing age, female sex and hypermetropia that correlate with ocular dimensions and a shallow anterior chamber. Age is thought to be correlated because the crystalline lens continues to grow throughout life thus making the anterior chamber shallower.

A recent systematic review failed to find any evidence supporting the theory that routine pupillary dilation with short acting mydriatics was a risk factor for acute angle closure glaucoma,[9] but there are numerous reports of angle closure attacks apparently provoked by various medications, including general anaesthesia, paroxitene and similar agents.

Treatment

Acute angle glaucoma leads to rapid loss of vision, initially from corneal oedema and subsequently from ischaemic optic neuropathy. Attempts are made to lower the IOP as quickly as possible and relieve pupil block by performing a peripheral iridectomy or iridotomy. The condition rarely spontaneously resolves so that placebo controlled trials could not be ethically conducted.

Recent suggestions for new interventions in acute angle closure include peripheral iridoplasty with the argon laser and early removal of the lens by phacoemulsification.

Chronic angle closure is often treated with medical agents similar to those used to treat open angle disease but iridotomy or iridectomy may be performed in order to deepen the peripheral anterior chamber. Some advocate earlier removal of the lens to deepen the anterior chamber.

Question

What are the effects of medical treatment for acute angle closure glaucoma?

The evidence

Only one randomised controlled trial (RCT) exists in the literature on the medical treatment of angle closure glaucoma that relates to the use of pilocarpine inserts versus intensive topical pilocarpine in the initial control of the IOP. The RCT (77 eyes) compared three groups: initial treatment with low-dose pilocarpine (2% pilocarpine drops applied to the eye twice in one hour), intensive pilocarpine (4% pilocarpine drops applied to the eye every five minutes for one hour or more) and pilocarpine ocular inserts (releasing 40 micrograms pilocarpine per hour).[10] All of the people in the RCT also received treatment with intravenous acetazolamide (500 mg intravenously). The RCT found no significant difference in the intraocular pressures after two hours and reported that ocular inserts were associated with local discomfort.

Comment

There is a strong consensus that medical treatments which involve pressure lowering drugs (especially those that can be given parenterally such as intravenous acetazolamide) are effective in acute angle closure glaucoma. We found no evidence from RCTs to support this view but management protocols are published having been refined through audit cycles.[11] The use of pilocarpine is somewhat paradoxical since it is known to cause further shallowing of the anterior chamber[12] but probably works by helping to open the angle by tensing the iris diaphragm and pulling on the scleral spur. It may also help to resolve relative pupil block. The use of osmotic agents in refractory attacks is somewhat controversial and intravenous mannitol is used less frequently than in the past because of the potential to harm the patient. Oral glycerol is still used by some.

Question

What is the effectiveness of medical treatment for chronic angle closure glaucoma?

The evidence

There are no RCTs in the Cochrane central register of controlled trials (CENTRAL) addressing this question. It is possible that some of the studies on chronic glaucoma in general have included narrow angle glaucoma but this specific question has not been addressed.

Comment

This is a major concern, as chronic angle closure glaucoma is a difficult condition to manage, perhaps because there is a very poor evidence base. Pilocarpine is commonly used but, at least in theory, this may be causing harm in the long term. The effectiveness of newer agents in preventing optic nerve damage in the disease in not known though there is one RCT that compared the effects of latanoprost and timolol in lowering IOP in these patients.[13] Latanoprost was marginally better and there was no difference in reported adverse effects.

Question

What are the effects of surgical treatment for acute angle closure glaucoma?

The evidence

Surgical peripheral iridectomy has largely been replaced by Nd:YAG laser iridotomy. We found no systematic review but found one RCT (48 people with uniocular acute angle closure glaucoma) that compared peripheral iridectomy versus Nd:YAG laser iridotomy.[14] The trial found no significant difference in visual acuity (0·30 logMAR units with peripheral iridectomy versus 0·57 logMAR units with laser iridotomy; statistical analysis not provided), and no significant difference in intraocular pressure (intraocular pressure <21 mmHg: 15/21 (70%) with peripheral iridectomy v 19/27 (72%) with laser iridotomy; RR 1·02, 95% CI 0·71–1·46) after three years.

Although it is widely accepted that prophylactic treatment should be delivered to the second eye in a patient who presents with acute angle closure in one eye, we found no RCT evidence to support this. Surgical iridectomy involves opening the eye and hence the theoretical risk of serious complications, including intraocular infection or haemorrhage. One trial compared Nd:YAG laser to surgical iridectomy as a prophylactic measure to the second eye.[15] There was no difference in effectiveness or safety observed in the study, although patients preferred the more convenient laser treatment.

Laser iridotomy can cause bleeding from the iris, pressure spikes and corneal oedema, and both Nd:YAG and argon laser iridotomy can produce focal lens opacity.[16] In one RCT comparing Nd:YAG and Argon laser, iris haemorrhage was more common with the Nd:YAG laser, but pupil distortion, iritis and late blockage were more common with the argon laser.[17] The mean number of laser burns required to penetrate the iris was six with the Nd:YAG laser and 73 with the argon laser.

Comment

Nd:YAG laser is almost exclusively used to perform peripheral iridotomy now, though some practitioners advocate the pretreatment of an iris with thick peripheral folds with argon laser to facilitate the subsequent penetration of the YAG. There is no trial evidence to support this view.

Question

What is the effectiveness of medications to reduce the risk of intraocular pressure spikes after YAG laser iridotomy?

The evidence

It is common practice to instil apraclonidine 0·5% or 1% either before or after YAG laser iridotomy to reduce the risk of IOP spikes. There is one double masked RCT in the Cochrane CENTRAL register in which patients requiring YAG laser iridotomy were randomised to apraclonidine combined with pilocarpine or placebo.[18] Apraclonidine was effective in reducing the IOP spikes, which were more common in people with chronic angle closure glaucoma. There is one additional trial that reports a comparison of 0·5% and 1% apraclonidine, showing no difference in effectiveness in preventing pressure spikes after iridotomy for narrow angles.[19]

Question

What is the effectiveness of argon laser iridoplasty in the treatment of acute angle closure glaucoma?

The evidence

This treatment has been advocated in Chinese populations where this condition is more common. There is one RCT in the Cochrane CENTRAL register in which 73 eyes of 64 consecutive patients presenting with acute angle closure glaucoma were randomised to early argon laser iridoplasty or conventional medical treatment followed by laser iridotomy.[20] Iridoplasty was successful in achieving more rapid control of IOP but there was no difference in IOP at two hours. There were no adverse effects reported in the short term for the new treatment.

Comment

Patients were matched in this trial for possible confounding effects. Long-term outcome has not been reported and no information on visual outcome has been provided.

Question

What is the effectiveness of surgical treatments for chronic angle closure glaucoma?

The evidence

There are no RCTs in the Cochrane CENTRAL register that deal with this question.

Comment

Laser iridotomy is quite frequently performed in patients with chronic closed angle glaucoma, especially if it is believed that there is an element of pupil block in the closure. When this is the case, the pressure falls somewhat but often, the meshwork is already damaged and laser iridotomy has little effect. In some cases, it may make control of IOP more difficult. Dealing with the cataract later may also be made more difficult if the laser results in the formation of posterior synaechiae.

Some advocate earlier removal of the lens when the angle is narrow to create more space in the anterior segment but there have been no prospective RCTs to test this hypothesis.

Conclusions

Angle closure glaucoma contributes a very significant proportion of the global burden of glaucoma and glaucoma blindness. The Chinese population in whom this form dominates is one reason for this. The fact that it can be a much more aggressive and devastating condition is another real concern. A trial is ongoing in Mongolia to see whether it is possible to reduce the burden of blindness with prophylactic surgical iridectomy.[21] The state of the evidence base seems considerably less well developed than it is for open angle glaucoma.

Implications for practice

Management of acute angle closure should normally follow strict guidelines to ensure that the condition is efficiently and rapidly treated and that the second eye is also dealt with. Although there is no trial evidence for this, clinical experience that angle closure is a bilateral disease is so well established that the opportunity to prevent an attack in the second eye should always be taken.

Management of chronic angle closure is much more difficult, especially when it occurs in an eye bordering on the nanophthalmic. These eyes are difficult to control medically, and surgically are often fraught with difficulty including the possibility of inducing malignant glaucoma. The best principle to follow in these cases is to try to avoid doing harm by minimising interventions and opting for surgery only when everyone concerned clearly understands the trade-off between risk and benefit.

Implications for research

There is an urgent need for more evidence in all aspects of angle closure glaucoma. Laser iridoplasty looks promising in the management of acute disease and possibly also in chronic conditions though more evidence is needed. More evidence is needed on the management of chronic narrow angle glaucoma. Perhaps the most urgently needed study is

of early treatment with lens extraction, especially as there is now evidence that glaucoma treatments cause cataract. What is also needed are better diagnostic means to determine the relevance of narrow angles in patients with glaucoma so that the appropriate treatment can be instituted.

Acknowledgements

This chapter is based on that already published in *Clinical Evidence* (Shah R, Wormald R. Acute angle closure glaucoma. *Clinical Evidence* (June issue 7). London: BMJ Publishing Group, 2002) by the same authors. Major changes have been made for this edition. The original chapter was, however, written by Professor Colm O'Brien and Mr Jeremy Diamond, whose contribution is gratefully acknowledged.

References

1. Foster PJ, Buhrmann R, Quigley HA, Johnson GJ. The definition and classification of glaucoma in prevalence surveys. *Br J Ophthalmol* 2002;**86**(2):238–42.
2. Lai JS, Liu DT, Tham CC *et al.* Epidemiology of acute primary angle closure in the Hong Kong Chinese population: prospective study. *Hong Kong Med J* 2001;**7**(2):118–23.
3. Wong TY, Foster PJ, Seah SK, Chew PT. Rates of hospital admissions for primary angle closure glaucoma among Chinese, Malays, and Indians in Singapore. *Br J Ophthalmol* 2000;**84**(9):990–2.
4. Bonomi L, Marchini G, Marraffa M *et al.* Epidemiology of angle-closure glaucoma: prevalence, clinical types, and association with peripheral anterior chamber depth in the Egna-Neumarket Glaucoma Study. *Ophthalmology* 2000;**107**(5):998–1003.
5. Foster PJ, Oen FT, Machin D *et al.* The prevalence of glaucoma in Chinese residents of Singapore: a cross-sectional population survey of the Tanjong Pagar district. *Arch Ophthalmol* 2000;**118**(8):1105–11.
6. Foster PJ, Baasanhu J, Alsbirk PH, Munkhbayar D, Uranchimeg D, Johnson GJ. Glaucoma in Mongolia. A population-based survey in Hovsgol province, northern Mongolia. *Arch Ophthalmol* 1996;**114**(10): 1235–41.
7. Foster PJ, Devereux JG, Alsbirk PH *et al.* Detection of gonioscopically occludable angles and primary angle closure glaucoma by estimation of limbal chamber depth in Asians: modified grading scheme. *Br J Ophthalmol* 2000;**84**(2):186–92.
8. Dandona L, Dandona R, Mandal P *et al.* Angle-closure glaucoma in an urban population in southern India. The Andhra Pradesh eye disease study. *Ophthalmology* 2000;**107**(9):1710–16.
9. Pandit RJ, Taylor R. Mydriasis and glaucoma: exploding the myth. A systematic review. *Diabetic Med* 2000;**17**:693–9.
10. Edwards RS. A comparative study of Ocusert Pilo 40, intensive pilocarpine and low-dose pilocarpine in the initial treatment of primary acute angle-closure glaucoma. *Curr Med Res Opin* 1997;**13**: 501–9.
11. Choong YF, Irfan S, Menage MJ. Acute angle closure glaucoma: an evaluation of a protocol for acute treatment. *Eye* 1999;**13**(5): 613–16.
12. Yang CC, Chou SC, Hung PT, Yang CH, Hung L, Tsai CB. Anterior chamber angles shallowing and intraocular pressure after topical pilocarpine. *J Ocul Pharmacol Ther* 1997;**13**(3):219–24.
13. Aung T, Wong HT, Yip CC, Leong JY, Chan YH, Chew PT. Comparison of the intraocular pressure-lowering effect of latanoprost

and timolol in patients with chronic angle closure glaucoma: a preliminary study. *Ophthalmology* 2000;**107**(6):1178–83.

14. Fleck BW, Wright E, Fairley EA. A randomized prospective comparison of operative peripheral iridectomy and Nd:YAG laser iridotomy treatment of acute angle closure glaucoma: 3 year visual acuity and intraocular pressure control outcome. *Br J Ophthalmol* 1997;**81**:884–8.

15. Fleck BW, Dhillon B, Khanna V *et al.* A randomised, prospective comparison of Nd:YAG laser iridotomy and operative peripheral iridectomy in fellow eyes. *Eye* 1991;**5**:315–21.

16. Pollack IP, Robin AL, Dragon DM *et al.* Use of neodymium:YAG laser to create iridotomies in monkeys and humans. *Trans Am Ophthalmol Soc* 1984;**82**:307–28.

17. Moster MR, Schwartz LW, Spaeth GL *et al.* Laser iridectomy. A controlled study comparing argon and neodymium:YAG. *Ophthalmology* 1986;**93**:20–4.

18. Fernandez-Bahamonde JL, Alcaraz-Michelli V. The combined use of apraclonidine and pilocarpine during laser iridotomy in a Hispanic population. *Ann Ophthalmol* 1990;**22**(12):446–9.

19. Rosenberg LF, Krupin T, Ruderman J *et al.* Apraclonidine and anterior segment laser surgery. Comparison of 0·5% versus 1·0% apraclonidine for prevention of postoperative intraocular pressure rise. *Ophthalmology* 1995;**102**(9):1312–18.

20. Lam DS, Lai JS, Tham CC, Chua JK, Poon AS. Argon laser peripheral iridoplasty versus conventional systemic medical therapy in treatment of acute primary angle-closure glaucoma: a prospective, randomized, controlled trial. *Ophthalmology* 2002;**109**(9):1591–6.

21. Nolan WP, Baasanhu J, Undraa A *et al.* Screening for primary angle closure glaucoma in Mongolia: a randomised controlled trial to determine whether screening and prophylactic treatment will reduce the incidence of primary angle closure glaucoma in an east Asian population. *Br J Opthalmol* 2003;**87**(3):271–4.

31 Modification of wound healing in glaucoma drainage surgery

JF Kirwan, Richard Wormald

Background

Glaucoma drainage surgery has a pivotal role in the management of glaucoma. In the developing world, it is the mainstay of treatment and in richer countries it is used in aggressive disease and where other therapies fail.

The most common procedure performed is trabeculectomy, a guarded filtration procedure. In older Europeans with primary open angle glaucoma, trabeculectomy has a success rate of at least 80%, and in individuals undergoing surgery early in the clinical course without extensive prior use of medical therapy the results are even better.[1]

However, it is clear that there are groups of patients with a poorer prognosis for surgery. Risk factors for failure of glaucoma drainage surgery include young age (particularly children), black African ethnic origin, prior medical therapy with adrenergic agents and pilocarpine, previous failed glaucoma drainage surgery, aphakia and previous cataract surgery, uveitis, angle recession glaucoma (secondary to trauma) and anterior segment neovascularisation.[2] These factors are thought to be additive. In an effort to improve results, especially where risk of failure is increased, investigators have studied the use of antiproliferative agents to inhibit postoperative scarring in the sub-conjunctival space.

Postoperative corticosteroids have been clearly shown to improve results after surgery and are used routinely. In their relatively small RCT, Starita et al.[3] showed a significantly better success rate with postoperative topical steroids that persisted at both 5 and 10-year follow up.

Beta radiation was first used for glaucoma drainage surgery over 60 years ago but has not gained widespread use.[4] The use of 5-fluorouracil, given as multiple postoperative injections, was first described in 1984[5] while mitomycin C as a peroperative topical application was first described by Chen et al. in 1990,[6] who reported using it in a case series going back to 1981. Subsequently, intra-operative 5-fluorouracil and mitomycin C have been widely, although variably, used.[7,8]

Question

Do postoperative injections of 5-fluorouracil improve results in high-risk glaucoma drainage surgery, primary glaucoma drainage surgery or combined cataract and glaucoma drainage surgery?

The evidence

A systematic review by Wormald et al. has addressed these questions.[9] A total of nine trials were found, but most were not of high quality. The main outcomes examined were "clinical failure" (i.e. the need to repeat surgery due to loss of intraocular pressure control) and mean postoperative intraocular pressure at one year. A requirement for the use of medical therapy was not a definition of failure.

For cases with a high risk of failure, the review found data from two studies with a total of 239 participants: a large multi-centre study and a smaller study.[10,11] The smaller study[11] showed a considerably larger effect. Patients who had undergone previous failed glaucoma drainage surgery or cataract extraction were included. The main exclusion criterion was prior exposure to 5-fluorouracil. The data suggested a 60% reduction in the risk of failure: from 43% to 19%. The relative risk (RR) estimate was 0·4 (95% CI 0·16–0·90). The summary number needed to treat (NNT) estimate was four cases (95% CI 3–8). Mean intraocular pressure (IOP) was only reported in the smaller study, where there was a 16 mmHg lower mean IOP in treated subjects.

For primary trabeculectomy, which was defined as an initial surgical procedure in subjects with uncontrolled open angle glaucoma, the systematic review found two studies with a total of 112 participants using the dosing regimen as originally described[12,13] and two studies using a less intensive regimen with a total of 120 randomised subjects.[14,15] The systematic review found a reduction in risk of failure from 18% to 3%, which represents a 76% reduction in risk. The RR estimate was 0·24 (95% CI 0·08–0·74). The summary

NNT estimate was five cases (95% CI 3–12). The constituent trials in the systematic review were small and produced no statistically significant results. The mean postoperative intraocular pressure was 5 mmHg lower in the subjects treated with 5-fluorouracil. The trial by Chaudhry *et al.* demonstrated no significant difference in success rates (defined as IOP <21 mmHg on no medications in this study) or degree of IOP reduction.[15]

For combined cataract extraction and glaucoma drainage surgery, a total of 142 subjects were randomised in three trials.[16–18] The point estimate of relative risk reduction was 0·42, equivalent to a 58% reduction in the risk of failure. However, the confidence intervals are very broad and firm conclusions cannot be drawn. This is primarily because there was a very low failure rate in both arms of each study. The mean postoperative IOP was significantly lower in two of the studies.[16,18] However, the mean IOP values were very different in the three studies so a pooled estimate was not available.

Question

What are the adverse effects of postoperative 5-fluorouracil?

The evidence

The systematic review considered adverse effects for all trials. Use of postoperative 5-fluorouracil was associated with a significantly increased risk of postoperative wound leak with a point estimate of risk 1·7 (95% CI 1·04–2·64). Hypotony was only found in the cases undergoing primary trabeculectomy, with a significantly increased risk in subjects treated with 5-fluorouracil. The point estimate was 7·4 (95% CI 1·2–45·0) with a number needed to harm (NNH) of 56 subjects (95% CI 24–518). No cases of endophthalmitis were reported in any trial. Expulsive haemorrhage was only reported in one trial with no difference between the treated and control subjects.[19] There was no convincing evidence that 5-fluorouracil increased the risk of a shallow anterior chamber, although the event rate was low. The risk of corneal epithelial toxicity is increased by treatment with 5-fluorouracil. The point estimate of risk was 6·2 (95% CI 3·9–9·7). Postoperative cataract was reported by Chaudhry,[15] which found this in 16% of treated eyes compared with 3% of control eyes. Despite this being a large effect, it was not statistically significant.

Comment

The routine use of a course of injections of 5-FU is less frequent now. Additional *ad hoc* injections for an apparently failing bleb are quite commonly practised in some clinics although there is no good evidence to support its use.

There is a major gap in the evidence with regard to any attempt to measure patient-orientated outcomes. Frequent postoperative sub-conjunctival injections are potentially unpleasant for patients and the keratopathy associated with 5-FU is painful. It is probably because of this that clinicians now prefer to use 5-FU or mitomycin peroperatively.

None of the trials have sufficient long-term follow up to provide evidence of the risk of longer term complications such as hypotony secondary to late leakage from a thin walled bleb and endophthalmitis.

Question

Does intraoperative 5-fluorouracil improve results in primary glaucoma drainage surgery compared with surgery without an antimetabolite?

The evidence

To date, data are only available for primary glaucoma drainage surgery. There is no published systematic review but three published trials were found: two from Africa, by Egbert *et al.*[20] and Yorston and Khaw.[21] and Khaw and one from the United Kingdom by Leyland *et al.*[22] Success was defined in all trials by intraocular pressure criteria of antiglaucoma drugs. In Africa, this is an essential requirement due to inherent problems in treating glaucoma medically.[23]

The Egbert *et al.* study[20] reported short-term follow up, with a minimum of 90 days of follow up required for inclusion. A significant effect of 5-fluorouracil was reported with a failure rate of 13% for 5-fluorouracil and 45% for controls (defined as an IOP >21 mmHg). Of 61 eligible eyes, 55 were included in the analysis (24 after 5-fluorouracil and 31 controls). Case selection was mixed; only 75% had primary open angle glaucoma (POAG) and were undergoing a first procedure for glaucoma. The trial showed a clear advantage for the use of 5-fluorouracil, although given the small sample size, eclectic case selection and short follow up, the results can not be considered definitive.

Yorston and Khaw[21] performed a randomised controlled trial of 5-fluorouracil versus standard trabeculectomy in Kenya. Of 68 patients with POAG, 56 (85%) were followed for a minimum of six months and 30 followed for two or more years (44%). A significant effect of 5-fluorouracil was found with 88·8% of 5-fluorouracil subjects and 70·6% of controls having an IOP <22 mmHg at two years. At six months, the mean postoperative IOPs were 16·9 mmHg (5-fluorouracil) and 17·4 (controls). Complications were similar in both groups, with subsequent cataract being the most important complication. The effect of 5-fluorouracil seems to be a prolongation of success in this population rather than a lower IOP. The authors commented on an increased incidence of cystic blebs (which may predispose to postoperative infection) in the 5-fluorouracil group in the early postoperative period, but this effect diminished with time. The authors estimated that the cost of 5-fluorouracil was £1·25 per failure prevented (NNT 6). For both African studies, loss to follow up was significant, which may limit the conclusions that can be drawn.

Leyland *et al.*'s study was performed on subjects undergoing a first glaucoma drainage surgery where the risk of failure was not considered to be particularly high. There were no significant differences between the treated and control groups, although the study had limited power (approximately 20%) to detect a 10% difference in success rate between the two groups as the success rate was high in both arms.[22]

Question

What are the adverse effects of intraoperative 5-fluorouracil?

The evidence

No excess complications were reported in the Egbert *et al.* or the Leyland *et al.* study, although a non-significant increase in bleb leaks was reported in the former study (four of 24 eyes *v* two of 31 eyes). Yorston and Khaw reported an excess of shallow anterior chambers in the early postoperative period, with thin walled drainage blebs at three months, but no numbers were reported. There were no cases of hypotony reported, but hypotony appears to be rare in Africans.[24]

Comment

So far there have been few trials and no systematic review providing a summary of the evidence for this fairly common practice. Some surgeons are happy to use topical 5-FU in primary trabeculectomy without excess risk factors for failure although the trade off of risk and benefit for this practice is not certain.

One further large trial will soon be completed in the UK and two others have been completed in Chile and Singapore but have not yet been published. A Cochrane systematic review is also near completion.

Question

Does intraoperative mitomycin C improve results in high-risk glaucoma drainage surgery, primary glaucoma drainage surgery and combined cataract and glaucoma drainage surgery?

The evidence

This question has been addressed in a Cochrane review by Wilkins *et al.*[25] The review included 11 trials covering 698 subjects. As for the review on postoperative 5-fluorouracil, the main outcome measurements were the proportion of successful cases (unsuccessful cases defined by uncontrolled intraocular pressure or repeat surgery).

For subjects with a high risk of failure, there were four trials with 193 subjects.[26–29] Two trials included high-risk subjects and one included subjects undergoing combined glaucoma and cataract extraction who were already at high risk of surgical failure due to previous failed surgery. One trial specifically included subjects with secondary glaucomas. The trials showed a significantly reduced risk of failure at 12 months: summary odds ratio (OR) 0·32, 95% CI 0·2–0·53. The summary NNT estimate was 3 (95% CI 2–4). Three trials reported IOP data; the summary mean IOP difference was 5·31 mmHg (95% CI 3·85–6·76 mmHg).

Three trials were found for combined cataract extraction and glaucoma surgery.[30–32] A total of 167 participants were randomised. No benefit of mitomycin C was found. For IOP two trials reported significantly lower IOP and one did not. The combined result suggested a mean difference in IOP reduction of 3·34 mmHg (95% CI 2·51–4·16 mmHg).

For primary trabeculectomy a total of 338 participants undergoing a first glaucoma surgical procedure were randomised in four trials.[33–36] In the largest trial,[36] subjects were randomised to placebo or to one of three dosing regimens of mitomycin C (0·2 mg/ml for two minutes, 0·2 mg/ml for four minutes or 0·4 mg/ml for two minutes). A summary OR of 0·29 (95% CI 0·16–0·53) was found. The summary NNT estimate was five (95% CI 4–8). Two trials reported IOP data at 12 months. The pooled estimate was a mean difference of 5·41 mmHg (95% CI 3·48–7·34 mmHg).

Question

What are the adverse effects of intraoperative mitomycin C?

The evidence

From data in the review, mitomycin C was associated only with an excess risk of cataract and the NNH was 15.[25] Robin *et al.*'s trial found an increased risk of cataract with longer mitomycin C treatment times.[36] Specifically, use of mitomycin C was not associated with an increased rate of endophthalmitis, hypotony, wound leak or shallow anterior chamber. However, the event rates of these complications were low.

Comment

The majority of trials in this review[25] were not judged to be of high quality though there were more better quality studies than in the 5-FU review.

The absence of effect in triple procedures is explained by the fact that IOPs were low in many patients entering the trials. Drainage was performed to reduce the risk of postoperative IOP spikes although this was not measured as an outcome.

Many recognise the increasing incidence of hypotony, wound leak and endophthalmitis as important late complications of the use of mitomycin C although none of the trials have long enough follow up to address these important issues. Retrospective studies have quantified the risks but active surveillance is needed to monitor this problem prospectively.

Question

What are the comparative effects of mitomycin C and 5-fluorouracil in the modification of wound healing after glaucoma surgery?

The evidence

There is no systematic review but there are five randomised controlled trials comparing mitomycin C and 5-FU in adults and one in paediatric glaucoma. Two trials dealt with patients at high risk of failure, one with pseudophakic patients, one with black West African patients and two with primary trabeculectomy.

The first comparative trial was by Kitazawa *et al.*,[37] in which 32 patients had one eye randomised either to mitomycin C 0·2 mg/ml applied during surgery or 10 postoperative injections of 5-fluorouracil over two weeks. All eyes had a poor surgical prognosis; follow up was between seven and 12 months. Eighty-eight per cent of eyes treated with mitomycin C compared to 47% of eyes treated with 5-FU achieved an IOP less than 20 mmHg. Corneal complications were more common in the 5-FU group while other complications were similar in both groups.

Lamping and Belking compared postoperative 5-FU injections and peroperative mitomycin C in patients who had previously undergone extracapsular cataract extraction and posterior chamber lens implantation.[38] Eighty eyes in 74 patients were randomised and followed up for 12 months. IOPs were significantly lower in the mitomycin C group and there was no difference in complications.

Katz *et al.* compared postoperative 5-FU with intra-operative mitomycin in eyes at high risk of failure.[39] Nineteen eyes in 19 patients were randomised to 5-FU compared with 20 eyes in 20 patients randomised to mitomycin C. They were followed up for 26–38 months. Postoperative exclusions meant that the analysis was not intention to treat. Pressures were found to be significantly lower in the mitomycin C group. Complications were similar in both groups except for a more frequent occurrence of Tenon's cysts in the mitomycin C group.

Researchers in all of these initial studies concluded that mitomycin C was as or more effective than postoperative 5-FU injections with similar or indeed fewer complications.

Kuldev Singh and colleagues went on to compare intraoperative 5-FU with mitomycin C in a West African population.[40] These patients were undergoing a primary procedure without prolonged previous exposure to topical medications. The intervention was either 50 mg/ml 5-FU for five minutes or mitomycin C 0·5 mg/ml for 3·5 minutes, applied to the exposed sclera with a soaked sponge. One eye of each of the 85 patients was randomised and followed for at least four months (CI 4–19, mean 10 months). Mitomycin C achieved a significantly higher success rate (proportion of IOP <21 mmHg) and lower mean IOP though the difference in patients achieving an IOP of <15 mmHg was not significant. There was no reported difference in complication rates and a further paper reported that for longer term follow up of patients in this and another trial, there was no difference in risk of hypotony, which occurred in two of 101 participants.[24]

The same group went on to conduct a similar trial in California.[41] The dose of 5-FU was the same but mitomycin C was applied for two minutes at a concentration of 0·4 mg/ml. One eye of 113 patients were randomised and followed for an average of 309 days for the 5-FU group and 339 days for the mitomycin C group. Predefined target IOPs were met a little more frequently in the mitomycin C group but did not reach statistical significance. Complications were again similar in both groups.

The most recent study reported was from Indiana.[42] This also compared the two agents in primary trabeculectomy. One hundred and fifteen eyes of 103 patients were randomised in a double-masked manner either to 50 mg/ml 5-FU for five minutes or 0·2 mg mitomycin C for two minutes. Outcomes were measured at six and 12 months in terms of success defined by various different IOP cut-off points. None of the outcomes was statistically different at either time point. Complications occurred more frequently in the mitomycin C group but this was not satisfactory.

Comment

It seems somewhat counter intuitive that peroperative 5-FU seems to be as effective as mitomycin C in primary trabeculectomy while postoperative injections (overall a considerably higher dose) is less effective in eyes at higher baseline risk of failure. Dose and duration of application of mitomycin C has tended to become less with the passage of time, perhaps because of the recognition of the much longer term complications now being reported. The trials have been conducted over more than a 10-year time span and there has been a noticeable improvement both in the standard of conduct and reporting of the trials over that period. As is so often observed, the size of the observed effect becomes less as the quality of the clinical experiments improve.

Question

Is beta radiation effective in improving the results of glaucoma drainage surgery?

Three trials were found that have examined the effect of beta radiation in improving the outcome of glaucoma drainage surgery. Two of these included white patients undergoing primary trabeculectomy and the other recruited Chinese subjects. Barnes *et al.* used 750 cGy just before surgery with 65 subjects.[43] The mean IOP reduction was very similar in both treated and control subjects, success was achieved in 100% of treated subjects and 88% of control subjects (intraocular pressure <21 mmHg with or without medication). Mean reductions in IOP of 10·3 mmHg and 9·3 mmHg were found in treated and control subjects.

Rehman *et al.* used a very similar methodology in a similar patient population, except that treatment was applied on completion of surgery and it was double masked; 61 subjects were treated.[44] The success rate was 100% in treated eyes and 95% in untreated eyes using the above criteria. For success without medication, the respective success rates were 90% and 86%. Complications were similarly prevalent in both groups in both trials.

Lai and Ho reported data from a Chinese population of 101 subjects with 1000 cGy applied on completion of surgery.[45] They reported success rates of 90% in treated subjects and 74% in control subjects. This difference was found to be significant. No excess of complications were reported in the subjects treated with beta radiation, although follow up was limited to one year (personal communication). Mean IOP data were not available. All three trials were of reasonable quality.

A further study by O'Donoghue *et al.*[46] compared beta radiation with postoperative 5-fluorouracil injections in high-risk subjects. Follow up was short, for a minimum of eight months and 70 subjects were studied. Success rates of 76% for the subjects treated with beta radiation and 79% for the subjects treated with 5-fluorouracil were reported (IOP >21 mmHg without medications). There was a trend for the subjects treated with beta radiation to have more favourable bleb morphology, while corneal toxicity was more common

in the subjects treated with 5-fluorouracil (88% *v* 7%). Again, no patient-orientated outcome was reported but it might be supposed that those without injections had a less traumatic experience.

Comment

Beta radiation seems to be a relatively cheap and simple alternative to antimetabolites but when comparing costs, the process of safely storing the radioactive source needs to be taken into account. Neither mitomycin C nor 5-FU are very costly. There may be specific advantages for use of these treatments in the developing world and there is an ongoing trial addressing this question in South Africa.

It may be that adverse outcomes are less severe after beta radiation compared to mitomycin C, but this study has not yet been done. Follow up would need to be long term to capture late adverse events.

Implications for practice

The evidence base for the modification of wound healing in glaucoma surgery is relatively well populated with trials though it remains hard to be clear about the trade-off between risk and benefit in the different risk groups. Everyone's ideal is to achieve a successful procedure first time round but the enthusiasm to achieve this must be tempered by the awareness of late complications. So far, we lack sufficient quantifiable estimates of risk and benefit for the different agents in use. It is interesting that more recent studies suggest that the clinical effectiveness of 5-FU and mitomycin C is not very different, while most of the reports of late complications relate to mitomycin C.

The evidence presented here can be used to guide clinicians to make the best judgement about choice of treatment for individual patients. This will always need to be a carefully balanced and properly informed choice for both patient and clinician.

Implications for research

In cell culture, there are enormous differences between 5-FU and mitomycin C. The latter is far more toxic, although 5-FU is also a poison.

Wound healing research has identified key growth factors in the healing of trabeculectomy drainage blebs, particularly transforming growth factor beta. Monoclonal antibodies to this have now been commercially produced and the results of a phase I/IIa trial are encouraging.[47] Clearly the costs of producing such an agent will be high, but if it can be shown to reduce long-term complications safely, while preserving or improving effectiveness, then savings may accrue with time.

Glaucoma is a long-term disease and therefore effectiveness studies have to address long-term safety and effectiveness. We found only one study in this review that managed 10-year outcomes.[3] This may need to become a minimum aim in future research.

References

1. Broadway DC, Grierson I, O'Brien C, Hitchings RA. Adverse effects of topical antiglaucoma medication. II. The outcome of filtration surgery. *Arch Ophthalmology* 1994;**112**(11):1446–54.
2. Ritch R, Shields MB *et al. The Glaucomas.* St Louis: Mosby, 1996.
3. Starita RJ, Fellman RL, Spaeth GL, Poryzees EM, Greenidge KC, Traverso CE. Short- and long-term effects of postoperative corticosteroids on trabeculectomy. *Ophthalmology* 1985;**92**(7):938–46.
4. Iliff CE. Surgical control of glaucoma in the negro. *Am J Ophthalmol* 1944;**27**:731–8.
5. Heuer DK, Parrish RK 2nd, Gressel MG, Hodapp E, Palmberg PF, Anderson DR. 5-fluorouracil and glaucoma filtering surgery. II. A pilot study. *Ophthalmology* 1984;**91**(4):384–94.
6. Chen CW, Huang HT, Bair JS, Lee CC. Trabeculectomy with simultaneous topical application of mitomycin C in refractory glaucoma. *J Ocul Pharmacol* 1990;**6**(3):175–82.
7. Chen PP, Yamamoto T, Sawada A, Parrish RK 2nd, Kitazawa Y. Use of antifibrosis agents and glaucoma drainage surgery in the American and Japanese Glaucoma Societies. *J Glaucoma* 1997;**6**(3):192–6.
8. Edmunds B, Thompson JR, Salmon JF, Wormald RP. The National Survey of Trabeculectomy. II. Variations in operative technique and outcome. *Eye* 2001;**15**(4):441–8.
9. Wormald R, Wilkins MR, Bance C. Post operative 5-fluorouracil for glaucoma surgery (Cochrane Review). In: Cochrane Collaboration: *Cochrane Library.* Issue 2. Oxford: Update Software, 2003.
10. Fluorouracil Filtering Surgery Study Group. Fluorouracil Filtering Surgery one-year follow-up. The Fluorouracil Filtering Surgery Study Group. *Am J Ophthalmol* 1989;**108**(6):625–35.
11. Ruderman JM, Welch DB, Smith MF, Shoch DE. A randomized study of 5-fluorouracil and filtration surgery. *Am J Ophthalmol* 1987;**104**(3):218–24.
12. Ophir A, Ticho U. A randomized study of trabeculectomy and subconjunctival administration of fluorouracil in primary glaucomas. *Arch Ophthalmology* 1992;**110**(8):1072–5.
13. Goldenfeld M, Krupin T, Ruderman JM *et al.* 5-Fluorouracil in initial trabeculectomy. A prospective, randomized, multicenter study. *Ophthalmology* 1994;**101**:1024–9.
14. Loftfield K, Ball SF. 5-FU in primary trabeculectomy: a randomised trial. *Invest Ophthalmol Vis Sci* 1991;**32**(4):745.
15. Chaudhry IA, Pasha MA, O'Connor DJ, Weitzman ML, Caprioli J. Randomized, controlled study of low-dose 5-fluorouracil in primary trabeculectomy. *Am J Ophthalmol* 2000;**130**(6):700–3.
16. O'Grady JM, Juzych MS, Dhin DH, Lemon LC, Swendris RP. Trabeculectomy, phacoemulsification, and posterior chamber lens implantation with and without 5-fluorouracil. *Am J Ophthalmol* 1993;**116**(5):594–9.
17. Wong PC, Ruderman JM, Krupin T *et al.* 5-Fluorouracil after primary combined filtration surgery. *Am J Ophthalmol* 1994;**117**(2):149–54.
18. Gandolfi SA, Vecchi M. 5-Fluorouracil in Combined Trabeculectomy and Clear-cornea Phacoemulsification with Posterior Chamber Intraocular Lens Implantation. *Ophthalmology* 1997;**104**:181–6.
19. Fluorouracil Filtering Surgery Study Group. Risk factors for suprachoroidal hemorrhage after filtering surgery. The Fluorouracil Filtering Surgery Study Group. *Am J Ophthalmol* 1992;**113**(5):501–7.
20. Egbert PR, Williams AS, Singh K, Dadzie P, Egbert TB. A prospective trial of intraoperative fluorouracil during trabeculectomy in a black population. *Am J Ophthalmol* 1993;**116**(5):612–16.
21. Yorston D, Khaw PT. A randomised trial of the effect of intraoperative 5-FU on the outcome of trabeculectomy in east Africa. *Br J Ophthalmol* 2001;**85**(9):1028–30.
22. Leyland M, Bloom P, Zinicola E, McAlister J, Rassam S, Migdal C. Single intraoperative application of 5-Fluorouracil versus placebo in low-risk trabeculectomy surgery: a randomized trial. *J Glaucoma* 2001;**10**(6):452–7.
23. Schwab L, Steinkuller PG. Surgical treatment of open angle glaucoma is preferable to medical management in Africa. *Soc Sci Med* 1983;**17**(22):1723–7.
24. Singh K, Byrd S, Egbert PR, Budenz D. Risk of hypotony after primary trabeculectomy with antifibrotic agents in a black west African population. *J Glaucoma* 1998;**7**(2):82–5.
25. Wilkins MR, Indar A, Wormald R. Intra-operative mitomycin C for glaucoma surgery. In: Cochrane Collaboration. *Cochrane Library.* Issue 2. Oxford: Update Software, 2003.
26. Turacli E, Gunduz K, Aktan G, Tamer C. A comparative clinical trial of mitomycin C and cyclosporin A in trabeculectomy. *Eur J Ophthalmol* 1996;**6**(4):398–401.
27. Wu L, Yin J. The effect of mitomycin C on the filtration surgery of glaucoma with poor prognosis. *Chung Hua Yen Ko Tsa [Chinese J Ophthalmol]* 1996;**32**(1):32–4.
28. Andreanos D, Georgopoulos GT, Vergados J, Papaconstantinou D, Liokis N, Theodossiadis P. Clinical evaluation of the effect of mitomycin-C in re-operation for primary open angle glaucoma. *Eur J Ophthalmol* 1997;**7**(1):49–54.
29. Shin DH, Kim YY, Sheth N *et al.* The role of adjunctive mitomycin C in secondary glaucoma triple procedure as compared to primary glaucoma triple procedure. *Ophthalmology* 1998;**105**(4):740–5.
30. Shin DH, Simone PA, Song MS *et al.* Adjunctive subconjunctival mitomycin C in glaucoma triple procedure. *Ophthalmology* 1995;**102**(10):1550–8.
31. Cohen JS, Greff LJ, Novack GD, Wind BE. A placebo-controlled, double-masked evaluation of mitomycin C in combined glaucoma and cataract procedures. *Ophthalmology* 1996;**103**(11):1934–42.
32. Carlson DW, Alward WL, Barad JP, Zimmerman MB, Carney BL. A randomized study of mitomycin augmentation in combined phacoemulsification and trabeculectomy. *Ophthalmology* 1997;**104**(4):719–24.
33. Costa VP, Comegno PE, Vasconcelos JP, Malta RF, Jose NK. Low-dose mitomycin C trabeculectomy in patients with advanced glaucoma. *J Glaucoma* 1996;**5**(3):193–9.
34. Szymanski A, Gierek-Lapinska A, Koziak M, Gierek-Ciaciura S. A fluorophotometric study of corneal endothelium after trabeculectomy using different concentrations of Mitomycin-C. *Int Ophthalmol* 1996;**20**(1–3):95–9.
35. Martini E, Laffi GL, Sprovieri C, Scorolli L. Low-dosage mitomycin C as an adjunct to trabeculectomy. A prospective controlled study. *Eur J Ophthalmol* 1997;**7**(1):40–8.
36. Robin AL, Ramakrishnan R, Krishnadas R *et al.* A Long-term Dose-Response Study of Mitomycin in Glaucoma Filtration Surgery. *Arch Ophthalmol* 1997;**115**:969–74.
37. Kitazawa Y, Kawase K, Matsushita H, Minobe M. Trabeculectomy with mitomycin. A comparative study with fluorouracil. *Arch Ophthalmol* 1991;**109**(12):1693–8.
38. Lamping KA, Belkin JK. 5-Fluorouracil and mitomycin in pseudophakic patients. *Ophthalmology* 1995;**102**(1):70–5.
39. Katz GJ, Higginbotham EJ, Lichter PR *et al.* Mitomycin C versus 5-fluorouracil in high-risk glaucoma filtering surgery. Extended follow up. *Ophthalmology* 1995;**102**(9):1263–9.
40. Singh K, Egbert PR, Byrd S *et al.* Trabeculectomy with intraoperative 5-fluorouracil versus mitomycin C. *Am J Ophthalmol* 1997;**123**(1):48–53.
41. Singh K, Mehta K, Shaikh NM *et al.* Trabeculectomy with intraoperative mitomycin C versus 5-fluorouracil. Prospective randomised clinical trial. *Ophthalmology* 2000;**107**(12):2305–9.
42. WuDunn D, Cantor LB, Palanca-Capistrano AM *et al.* A prospective randomised controlled trial comparing intraoperative 5-fluorouracil versus mitomycin C in primary trabeculectomy. *Am J Ophthalmol* 2002;**134**:521–8.
43. Barnes RM, Mora JS, Best SJ *et al.* Beta radiation as an adjunct to low-risk trabeculectomy. *Clin Exp Ophthalmol* 2000;**28**(4):259–62.

44. Rehman SU, Amoaku WM, Doran RM, Menage MJ, Morrell AJ. Randomized controlled clinical trial of beta irradiation as an adjunct to trabeculectomy in open-angle glaucoma. *Ophthalmology* 2002; **109**(2):302–6.

45. Lai J, Ho C. Trabeculectomy combined with beta irradiation in uncomplicated primary open angle glaucoma. *Invest Ophthalmol Vis Sci* 1994;**34**:1432.

46. O'Donoghue EP, Ridgway AEA. Strontium 90 *v* 5-FU as adjunct to surgery for patients at high risk of trabeculectomy failure: A prospective randomised trial. *Invest Ophthalmol Vis Sci* 1994; **35**:1432.

47. Siriwardena D, Khaw PT, King AJ *et al.* Human antitransforming growth factor beta(2) monoclonal antibody – a new modulator of wound healing in trabeculectomy: a randomised placebo controlled clinical study. *Ophthalmology* 2002;**109**(3):427–31.

Section VIII

Cataract

Emma Hollick, Editor

Cataract: mission statement

Age-related cataract remains the commonest cause of blindness throughout the world and cataract surgery forms the major surgical workload of eye departments. Recent advances in surgical technique, equipment and intraocular lenses have significantly affected the way surgery is being performed. This section presents the evidence available on some important aspects of cataract surgery, with the objective of assessing the degree to which modern cataract surgical practice is based on high quality evidence from randomised controlled trials (RCTs). The findings of recent RCTs on cataract surgery found in the Cochrane Eyes and Vision Group register and published systematic reviews of trials are described.

Clinical assessments of different cataract surgical techniques are described in Chapter 32. Evidence for any benefit of phacoemulsification over extracapsular cataract extraction is discussed. The effect of different viscoelastics, incisions, phacoemulsification techniques and incision closure techniques are described. Chapter 33 looks at studies of intraocular lens biocompatibility. The areas investigated are the influence of intraocular lens type on anterior chamber inflammation, surface cytology, anterior capsule reaction, lens implant decentration, posterior capsule opacification and postoperative vision. Chapter 34 evaluates the evidence of whether the use of multifocal intraocular lenses offers benefits over the current standard treatment of monofocal intraocular lens implantation. RCTs examining the perioperative management of cataract surgery are described in Chapter 35. This chapter sets out the evidence available in the following areas: prevention and treatment of cystoid macular oedema, prevention and treatment of endophthalmitis, and postoperative anti-inflammatory treatment.

Throughout this section gaps in the evidence are highlighted. It is apparent that standardised and objective outcome measures are required to improve the quality of future RCTs. The implications for future research are also addressed.

32 Cataract surgical techniques

Jodhbir S Mehta

Background

Cataract surgery forms the major surgical workload of eye departments throughout the world. Technological advances in equipment, as well as intraocular lens design and drugs, have affected the way surgery is being performed, particularly over the past ten years.

Treatment options

Extracapsular extraction with intraocular lens implantation became the panacea in treatment for cataract patients. However, even though spherical equivalent neutrality could be achieved, problems with postoperative astigmatism remained.

Phacoemulsification emerged as an alternative method for cataract removal, through a small incision in a "closed environment". Although initially viewed with scepticism, almost 90% of cataract surgery is now performed by this technique.

This chapter aims to present evidence available on surgical techniques involved in cataract removal. The randomised controlled trials (RCTs) discussed are concerned with phacoemulsification, including its comparison with extracapsular cataract extraction (ECCE). Studies which looked solely at ECCE surgery have not been included.

Question

What is the difference in effect on surgical outcome between phacoemulsification and extracapsular cataract extraction?

The evidence

There are nine RCTs that have compared the effects of phacoemulsification (phaco) and ECCE (Table 32.1).[1–9] There is evidence for significantly greater postoperative inflammation following ECCE than phaco.[1–3] Landau and Laurell showed less "in the bag" placement of IOL (intraocular lens implant) haptics following ECCE.[4] A better uncorrected visual acuity (UCVA) was shown in patients who underwent phaco compared to ECCE.[1,2,5–7] These studies, however, differ in the length of time in which there is a statistical benefit in UCVA. No statistical difference was noted in endothelial cell loss between the groups, but the coefficient of variation of endothelial cells was higher following ECCE, as was corneal thickness.[1,5] Two RCTs have looked at intraocular pressure levels (IOP) after surgery with differing results.[8,9] The IOP at six hours post operatively was higher in the ECCE group in Bömer *et al.*'s study,[9] and higher in the phaco group in Jürgens *et al.*'s study.[8] Two RCTs showed significantly less posterior capsule opacification following phaco than ECCE.[2,7]

No statistical difference was shown between the two techniques with respect to progression of diabetic retinopathy or presence of clinical significant macula oedema following surgery,[2] or of the cost of the two techniques with respect to the resources used.[7]

Comment

Overall, the evidence suggests that phacoemulsification has a number of advantages over ECCE; in particular reduced postoperative inflammation, better IOL placement, better UCVA, less posterior capsular opacification and reduced corneal swelling.

Question

What is the effect of different viscoelastics on surgical outcomes?

The evidence

The consequences of using various viscoelastics may be examined by analysing the IOP and endothelial cell function and morphology (Table 32.2). Comparison between studies was difficult since there was incomplete information as to whether patients were given preoperative, intraoperative, or postoperative medication in all cases, which would have had an effect on the postoperative IOP readings.

Three RCTs have compared the use of hydroxypropyl methylcellulose (HPMC) based products with Healon.[10–12] Significantly higher IOP was seen in the Healon group at 24 hours in one study.[10] However, the other two RCTs showed

Table 32.1 Effect of phacoemulsification or ECCE on surgical outcomes

Authors	Methods	Intervention	Participants	Outcomes	Results	Notes
Laurell et al., 1998[1]	RCT FU 3/7, 3/12, 12/12, 24/12	Phaco (5·2 mm incision, scleral tunnel) v ECCE (11 mm incision) and sutures PMMA lens Sutureless phaco	Phaco – 20 eyes ECCE – 20 eyes	LFP ACF Pachymetry VA	• DCF/flare intensity stat sig less in phaco group at 3/7 and 3/12 (P = 0·008), after no SSD • Stat sig better UCVA phaco group at 3/7 (P = 0·013) but BCVA and corneal thickness not SSD 2 groups at any FU	• One surgeon • Postop ST and guttae steroids • 5 eyes ECCE 3/7 no readings LFP/Pachy/VA • No brown irises
Dowler et al., 2000[2]	RCT FU 1–2 days 1, 6 wks, 3, 9, 12, 18, 24 months	Phaco (3·2 mm incision silicone IOL) v ECCE (PMMA lens, 5 × 10/0 nylon stitch) Diabetics	Phaco – 46 eyes (12 no DR) ECCE – 46 eyes (15 no DR)	LogMar VA CSME DR progression SLIS PCO	• Stat sig greater SLIS in ECCE group 1/52 FU (P = 0·0004) • Greater PCO rate ECCE group (P = 0·01). No SSD in presence of CSME/DR progression or develop of high risk DR between groups • Stat sig worse VA in ECCE group with DR at 1yr (P = 0·01) • CSME present at surgery most sig indicator of VA at 1yr regardless of surgical group	• Paired eyes 1yr apart
Chee et al., 1999[3]	RCT FU 1, 4, 8, 15, 30, 60, 90 days	Phaco (scleral tunnel, 6 mm) v ECCE Pigmented Irides PMMA lens	ECCE – 16 eyes Phaco – 18 eyes	LFP SLIS VA	• Stat sig greater flare and SLIS ECCE group up to day 60 (P = 0·016) • No SSD in UCVA at 2/12 FU both groups	• 2 surgeons • g NSAID preop, postop SC and guttae steroids
Landau and Laurell, 1999[4]	RCT FU 2 yrs	Phaco (5·2 mm incision, CCC, scleral tunnel, sutureless) v ECCE (11 mm incision, linear capsulotomy) and sutures PMMA lens	Phaco – 18 eyes ECCE – 17 eyes	IOL position by UBM LFP	• Stat sig higher "in bag" placement of haptics in phaco cases (P = 0·01) • AC depth stat sig shallower in ECCE group • No SSD in LFP/AC angle/iris thickness between groups	• Small no. • Effect on VA?
Ravalico et al., 1997[5]	RCT FU 7 and 30 days	Phaco (5·5 mm, 10/0 nylon) v ECCE (10 mm limbal incision, CCC, 10/0 nylon) PMMA lens	Phaco – 20 eyes ECCE – 20 eyes	SM Pachymetry ACF VA	• BCVA stat sig better phaco than ECCE 7/7 (P <0·01) no SSD 30/7 • No SSD in EC loss. CV stat sig higher ECCE group (P <0·01) • Stat sig increase corneal thickness/EC permeability ECCE group at 30/7 (P <0·01)	• Same surgeon • g NSAID preop postop SC and guttae steroids

(Continued)

Table 32.1 (Continued)

Authors	Methods	Intervention	Participants	Outcomes	Results	Notes
Leen et al., 1993[6]	RCT FU 3/12	Phaco (Scleral flap, Superior, 2 mm post limbus) v ECCE (Limbal incision, 11 mm – nuclear expression)	Phaco – 85 eyes ECCE – 31 eyes	Keratometry VA	• Stat sig better UCVA ($P = 0.005$) and SIA ($P = 0.044$) at 1/12 phaco group, no SSD any group at 3/12 • Phaco groups stat sig higher no. eyes cyl ≤1.5 D at 1/12 ($P = 0.05$) no SSD 3/12	• 90% power • ? initial investment
Minassian et al., 2001[7]	RCT FU 3, 6/52, 3, 6, 12 months	Phaco (3.2 m, OSA, silicone lens) v ECCE (12–14 mm incision, 7 mm PMMA lens, nylon sutures)	ECCE – 232 eyes Phaco – 244 eyes	VA Refraction Astigmatism Complication rates PCO Resource use Costs	• Stat sig more surgical complications ($P < 0.0001$) and PCO ($P = 0.014$) within 1 yr after surgery in ECCE group, and postop astigmatism sig less frequent in phaco group. • Higher proportion better UCVA of 6/9 or better in phaco group ($P < 0.0001$) • Average cost similar both groups.	
Jürgens et al., 1997[8]	RCT FU 3/6/24/ 72 hrs and 7 days	ECCE (10.5 mm limbal incision, PMMA lens, 5 × 10/0 nylon stitch) v Phaco (3.2 mm incision silicone IOL, 1 × 10/0 nylon stitch)	ECCE – 36 eyes (18 Healon, 18 Healon GV) Phaco – 22 eyes (11 Healon, 11 Healon GV)	IOP	• Stat sig higher IOP phaco group at 6 hrs ($P < 0.05$), no SSD after. • Stat sig higher IOP in ECCE and Healon GV than ECCE and Healon at 6 hrs	• i.c. Ach • No anti-glaucoma Tx postop • Small no.
Bömer et al., 1995[9]	RCT FU 3/6/24 hrs	Phaco (7 mm × 3.5 mm scleral tunnel) v ECCE (11 mm incision) 10/0 nylon	Phaco – 108 eyes 47 Sutureless 61 with suture ECCE – 12 eyes	IOP	IOP highest at 6 hr FU but stat sig higher in ECCE group ($P = 0.016$) but no SSD at 24 hrs.	• Very small no. • Postop anti-glaucoma Tx

Phaco, phacoemulsification and intraocular lens implant; PCO, posterior capsule opacification; IOL, intraocular lens implant; ECCE, extracapsular cataract extraction via nuclear expression and intraocular lens implant; CCC, continuous curvilinear capsulorhexis; LFP, laser flare photometry; SLIS, Slit amp inflammatory score = subjective AC cells and flare; BAB, blood aqueous barrier; SSD, statistical significant difference; ACF, anterior chamber fluorophotometry; AC, anterior chamber; ST, subtenons; SC, Subconj; DCF, median diffusion coefficient for fluorescein leakage through BAB; IOP, intraocular pressure measurement by Goldmann tonometry; UCVA, uncorrected visual acuity; BCVA, best corrected visual acuity; UBM, ultrasound biomicroscopy; SM, specular microscopy; CV, coefficient of variation of endothelial cells; PH, % hexagons; EC, endothelial cell; CSME, clinically significant macular oedema; DR, diabetic retinopathy; OSA, incision on steepest axis of astigmatism; SIA, surgically induced astigmatism

no difference[11,12] but the first had very few patients who underwent phacoemulsification and the second used pneumotonograph for IOP measurements, which could explain the different outcomes. There was a significant increase in corneal thickness at one day postoperatively in an HPMC group compared to Healon but no difference thereafter.[12]

Four RCTs have compared cohesive with dispersive agents.[13–16] No significant difference in IOP at 24 hours postoperatively or endothelial cell dysfunction/loss was seen between Amvisc Plus and Viscoat.[13] However, IOP was significantly higher at six hours postoperatively in a Viscoat group compared to Healon 5.[14] Miller showed significantly more time was needed to remove Viscoat than Healon GV, but no significant difference was noted in endothelial cell dysfunction between the two groups.[15] Koch *et al.* only showed a significant increase in corneal thickness with Healon compared with Viscoat at day one postoperatively.[16]

Three RCTs have looked at different Healon-based derivatives.[8,17,18] Higher IOP was seen at six hours with Healon GV compared to Healon in Jürgens *et al.*'s study,[8] but no significant difference was seen in Kohnen *et al.*'s.[17] However, in Kohnen *et al.*'s study preoperative diamox was given. No statistical difference was seen in IOP or corneal thickness postoperatively between patients using Healon or Microvisc.[18]

Comment

The evidence suggests that HPMC might produce a lower IOP but more corneal swelling after surgery than Healon. Evidence suggested Viscoat caused raised IOP at 24 hours postoperatively and was more difficult to remove than cohesive agents. Higher viscosity healonoids appear to cause a greater IOP rise at 24 hours.

Question

What is the effect of scleral tunnel depth on surgical outcome?

The evidence

Two RCTs have examined the effect of scleral tunnel depth (Table 32.3).[19,20] There was a significantly higher incidence of hyphaema in the deeper scleral tunnel group,[19] but no difference was noted in surgically induced astigmatism or wound strength between the two depths.[20]

Question

What is the effect of a corneal/scleral/limbal located phaco incision on surgical outcome?

The evidence

Four RCTs have compared the effects of scleral tunnel incisions with clear corneal incision,[21–24] and four with limbal based incisions[25–28] (Table 32.4). In comparing the scleral tunnel incision with the clear corneal (superior or temporal), there was no significant difference in visual acuity between groups postoperatively.[21,23,24] There was less alteration in blood aqueous barrier at three days postoperatively and lower IOP at six hours postoperatively with clear corneal incisions than with scleral tunnel incisions.[21] Analysis of astigmatism has produced conflicting results with two studies showing less astigmatism,[22,23] but Olsen *et al.* showing greater induced astigmatism in the corneal groups.[24] Direct comparison of these studies, however, was not possible since Kurimoto *et al.*[22] looked at absolute postoperative astigmatism, Cillino *et al.*[23] examined polar values and Olsen *et al.* examined the changes by vector analysis.

No statistically significant difference was noted in the surgically induced astigmatism between limbal incisions and scleral tunnels after one week.[25–27] Gimbel *et al.*'s study comparing a scleral flap to acute bevelled cataract incision showed greater astigmatism in the latter group, but this may be explained by the effect of sutures rather than location of incision (Table 32.5).[26] There was no difference in wound strength between limbal and tunnel groups (whether temporal or superior) after one day.[27] There was a lower IOP rise in the tunnel groups at six hours than in limbal, but no difference thereafter.[28]

Comment

Evidence suggests clear corneal incisions caused reduced inflammation and IOP compared to scleral tunnels. No advantage was seen with respect to the UCVA, and the results were equivocal for astigmatism. Between limbal and scleral tunnels there was no difference in surgically induced astigmatism or wound strength. There was a lower IOP initially in the scleral tunnel group.

Question

What is the effect of incision location on surgical outcome?

The evidence

Studies pertaining to the effect of incision location are tabulated in Table 32.6, all of which examine the effect of location of scleral tunnels.[27,29–31] Direct inter-study comparison is difficult since the size of the flaps varies between studies, as does the surgical technique. However, the data suggest a significant reduction in surgically induced

Table 32.2 Effect of different viscoelastics on surgical outcome

Authors	Methods	Intervention	Participants	Outcomes	Results	Notes
Lüchtenberg et al., 2000[10]	RCT FU 24 hrs	Adatocel v Amvisc Plus v Healon	Adatocel – 50 eyes Amvisc Plus – 50 eyes Healon – 50 eyes Phaco only	IOP	• No SSD IOP at 6 hrs post op between groups • 24 hrs IOP stat sig higher Healon group (P = 0·003) than Adatocel/Amvisc Plus	• Small no. phaco group
Smith and Lindstrom, 1991[11]	RCT FU 3/12	Occucoat v Healon	Occucoat – 166 eyes Healon – 56 eyes Phaco/ECCE and IOL	ECC by SM IOP	• No SSD in IOP between groups • No SSD ECC loss between groups or phaco/ECCE	
Pedersen, 1990[12]	RCT FU 5/52	Adatocel v Healon	Adatocel – 35 eyes Healon – 35 eyes Phaco only	Pachymetry IOP*	• Stat sig increase corneal thickness at 24 hrs Adatocel group (P<0·05), no SSD at 5/52 • No SSD in IOP 24 hrs – 5/52	• ? Anti-glaucoma Tx postop • Healon better protection for phaco • Single surgeon
Probst and Nichols, 1993[13]	RCT FU 2/12	Amvisc Plus v Viscoat	Amvisc Plus – 25 eyes Viscoat – 25 eyes	IOP ECC by SM Pachymetry	• No SSD in SM/pachymetry between 2 groups • No SSD IOP at 24 hrs, 1/52, 8/52 between 2 groups	• Anti-glaucoma Tx postop • Same surgeon • Ach intraop
Rainer et al., 2000[14]	RCT FU 1/52	Healon 5 v Viscoat	Healon 5 – 35 eyes Viscoat – 35 eyes	IOP	• IOP stat sig. higher Viscoat group at 6 hrs (P<0·0001), at 20 hr/24 hr and 1/52 no SSD	• No anti-glaucoma Tx postop • Same surgeon • 30% Viscoat Tx at 6 hrs
Miller and Colvard, 1999[15]	RCT FU 2/52	Healon GV v Viscoat	Healon GV – 70 eyes Viscoat – 70 eyes Phaco only	SM Pachymetry Operating Time	• Stat sig more time needed to remove Viscoat (P<0·001) • No SSD in corneal thickness, ECC and mean cell size 2 groups 24 hrs, 2/52 post op • Viscoat better maintaining cell hexagonality	• Single surgeon • No anti-glaucoma Tx postop

(Continued)

Table 32.2 (Continued)

Authors	Methods	Intervention	Participants	Outcomes	Results	Notes
Koch et al., 1993[16]	RCT FU 1/7, 1/52, 1, 2, 4/12	Healon v Viscoat	Healon – 29 eyes Viscoat – 30 eyes Phaco only	VA SM Pachymetry	• Stat sig less corneal thickness Viscoat group 1/7 ($P<0·05$) not SSD 1/52 • Stat sig less superior EC loss Viscoat group at 4/12 ($P<0·01$) • No SSD in CV/PH, central EC loss 2 groups at any visit	• Single surgeon • i.c. Ach • No anti-glaucoma Tx postop
Jürgens et al., 1997[8]	RCT FU 3/6/24/72 hrs and 7 days	Healon v Healon GV	Healon – 37 eyes (Phaco 11, ECCE 18) Healon GV – 37 eyes (Phaco 11, ECCE 18)	IOP	• Stat sig higher IOP Healon GV at 6 hrs, ($P<0·05$), no SSD after • No SSD between groups in pts who had IOP >30 mmHg • Stat sig higher IOP in ECCE and Healon GV than ECCE and Healon at 6 hrs	• i.c. Ach. • No anti-glaucoma Tx postop • Small no.
Kohnen et al., 1996[17]	RCT FU 6/24/36/48 hrs and 1/12	Healon v Healon GV	Healon – 30 eyes Healon GV – 30 eyes Phaco only	IOP Removal times (20 sec or 40 sec)	• No SSD in IOP mean in 2 groups at all times but SD higher in Healon GV at 6/24 hrs only • No difference between 20/40 sec removal times for Healon or Healon GV • No SSD in IOP between 20/40 sec groups	• Preop Diamox 12 hrs before. • No anti-glaucoma Tx postop • Single surgeon.
Arshinoff and Hofmann, 1997[18]	RCT FU 6/24 hrs 5/7, 1 and 6/12	Healon v Microvisc	Healon – 49 eyes Microvisc – 51 eyes Phaco only	Pachymetry IOP VA	• No SSD in IOP/VA between 2 groups at any post op period. No SSD in corneal thickness between 2 groups at all visits but stat sig increase at 24 hrs both groups compared pre op, no SSD at 5/7.	• Single surgeon • i.c. Ach. • No anti-glaucoma Tx postop

IOP, intraocular pressure measurement by Goldmann tonometry; IOP*, intraocular pressure measurement by pneumotonograph; HPMC, Hydroxypropyl methylcellulose; SM, specular microscopy; SD, standard deviation; SSD, statistical significant difference; CV, coefficient of variation; PH, % hexagons, EC, Endothelial cell; ECC, endothelial cell count; Occucoat, 2% HPMC in balanced salt solution (viscosity 4000 centipose (cps) at 0 shear rate); Viscoat, 4% sodium chondroitin sulfate – 3% sodium hyaluronate (ratio 1:3) (viscosity 40 000 cps at 0 shear rate); Healon, 1% sodium hyaluronate (osmolality, 302 mosm/kg/H$_2$O) (viscosity 200 000 cps at 0 shear rate); Healon 5, 2·3% sodium hyaluronate (viscosity 7 000 000 cps at 0 shear rate), Amvisc Plus, 1·6% sodium hyaluronate (osmolality, 340 mosm/kg/H$_2$O) (Dynamic viscosity of 55 000 cps at 25°C, 2/sec shear rate), Adatocel, 2% HPMC in Ringer-lactate (osmolality, 300 mosm/kg/H$_2$O); Healon GV, 1·4% sodium hyaluronate (viscosity 2 000 000 cps at 0 shear rate); Microvisc, 1% sodium hyaluronate (viscosity 1 000 000 cps at 0 shear rate)

Table 32.3 Effect of scleral tunnel depth on surgical outcome

Authors	Methods	Intervention	Participants	Outcomes	Results	Notes
John et al., 1992[19]	RCT FU 1/7, 4/12	Phaco, incision (6 mm × 3 mm post to limbus): Deep scleral tunnel (0·27 mm) v Superficial pocket (0·17 mm) Closed continuous suture, 10/0 nylon	Deep – 66 eyes Superficial – 63 eyes	Incidence hyphaema VA IOP	• Stat sig higher incidence of hyphaema in deep group (P<0·001) • No SSD in IOP/VA between groups	• Anticoagulation stopped • ? 1 surgeon variation technique
Anders et al., 1995[20]	RCT FU 1/7, 1–4/52, 8/12	Phaco all eyes, no sutures: scleral incision (trapezoid 7 mm × 1 mm post surgical limbus): 300 μm v 500 μm	180 eyes randomised	Wound strength by OD SIA	• No SSD in SIA between 2 groups (SIA stabilise after 4/52 in 500 μm group, 1/7 in 300 μm not SSD) • No SSD in wound strength between the 2 groups	

Phaco, phacoemulsification and intraocular lens implant; UCVA, uncorrected visual acuity; BCVA, best corrected visual acuity; SSD, statistical significant difference; OD, ophthalmodynamometer; SIA, surgically induced astigmatism

Table 32.4 Effect of corneal or scleral incision on surgical outcome

Authors	Methods	Intervention	Participants	Outcomes	Results	Notes
Dick et al., 2000[21]	RCT FU 6 hrs,1/7, 2/7,3/7 and 5/12	Temporal incision: Clear corneal (CC) (3·2 mm) v scleral tunnel (SC) (1·5 mm post limbus, 3·2 mm) Phaco and silicone IOL	CC – 50 eyes SC – 50 eyes All Caucasian	Flare by LFP IOP VA	• Alteration in BAB stat sig lower with clear corneal incision in first 3/7 postop ($P<0.0001$). No SSD at 5/12 • IOP stat sig lower CC at 6 hrs ($P<0.0001$), no SSD after • No SSD in UCVA/BCVA between 2 groups	• Diclofenac preop od • Subconj and g pred postop
Kurimoto et al., 1999[22]	RCT FU 1, 3, 10, 30 and 100 days	Phaco: Clear corneal (CC) (4·1mm) OSA v BENT scleral tunnel (1·5 mm post limbus x 4·1mm)	CC – 29 eyes BENT – 29 eyes	Astigmatism	• Postop astig less in CC than n BENT group, only stat sig at 30 days ($P<0.05$)	
Cillino et al., 1997[23]	RCT FU 1/7, 2 and 8/52	Phaco, no stitch: Temporal (corneal, 5·2 mm incision) v Superior (linear, 5 × 1 mm post to limbus) PMMA lens both groups	Temporal – 40 eyes Superior – 40 eyes	Astigmatism VA	• No SSD in net astig between groups SSD in mean SIA since WR in temporal group and AR in superior grcup • No SSD in UCVA (better VA in temporal group 2/52 not SSD)	
Olsen et al., 1997[24]	RCT FU 1/7, 1/52, 6/12	Phaco: Clear corneal (CC) v Scleral tunnel (SC) (2 mm post limbus) Incisions 3·5–4 mm length, OSA	CC – 50 eyes SC – 50 eyes	Astigmatism CT VA	• Stat more SIA (both RA anc IRA) in CC group up to 6/12 ($P<0.01$) • No SSD in VA 2 groups	• Error if use SIA not at 90°
Hunold et al., 1995[25]	RCT FU 1/7, 2/52, 1, 3, 6 months	Phaco, superior: scleral tunnel (5 mm × 2 mm post limbus, frown incision, 1 stitch) v limbal incision (5 mm, continuous X suture)	Limbal – 21 eyes Tunnel – 23 eyes	Astigmatism UCVA	• No SSD in cyl in all FU groups • No SSD in vector, UCVA be:ween groups	

(Continued)

Table 32.4 (Continued)

Authors	Methods	Intervention	Participants	Outcomes	Results	Notes
Gimbel et al., 1995[26]	RCT FU 2 days, 2 wks, 6 and 12 months	Phaco, superior: Scleral flap (6 mm × 2·5 mm frown incision, horizontal suture gp1) v acute beveled incision (ABI, 6 mm incision, limbal, gp 2, running suture) Suture 10/0 prolene All WR astig preop	Acute bevelled incision – 28 eyes Horizontal suture – 35 eyes	Astigmatism	• Stat sig increase in keratometric cyl in gp 2 ($P = 0·005$), no SSD gp 1 compared with preop levels at 2/12 • No SSD at 1yr between groups • No SSD in SIA up to 1yr postop, but no. of eyes with induced ATR cyl stat sig higher than number with WR for both groups ($P < 0·1$)	
Anders et al., 1997[27]	RCT FU 1/7, 1–4/52, 8/12	Phaco, superior, no sutures: limbal incision (7 mm, trapezoid) v scleral incision (trapezoid 7 mm × 1 mm postsurgical limbus) Phaco, temporal, no sutures: Limbal incision (7 mm, trapezoid) v Scleral incision (trapezoid 7 mm × 1 mm postsurgical limbus)	180 eyes randomised	Wound strength by OD SIA	• Stat sig greater SIA at 1/7 ($P = 0·005$) in limbal group than scleral, no SSD after in superior group • Stat sig greater wound strength 1/7 FU scleral incision ($P = 0·001$) but no SSD after, in superior group • Stat sig greater SIA in limbal group than scleral at 1/52 ($P < 0·001$) but not SSD after, in temporal group • No SSD wound strength between 2 groups	
Börner et al., 1995[28]	RCT FU 3, 6, 23 hrs	Phaco superior incision i.c. Ach incision: 7 mm limbal (5 × 10/0 nylon) v scleral tunnel (7 mm × 2 mm scleral flap, no sutures)	Limbal – 56 eyes Tunnel – 44 eyes	IOP	• Stat sig lower IOP for tunnel group at 6 hrs ($P = 0·0009$), no SSD after • Stat sig more IOP >30 in suture group, over FU	• 7 different surgeons • occ pilo at end

LFP, laser flare photometry; BAB, blood aqueous barrier; SSD, statistical significant difference; IOP, intraocular pressure measurement by Goldmann tonometry; UCVA, uncorrected visual acuity; BCVA, best corrected visual acuity; CT, corneal topography; OSA, incision on steepest axis of astigmatism; SIA, surgically induced astigmatism; RA, regular astigmatism; IRA, irregular astigmatism; BENT, between nine and twelve o'clock; OD, ophthalmodynamometer

Table 32.5   Effect of incision size on postoperative outcome

Authors	Methods	Intervention	Participants	Outcomes	Results	Notes
El-Maghraby et al., 1993[32]	RCT FU 2/12	Scleral flap 2·5 mm post limbus: 3·5 mm v 5·5 mm v 6·5 mm	151 eyes	Astigmatism VA	• 3·5 mm less early SIA (F <0·02) and more rapid VA rehab (P <0·05). 5·5/6 mm more early total keratometric cyl and SIA.	
Grabow et al., 1991[33]	RCT FU 3/12	Scleral flap 2 mm post surgical limbus: 4 mm v 5·2 mm v 7 mm	4 mm – 280 eyes 5·2 mm – 215 eyes 7 mm – 20 eyes	Astigmatism VA	• No SSD in SIA among 3 groups at 3/12 • Earlier VA recovery in 4/5·2 mm groups • 4 mm stat sig better UCVA at 3/12	
Martin et al., 1993[34]	RCT FU 6/12	Scleral flap, 3 mm post limbus: 3·2 mm v 5 mm v 6 mm	3·2 mm – 68 eyes 5 mm – 60 eyes 6 mm– 68 eyes	Keratometry VA	• 3 groups no SSD in SIA • UCVA only SSD (P<0·01) 2/7 later no SSD	
Olson et al., 1998[35]	RCT FU 36/12	Scleral flap, superior, 1·5 mm post to limbus: 3·2 mm v 5·5 mm	3·2 mm – 55 eyes 5·5 mm – 56 eyes	Keratometry VA	• 3·2 mm group stat sig reduced SIA and better UCVA (P<0·001). BCVA equal 2 groups. WW stat sig commoner in 3·2 mm group	• Different lenses • PCO rates
Leen et al., 1993[6]	RCT FU 3/12	Scleral flap, superior, 2 mm post limbus: 4 mm, 6 mm Limbal incision: 11 mm – nuclear expression 10/0 nylon sutures radial 4 mm (1), 6 mm (2), 11 mm(6–9)	4 mm – 26 eyes 6 mm – 59 eyes 11 mm – 31 eyes	Keratometry VA	• 4 mm stat sig better UCVA and SIA at 1/12, no SSD any group at 3/12	• No suture removed during study
Levy et al., 1994[36]	RCT FU 6/12	Scleral flap, superior, 3 mm post to limbus: 3·5 mm v 5·1 mm	3·5 mm – 40 eyes 5·1 mm – 40 eyes	Keratometry VA	• 3·5 mm less SIA (P = 0·046), better UCVA (P<0·01) at 3/12, afterwards no SSD between groups	• Different lenses
Mendivil, 1996[37]	RCT FU 6/12	Scleral flap, superior, 3 mm post to surgical limbus: 3·2 mm v 4·0 mm 1 × 10/0 nylon radial suture all cases	3·2 mm – 58 eyes 4 mm – 59 eyes	Keratometry VA	• No SSD in UCVA, SIA 2 groups	
Gimbel et al., 1992[38]	RCT FU 1/7, 2–3 wks, 2/3/6/ 12/24 months	Scleral flap, superior: 6·5 mm v 7·5 mm Phaco, 4 different suture material, sutured continuous	6·5 mm – 90 eyes 7·5 mm – 110 eyes	SIA	• SIA and net postop astigmatism not SSD between 2 groups	

(Continued)

Table 32.5 (Continued)

Authors	Methods	Intervention	Participants	Outcomes	Results	Notes
Dam-Johansen and Olsen, 1997[39]	RCT FU 1/7, 1,2/52 1,4/12	Scleral tunnel, superior, 2 mm post limbus: 4 mm (1 10/0 nylon suture) v 6 mm (2 X 10/0 nylon suture) No sutures removed	4 mm – 98 eyes 6 mm – 99 eyes	SIA	• SSD SIA between 2 groups at 4/12 (*P*<0·01). 6 mm induced sig more cases of AR at an earlier time than the 4 mm group (*P*<0·02).	• One surgeon
Davison, 1993[40]	RCT FU 1/7, 2/52, 1 yr	Scleral tunnel, superior linear groove 3 mm post to limbus: 4 mm (folded silicone lens) v 5·5 mm (PMMA lens) 2 × pattern 10/0 nylon for all cases No sutures cut during FU	4 mm – 93 eyes 5·5 mm – 98 eyes	Astigmatism UCVA Hyphaema	• At 2/52 no SSD in mean SIA between groups. WR shifts seen in both groups. No SSD in mean SIA at 1 yr between groups. AR shifts seen in both groups. No SSD in UCVA between 2 groups. Stat sig higher incidence 1/7 hyphaema in 5·5 mm group	• One surgeon
Oshika et al., 1994[41]	RCT FU 6/12	Scleral flap, superior, 2·5 mm post surgical limbus: 3·2 mm v 5·5 mm	3·2 mm – 93 eyes 5·5 mm – 89 eyes	Keratometry VA CT Aqueous flare SM FP	• 3·2mm stat sig (*P*<0·01) better UCVA 1/12 postop no SSD after in 2 groups • SIA less 3·2 mm than 5 mm up to 6/12 (overall small). 3·2 mm stat sig more pts cyl ≤1·5 D at 1/12 (*P*<0·05). 3·2 mm stat sig less WRF on CT (*P*<0·01). Aq flare/cell stat sig less 3·2 mm at 1/52 (*P*<0·05), after no SSD. No SSD FP, SM at 3/12	
Hayashi et al., 1995[42]	RCT FU 6/12	Scleral flap, BENT, 2 mm post ant. margin limbal arcade: 3·2 mm v 4 mm v 5 mm	200 eyes: 3·2 mm – 64 eyes 4 mm – 65 eyes 5 mm – 71 eyes	CT Keratometry	• SIA less with 3·2 mm. 3·2 mm no change central cornea, 4/5 mm focal steepening • 3·2 mm corneal shape recover by 1/12, 4/5 mm not fully recover 6/12	
Diestelhorst et al., 1996[43]	RCT FU 5/7	Scleral flap, superior: 3 mm v 6 mm	3 mm – 20 eyes 6 mm – 19 eyes	FP VA	• No SSD in BAB disruption between 2 groups	• NSAID only postop

(Continued)

Table 32.5 (Continued)

Authors	Methods	Intervention	Participants	Outcomes	Results	Notes
Kohnen et al., 1995[44]	RCT FU 6/12	Corneal incision, temporal 2 step: 3·5 mm v 4 mm v 5 mm (1 radial suture 10/0 nylon)	3·5 mm – 20 eyes 4 mm – 20 eyes 5 mm – 20 eyes	Keratometry CT	• SIA stat sig lower in 3·5 mm than 4/5 mm (P <0·05) at 6/12. Temporal incision minimal SIA over 6/12	
Dick et al., 1996[45]	RCT FU 4/7, 6, 12 months	Clear corneal incision, temporal 2 step: 3·5 mm (sutureless and injector foldable silicone lens) v 5 mm (radial suture, PMMA lens)	3·5 mm – 28 eyes 5 mm – 30 eyes	EC loss by SM	• No SSD in PH/CV between 2 groups at FU • Mean EC loss 3·5 mm ess than 5·0 mm at 1 yr but not stat sig	• One surgeon
Holweger and Marefat, 1997[46]	RCT FU 8/12	Clear corneal temporal incision: 3·5 mm (sutureless) v 5 mm (1 suture 10/0 vicryl)	3·5 mm – 100 eyes 5 mm – 100 eyes	CT ECC IOL centration	• No SSD in CT/ECC changes between groups at 8/12 (smallest change cyl 3·5 mm group). No diff in IOL centration between groups	• 3·5 mm silicone • 5 mm PMMA

SIA, surgically induced astigmatism; UCVA, uncorrected visual acuity; BCVA, best corrected visual acuity; BENT, between nine and twelve o'clock; AR, against the rule astigmatism; WR, with the rule astigmatism; WW, with the wound astigmatism; WRF, wound related flattening; SSD, statistical significant difference; CT, corneal topography; SM, specular microscopy; FP, Fluorophotometry; BAB, blood aqueous barrier; D&C, divide and conquer; EC, endothelial cell; ECC, endothelial cell count; CV, coefficient of variation of endothelial cells; PH, % hexagonal endothelial cells

astigmatism in the temporal and BENT (BEtween Nine and Twelve o'clock) location compared to superior incisions.[27,29,30] However, no difference was noted in visual acuity.[29,30] One study examined wound strength and found no significant difference between temporal or superior scleral flaps.[27]

The evidence suggests reduced surgically induced astigmatism in the temporal and BENT groups compared to superior incisions but no difference in wound strength or visual acuity.

Question

What is the effect of phaco incision size on surgical outcomes?

The evidence

Thirteen RCTs have examined the effect of the different size of scleral flaps[6,32–43] while three have concentrated on clear corneal incisions (Table 32.5).[44–46] Inter-study comparison of the scleral flap groups are problematic since apart from the variation in sizes of incision studied, the use of sutures and their tightness will have an effect on astigmatic outcome measures. However, evidence from the studies suggested that smaller incisions were associated with statistically less surgically induced astigmatism and an earlier rehabilitation in visual acuity, particularly uncorrected visual acuity.[6,32–41]

Further outcome measures in patients who had variation in the size of their scleral tunnels included a higher incidence of hyphaemas in larger incision group,[40] significantly lower aqueous humour cell count and flare at one week postoperatively,[41] less wound-related flattening at three months,[41] and fewer central corneal changes on corneal topography in the smaller incision group.[42] No statistical difference was noted with respect to specular microscopy or fluorophotometry between different incision sizes.[41,43]

For corneal incisions the influence of incision size on outcome appears to be similar to scleral tunnels. There was significantly less astigmatism in the smaller incision group after six months.[44] There was no statistical difference in endothelial cell morphology or endothelial cell loss,[45,46] or corneal topography changes between incision sizes studied.[46]

Comment

Overall, the evidence suggests that smaller scleral tunnel incisions were associated with less astigmatism, improved earlier UCVA, reduced incidence of hyphaemas, less

postoperative inflammation, less wound-related flattening, and less change in the central cornea on corneal topography compared to large incisions. Smaller corneal incisions were also associated with reduced astigmatism compared to larger ones.

Question

What is the effect of different phacoemulsification techniques on surgical outcome?

The evidence

Four studies have looked at different techniques for nuclear fractis (Table 32.7).[16,47–49] Less corneal endothelial cell loss was shown to occur when performing phaco in the posterior chamber as opposed to iris plane.[16] A comparison of divide and conquer to three other techniques, showed less endothelial cell loss at one month compared to Chip and Flip but this was not significant at three months.[47] "Reversed Tip and Snip" showed significantly less endothelial cell loss compared with divide and conquer at three months.[48] "Phaco chop" showed significantly less phaco time, less phaco power and less equivalent phaco time in comparison to divide and conquer.[49] However, there was no difference between the two groups with respect to complications or postoperative visual acuity.

Comment

The evidence suggests that endocapsular phaco surgery is safer than iris plane, and that there are advantages of the newer nuclear fractis techniques.

Question

What is the effect of sutures on phaco incision closure?

The evidence

Table 32.8 summarises RCTs on the effect of sutures on phaco incision closure, which have looked at scleral tunnels (Table 32.8).[25,28,26,39,50–55] Intraoperative variations, such as linear versus frown incision, amount of cautery and size of incision (4–7 mm), make it difficult to compare the studies directly using the size of postoperative astigmatism as a outcome measure.

In comparing studies that examined the effect of no suture *v* one suture (in all cases 10/0 nylon, eight studies),[25,28,39,50–54] only one study showed any difference between the two groups with respect to the amount of

Table 32.6 Effect of incision location on surgical outcome.

Authors	Methods	Intervention	Participants	Outcomes	Results	Notes
Kawano et al, 1993[29]	CCT Phaco and 6 mm lens FU 24/52	Scleral pocket, 6·5 × 2 mm: BENT v Superior	BENT – 121 eyes Superior – 59 eyes	Astigmatism VA	• SIA less BENT than superior ($P = 0.001$) at 1/52, not SSD 24/52 • UCVA stat sig better 1/52, not SSD 24/52	
Wirbelauer et al, 1997[30]	RCT FU 5/12 Phaco and PMMA lens	Scleral pocket, 7 × 2 mm: superior v temporal v modified BENT	63 eyes	Astigmatism VA	• Reduced SIA in modified BENT ($P = 0.0001$) • Superior group largest SIA	
Mendivil, 1996[31]	RCT Phaco and 5 mm lens FU 6/12	Scleral pocket, 4 × 3 mm; superior v lateral	168 eyes randomised	Astigmatism VA CT	• No difference UCVA • SIA superior group assoc. AR • SIA lateral group assoc. WR	
Anders et al, 1997[27]	RCT FU 1/7, 1–4/52, 8/12	Scleral (trapezoid) incision (7 mm × 1 mm postsurgical limbus): Superior v temporal limbal incision (trapezoid) (7 mm): superior v temporal No sutures	180 eyes randomised	Wound strength by OD SIA	• No SSD in limbal incisior s sup v temp, up to 4/52. Stat sig less SIA in temporal than sup at 8/12 scleral group ($P = 0.001$). • SIA highest with superior limbal incisions at 8/12 • No SSD in scleral incision with regard to wound strength • Stat sig stronger wound temporal limbal than superior at 1/52 ($F = 0.003$)	No details on no.

SIA, surgically induced astigmatism; BENT, between nine and twelve o'clock; UCVA, uncorrected visual acuity; AR, against the rule astigmatism; WR, with the rule astigmatism; OD, ophthalmodynamometer; CT, corneal topography

Table 32.7 Effect of phacoemulsification technique on surgical outcome

Authors	Methods	Intervention	Participants	Outcomes	Results	Notes
Koch et al., 1993[16]	RCT FU 1/7, 1/52, 1, 2, 4/12	Iris plane (IP) phaco v C&F Phaco (PC)	IP – 26 eyes PC – 33 eyes	VA SM Pachymetry	• Central EC loss stat sig greater in IP group at 4/12 (P <0·12) • Reduced increase n CV/PH centrally in PC group (P <0·02).	• Single surgeon i.c. Ach. • No anti-glaucoma Tx postop
Kosirukvongs et al, 1997[47]	RCT FU 3/12	D&C v C&F	D&C – 22 eyes C&F – 19 eyes	ECC Corneal thickness	• Greater EC loss C&F group at 1/12 (P = 0·05), not sig 3/12 • Increase cell shape variation C&F group (P = 0·03) • No SSD in corneal thickness any FU	Small no.
Kohlhaas et al, 1997[48]	RCT FU 3/12	D&C v Reverse Tip & Snip	30 eyes each group	ECC	• Reverse Tip & Snip less cell loss than D&C (P <0·001)	
Wong et al., 2000[49]	RCT FU 2/52	Phaco Chop v D&C	D&C – 55 eyes Phaco Chop – 62 eyes	Phaco time/ power Equivalent phaco time VA Intraop complications Operating time	• Phaco Chop less phaco time (P <0·0001), EPT (P <0·0001) • No diff complications • Phaco Chop shorter operating time	

D&C, divide and conquer; C&F, chip and flip; EPT, equivalent phaco time; EC, endothelial cell; ECC, endothelial cell count; SM, specular microscopy; CV, coefficient of variation of endothelial cells; PH, % hexagons

surgically induced astigmatism, which was significant at one week postoperative but not at three months.[50] However, three studies showed earlier stabilisation of astigmatism in the sutureless incision group.[41,51,52] Analysis of surgical outcomes for which there was no statistical difference included computerised videokeratography,[53] uncorrected visual acuity,[25] and intraocular pressure.[28]

One study looked at the effect of suture adjustment intra-operatively, and suggested less variation in postoperative astigmatism between the adjusted and unadjusted groups up to two years but this was not statistically significant.[54]

Azar *et al.* compared sutureless incisions to closure with one and three sutures.[55] They suggested that one stitch closure in a 5·5 mm scleral flap incision was the most astigmatic neutral closure.[55] Gimbel *et al.* compared sutureless closure with three different suture closures and suggested that horizontal suture closure of a 6 mm flap was the most astigmatic neutral closure.[26]

Comment

Overall, the evidence suggests a minimal difference in induced astigmatism between sutureless and one suture groups, but earlier stablisation of astigmatism in the sutureless group.

Question

What is the effect of different suture material or technique on incision closure?

The evidence

Three RCTs have examined the effect of different suture materials on incision closure[38,56,57] and one has examined different techniques of suture tying (Table 32.9).[46] Two studies have looked at scleral tunnel incisions,[38,56] one at clear corneal incisions[46] and one is an objective comparison in a mixture of cases of phaco, ECCE, and intracapsular cataract extractions.[57] Mersilene, 9/0 and 10/0 nylon induced statistically more with the rule astigmatism than Prolene and Novafil at day one.[38,56] However, by two months there was no statistical difference in the astigmatism or UCVA between the groups.[38]

Following clear corneal incisions, no statistical difference in corneal topography was noted between one radial suture and one X suture after eight months.[48]

Comment

Mersilene, 9/0 and 10/0 nylon induced more astigmatism than Prolene and Novafil in the short term. No topographical difference was seen between one radial suture or X suture in incision closure.

Question

What alternatives are there to sutures for incision closure?

The evidence

Table 32.10 tabulates RCTs investigating the effect of incision closure by alternative materials.[50,58–60] Three studies compare the effect of scleral tunnel closure with a tissue adhesive (fibrin in two studies, cyanoacrylate in one) to closure with one suture. Cyanoacrylate was shown to be safe and equally as effective as suturing with respect to postoperative astigmatism.[50] Both the fibrin studies showed that fibrin was safe and induced significantly less postoperative astigmatism than a single suture. However, no difference was noted in final best-corrected visual acuity between the fibrin group and sutured group.[58,59] There was no discussion about the costs of these materials.

One study examined conjunctival closure either manually or after saline injection. Subjective evidence suggested better closure with saline injection after one week but no difference after one month.[60]

Comment

The evidence suggests adhesive closure is equal to or better than single suture closure with respect to postoperative astigmatism.

Summary

These studies have provided evidence for the benefits of sutureless or single suture closure, small astigmatic neutral incisions, and temporal clear corneal incisions. The evidence from specific surgical techniques along with evidence from Table 32.1 indicates the advantages of phacoemulsification over ECCE. Viscoelastic technology has also improved to enhance the effectiveness of endothelial protection during phacoemulsification. However, only one randomised controlled trial examined the cost-effectiveness of the two procedures. In developing countries where phacoemulsification is now being performed in major cities, the initial investment needed to buy equipment may well put phaco out of the reach of the masses of the rural population who are "blinded" with cataracts. However, distinct advantages such as the reduced rate of posterior capsular opacification, fewer surgical complications, and better UCVA, may well make the initial investment financially viable in the long term.

Table 32.8 Effect of sutures on phaco incision closure

Authors	Methods	Intervention	Participants	Outcomes	Results	Notes
Alió et al., 1996[50]	RCT FU 1, 12/52	Superior, 6·5 mm × 2·5 mm behind limbus, frown incision scleral tunnel: closure with suture (1 × 10/0 nylon, horizontal anchor) v sutureless	Suture – 105 eyes Sutureless – 101 eyes	Astigmatism	• Stat sig more astigmatism in sutureless group ($P < 0.01$) at 1/52, no SSD at 12/52	• One surgeon
Dam-Johansen and Olsen, 1997[39]	RCT FU 1/7, 1, 2/52 1, 4/12	Scleral tunnel, superior, 2 mm post limbus: 4 mm (1 10/0 nylon suture) v 4 mm (sutureless). No sutures removed	Suture – 49 eyes Sutureless – 49 eyes	SIA	• No SSD in SIA between both groups but single stitch had larger induced cyl. • Initial WR shift, in suture group at 1/52 then followed astigmatism of sutureless group but not SSD	• One surgeon
Mendivil, 1997[51]	RCT FU 1, 2 wks, 1, 3, 6 months	Superior, 3·2 mm × 3 mm post surgical limbus, linear incision scleral tunnel: closure with suture (1 × 10/0 nylon, radial) v sutureless	Suture – 58 eyes Sutureless – 48 eyes	Astigmatism UCVA	• No SSD in UCVA between groups all FU visits. AR present in both eyes postop but no SSD between groups any FU visit • SIA stabilised quicker in sutureless group, not SSD	
Lyhne and Corydon, 1996[52]	RCT FU 1/52 1, 3 and 6/12	Superior, 5·2 mm × 2 mm behind limbus, linear incision scleral tunnel: Adjusted (intra op cyl. 1D WR Cross Suture) v 1 × unadjusted cross suture v no suture (suture 10/0 nylon)	Adj suture – 25 eyes Unadj suture – 24 eyes Sutureless – 26 eyes	Astigmatism Size SIA Time for stability	• No SSD in post op cyl between 3 groups • No SSD in SIA at 3/12 between groups but sutureless reach value 1/52 and stable after • Sutured stat sig change 1/52–3/12 ($P < 0.01$) • Most variation unadj group though not SSD	• No cutting of sutures • One surgeon
El Kasaby et al., 1995[53]	RCT FU 6/52	Superior, 6 mm × 2 mm behind limbus, frown incision scleral tunnel: Closure with suture (1 × 10/0 nylon, horizontal mattress) v sutureless	Suture – 15 eyes Sutureless – 15 eyes	CVK SIA	• No SSD in complications/AR between groups. Flattening along 90° meridian more without suture but not SSD • No SSD in mean corneal power at 90° meridian	• One surgeon
Hunold et al., 1995[25]	RCT FU 1/7, 2/52, 1, 3, 6 months	Superior, scleral tunnel (5 mm × 2 mm post limbus, frown incision): 1 stitch v sutureless	1 stitch – 23 eyes Sutureless – 23 eyes	Astigmatism UCVA	• No SSD in cyl in all FU groups • No SSD in vector, UCVA between groups	

(Continued)

Table 32.8 (Continued)

Authors	Methods	Intervention	Participants	Outcomes	Results	Notes
Börner et al., 1995[28]	RCT FU 3/6/24 hrs	Superior, 7 mm × 3·5 mm scleral tunnel: Suture (1×10/0 nylon) v sutureless	Suture – 61 eyes Sutureless – 47 eyes	IOP	• IOP highest at 6 hrs but no SSD between groups	• Multiple surgeons
Lyhne and Corydon, 1998[54]	RCT FU 6/12, 1, 2 yrs	Superior, 5·2 mm × 2 mm post limbus, linear incision scleral tunnel: Adjusted (intra op cyl. 1D WR cross suture) versus 1× unadjusted cross suture v sutureless (suture 10/0 nylon)	Adj suture – 25 eyes Unadj suture – 24 eyes Sutureless – 26 eyes	Astigmatism Size SIA	• No SSD in postop cyl (6/12 – 24/12) between groups but more fluctuation in unadj group. No SSD in SIA at 2 yr FU, but unadj group further AR drift between 1–2 yrs, other groups stable (adj 6/12, sutureless 1/52)	• No cutting of sutures • One surgeon
Azar et al., 1997[55]	RCT FU 1/7, 1, 4, 8 wks, 6, 12 months	Superior, 5·5 mm × 1·5 mm post surgical limbus, scleral tunnel: sutureless v 1 suture (radial) v 3 sutures (radial) (suture = 10/0 nylon)	Sutureless – 50 eyes 1 suture – 40 eyes 3 sutures – 41 eyes	SIA VA	• Stat sig better UCVA in no and 1 suture group than 3 sutures at 1/52 no SSD after • No SSD in surgically induced SphEq at all visits • Mean keratometric astig stat sig greater 3 sutures ($P = 0.07$) postop, no SSD 8/52 • Stat sig higher AR shift in sutureless group and sig WR in 3 sutures group 8/52 postop ($P<0.05$) no SSD after	• Two surgeons • PMMA lens • No sutures cut. 1 suture lowest % WR (4/52) and without sig AR shift
Gimbel et al., 1995[26]	RCT FU 2 days, 2 wks, 6 and 12 months	Superior scleral tunnel: 1. Sutureless (6 mm × 2·5 mm frown incision, gp 1) versus 2. Horizontal suture (6 mm × 2·5 mm frown incision, gp 2) versus 3. Horizontal and running (HR) suture (6 mm × 2·5 mm frown incision, gp 3) versus 4. Acute beveled incision (ABI, 6 mm incision limbal, running suture, gp 4) (suture 10/0 Prolene) All WR astig preop	Sutureless – 34 eyes Horizontal suture – 35 eyes Horizontal and running – 31 eyes Acute beveled incision – 28 eyes	Astigmatism	• Stat sig reduction in keratometric cyl gp1 at 2/12, stat sig increased in gp 3 ($P = 0.020$) and 4 ($P = 0.005$), no SSD group 2 with preop levels. No SSD at 1 yr between groups • No SSD in SIA up to 1 yr postop, but no. of eyes with induced ATR cyl stat sig higher than number with WR for all 4 groups ($P<0.01$)	• One surgeon

Phaco, phacoemulsification and intraocular lens implant; UCVA, uncorrected visual acuity; BCVA, best corrected visual acuity; SSD, statistical significant difference; CVK, computerised videokeratography; AR, against the rule astigmatism; WR, with the rule astigmatism; Cyl, cylinder; EC, endothelial cell; ECC, endothelial cell count; CT, corneal topography; SM, specular microscopy; vicryl, polglactin; SphEq, spherical equivalent

Table 32.9 Effect of suture variation on incision closure

Authors	Methods	Intervention	Participants	Outcomes	Results	Notes
Mendivil, 1997[56]	RCT FU 1, 2 weeks and 6, 12 months	Phaco (superior, 4 mm × 3 mm posterior to surgical limbus scleral tunnel) closure 1 suture: 10/0 Ethilon monofilament v 9/0 Ethilon monofilament. No cautery. Tightness controlled	10/0 – 47 eyes, 9/0 – 49 eyes	UCVA Astigmatism	• No SSD in UCVA between groups postop • SSD between groups in mean postop astigmatism • AR with 10/0 and WR with 9/0 in all FU visits ($P<0·05$)	• Same surgeon • Sutures not cut • IOP equal after suture with Schiotz
Gimbel et al, 1992[38]	RCT FU 1/7, 2–3 wks, 2/3/6/12/24 months	Phaco (6·5/7·5 mm scleral tunnel, superior incision) closure: 10/0 nylon monofilament v 10/0 Prolene v 11/0 Mersilene v 10/0 Novafil. Light cautery, continuous shoelace closure	Nylon – 50 eyes, Prolene – 52 eyes, Mersilene – 48 eyes, Novafil – 50 eyes	VA SIA Visual rehab	• No SSD in UCVA among groups any FU visit. At 1/7 nylon and Mersilene stat sig more WR and SIA than Prolene/ Novafil ($P<0·01$) • WR decayed faster for nylon > Mersilene over 3/12. At 2/12 no SSD between groups • AR shift seen in Prolene (1/12), Novafil (2/12), Nylon (5/12), Mersilene (8/12) • Decay stable Prolene (5/12), Novafil and Mersilene 1 yr but Nylon sig AR shift between 1–2 yrs	• Different knot tying
Blaydes and Berry, 1979[57]	RCT FU 24 hrs, 1, 2, 3, 4, 5 wks	Phaco (2 sutures – 1 mono,1 braid) ICCE/ECCE (9 sutures – 2 mono, 2 braid poly 910 and 5 10/0 nylon) 9/0 Monofilament polyglactin 910 versus 9/0 Braid polyglactin 910	150 eyes, 9/0 mono and 9/0 braid in all	Pliability Knot Pull-through Strength Disappearance Reaction Wound healing	• Monofilament stiffer • Good knots both materials • More drag with braid • Both high tensile strength • Mono ~36 days, Braid ~30 days • Minimal both materials • Excellent both materials	• Same surgeon
Holweger and Marefat, 1997[46]	RCT FU 8/12	Phaco (5 mm clear corneal incision, temporal, 1 suture10/0 vicryl, PMMA lens): Radial stitch versus X stitch	Radial – 25 eyes, X stitch – 25 eyes	CT	• No SSD in CT changes between 2 groups at 8/12 • Small WR shift in X stitch group	

ICCE, intracapsular extraction, ECCE, extracapsular cataract extraction via nuclear expression and intraocular lens implant; Phaco, phacoemulsification and intraocular lens implant; UCVA, uncorrected visual acuity; BCVA, best corrected visual acuity; SSD, statistical significant difference; SIA, surgically induced astigmatism; Ethilon, monofilament nylon polyamide-6; polyglactin 910 (vicryl), copolymer of lactide and glycolide; Prolene, polypropylene; Mersilene, polyester; Novafil, polyethylene; AR, against the rule astigmatism; WR, with the rule astigmatism; CT, corneal topography

Table 32.10 Effect on phaco incision closure by alternative materials

Authors	Methods	Intervention	Participants	Outcomes	Results	Notes
Alió et al., 1996[50]	RCT FU 1, 12/52	6·5 mm × 2·5 mm post limbus scleral tunnel, frown incision closure; with suture (1 ×10/0 nylon) v without suture v cyanoacrylate adhesive	With suture – 105 eyes without suture – 101 eyes Adhesive – 103 eyes	Astigmatism	• No SSD between suture and adhesive groups • Stat sig more astigmatism in without suture group than others at 1/52, (P<0·1) no SSD at 12/52	• One surgeon
Mester et al., 1993[58]	RCT FU 1, 7 days 6 months	6 mm × 2·5 mm post limbus scleral tunnel closure: Tissucol (fibrin) v single stitch (10/0 nylon)	Fibrin – 167 eyes Stitch – 218 eyes	Astigmatism VA	• SIA smaller in fibrin group at 6/12 FU (P<0·05) • No SSD in BCVA between groups	
Mulet et al., 1997[59]	RCT	6 mm × 2 mm post limbus scleral tunnel closure: Tissucol (fibrin) v single stitch (10/0 nylon)	Fibrin – 28 eyes Stitch – 28 eyes	Astigmatism	• Stat sig less astigmatism in fibrin group (P<0·05)	
Meacock et al., 1996[60]	RCT FU 1,7, 28 days	5 mm scleral tunnel conjunctival closure: manually v saline injection	Manually – 22 eyes Saline injection – 16 eyes	Bare sclera	• Stat sig better conj wound closure in saline injected group up to 7 days FU • No SSD at 28 days	

Phaco, phacoemulsification and intraocular lens implant; UCVA, uncorrected visual acuity; BCVA, best corrected visual acuity; SSD, statistical significant difference; SIA, surgically induced astigmatism; Tissucol, fibrin sealant 2 components protein/apoprotein and thrombin/$CaCl_2$

References

1. Laurell CG, Zetterström C, Philipson B *et al.* Randomized study of the blood–aqueous barrier reaction after phacoemulsification and extracapsular cataract extraction. *Acta Ophthalmol Scand* 1998;**76**: 573–8.

2. Dowler JG, Hykin PG, Hamilton AM. Phacoemulsification versus extracapsular cataract extraction in patients with diabetes. *Ophthalmology* 2000;**107**:457–62.

3. Chee SP, Ti SE, Sivakumar M *et al.* Postoperative Inflammation: extracapsular cataract extraction versus phacoemulsification. *J Cataract Refractive Surg* 1999;**25**:1280–5.

4. Landau IE, Laurell C-G. Ultrasound biomicroscopy examination of intraocular lens haptic position after phacoemulsification with continuous curvilinear capsulorhexis and extracapsular cataract extraction with linear capsulotomy. *Acta Ophthalmol Scand* 1999; *77*:394–6.

5. Ravalico G, Tognetto D, Palomba MA *et al.* Corneal endothelial function after extracapsular cataract extraction and phacoemulsification. *J Cataract Refractive Surg* 1997;**23**:1000–5.

6. Leen MM, Ho CC, Yanoff M. Association between surgically-induced astigmatism and cataract incision size in the early postoperative period. *Ophthalmic Surg* 1993;**24**:586–92.

7. Minassian DC, Rosen P, Dart JKG *et al.* Extracapsular cataract extraction compared with small incision surgery by phacoemulsification: a randomized trial. *Br J Ophthalmol* 2001;**85**: 822–9.

8. Jürgens I, Matheu A, Castilla M. Ocular hypertension after cataract surgery: a comparison of three surgical techniques and two viscoelastics. *Ophthalmic Surg Lasers* 1997;**28**:30–6.

9. Bömer TG, Lagreze WD, Funk J. Intraocular Pressure Rise after Cataract Extraction – Influence of Surgical Technique, Surgeon's Experience and Prophylactic Medication. A Prospective, Randomized Double-Blind Study. *Klinische Monatsblatter Für Augenheilkunde* 1995;**206**:13–9.

10. Lüchtenberg M, Luchtenberg C, Lang M *et al.* Intraocular pressure after IOL implantation by using three different types of viscoelastics. *Ophthalmology* 2000;**97**:331–5.

11. Smith SG, Lindstrom RL. 2% Hydroxypropyl methylcellulose as a viscous surgical adjunct. A multicenter prospective randomized trial. *J Cataract Refractive Surg* 1991;**17**:839–42.

12. Pedersen OO. Comparison of the protective effects of methylcellulose and sodium hyaluronate on corneal swelling following phacoemulsification of senile cataracts. *J Cataract Refractive Surg* 1990;**16**:594–6.

13. Probst LE, Nichols BD. Corneal endothelial and intraocular pressure changes after phacoemulsification with Amvisc Plus and Viscoat. *J Cataract Refractive Surg* 1993;**19**:725–30.

14. Rainer G, Menapace R, Findl O *et al.* Intraocular pressure after small incision cataract surgery with Healon 5 and Viscoat. *J Cataract Refractive Surg* 2000;**26**:271–6.

15. Miller KM, Colvard DM. Randomized clinical comparison of Healon GV and Viscoat. *J Cataract Refractive Surg* 1999;**25**:1630–6.

16. Koch DD, Liu JF, Glasser DB *et al.* A comparison of corneal endothelial changes after use of Healon or Viscoat during phacoemulsification. *Am J Ophthalmol* 1993;**115**:188–201.

17. Kohnen T, von Ehr M, Schutte E *et al.* Evaluation of intraocular pressure with Healon and Healon GV in sutureless cataract surgery with foldable lens implantation. *J Cataract Refractive Surg* 1996;**22**: 227–37.

18. Arshinoff SA, Hofmann I. Prospective, randomized trial of Microvisc and Healon in routine phacoemulsification. *J Cataract Refractive Surg* 1997;**23**:761–5.

19. John ME, Randall LN, Boleyn BA *et al.* Effect of a superficial and a deep scleral pocket incision on the incidence of hyphema. *J Cataract Refractive Surg* 1992;**18**:495–9.

20. Anders N, Pham DT, Wollensak J. Wound Strength in self-sealing cataract surgery depending on the site and the depth of the Incision. *Klinische Monatsblatter Für Augenheilkunde* 1995;**206**:442–5.

21. Dick HB, Schwenn O, Krummenauer F *et al.* Inflammation after sclerocorneal versus clear corneal tunnel phacoemulsification. *Ophthalmology* 2000;**107**:241–7.

22. Kurimoto Y, Komurasaki Y, Yoshimura N *et al.* Corneal astigmatism After cataract surgery with 4·1 mm BENT scleral and 4·1 mm plus meridian corneal incisions. *J Cataract Refractive Surg* 1999;**25**: 427–31.

23. Cillino S, Morreale D, Mauceri A *et al.* Temporal versus superior approach phacoemulsification: Short-term postoperative astigmatism. *J Cataract Refractive Surg* 1997;**23**:267–71.

24. Olsen T, Dam Johansen M, Bek T *et al.* Corneal versus scleral tunnel incision in cataract surgery: a randomized study. *J Cataract Refractive Surg* 1997;**23**:337–41.

25. Hunold W, Auffarth GU, Bailitis S *et al.* No-stitch tunnel incision versus corneoscleral incision. A prospective, randomized study. *Ophthalmology* 1995;**92**:274–9.

26. Gimbel HV, Sun R, DeBroff BM. Effects of wound architecture and suture technique on postoperative astigmatism. *Ophthalmic Surg Lasers* 1995;**26**:524–8.

27. Anders N, Pham DT, Antoni HJ *et al.* Postoperative astigmatism and relative strength of tunnel incisions: a prospective clinical trial. *J Cataract Refractive Surg* 1997;**23**:332–6.

28. Bömer TG, Lagreze WD, Funk J. Intraocular pressure rise after phacoemulsification with posterior chamber lens implantation: effect of prophylactic medication, wound closure, and surgeon's experience. *Br J Ophthalmol* 1995;**79**(9):809–13.

29. Kawano K. Modified corneoscleral incision to reduce postoperative astigmatism after 6 mm diameter intraocular lens implantation. *J Cataract Refractive Surg* 1993;**19**:387–92.

30. Wirbelauer C, Anders N, Pham DT *et al.* Effect of incision location on preoperative oblique astigmatism after scleral tunnel incision. *J Cataract Refractive Surg* 1997;**23**:365–71.

31. Mendivil A. Comparative study of astigmatism through superior and lateral small incisions. *Eur J Ophthalmol* 1996;**6**:389–92.

32. El Maghraby A, Anwar M, el Sayyad F *et al.* Effect of incision size on early postoperative visual rehabilitation after cataract surgery and intraocular lens implantation. *J Cataract Refractive Surg* 1993; **19**:494–8.

33. Grabow HB. Early Results of 500 Cases of No-Stitch cataract surgery. *J Cataract Refractive Surg* 1991;**17**(Suppl):726–30.

34. Martin RG, Sanders DR, Miller JD *et al.* Effect of cataract wound incision size on acute changes in corneal topography. *J Cataract Refractive Surg* 1993;**19**(Suppl):170–7.

35. Olson RJ, Crandall AS. Prospective randomized comparison of phacoemulsification cataract surgery with a 3·2-mm *v* a 5·5-mm sutureless incision. *Am J Ophthalmol* 1998;**125**:612–20.

36. Levy JH, Pisacano MD, Chadwick BS. Astigmatic changes after cataract surgery with 5·1 mm and 3·5 mm sutureless incisions. *J Cataract Refractive Surg* 1994;**20**:630–3.

37. Mendivil A. Intraocular lens implantation through 3·2 versus 4·0 mm incisions. *J Cataract Refractive Surg* 1996;**22**:1461–4.

38. Gimbel HV, Raanan DG, DeLuca M. Effect of suture material on postoperative astigmatism. *J Cataract Refractive Surg* 1992;**18**:42–50.

39. Dam-Johansen M, Olsen T. Induced astigmatism after 4 and 6 mm scleral tunnel incision. A randomized study. *Acta Ophthalmo Scand* 1997;**75**:669–74.

40. Davison JA. Keratometric comparison of 4·0 mm and 5·5 mm scleral tunnel cataract incisions. *J Cataract Refrac Surg* 1993;**19**:3–8.

41. Oshika T, Tsuboi S, Yaguchi S *et al.* Comparative study of intraocular lens implantation through 3·2 and 5·5 mm incisions. *Ophthalmology* 1994;**101**(7):1183–90.

42. Hayashi K, Hayashi H, Nakao F *et al.* The correlation between incision size and corneal shape changes in sutureless cataract surgery. *Ophthalmology* 1995;**102**:550–6.

43. Diestelhorst M, Dinslage S, Konen W *et al.* Effect of 3·0 mm tunnel and 6·0 mm corneoscleral incisions on the blood–aqueous barrier. *J Cataract Refractive Surg* 1996;**22**:1465–70.

44. Kohnen T, Dick B, Jacobi KW. Comparison of the induced astigmatism after temporal clear corneal tunnel incisions of different sizes. *J Cataract Refractive Surg* 1995;**21**:417–24.

45. Dick HB, Kohnen T, Jacobi FK, Jacobi KW. Long-term endothelial cell loss following phacoemulsification through a temporal clear corneal incision. *J Cataract Refractive Surg* 1996;**22**:63–71.

46. Holweger RR, Marefat B. Corneal changes after cataract surgery with 5·0 mm sutured and 3·5 mm sutureless clear corneal incisions. *J Cataract Refractive Surg* 1997;**23**:342–6.

47. Kosrirukvongs P, Slade SG, Berkeley RG. Corneal endothelial changes after divide and conquer versus chip and flip phacoemulsification. *J Cataract Refractive Surg* 1997;**23**:1006–12.

48. Kohlhaas M, Klemm M, Kammann J *et al.* Endothelial cell loss after phacoemulsification – a comparison between the "Reversed Tip and Snip" technique and "Divide and Conquer" technique. *Klinische Monatsblatter Für Augenheilkunde* 1997;**210**(2):82–5.

49. Wong T, Hingorani M, Lee V. Phacoemulsification time and power requirements in phaco chop and divide and conquer nucleofractis techniques. *J Cataract Refractive Surg* 2000;**26**:1374–8.

50. Alio J L, Mulet ME, Garcia JC. Use of cyanoacrylate tissue adhesive in small-incision cataract surgery. *Ophthalmic Surg Lasers* 1996; **27**:270–4.

51. Mendivil A. Frequency of induced astigmatism following phacoemulsification with suturing versus without suturing. *Ophthalmic Surg Lasers* 1997;**28**(5):377–81.

52. Lyhne N, Corydon L. Astigmatism after phacoemulsification with adjusted and unadjusted sutured versus sutureless 5·2 mm superior scleral incisions. *J Cataract Refractive Surg* 1996;**22**:1206–10.

53. El Kasaby HT, McDonnell PJ, Deutsch J. Videokeratography: a comparison between 6 mm sutured and unsutured incisions for phacoemulsification. *Eye* 1995;**9**:719–21.

54. Lyhne N, Corydon, L. Two year follow up of astigmatism after phacoemulsification with adjusted and unadjusted sutured versus sutureless 5·2 mm superior scleral incisions. *J Cataract Refract Surg* 1998;**24**:1647–51.

55. Azar DT, Stark WJ, Dodick J *et al.* Prospective, randomized vector analysis of astigmatism after three-, one-, and no-suture phacoemulsification. *J Cataract Refractive Surg* 1997;**23**:1164–73.

56. Mendivil A. Effect of nylon suture diameter on induced astigmatism after phacoemulsification. *J Cataract Refract Surg* 1997;**23**: 1196–9.

57. Blaydes JE, Berry J. A comparative evaluation of 9-0 monofilament and 9-0 braid polyglactin 910 in cataract surgery (intracapsular, extracapsular, and phacoemulsification). *Ophthalmic Surg* 1979;**10**:49–54.

58. Mester U, Zuche M, Rauber M. astigmatism after phacoemulsification with posterior chamber lens implantation: small incision technique with fibrin adhesive for wound closure. *J Cataract Refractive Surg* 1993;**19**:616–9.

59. Mulet Homs ME, Alio Y, Sanz JL *et al.* Efficacy of fibrinogen as bioadhesive in cataract surgery through scleral tunnel. *Archivos De La Sociedad Espanola De Oftalmologia* 1997;**72**:427–30.

60. Meacock WR, Chittenden H, Govan J. Conjunctival wound closure by saline injection in sutureless, scleral tunnel incision phacoemulsification. *J Cataract Refractive Surg* 1996;**22**:1240–1.

33 Intraocular lens implant biocompatibility

Emma Hollick

Background

There are three major aspects to intraocular lens implant (IOL) biocompatibility within the human eye. These are the effect of the IOL on the blood aqueous barrier, the cellular reaction on the anterior surface of the IOL, and the effect on the lens capsule. Blood aqueous barrier changes can be assessed by the measurement of anterior chamber flare and cell levels using the laser flare and cell meter. Cells on the anterior surface of the implant can be examined *in vivo* postoperatively using specular microscopy and have been used extensively as a means of assessing the foreign body response to IOL. Postoperatively the cytology on the anterior surface of the lens implant is made up of three distinct cell populations: small cells, epithelioid/giant cells and lens epithelial cells. The effect of the IOL on the capsule consists of lens epithelial cell proliferation and metaplasia leading to anterior and posterior capsular opacification, and IOL decentration, all of which can affect visual outcome.

In this chapter the evidence for the effectiveness of different IOL designs and materials on biocompatibility is presented.

Question

Does the IOL type have an influence on the amount of blood aqueous barrier breakdown?

The evidence

Seven randomised controlled trials (RCTs)[1–7] have commented on the amount of blood aqueous barrier breakdown with different IOL types (Table 33.1). Two studies showed that the heparin-surface-modified (HSM) polymethylmethacrylate (PMMA) lenses had a lower postoperative flare reaction than unmodified PMMA,[1,2] and one showed no differences in the laser flare measurements between HSM and PMMA lenses at any stage.[3]

Two studies looked at laser meter readings of flare and cells after phacoemulsification with the implantation of either a silicone or a PMMA IOL.[4,5] One showed a

difference in postoperative flare and cell measurements and the other did not. A smaller incision was used for the silicone IOL. Two studies compared HSM-PMMA and hydrophobic acrylic (AcrySof) IOLs in patients with diabetes and found no significant difference in the postoperative flare readings.[6,7] With modern foldable lenses and good surgery postoperative blood aqueous barrier changes are largely influenced by the surgical technique and any effect of the IOL type on flare and cells is probably negligible.

Question

Does heparin-surface-modification have an influence on the amount of cells on the anterior surface of the IOL? What about the amount of IOL surface cells with foldable IOLs?

The evidence

The use of heparin-surface-modification of PMMA lens implants has been shown to reduce the postoperative cellular reaction on the surface of the lens implant after cataract surgery.[3,8–14] These studies are summarised in Table 33.2. None of the studies showed any significant difference between the two groups with respect to the visual acuity of the patients.

There are four studies comparing foldable and PMMA IOLs with respect to the cellular reaction on the surface of the IOL (Table 33.3).[15–18] In the first study by Hollick *et al.* the first-generation silicone IOL appeared to be the least biocompatible, and the hydrophobic acrylic the most.[15] In the second study by Hollick *et al.* the hydrophilic acrylic IOL (Hydroview) appeared to be very biocompatible compared to PMMA and a second-generation silicone lens, but was associated with an unusual lens epithelial cell (LEC) response.[16] Many LECs were found on the anterior surface of the Hydroview IOL and these did not regress as they do on other IOL types.

In Ravalico *et al.*'s study the conventional PMMA material exhibited the most cellular adhesion of the groups.[17] The authors suggest that second-generation silicone and hydrophilic acrylic IOLs appear to be more biocompatible

Table 33.1 Influence of IOL type on blood aqueous barrier breakdown

Authors	Methods	Interventions	Participants	Outcomes	Results	Notes
Martin and Sanders, 1992[4]	RCT Phaco 1 year FU	One-piece Starr silicone v PMMA	n = 112 Age-related cataract only	Laser flare and cells at 1 day, 3 months, and 1 year (VA, astigmatism)	Lower flare and cells with silicone at day 1	Smaller incision used for silicone
Martin et al., 1992[5]	RCT Phaco 3 months FU	Three-piece Allergan silicone v PMMA	n = 112 Age-related cataract only	Laser flare and cells at 1 day and 3 months (VA, astigmatism, endothelial cell count)	No difference in flare and cells	Smaller incision used for silicone
Mester et al., 1998[1]	RCT Fellow eye study 3 months FU	HSM-PMMA v unmodified PMMA	n = 100 High-risk eyes (diabetes, glaucoma, pseudoexfoliation, uveitis)	Laser flare and cells at 1 day, 1 and 6 weeks, 3 months	Lower flare with HSM-PMMA at 6 weeks and 3 months	
Shah and Spalton, 1995[3]	RCT ECCE 1 year FU	HSM-PMMA v unmodified PMMA	n = 54 Age-related cataract only British	Laser flare and cells at 1, 2, 7 days, 1, 3, 6, 12 months (fluorophotometry, cytology specular microscopy, endothelial cell count)	No difference in flare or cells	
Umezawa and Shimizu, 1993[2]	RCT Phaco 1 year FU	HSM-PMMA v SP-PMMA v unmodified PMMA	n = 90 Age-related cataract only Transnational	Laser flare and cells at 1 and 2 weeks, 1 and 12 months (fibrin, CMO, ACO, PCO)	Lower flare with HSM-PMMA at 1 and 2 weeks, 1 month and 1 year	
Gatinel et al., 2001[6]	RCT Phaco 8 months FU	HSM-PMMA v hydrophobic acrylic (AcrySof)	n = 44 Diabetic patients French	Laser flare and cells at 1, 7, 30, and 240 days	No significant difference in flare	6 mm incision for both IOLs
Krepler et al., 2001[7]	RCT Phaco 3 months FU	HSM-PMMA v hydrophobic acrylic (AcrySof)	n = 62 Diabetic patients with NPDR Austrian	Laser flare and cells at 1, 7, 30, and 90 days	No significant difference in flare	Smaller incision for AcrySof

HSM, heparin-surface-modified; SP, surface passivated; FU, follow up; VA, visual acuity; CMO, cystoid macular oedema; ACO, anterior capsular opacification; PCO, posterior capsular opacification; NPDR, (non-proliferative diabetic retinopathy) other outcome measures; cs, contrast sensitivity BAT, brightness acuity testing

than the three PMMA lens types. In Sveinsson and Seland's study the amount of IOL precipitates, which were most likely to be epithelioid cells and giant cells, were the same on the hydrophilic acrylic and PMMA IOLs.[18]

Three studies compare different foldable IOLs (Table 33.4).[19–21] These found IOL-related differences in the cellular reaction after cataract surgery. The incidence of lens epithelial cells was highest in the Hydroview group, and more giant cells were seen with hydrophobic acrylic IOLs.

Comment

To summarise, the foldable IOLs, with the exception of first-generation silicone lenses, appear to be at least as biocompatible in terms of surface cytology as PMMA, if not more biocompatible. The second-generation silicone IOLs with a sharp edge appear to have a particularly low incidence of all cell types.

Question

Does IOL material have an influence on the anterior capsule reaction?

The evidence

The changes in the anterior capsule occurring after cataract surgery consist of opacification and fibrosis, which can lead to capsulorhexis contraction (phimosis), IOL decentration and tilt. These are caused by LECs undergoing fibroblastic transformation when the anterior capsule comes into contact with the IOL, and can be considered to be an index of biocompatibility. These changes have been shown to be influenced by the type of IOL used. Five studies have looked at anterior capsule opacification (ACO) (Table 33.5).[2,19,21,22] Two studies have shown less ACO with HSM-PMMA lenses than unmodified PMMA at three months.[2,22] In Tognetto and colleagues' study comparing three hydrophilic acrylic IOLs, a significantly higher rate of ACO was found with the ACR6D lens.[21] Miyake *et al.* showed less ACO with hydrophobic acrylic AcrySof IOLs than second-generation silicone, and less with the Memory hydrophilic acrylic lens compared to AcrySof.[22] They suggest that the more hydrophobic lenses induce more ACO. In the Abela-Formanek study the hydrophobic acrylic AR40 lens showed the most ACO, followed by silicone, then Hydroview, AcrySof, with the least ACO with MemoryLens.[19] With the exception of AcrySof, ACO was more predominant in the hydrophobic IOL groups.

The second change in the anterior capsule reflecting IOL biocompatibility is the contraction of the capsulorhexis opening. Three RCTs have studied this and these are

summarised in Table 33.5.[23–25] It appears that the contraction of the anterior capsule opening is greatest with silicone IOLs, with relative stability of the anterior capsule on the surface of AcrySof IOLs.

Decentration of IOLs has been investigated in four RCTs, which are summarised in Table 33.6.[26–29] All surgeries consisted of phacoemulsification after an intact continuous curvilinear capsulorhexis (CCC), with the IOL located in the capsular bag. The study by Dick *et al.* revealed very little difference in decentration between plate-haptic silicone, silicone disc lens and PMMA.[26] Hayashi *et al.*'s study suggests that when the IOL is placed within the capsular bag there is a small degree of tilt and decentration just after surgery, but this does not increase significantly with time in any of the three IOLs.[27] The results were similar in Jung *et al.*'s and Wang *et al.*'s studies, showing no significant increase in decentration and tilt up to two months and six months after surgery respectively, and no difference between the hydrophobic acrylic and silicone IOLs used in Jung *et al.*'s study and the silicone and PMMA IOLs in Wang *et al.*'s.[28,29]

Comment

The hydrophilicity of the IOL appeared to have a loose association with the amount of ACO. Contraction of the capsulorhexis opening was greatest with silicone IOLs. All the IOLs studied showed good stability within the bag with an intact capsulorhexis.

Question

What influence does design and surface modification of PMMA lenses have on posterior capsule opacification?

The evidence

Eighteen RCTs have looked at the effect of IOL type on the amount of PCO.[6,10,18,19,30–44] Many of these suffer from the disadvantage of not having an objective measure of PCO, and relying on Nd:YAG laser posterior capsulotomy rates as an indirect measure of PCO, or using subjective grading techniques.[6,10,18,19,30–34,38,39,44] More recently some objective measures for quantifying PCO have been developed.[35–37,40–43]

The first group of papers looked at various PMMA designs and modifications to investigate their effect on PCO.[10,30–34] Their results are presented in Table 33.7. Three of the studies looked at the effect of heparin-surface-modification on PCO, and their conclusions differ. In Lai and Fan's paper there was a trend to lower PCO with HSM but this was not significant.[10] In Winter-Nielson *et al.*'s study there was no difference in the frequency of PCO between patients with

Table 33.2 IOL surface cytology with heparin-surface-modified and unmodified PMMA IOLs

Authors	Methods	Interventions	Participants	Outcomes	Results
Borgioli et al., 1992[6]	RCT 1 year FU ECCE	HSM-PMMA v unmodified PMMA	n = 524 Age-related cataract only Transnational	Slit lamp: cellular deposits present on IOL at 1 day, 2 weeks, 3 and 12 months (VA, complications)	HSM 29·8% v PMMA 48·8% at some point post op, $P<0·001$. Difference most pronounced at 3 months
Condon et al., 1995[7]	RCT 1 year FU ECCE	HSM-PMMA v unmodified PMMA	n = 239 Diabetes and/or glaucoma German	Specular microscopy: giant cells and cellular deposits at 1 week, 1, 3, 6 and 12 months	Fewer giant cells on HSM than PMMA at all FU points No difference between IOLs for cellular deposits
Lai and Fan, 1996[10]	RCT 1 year FU ECCE	HSM-PMMA v unmodified PMMA	n = 99 Age-related cataract only Asian	Slit lamp: cellular deposits present on IOL at 1 and 2 weeks, 3 and 12 months (VA, PCO)	Less cellular deposits on HSM at 3 and 12 months HSM 27% v PMMA 64% at some point postop, $P=0·001$. Difference most pronounced at 3 months
Philipson et al., 1992[11]	RCT 3 months FU ECCE	HSM-PMMA v unmodified PMMA	n = 266 Age-related cataract only Swedish	Slit lamp: cellular deposits present on IOL at 1 day, 1 week, 1 and 3 months (VA, adverse effects)	HSM 13·5% v PMMA 26·7% at 3 months, $P=0·016$. No significant difference at 1 week or 1 month
Shah and Spalton, 1995[3]	RCT 1 year FU ECCE	HSM-PMMA v unmodified PMMA	n = 54 Age-related cataract only British	Specular microscopy: small and giant cells at 1, 3, 6 and 12 months (Laser flare and cells)	% not discussed in text. Graphs show significantly lower small cell response with HSM at 1 month, and giant cell response with HSM at 1, 3, 6, and 12 months
Trocme and Li, 2000[12]	RCT 1 year FU Phaco	HSM-PMMA v unmodified PMMA	n = 367 Age-related cataract and/or diabetes or glaucoma American	Specular microscopy: giant cells Slit lamp: cellular deposits At 1 week, 1, 3, 6 and 12 months (VA)	% not discussed in text. Significantly fewer giant cell and cellular deposits with HSM at 3 months, $P<0·05$. Also significantly fewer giant cells at 1 week, 1 and 6 months for routine patients, and all visits for diabetic patients
Ygge et al., 1990[13]	RCT 4 weeks FU ECCE	HSM-PMMA v unmodified PMMA	n = 53 Age-related cataract only Swedish	Specular microscopy: small and giant cells at 1 and 4 weeks	HSM small cells in all cases: 25·4 cells/mm^2 at 1 week, 13·3 cells/mm^2 at 4 weeks. No giant cells at 1 or 4 weeks. PMMA small cells in all cases: 43·2 cells/mm^2 at 1 week, 378 cells/mm^2 at 4 weeks. Giant cells in 2/30 at 1 week, 18/30 at 4 weeks. Significantly less small cells for HSM
Zetterstrom et al., 1992[14]	RCT 1 year FU ECCE	HSM-PMMA v unmodified PMMA	n = 40 Pseudoexfoliation Swedish	Slit lamp: cellular deposits present on IOL at 1 day, 1 week, 3, 6 and 12 months (VA)	Less cell deposits with HSM at 3, 6 and 12 months, $P<0·001$. Cell deposits on 21% of HSM and 94% of PMMA at some point postop

For abbreviations see Table 33.1.

Table 33.3 Surface cytology with foldable IOLs compared to PMMA

Authors	Methods	Interventions	Participants	Outcomes	Results		
					Small cells	Giant/epithelioid cells	Notes
Hollick et al., 1998[15]	RCT 2 years FU ECCE	1 Hydrophobic acrylic (Alcon AcrySof) = A 2 Silicone (Iolab L141U) = S 3 PMMA = P	n = 90 Age-related cataract only British	Specular microscopy: small cells and giant on IOL at days 1, 7, 30, 90, 180, 360, 720	S had highest small cell grades (P=0.02) A – 19/30 S – 27/30 P – 15/30	No giant cells on A (P=0.003) A – 0/30 S – 0/30 P – 2/30	
Hollick et al., 1999[16]	RCT 1 year FU Phaco	1 Hydrophilic acrylic (Storz Hydroview) = H 2 Silicone (Allergan SI 30) = S 3 PMMA = P	n = 90 Age-related cataract only British	Specular microscopy: small cells, giant and lens epithelial cells on IOL at days 1, 7, 30, 90, 180, 360	At 1/12: (P=0.01) H – 4/30 S – 15/30 P – 11/30 Shorter duration and lower grade on H	At 1/12: (P<0.01) H – 0/30 S – ?/30 P – 1/30 Longer duration and higher grade on P	Lens epithelial cells at 1/12: (P<0.01) H – 20/30 S – 0/30 P – 12/30 Longer duration on H
Ravalico et al., 1997[17]	RCT 6 months FU Phaco	1 Hydrophilic acrylic (logel) = H 2 Silicone (Allergan SI 30) = S 3 PMMA = P 4 Surface-passivated PMMA = SP 5 PMMA = HSM	n = 50 Age-related cataract only Italian	Specular microscopy: small cells and giant on IOL at days 7, 30, 90, 180	At 1/12: (P<0.001) H – 10/10 S – 10/10 P – 10/10 SP – 10/10 HSM – 10/10 Lowest density on S Medium density on H, SP, HSM Highest density on P	At 1/12: (P<0.001) H – 0/10 S – 0/10 P – 8/10 SP – 2/10 HSM – 1/10 None on H and S Low density on SP, HSM Highest density on P	
Sveinsson and Seland, 1990[18]	RCT 1 year FU ECCE	1 Hydrophilic acrylic (logel) = H 2 PMMA = P	n = 40 Age-related cataract only, except one with congenital cataract Norwegian	Slit lamp: IOL precipitates at days 7, 30, 180, 360	"IOL precipitates" discussed	"IOL precipitates" at 6/12 (P=NS) H – 1/19 P – 11/16 Similar grades	No difference in posterior synechiae.

Table 33.4 Surface cytology with foldable IOLs

Authors	Methods	Interventions	Participants	Outcomes	Results		
					Small cells	Giant/epithelioid cells	Notes
Abela-Formanek et al, 2002[19]	RCT 1 year FU Phaco	1 Hydrophilic acrylic (Hydroview) = H 2 Hydrophilic acrylic (MemoryLens) = M 3 Hydrophobic acrylic (AcrySof) = A 4 Hydrophobic acrylic (AMO Sensar AR40) = AS 5 Silicone square edge (CeeOn 920) = Sr 6 Silicone round edge (CeeOn 911A) = Ss	n = 190 Age-related cataract only Austrian	Specular microscopy: small cells and epithelioid/giant cells on IOL at days 1, 7, 30, 90, 180, 360 (ACO, PCO)	% at 1 year: H – 0 M – 54 A – 7 AS – 4 Sr – 12 Ss – 22 M had significantly more small cells	% at 1 year: H – 4 M – 8 A – 17 AS – 30 Sr – 4 Ss – 0 Lowest incidence of giant cells on Sr and Ss (P = 0·C044)	% Lens epithelial cells at 1 year: H – 85 M – 27 A – 4 AS – 3 Sr – 0 Ss – 0 (P = 0·0001)
Mullner-Eidenbock et al, 2001[20]	RCT 6 months FU Phaco	1 Hydrophilic acrylic (Hydroview) = H 2 Hydrophobic acrylic (AcrySof) = A 3 Hydrophilic acrylic (MemoryLens) = M 4 Silicone (CeeOn) = S	n = 100 Age-related cataract only Austrian	Specular microscopy: small cells, epithelioid/giant cells and lens epithelial cells on IOL at days 1, 7, 30, 90, 180	% at 1/12: H – 40 A – 46 M – 60 S – 40	% at 1/12: H – 0 A – 17 M – 20 S – 8	% Lens epithelial cells at 1/12: H – 92 A – 75 M – 76 S – 40 Higher grades on H
Tognetto et al, 2002[21]	RCT 6 months FU Phaco	Hydrophilic acrylics 1 Hydroview = H 2 Cornea ACR6D = C 3 Ioltech Stabibag = I	n = 73 Age-related cataract only Italian	Specular microscopy: small, epithelioid, giant and lens epithelial cells on IOL at days 7, 30, 90, 180 (ACO)	% at 1/12: H – 34·7 C – 33·3 I – 66·6 I had significantly higher grades	Low grade in all 3 groups with similar proportions	Significantly more LECs with H and C than I

Table 33.5 Influence of IOL type on anterior capsular opacification and contraction of the capsular opening

Authors	Methods	Interventions	Participants	Outcomes	Results
Miyake et al, 1996[22]	Randomised fellow eye study 3 months FU Phaco	1 HSM-PMMA 2 Unmodified PMMA	n = 28 Age-related cataract only Japanese	Slit lamp grading of ACO at 1 and 3 months (Laser flare and cells)	No significant difference at 1 month Less ACO with HSM than PMMA at 3 months (no sig. diff. in flare cells at 1/12. Lower flare cells with HSM at 3/12)
Miyake et al, 1996[22]	Randomised fellow eye study 3 months FU Phaco	1 Hydrophobic acrylic (Alcon AcrySof) = A 2 Silicone (second-gen) = S 3 Memory = M	n = 120 Age-related cataract only Japanese	Slit lamp grading of ACO at 1 and 3 months (laser flare and cells)	No significant difference at 1 month Less ACO with A than S, and M than A at 3 months (At 1 and 3 months flare cells lower in A than S. No sig. diff. between M and A)
Umezawa and Shimizu, 1993[2]	RCT 1 year FU Phaco	1 HSM-PMMA 2 SP-PMMA 3 Unmodified PMMA	n = 90 Age-related cataract only Transnational	Slit lamp grading of ACO at 3 months and 1 year	HSM-PMMA and SP-PMMA IOLs had less ACO than unmodified PMMA at 3 months. No difference at 1 year
Abela-Formanek et al, 2002[19]	RCT 1 year FU Phaco	1 Hydrophilic acrylic (Hydroview) = H 2 Hydrophilic acrylic (MemoryLens) = M 3 Hydrophobic acrylic (AcrySof) = A 4 Hydrophobic acrylic (AMO Sensar AR40) = AS 5 Silicone square edge (CeeOn 920) = Sr 6 Silicone round edge (CeeOn 911A) = Ss	n = 190 Age-related cataract only Austrian	Slit lamp grading of ACO at 1 year (specular microscopy, PCO)	% at 1 year: H – 74 M – 43 A – 48 AS – 100 Sr – 69 Ss – 88

(Continued)

Table 33.5 *(Continued)*

Authors	Methods	Interventions	Participants	Outcomes	Results
Tognetto et al., 2002[21]	RCT 6 months FU Phaco	Hydrophilic acrylics 1 Hydroview = H 2 Cornea ACR6D = C 3 Ioltech Stabibag = I	n = 73 Age-related cataract only Italian	Slit lamp grading of ACO at days 7, 30, 90, 180 (specular microscopy)	% at 1/12: H – 13·0 C – 50·0 I – 29·1
Ursell et al., 1997[23]	RCT 1 year FU ECCE Phaco	1 Hydrophobic acrylic (Alcon AcrySof) = A 2 Silicone (Iolab L141U) = S 3 PMMA = P	n = 90 Age-related cataract only British	Area inside CCC measured by image analysis at days 7, 30, 180, 360	Less change in CCC area with A than P and S, *P* = 0·0001.
Hayashi et al., 1997[24]	RCT 6 months FU Phaco	1 Hydrophobic acrylic (Alcon AcrySof) = A 2 Silicone (SI 30) = S 3 PMMA = P	n = 240 Age-related cataract only Japanese	CCC size measured with Anterior Eye Segment Analysis System at 1 week, 3, 6 and 12 months	More contraction of the CCC opening with S than A or P
Cochener et al, 1999[25]	RCT 5 months FU Phaco	1 PMMA = P 2 Second-gen. silicone (SI 40) = S	n = 42 Age-related cataract only French	CCC contraction rate measured by image analysis at days 1, 30, 150	More contraction of the CCC opening with S than P

For abbreviations see Table 33.1.

Table 33.6 IOL decentration

Authors	Methods	IOLs compared	Participants	Outcome (technique used to measure decentration)	Results	
					IOL decentration	IOL tilt
Dick et al., 1997[26]	RCT 2 years FU	1 Silicone (plate-haptic) = Sp 2 Silicone (disc, loop haptic) = Sd 3 PMMA = P	n = 67 No other ocular pathology German	Biomicroscopic assessment at 2 years (VA, IOP, posterior capsule examination, corneal topography)	% with no decentration: Sp – 66, Sd – 72, P – 69 % with <1 mm decentration: Sp – 30, Sd – 20, P – 25 % with >1mm decentration: Sp – 4, Sd – 8, P – 6	Not measured
Hayashi et al., 1997[27]	RCT 1 year FU Phaco	1 Hydrophobic acrylic (Alcon AcySof) = A 2 Silicone (Allergan SI 30) = S 3 PMMA = P	n = 240 No other ocular pathology Japanese	Anterior Eye Segment Analysis System at 1 week and 1, 3, 6, 9 and 12 months: IOL decentration IOL tilt	Mean change at 1 year in mm ± SD: (P=0.35) A=0.31 ± 0.15 S=0.30 ± 0.16 P=0.27 ± 0.17 No increase between 1 week and 1 year	Mean change at 1 year in degrees ± SD: (P=0.81) A=2.71 ± 1.84 S=2.53 ± 1.36 P=2.62 ± 1.33 No increase between 1 week and 1 year
Jung et al., 2000[28]	RCT 2 months FU Phaco	1 Hydrophobic acrylic (Alcon AcrySof) = A 2 Silicone (Allergan Array multifocal) = S	n = 20 (40 eyes) No other ocular pathology Korean	Anterior Eye Segment Analysis System At 1 day and 1 and 2 months: IOL decentration IOL tilt	Mean change at 2 months in mm ± SD (P=0.08) A=0.20 ± 0.01 S=0.14 ± 0.01 No increase between 1 day and 2 months	Mean change at 2 months in degrees ± SD: (P=0.5) A=2.35 ± 1.53 S=2.06 ± 1.58 No increase between 1 day and 2 months
Wang et al., 1998[29]	RCT 6 months FU Phaco	1 Silicone (Allergan SI 30) = S 2 PMMA = P	n = 41 No other ocular pathology Chinese	Anterior Eye Segment Analysis System At 1 week and 1 and 6 months: IOL decentration IOL tilt	Mean change at 6 months in mm ± SD: (P=0.68) S=0.34 ± 0.2 P=0.30 ± 0.17 No increase between 1 week and 6 months	Mean change at 6 months in degrees ± SD: (P=0.81) S=3.61 ± 2.07 P=2.34 ± 1.69 No increase between 1 week and 6 months

modified and unmodified IOLs overall, but comparing the patients with laser-ridge (LR) IOLs, there was more PCO with modified LR IOLs compared to unmodified LR lenses.[33] In Zetterstrom's study on patients with pseudoexfoliation there was significantly less PCO and fewer YAGs with HSM lenses.[34]

Laser-ridge IOLs were investigated in three of the studies. Martin *et al.* showed that LR IOLs were associated with significantly more YAGs than biconvex, but not plano-convex IOLs, but they did not show any difference in PCO grades.[30] Westling and Calissendorff *et al.* showed that LR lenses had more PCO, but the same amount of YAG capsulotomies as PMMA lenses without a laser-ridge.[32] In Winter-Nielson *et al.*'s study there was no significant difference between biconvex and laser-ridge groups with respect to the need for YAG capsulotomy, but the heparin-surface-modified laser-ridge IOLs were associated with more YAGs compared to unmodified LR, HSM biconvex and unmodified biconvex IOLs.[33]

The convexity of the IOL optic was compared in three studies. In Martin *et al.*'s study biconvex IOLs were found to have lower YAG rates than plano-convex and laser-ridge IOLs.[30] In Sellman and Lindstroem's study IOLs with the convex surface posterior (PC) had less pearls than IOLs with the convex surface anterior (CP).[31] In Winter-Nielson *et al.*'s study there was no significant difference between biconvex and laser-ridge groups.[33] It has been proposed that the increased IOL surface contact with biconvex or IOLs with a posterior convex surface produce less PCO due to a barrier to lens epithelial cell migration.

Question

What influence do the lens design and material of foldable IOLs have on posterior capsule opacification?

The evidence

Eight of the twelve RCTs looking at this question (Table 33.8) compare one or two foldable IOLs to PMMA,[18,35–37,39–43] and the other four studies compare foldable IOLs.[19,38,42,44] All of the foldable IOLs were found to be associated with less PCO than PMMA except for one hydrophilic acrylic lens (Storz Hydroview). As we have seen when comparing the cytology on the surface of IOLs, this Hydroview IOL gets very few small cells and epithelioid cells on its surface but becomes covered with lens epithelial cells. It appears that the LECs grow onto the anterior surface and posterior capsule producing significant PCO.

The foldable IOLs associated with lowest rates of PCO in the studies are the second-generation silicone IOLs and the

AcrySof hydrophobic acrylic lens. In six studies the AcrySof IOL was associated with very low amounts of PCO and YAG capsulotomy rates.[19,35,36,38,40,43,44] Hayashi *et al.*'s study and the one by Pohjalainen *et al.* compared the AcrySof to a second-generation silicone IOL and found no significant difference in PCO.[35,43] Kucuksumer compared the hydrophobic AcrySof to a hydrophilic acrylic lens, the MemoryLens, and found that PCO was worse with the MemoryLens and YAG rates were higher.[38] In Abela-Formanek *et al.*'s study PCO was significantly greater with the hydrophilic, round edged IOLs (Hydroview, MemoryLens) than with hydrophobic sharp-edged IOLs (CeeOn 911A, AcrySof).[19] The difference in PCO between CeeOn 911A and AcrySof was not significant. In the hydrophobic acrylic group the AcrySof performed better than the round-edged AR40. In the second-generation silicone group, the CeeOn 911A performed better than the round-edged CeeOn 920.

The AcrySof IOL was the first foldable lens implant to be manufactured with a square optic edge. The square edge has come to be regarded as important in the prevention of PCO, by forming a barrier to LEC migration. The importance of the square-edge is supported by the study by Buehl *et al.* comparing two hydrophobic acrylic IOLs that were identical except for optic edge design.[42] The IOL with sharp posterior optic edge was associated with significantly less PCO than one with the round optic edges. Similarly in Abela-Formanek *et al.*'s study the CeeOn silicone IOL with a square-edge was associated with less PCO than the round-edged lens.[19]

The AcrySof material is more adhesive than other lens materials, which may also be important in the limitation of PCO and the stability of the anterior capsule on the surface of the IOL.[23] Hollick *et al.* showed that LECs that migrate onto the posterior capsule under the optic were more likely to regress in patients with AcrySof IOLs, whereas with first-generation silicone and PMMA IOLs these cells were more likely to progress.[45] They propose that this was most likely to be due to differences in the IOL material.

Comment

The hydrophobic IOLs tended to have a lower incidence of PCO than the hydrophilic ones, and IOLs with sharp-edged optics led to a lower incidence of PCO than round-edged IOLs. IOL material and optic edge design have a significant influence on PCO.

Question

What influence does IOL type have on visual acuity, contrast sensitivity, and glare?

Table 33.7 Posterior capsule opacification with PMMA IOLs

Authors	Methods	IOLs compared	Participants	Outcome (technique used to measure PCO)	Results
Lai and Fan, 1996[10]	RCT 1 year FU ECCE	1 HSM IOL = H 2 Unmodified IOL = P	n = 99 No other ocular pathology Malaysian	Clinical exam (not graded) at 1 year (cell deposits, VA)	At 1 year fibrosis present in: H = 58% (25/43), P = 77% (34/44); (P = NS) YAG required in: H = 1, P = 2 (P = NS)
Martin et al, 1992[30]	RCT 1 year FU Phaco	1 1-piece v 3-piece 2 Biconvex = B, plano-convex = PC, or laser-ridge = LR 3 Bag v sulcus	n = 600 No other ocular pathology American	Clinical PCO grade (0–3) at 1 year (VA, IOL centration, inflammation, complications at 1 day, 3 months, 1 year)	Moderate or severe PCO at 1 year in: 21% of bag IOLs v 53% of sulcus; (P < 0·001) PCO did not vary with IOL design YAG required at 1 year in: 16% of bag IOLs v 49% of sulcus; (P < 0·001). B = 23%, PC = 39%, LR = 34%; (P = 0·03)
Sellman and Lindstroem 1988[31]	RCT 1 year FU ECCE or phaco	1 Convex-plano = CP (anterior convex) 2 Plano convex = PC (posterior convex)	n = 505 No other ocular pathology Transnational	Clinical PCO grade (1–4) for fibrosis and Elschnig's pearls at 1 year (complications, slit lamp exam at 3 and 12 months)	Moderate or severe fibrosis at 1 year in: CP = 24%, PC = 44% (P = 0·48) Moderate or severe pearls at 1 year in: CP = 16·1%, PC = 7·1% (P = 0·03) No significant difference in YAG rates
Westling and Calissendorff, 1991[32]	RCT 1 year FU ECCE	1 Laser-ridge = LR 2 No laser-ridge = P	n = 319 No other ocular pathology Swedish	Clinical PCO grade (1–4) for fibrosis and Elschnig's pearls at 1 year (VA)	PCO present at 1 year in: LR = 50·4%, P = 35·7% (P = 0·0017) YAG required at 1 year in: LR = 17·7%, P = 17·7% (P = 0·99)
Winter-Nielson et al, 1998[33]	RCT 3 years FU ECCE with CCC	1 HSM biconvex = HB 2 Unmod. biconvex = B 3 HSM convex-plano with laser-ridge = HLR 4 Unmod. convex-plano with laser-ridge = LR	n = 250 No other ocular pathology Danish	Clinical PCO grade (1–4) for fibrosis and Elschnig's pearls; but only report YAG rates at 1, 2 and 3 years	Graphs in paper HLR required significantly more YAGs than other 3 groups; (P = 0·0004) No significant difference between B and HB HLR required significantly more YAGs than LR (P = 0·004) No significant difference between B and LR groups
Zetterstrom, 1993[34]	RCT 2 years FU ECCE	1 HSM = HSM 2 Unmod. PMMA = P	n = 40 Pseudoexfoliation Swedish	Clinical PCO grade (0–3) at 2 years (VA, cell deposits at 1 and 7 days, 3, 6 12, 24 months)	PCO at 2 years: None in H = 10/17, P = 1/15. Present in H = 6/17, P = 7/15 YAG in H = 1/17, P = 7/15 (P = 0·007)

For abbreviations see Table 33.1.

Table 33.8 Posterior capsule opacification with foldable IOLs compared to PMMA

Authors	Methods	IOLs compared	Participants	Outcome (technique used to measure PCO)	PCO
Abela-Formanek et al., 2002[19]	RCT 1 year FU Phaco	Hydrophilic acrylic 1 (Hydroview) = H 2 Hydrophilic acrylic (MemoryLens) = M 3 Hydrophobic acrylic (AcrySof) = A 4 Hydrophobic acrylic (AMO Sensar AR40) = AS 5 Silicone square edge (CeeOn 920) = Sr 6 Silicone round edge (CeeOn 911A) = Ss	n = 190 No other ocular pathology Austrian	Slit lamp grading at 1 year (specular microscopy, ACO)	% with no PCO in the central 3 mm at 1 year: H – 35, M – 39, A – 95, AS – 65, Sr – 68, Ss – 100 ($P = 0.0001$) % with no PCO external to the central 3 mm at 1 year: H – 0, M – 26, A – 95, AS – 23, Sr – 5, Ss – 94 ($P = 0.0001$)
Buehl et al., 2002[42]	RCT Paired eye study 1 year FU Phaco	Hydrophobic acrylic 1 Sensar OptiEdge AR40e (square-edge) 2 Sensar AR40 (round-edge)	n = 106 eyes (53 patients) No other ocular pathology Austrian	Image analysis of slit lamp and retroillumination images at 1 year Subjective PCO assessment at slit lamp at 1 week, 1 and 6 months and 1 year (VA, Nd:YAG capsulotomy incidence)	PCO score at 1 year: ($P < 0.001$) AR40e – 1.10 ± 0.22 (95% CI) AR40 – 2.19 ± 0.37 (95% CI) Nd:YAG in 1 eye with AR40
Hayashi et al., 1998[35]	RCT 2 years FU Phaco	1 Acrylic (AcrySof) = A 2 Silicone (SI 30) = S 3 PMMA IOL = P	n = 240 No other ocular pathology Japanese	Scheimpflug videophotography (central PCO density) at 2 years (VA)	Mean PCO score (SD): A = 16.0 (10.3), S = 12.0 (8.3), P = 26.3 (12.2) ($P < 0.001$) YAG in: A = 2.7% (2/73), S = 5.7% (4/70), P = 30.4% (21/69); ($P < 0.001$)
Hayashi, 2001[43]	RCT 2 years FU Phaco	1 Acrylic (AcrySof) = A 2 Silicone (SI 30) = S 3 PMMA IOL = P	n = 300 No other ocular pathology Japanese	Scheimpflug videophotography (PCO density) at 1 week, 3, 6, 12 and 24 months (VA, Nd:YAG capsulotomy incidence)	Mean PCO score at 2 years (SD): A = 11.7 (7.6), S = 14.1 (9.2), P = 23.2 (13.8); ($P < 0.001$) YAG by 2 years in: A = 4.2%, S = 14.4%, P = 28.9%
Hollick et al., 1999[36]	RCT 3 years FU ECCE (CCC)	1 Acrylic (AcrySof) = A 2 Silicone (first-gen.) = S 3 PMMA IOL = P	n = 90 No other ocular pathology British	Image analysis of retroillumination images (texture) at 6 months, 1, 2 and 3 years (VA)	Median % area of PCO: A = 10.2%, S = 39.9%, P = 56.1% ($P = 0.0001$) YAG in: A = 0% (0/19), S = 14% (3/22), P = 26% (6/23); ($P = 0.05$)

(Continued)

Table 33.8 *(Continued)*

Authors	Methods	IOLs compared	Participants	Outcome (technique used to measure PCO)	PCO
Hollick et al., 2000[37]	RCT 2 years FU Phaco	1 Hydrophilic acrylic (Hydroview) = H 2 Silicone (SI 30) = S 3 PMMA IOL = P	n = 90 No other ocular pathology British	Image analysis of retroillumination images (texture) at 1, 14, 30, 90, 180, 360, 720 days (VA, CS)	Median % area of PCO: H = 63, S = 17, P = 46; (P <0·0001) YAG in: H = 28, S = 0, P = 14; (P = 0·014)
Kucuksumer, 2000[38]	RCT 3 years FU Phaco	1 Acrylic (AcrySof) = A 2 Acrylic (MemoryLens) = M	n = 50 No other ocular pathology Turkish	Clinical PCO grade (1–4) taking VA into account at 1 and 3 years (VA, refraction)	Mean PCO grade at 3 years (SD): A = 0·16 (0·41), M = 1·76 (1·20) (P <0·001) YAG required in: A = 0%, M = 19% (P = 0·046)
Olson and Crandall, 1998[39]	RCT 3 years FU Phaco	1 Silicone (SI 30) = S 2 PMMA IOL = P	n = 119 No other ocular pathology American	Clinical PCO grade (0–4) taking VA into account at 3 years	Mean PCO grade: S = 0·88, P = 1·79 (P = 0·0001) YAGs required in: S = 24%, P = 33% (P = NS)
Pohjalainen et al., 2002[43]	RCT 2 years FU Phaco	1 Silicone (SI 30) = S 2 AcrySof IOL = A	n = 80 No other ocular pathology Finish	Clinical PCO grade (0–4) at 1–24 years	No PCO: S = 61%, A = 76% (P = NS) Clinically significant PCO (grade 3 and 4): S = 25%, A = 19% (P = NS) YAGs: S = 3%, A = 8% (P = NS)
Sveinsson and Seland, 1990[18]	RCT 1 year FU ECCE	1 Hydrophilic acrylic (Iogel) = H 2 PMMA IOL = P	n = 40 No other ocular pathology Norwegian	Slit lamp examination (PCO present or not) at 1 year (IOL precipitates, VA, complication)	PCO present in: H = 24%, P = 55%
Ursell et al., 1998[40]	RCT 2 years FU ECCE (CCC)	1 Acrylic (AcrySof) = A 2 Silicone (first-gen.) = S 3 PMMA IOL = P	n = 90 No other ocular pathology British	Image analysis of retroillumination images (texture) at 1, 14, 30, 90, 180, 360, 720 days	Median % area of PCO at 2 years: A = 11·8%, S = 33·5%, P = 43·7%; (P <0·001)
Wang and Woung, 2000[41]	RCT 1 year FU Phaco	1 Silicone (SI 30) = S 2 PMMA IOL = P	n = 40 No other ocular pathology Chinese	Image analysis of retroillumination images (intensity) at 1 year	No significant difference in central or peripheral opacity between S and P. Central 3 mm of posterior capsule significantly more "transparent" in S than P. YAG in: S = 0·05%, P = 0·05%

For abbreviations see Table 33.1.

Table 33.9 Influence of IOL type vision

Authors	Methods	Interventions	Participants	Outcomes	Results
Afsar et al., 1999[45]	RCT 2 months FU Phaco	1 Acrylic (AcrySof) = A 2 PMMA	n = 86 British	VA and CS at 2 months (refraction)	No significant difference
Anderson et al., 1994[46]	RCT 3 months FU Phaco	1 Oval optic PMMA 2 Round optic silicone	n = 182 American	Subjective visual disturbance at 1 and 3 weeks, and 3 months (refraction)	More with oval optic PMMA, $P = 0.03$
Johansen et al., 1997[47]	RCT 4 months FU Phaco	1 Silicone (SI 26) 2 PMMA	n = 91 Danish	VA and CS (Visitech sinusoidal gratings and Pelli-Robson) at 4 months	No significant difference in Snellen or Visitech Pelli-Robsen significantly lower for silicone $P = 1.67 \pm 0.11$, $S = 1.63 \pm 0.16$; $P < 0.01$
Kohnen et al., 1996[48]	RCT 6 weeks FU Phaco	1 AcrySof = A 2 Silicone (SI 40) = S 3 PMMA = P	n = 55 German	VA, BAT, CS (Regan chart), mesopic acuity (Rodenstock nyktometer) at 6 weeks	VA – no significant difference BAT – worse for S than for A CS – Lower for S than P No difference between P and A in any tests

For abbreviations see Table 33.1

The evidence

Four RCTs have vision as their primary outcome measure (Table 33.9), although their follow up was very short (six weeks to four months).[46–49] Afsar *et al.* found no significant difference in visual acuity or contrast sensitivity with AcrySof to PMMA, as would be expected at two months before the potential influence of PCO development.[46] Anderson *et al.* found that patients with oval-optic PMMA IOLs reported significantly more visual symptoms such as reflections, halos and ring around lights, than those with round-optic silicone IOLs.[47] They suggest that the oval IOL's truncated and thick edge may scatter light. In Johansen *et al.*'s study (comparing PMMA and silicone) and Kohnen *et al.*'s study (comparing PMMA, hydrophobic acrylic, and silicone), contrast sensitivity was lower for silicone IOLs than PMMA, with no significant difference between acrylic and silicone.[48,49] Neither study showed a significant difference in visual acuity between the groups. These comparisons suggest worse visual function results for silicone.

In the studies on PCO with foldable IOLs longer follow-up is reported and vision is discussed in the majority. In Hayashi *et al.*'s study comparing AcrySof, silicone and PMMA, visual loss of one or more lines was seen in 27·4% of those with AcrySof IOLs, 27·1% with silicone, and 63·8% with PMMA ($P < 0.001$).[35] In Hollick *et al.*'s study comparing AcrySof, silicone and PMMA, the visual acuity and contrast sensitivity were lowest for patients with PMMA IOLs, but this was not significant, perhaps due to the smaller numbers in this study.[36] In Hollick *et al.*'s study comparing Hydroview, silicone, and PMMA there was no significant difference in visual acuity at two years, but the patients with the silicone IOLs had significantly better contrast sensitivity.[37] Kucuksumer *et al.*'s study on AcrySof and MemoryLens showed no significantly better acuity at three years for AcrySof ($0·03 + -0·06$) than MemoryLens ($0·12 + -0·34$), $P = 0·02$.[38] In the study comparing PMMA and Iogel by Sveinsson and Seland, no significant difference was shown in the visual acuity between the two IOLs.[18]

Buehl *et al.*'s study comparing two hydrophobic acrylic IOLs, differing only in the shape of the posterior edge of the optic, showed no significant difference in visual acuity despite differences in PCO, which might be because the PCO had yet to spread across the central region.[42] There have been reports from non-randomised studies of edge glare from sharp IOL optic edges. The "half-rounded" edge profile of the AR40e (where the posterior edge is sharp and the anterior optic edge is round) did not cause more visual side effects than the round edge of the AR40 lens.

The early results suggest a possible worse visual outcome with silicone IOLs compared to PMMA and AcrySof, with similar results for PMMA (except for those with oval optics) and AcrySof. The long-term results show a different picture, largely reflecting which IOL type was associated with more PCO. In some studies no difference in acuity was shown despite differences in PCO, which may reflect the fact that acuity is a poor measure of the disability caused by PCO, and contrast sensitivity better; or may be due the small numbers of patients in some of these studies.

Implications for practice

It appears that there are two clinically important aspects to IOL biocompatibilty: the cytological reaction and the capsular reaction. An IOL may have excellent cytological biocompatibility, but poor capsular biocompatibility, such as the Hydroview IOL. The goal is to find an IOL which has both cytological and capsular biocompatibility. Material composition and design features, such as a sharp optic edge, appear to be important. The current hydrophobic IOLs offer good cytological and capsular biocompatibility. To date the second-generation silicone and the hydrophobic acrylic AcrySof IOLs appear to show the best overall performance. The least PCO was found with square-edged IOL designs such as the AcrySof and CeeOn 911A.

Implications for research

The debate continues over the relative influence of design and material on biocompatibility. A study comparing the hydrophobic IOLs with sharp optic edges made from different materials (such as AcrySof, Sensar OptiEdge AR40e and silicone CeeOn 911A), might help answer the question of whether the square edge is all important, or whether material also plays a role in determining the amount of PCO. Future research on IOLs should use an objective measure of PCO.

References

1. Mester U, Strauss M, Grewing R. Biocompatibility and blood aqueous barrier impairment in at-risk eyes with heparin-surface-modified or unmodified lenses. *J Cataract Refract Surg* 1998;**24**:380–4.
2. Umezawa S, Shimizu K. Biocompatibility of surface-modified intraocular lenses. *J Cataract Refract Surg* 1993;**19**:371–4.
3. Shah SM, Spalton DJ. Comparison of the postoperative inflammatory response in the normal eye with heparin surface modified and polymethylmethacrylate intraocular lenses. *J Cataract Refract Surg* 1995;**21**:579–85.
4. Martin RG, Sanders DR. Visual, astigmatic, and inflammatory results with the Starr AA-4203 single-piece foldable IOL: A randomised, prospective study. *Ophthalmic Surg* 1992;**23**:770–5.
5. Martin RG, Sanders DR, Van der Karr MA, DeLuca M. Effect of small incision intraocular lens surgery on postoperative inflammation and astigmatism: A study of the AMO SI-18NB small incision lens. *J Cataract Refract Surg* 1992;**18**:51–7.
6. Gatinel D, Lebrun T, Le Toumelin P, Chaine G. Aqueous flare induced by heparin-surface-modified poly(methylmethacrylate) and acrylic lenses implanted through the same-size incision in patients with diabetes. *J Cataract Refract Surg* 2001;**27**:855–60.

7. Krepler K, Ries E, Derbolav A, Nepp J, Wedrich A. Inflammation after phacoemulsification in diabetic retinopathy. *J Cataract Refract Surg* 2001;**27**:233–8.

8. Borgioli M, Coster DJ, Fan RF *et al.* Effect of heparin-surface-modification of polymethylmethacrylate intraocular lenses on signs of postoperative inflammation after extracapsular cataract extraction: One year results of a double-masked multicenter study. *Ophthalmology* 1992;**99**:1248–54.

9. Condon PI, Brancato R, Hayes P, Pouliquen Y, Saari KM, Wenzel M. Heparin surface modified IOLs compared with regular PMMA IOLs in patients with diabetes and/or glaucoma – one year results of a double blind randomised multi-independent trial. *Eur J Implant Refract Surg* 1995;**7**:194–201.

10. Lai YK, Fan RF. Effect of heparin-surface-modified polymethylmethacrylate intraocular lenses on the postoperative inflammation in an Asian population. *J Cataract Refract Surg* 1996;**22**(Suppl 1):830–4.

11. Philipson B, Fagerholm P, Calel B, Grunge A. Heparin surface modified intraocular lenses. Three month follow up of a randomised, double-masked clinical trial. *J Cataract Refract Surg* 1992;**18**:71–8.

12. Trocme SD, Li H. Effect of heparin-surface-modified intraocular lenses on postoperative inflammation after phacoemulsification: a randomised trial in a United States patient population. *Ophthalmology* 2000;**107**:1031–7.

13. Ygge J, Wenzel M, Philipson B, Fagerholm P. Cellular reactions on heparin surface-modified versus regular PMMA lenses during the first postoperative month; a double-masked and randomized study using specular microscopy. *Ophthalmology* 1990;**97**:1216–24.

14. Zetterstrom C, Lundvall A, Olivestedt G. Exfoliation syndrome and heparin surface modified intraocular lenses. *Acta Ophthalmol Copenh* 1992;**70**:91–5.

15. Hollick EJ, Spalton DJ, Pande MV, Ursell PG. Biocompatibility of PMMA, Silicone and Acrysof intraocular lenses: Randomised comparison of the cellular reaction on the anterior implant surface. *J Cataract Refract Surg* 1998;**24**:361–6.

16. Hollick EJ, Spalton DJ, Ursell PG. Surface cytology on intraocular lenses: Can increased biocompatibility have disadvantages? *Arch Ophthalmol* 1999;**117**:872–8.

17. Ravalico G, Baccara F, Lovisato A, Tognetto D. Postoperative cellular reaction on various intraocular lens materials. *Ophthalmology* 1997;**104**:1084–91.

18. Sveinsson O, Seland J. A randomised prospective clinical comparison of HEMA (IOGEL) and PMMA intraocular lenses. *Acta Ophthalmol* 1990;**68**(Suppl 195):43–7.

19. Abela-Formanek C, Amon M, Schild G, Schauersberger J, Heinze G, Kruger A. Uveal and capsular biocompatibility of hydrophilic acrylic, hydrophobic acrylic, and silicone intraocular lenses. *J Cataract Refract Surg* 2002;**28**:50–61.

20. Mullner-Eidenbock A, Amon M, Schauersberger J, Kruger A, Abela C, Petternel V, Zidek T. Cellular reaction on the anterior surface of 4 types of intraocular lenses. *J Cataract Refract Surg* 2001;**27**:734–40.

21. Tognetto D, Toto L, Ballone E, Ravalico G. Biocompatibility of hydrophilic intraocular lenses. *J Cataract Refract Surg* 2002;**28**:644–51.

22. Miyake K, Ota I, Miyake S, Maekubo K. Correlation between intraocular lens hydrophilicity and anterior capsule opacification and aqueous flare. *J Cataract Refract Surg* 1996;**22**:764–9.

23. Ursell PG, Spalton DJ, Pande MV. Anterior capsule stability in eyes with intraocular lenses made of poly(methyl methacrylate), silicone and AcrySof. *J Cataract Refract Surg* 1997;**23**:1532–8.

24. Hayashi K, Hayashi H, Nakao F, Hayashi F. Reduction in the area of the anterior capsule opening after polymethylmethacrylate, silicone, and soft acrylic intraocular lens implantation. *Am J Ophthalmol* 1997;**123**:441–7.

25. Cochener B, Jacq P, Colin J. Capsule contraction after continuous curvilinear capsulorhexis: polymethylmethacrylate verus silicone intraocular lenses. *J Cataract Refract Surg* 1999;**25**:1362–9.

26. Dick B, Kohnen T, Jacobi F, Jacobi KW. Long-term outcome after implantation of various intraocular lenses through a corneal tunnel. *Klinische Monatsblatter für Augenheilkunde* 1997;**211**:106–12.

27. Hayashi K, Harada M, Hayashi H, Nakao F, Hayashi F. Decentration and tilt of polymethylmethacrylate, silicone and acrylic soft intraocular lenses. *Ophthalmology* 1997;**104**:793–8.

28. Jung CK, Chung SK, Baek NH. Decentration and tilt: silicone multifocal versus acrylic soft intraocular lenses. *J Cataract Refract Surg* 2000;**26**:582–5.

29. Wang MC, Woung LC, Hu CY, Kuo HC. Position of polymethylmethacrylate and silicone intraocular lenses after phacoemulsification. *J Cataract Refract Surg* 1998;**24**:1652–7.

30. Martin RG, Sanders DR, Souchek J, Raanan MG, DeLuca M. Effect of posterior chamber intraocular lens design and surgical placement on postoperative outcome. *J Cataract Refract Surg* 1992;**18**:333–41.

31. Sellman TR, Lindstroem RL. Effect of plano convex posterior chamber lens on capsular opacification from Elschnig pearl formation. *J Cataract Refract Surg* 1988;**14**:68–72.

32. Westling AK, Calissendorff BM. Factors influencing the formation of posterior capsular opacities after extracapsular cataract extraction with posterior chamber lens implant. *Acta Ophthalmol Copenh* 1991;**69**:315–20.

33. Winter-Nielsen A, Johansen J, Pedersen GK, Corydon L. Posterior capsule opacification and neodymium: YAG capsulotomy with heparin-surface-modified intraocular lenses. *J Cataract Refract Surg* 1998;**24**:940–4.

34. Zetterstrom C. Incidence of posterior capsule opacification in eyes with exfoliation syndrome and heparin-surface-modified intraocular lenses. *J Cataract Refract Surg* 1993;**19**:344–7.

35. Hayashi K, Hayashi H, Nakao F, Hayashi F. Quantitative comparison of posterior capsular opacification after polymethylmethacrylate, silicone and soft acrylic intraocular lens implantation. *Arch Ophthalmol* 1998;**116**:1579–82.

36. Hollick EJ, Spalton DJ, Ursell PG *et al.* The effect of PMMA, silicone and polyacrylic intraocular lenses on posterior capsular opacification three years after cataract surgery. *Ophthalmology* 1999;**106**:49–54.

37. Hollick EJ, Spalton DJ, Ursell PG, Meacock WR, Barman SA, Boyce JF. Posterior capsular opacification with hydrogel, polymethylmethacrylate and silicone intraocular lenses: Two year results of a randomised prospective trial. *Am J Optthalmol* 2000;**129**:577–84.

38. Kucuksumer Y, Bayraktar S, Sahin S, Yilmaz OF. Posterior capsule opacification 3 years after implanation of an AcrySof and a MemoryLens in fellow eyes. *J Cataract Refract Surg* 2000;**26**:1176–82.

39. Olson R, Crandall A. Silicone versus polymethylmethacrylate intraocular lenses with regard to capsular opacification. *Ophthalmic Surg Lasers* 1998;**29**:55–8.

40. Ursell PG, Spalton DJ, Pande MV *et al.* Relationship between intraocular lens biomaterials and posterior capsule opacification. *J Cataract Refract Surg* 1998;**24**:352–60.

41. Wang MC, Woung LC. Digital retroilluminated photography to analyse posterior capsule opacification in eyes with intraocular lenses. *J Cataract Refract Surg* 2000;**26**:56–61.

42. Buehl W, Findl O, Menapace R *et al.* Effect of an acrylic intraocular lens with a sharp posterior optic edge on posterior capsular opacification. *J Cataract Refract Surg* 2002;**28**:1105–11.

43. Hayashi K, Hayashi H, Nakao F, Hayashi F. Changes in posterior capsule opacification after poly (methylmethacrylate), silicone, and acrylic intraocular lens implantation. *J Cataract Retract Surg* 2001;**27**:817–24.

44. Pohjalainen T, Vesti E, Uusitalo RJ, Laatiainen L. Posterior capsular opacification in pseudophakic eyes with silicone or acrylic intraocular lenses. *Eur J Ophthalmol* 2002;**12**:212–18.

45. Hollick EJ, Ursell PG, Pande M, Spalton DJ. Lens epithelial cell regression on the posterior capsule: a 2 year prospective randomised trial with three different intraocular lens materials. *Br J Ophthalmol* 1998;**82**:1182–8.

46. Afsar AJ, Patel S, Woods RL, Wykes W. A comparison of visual performance between a rigid PMA and a foldable acrylic intraocular lens. *Eye* 1999;**13**:329–35.

47. Anderson CJ, Sturm RJ, Shapiro MB, Ballew C. Visual disturbances associated with oval-optic polymethylmethacrylate and round-optic silicone intraocular lenses. *J Cataract Refract Surg* 1994;**20**:295–8.

48. Johansen J, Dam Johansen M, Olsen T. Contrast sensitivity with silicone and polymethylmethacrylate intraocular lenses. *J Cataract Refract Surg* 1997;**223**:1085–8.

49. Kohnen S, Ferrer A, Braweiler P. Visual function in pseudophakic eyes with polymethylmethacrylate, silicone and acrylic intraocular lenses. *J Cataract Refract Surg* 1996;**22**:1303–7.

34 Multifocal and monofocal intraocular lenses

Martin Leyland

Background

Current techniques of cataract surgery and IOL implantation allow accurate prediction of postoperative refraction such that there can now be a reasonable expectation of good uncorrected distance acuity. This has been driven partly by the change from cataract surgery using a large (10 mm) incision to small (3–4 mm) incision phacoemulsification surgery. Among other benefits, this change offers greater predictability of refractive outcomes, which is a necessary pre-requisite for good visual acuity without the need for glasses.[1,2]

Treatment options

Standard IOLs used have a fixed refractive power, so that the focal length is fixed (monofocal). This means that most patients will require a reading addition to their distance glasses.[3] While the majority of people undergoing cataract surgery may be happy to use reading glasses, a proportion are likely to seek good unaided near vision as well as distance vision. The need for reading glasses for near vision is unlikely to be considered an important issue at present in developing countries, where the burden of blindness due to cataract is very high.

One approach to improve near visual acuity is to modify the IOL. An IOL may provide near and distance vision if both powers are present within the optical zone. This has been attempted using diffractive optics or with zones of differing refractive power. Both types of IOL divide light up to focus at two (bifocal) or more (multifocal) points, so that both near and distant objects may be focussed on the retina. Optical evaluation of multifocal IOLs indicates that a two- to three-fold increase in the depth of field is achieved at the expense of a 50% reduction in the contrast of the retinal image.[4]

Question

Does the use of multifocal intraocular lenses offer benefits over the current standard treatment of monofocal intraocular lens implantation?

The evidence

A systematic review of randomised controlled trials of multifocal intraocular lenses was undertaken to determine whether their use offers benefits over the current standard treatment of monofocal intraocular lens implantation.[5] Eight RCTs were identified for inclusion in the review,[5–12] and the characteristics of these trials are summarised in Table 34.1.

Question

Does the use of multifocal intraocular lenses offer benefits over monofocal intraocular lenses for visual acuity (unaided and corrected)?

The evidence

Distance acuity was described in five trials as the proportion of participants achieving specified acuity levels (Figure 34.1). The proportion of participants achieving less than 6/6 unaided was not significantly different between multifocal and monofocal groups (Peto odds ratio 1·21, 95% CI 0·75–1·96). Three trials describe mean acuity rather than proportions (Figure 34.2). There was no evidence of any difference in acuity between multifocal and monofocal groups (standardised mean difference −0·03, 95% CI −0·24 −0·18).

Similarly, there was no difference between IOL types with respect to the proportion of participants achieving less than 6/6 best corrected visual acuity in seven studies (Peto odds ratio 1·43, 95% CI 0·99–2·09, Figure 34.3). There was no difference in mean best-corrected acuity in the three refractive IOL trials that reported this outcome (standardised mean difference 0·19, 95% CI −0·03–0·40, Figure 34.4).

Because of significant heterogeneity no meta-analysis was conducted on the data for near visual acuity. The six trials that reported this outcome found that near vision tended to improve with the use of a multifocal IOL (Figure 34.5).

Table 34.1 Characteristics of trials comparing multifocal to monofocal intraocular lenses

Trial	Method	Method quality*	Participants	Intervention	Outcomes
El-Maghraby et al, 1992[6]	Randomised Single centre Masking not stated Study duration 2 to 4 months	Jadad score 3 Allocation concealment adequate	Saudi Arabia 47% male Mean age 57 years Multifocal group: 39 Monofocal group: 38 Unilateral – fellow eye not blind	Rigid PMMA IOLs: 3M diffractive IOL (815LE) or 3M monofocal IOL (15LE) Phaco with can-opener capsulotomy	Distance acuity Near acuity
Steinert et al, 1992[10]	Randomised Multicentre Double-masked Study duration 3 to 6 months	Jadad score 5 Allocation concealment adequate	USA 42% male Mean age 72 years Multifocal group: 32 Monofocal group: 30 Unilateral – fellow eye phakic	Rigid PMMA IOLs: Allergan refractive IOL (MPC25NB) or Allergan monofocal IOL (PC25NB) Phaco, capsulotomy type not specified	Distance acuity Near acuity Depth of field Contrast sensitivity Glare Spectacle use Non-validated subjective assessment
Percival et al, 1993[8]	Randomised Single centre Masking not stated Study duration 4 to 6 months	Jadad score 2 Allocation concealment unclear	UK 42% male Mean age 77 years Multifocal group: 25 Monofocal group: 25 Unilateral – fellow eye phakic, most cataractous	Rigid PMMA IOLs: Allergan refractive IOL (MPC25) or Allergan monofocal IOL (PC25) Myopic astigmatism monofocal group ECCE with can-opener capsulotomy	Distance acuity Near acuity Depth of field Contrast sensitivity Spectacle use Non-validated subjective outcome Adverse phenomena
Rossetti et al, 1994[9]	Randomised Single centre Masking not stated Study duration 12 months	Jadad score 1 Allocation concealment unclear	Italy 41% male Mean age 71 years Multifocal group: 38 Monofocal group: 42 Unilateral – fellow eye phakic with no significant cataract	Rigid PMMA IOLs: 3M diffractive IOL (unspecified) or 3M monofocal IOL (unspecified) ECCE, capsulotomy type not specified	Distance acuity Near acuity Contrast sensitivity Spectacle use Non-validated subjective assessment of visual quality questionnaire Adverse phenomena
Allen et al, 1996[5]	Randomised Multicentre Open/unmasked Study duration 5 to 6 months	Jadad score 1 Allocation concealment adequate	Europe 49% male Mean age 66 years Multifocal group: 79 Monofocal group: 70 Unilateral – status of fellow eye not reported	Rigid PMMA IOLs: Pharmacia diffractive IOL (808X) or Pharmacia monofocal IOL (808D) Phaco and ECCE Capsulotomy not specified	Distance acuity Near acuity Contrast sensitivity Spectacle use Non-validated questionnaire Adverse phenomena

(Continued)

Table 34.1 (Continued)

Trial	Method	Method quality*	Participants	Intervention	Outcomes
Javitt et al., 2000[7]	Randomised Multi-centre Double-masked Study duration 3 to 6 months	Jadad score 5 Allocation concealment adequate	USA, Germany and Austria 44% male Mean age not given, 50% 65–74 years Multifocal group: 124 Monofocal group: 111 Bilateral surgery	Foldable 3-piece silicone optic, PMMA haptic IOLs: Allergan refractive IOL (SA40N) or Allergan monofocal IOL (SI40NB) phaco with continuous circular capsulorhexis	Distance acuity Near acuity Validated questionnaire (modified cataract TyPE) Validated quality of life questionnaire
Kamlesh et al., 2001[14]	Randomised Single centre Study duration 3 months	Jadad score 1 Allocation concealment unclear	India Gender not given Mean age 55·7 yrs (multifocal), 53·5 yrs (monofocal) No none-cataract pathology Astigmatism less than 1·5 dioptres Unilateral surgery	Domilens aspheric refractive IOL (Progress 3) or monofocal IOL (Flex 65) ECCE with envelope capsulotomy Refractive aim not stated	Distance acuity Near acuity Depth of field Contrast sensitivity Spectacle use Non-validated subjective outcome Adverse phenomena
Leyland et al., 2002[12]	Randomised Double-masked trial of bilateral multifocal, bifocal, or monofocal intraocular lenses	Jadad score 5 Allocation concealment adequate	UK Over 50 years of age Bilateral cataract No none-cataract pathology Less than 1·5 dioptres astigmatism Bilateral surgery	Multifocal (refractive, 2 designs) or monofocal IOL implantation Surgical intervention: Bilateral small incision phaco and IOL, aiming for emmetropia	Distance acuity Near acuity Depth of field Contrast sensitivity Spectacle use Validated questionnaire (modified cataract type E) Adverse phenomena

*Methodological quality was scored from 0 to 5 (Jadad, 1996)[13], with 5 points indicating the best methodology.
Abbreviations: IOL, intraocular lens; PMMA, polymethylmethacrylate; ECCE, extracapsular cataract extraction

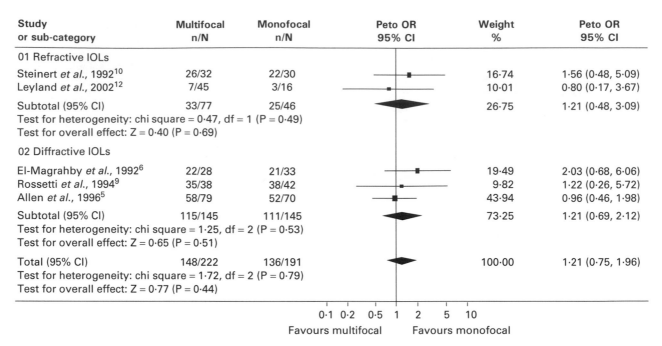

Study or sub-category	Multifocal n/N	Monofocal n/N	Peto OR 95% CI	Weight %	Peto OR 95% CI
01 Refractive IOLs					
Steinert *et al.*, 1992[10]	26/32	22/30		16·74	1·56 (0·48, 5·09)
Leyland *et al.*, 2002[12]	7/45	3/16		10·01	0·80 (0·17, 3·67)
Subtotal (95% CI)	33/77	25/46		26·75	1·21 (0·48, 3·09)
Test for heterogeneity: chi square = 0·47, df = 1 (P = 0·49)					
Test for overall effect: Z = 0·40 (P = 0·69)					
02 Diffractive IOLs					
El-Magrahby *et al.*, 1992[6]	22/28	21/33		19·49	2·03 (0·68, 6·06)
Rossetti *et al.*, 1994[9]	35/38	38/42		9·82	1·22 (0·26, 5·72)
Allen *et al.*, 1996[5]	58/79	52/70		43·94	0·96 (0·46, 1·98)
Subtotal (95% CI)	115/145	111/145		73·25	1·21 (0·69, 2·12)
Test for heterogeneity: chi square = 1·25, df = 2 (P = 0·53)					
Test for overall effect: Z = 0·65 (P = 0·51)					
Total (95% CI)	148/222	136/191		100·00	1·21 (0·75, 1·96)
Test for heterogeneity: chi square = 1·72, df = 2 (P = 0·79)					
Test for overall effect: Z = 0·77 (P = 0·44)					

0·1 0·2   0·5   1   2   5   10

Favours multifocal   Favours monofocal

Figure 34.1 Distance visual acuity – less than 6/6 unaided

Study or sub-category	N	Multifocal Mean (SD)	N	Monofocal Mean (SD)	SMD (fixed) 95% CI	Weight %	SMD (fixed) 95% CI
01 Refractive IOLs							
Steinert *et al.*, 1992[10]	32	−6·33 (1·73)	30	−6·37 (1·93)		18·23	0·02 (−0·48, 0·52)
Javitt and Steinert, 2000[7]	123	−7·78 (1·21)	109	−7·66 (1·36)		67·95	−0·09 (−0·35, 0·16)
Leyland *et al.*, 2002[15]	45	0·08 (0·13)	16	0·05 (0·15)		13·83	0·22 (−0·35, 0·79)
Subtotal (95% CI)	200		155			100·00	−0·03 (−0·24, 0·18)
Test for heterogeneity: chi square = 1·00, df = 1 (P = 0·61)							
Test for overall effect: Z = 0·27 (P = 0·79)							
02 Diffractive IOLs							
Subtotal (95% CI)	0		0				Not estimable
Test for heterogeneity: not applicable							
Test for overall effect: not applicable							
Total (95% CI)	200		155			100·00	−0·03 (−0·24, 0·18)
Test for heterogeneity: chi square = 1·00, df = 2 (P = 0·61)							
Test for overall effect: Z = 0·27 (P = 0·79)							

−10   −5   0   5   10

Favours multifocal   Favours monofocal

Figure 34.2 Distance visual acuity – mean unaided

Comment

There was no difference between multifocal and monofocal IOL groups with respect to distance visual acuity. Unaided near vision is critical to the assessment of multifocal efficacy, but was reported in a manner that makes comparison between trials difficult. It is not made clear in most trials whether the reported print size read has been corrected for reading distance so as to allow a near acuity to be calculated. Only two trials explicitly report near acuity.[7,13] A further problem is the use of Jaeger cards. These are not standardised between manufacturers, so that J3 from one trial cannot be

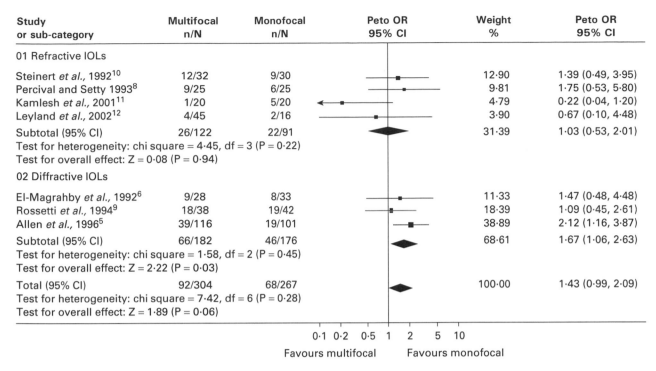

Study or sub-category	Multifocal n/N	Monofocal n/N	Peto OR 95% CI	Weight %	Peto OR 95% CI
01 Refractive IOLs					
Steinert *et al.,* 1992[10]	12/32	9/30		12·90	1·39 (0·49, 3·95)
Percival and Setty 1993[8]	9/25	6/25		9·81	1·75 (0·53, 5·80)
Kamlesh *et al.,* 2001[11]	1/20	5/20		4·79	0·22 (0·04, 1·20)
Leyland *et al.,* 2002[12]	4/45	2/16		3·90	0·67 (0·10, 4·48)
Subtotal (95% CI)	26/122	22/91		31·39	1·03 (0·53, 2·01)
Test for heterogeneity: chi square = 4·45, df = 3 (P = 0·22)					
Test for overall effect: Z = 0·08 (P = 0·94)					
02 Diffractive IOLs					
El-Magrahby *et al.,* 1992[6]	9/28	8/33		11·33	1·47 (0·48, 4·48)
Rossetti *et al.,* 1994[9]	18/38	19/42		18·39	1·09 (0·45, 2·61)
Allen *et al.,* 1996[5]	39/116	19/101		38·89	2·12 (1·16, 3·87)
Subtotal (95% CI)	66/182	46/176		68·61	1·67 (1·06, 2·63)
Test for heterogeneity: chi square = 1·58, df = 2 (P = 0·45)					
Test for overall effect: Z = 2·22 (P = 0·03)					
Total (95% CI)	92/304	68/267		100·00	1·43 (0·99, 2·09)
Test for heterogeneity: chi square = 7·42, df = 6 (P = 0·28)					
Test for overall effect: Z = 1·89 (P = 0·06)					

0·1 0·2 0·5 1 2 5 10

Favours multifocal   Favours monofocal

Figure 34.3 Distance visual acuity – less than 6/6 best corrected

Study or sub-category	N	Multifocal Mean (SD)	N	Monofocal Mean (SD)	SMD (fixed) 95% CI	Weight %	SMD (fixed) 95% CI
01 Refractive IOLs							
Steinert *et al.,* 1992[10]	32	−7·67 (1·25)	30	−8·19 (1·49)		18·02	0·37 (−0·13, 0·88)
Javitt, and Steinert, 2000[7]	123	−8·40 (0·97)	109	−8·46 (0·94)		68·46	0·06 (−0·20, 0·32)
Leyland *et al.,* 2002[15]	45	0·05 (0·10)	16	−0·01 (0·11)		13·52	0·58 (−0·00, 1·16)
Subtotal (95% CI)	200		155			100·00	0·19 (−0·03, 0·40)
Test for heterogeneity: chi square = 3·17, df = 2 (P = 0·21)							
Test for overall effect: Z = 1·73 (P = 0·08)							
02 Diffractive IOLs							
Subtotal (95% CI)	0		0				Not estimable
Test for heterogeneity: not applicable							
Test for overall effect: not applicable							
Total (95% CI)	200		155			100·00	−0·19 (−0·03, 0·40)
Test for heterogeneity: chi square = 3·17, df = 2 (P = 0·21)							
Test for overall effect: Z = 1·73 (P = 0·08)							

−10 −5 0 5 10

Favours multifocal   Favours monofocal

Figure 34.4 Distance visual acuity – mean best corrected

assumed to equal J3 from another. Despite these caveats, it is clear that unaided near acuity is improved by the use of multifocal IOLs. It is important to remember, however, that monofocal IOL near acuity can be restored by the use of reading glasses.

Question

Does the use of multifocal intraocular lenses offer benefits over monofocal intraocular lenses in terms of spectacle dependence?

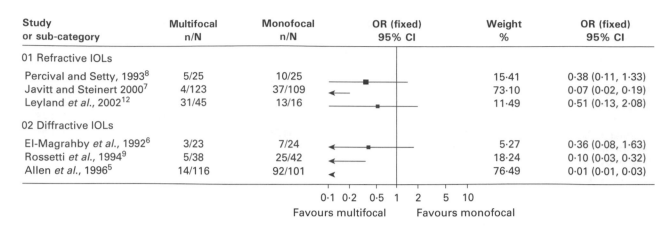

Study or sub-category	Multifocal n/N	Monofocal n/N	OR (fixed) 95% CI	Weight %	OR (fixed) 95% CI
01 Refractive IOLs					
Percival and Setty, 1993[8]	5/25	10/25		15·41	0·38 (0·11, 1·33)
Javitt and Steinert 2000[7]	4/123	37/109		73·10	0·07 (0·02, 0·19)
Leyland *et al.*, 2002[12]	31/45	13/16		11·49	0·51 (0·13, 2·08)
02 Diffractive IOLs					
El-Magrahby *et al.*, 1992[6]	3/23	7/24		5·27	0·36 (0·08, 1·63)
Rossetti *et al.*, 1994[9]	5/38	25/42		18·24	0·10 (0·03, 0·32)
Allen *et al.*, 1996[5]	14/116	92/101		76·49	0·01 (0·01, 0·03)

0·1   0·2   0·5   1   2   5   10
Favours multifocal   Favours monofocal

Figure 34.5   Near visual acuity – less than J3/J4 unaided

Table 34.2   Summary of subjective outcome ("patient satisfaction") data

Study	Validated measure?	Outcome	Multifocal	Monofocal
El-Maghraby *et al.*, 1992[6]	Not measured	–	–	–
Steinert *et al.*, 1992[10]	No; standard questionnaire	Mean satisfaction 1–7 (1 = best, 7 = worst) (SD)	1·77 (1·36)	1·35 (0·80)
Percival and Setty, 1993[8]	No; method not reported	Percentage satisfied	96%	92%
Rossetti *et al.*, 1994[9]	No; method not reported	Percentage satisfied or highly satisfied	68%	78%
Allen *et al.*, 1996[5]	No; method not reported	Overall visual satisfaction good	95%	93%
Javitt and Steinart, 2000[7]	Yes; TyPE questionnaire	Mean overall visual satisfaction 0–10 (0 = worst, 10 = best)	8·4	7·9
Kamlesh *et al.*, 2001[11]	No; standard questionnaire	Percentage rating vision as good	70%	80%
Leyland *et al.*, 2002[12]	Yes; TyPE questionnaire	Median overall visual satisfaction 0–10 (0 = worst; 10 = best)	–	–

The evidence

In all RCTs the majority of multifocal IOL participants still used spectacles for some tasks – usually for reading small print. Freedom from spectacles was, however, more frequent with multifocal than monofocal IOLs in seven trials

(Peto odds ratio for spectacle dependence 0·15, 95% CI 0·11–0·22, Figure 34.6).

Comment

Spectacle independence is more likely to be achieved with use of the multifocal IOL than monofocal IOLs.

Study or sub-category	Multifocal n/N	Monofocal n/N	Peto OR 95% CI	Weight %	Peto OR 95% CI
01 Refractive IOLs					
Steinert et al., 1992[10]	22/31	25/28		7·77	0·33 (0·09, 1·16)
Percival and Setty, 1993[8]	14/25	23/25		7·87	0·16 (0·05, 0·56)
Javitt and Steinert 2000[7]	84/124	102/109		30·07	0·20 (0·11, 0·38)
Kamlesh et al., 2001[11]	9/20	19/20		6·90	0·10 (0·03, 0·37)
Leyland et al., 2002[12]	32/45	16/16		6·45	0·18 (0·05, 0·73)
Subtotal (95% CI)	161/245	185/198		59·06	0·19 (0·12, 0·30)
Test for heterogeneity: chi square = 1·78, df = 4 (P = 0·78)					
Test for overall effect: Z = 7·13 (P < 0·00001)					
02 Diffractive IOLs					
Rossetti et al., 1994[9]	20/38	39/42		12·54	0·13 (0·05, 0·35)
Allen et al., 1996[5]	72/116	97/98		28·41	0·11 (0·06, 0·21)
Subtotal (95% CI)	92/154	136/140		40·94	0·11 (0·07, 0·20)
Test for heterogeneity: chi square = 0·07, df = 2 (P = 0·79)					
Test for overall effect: Z = 7·73 (P < 0·00001)					
Total (95% CI)	253/399	321/338		100·00	0·15 (0·11, 0·22)
Test for heterogeneity: chi square = 3·76, df = 6 (P = 0·71)					
Test for overall effect: Z = 10·42 (P < 0·00001)					

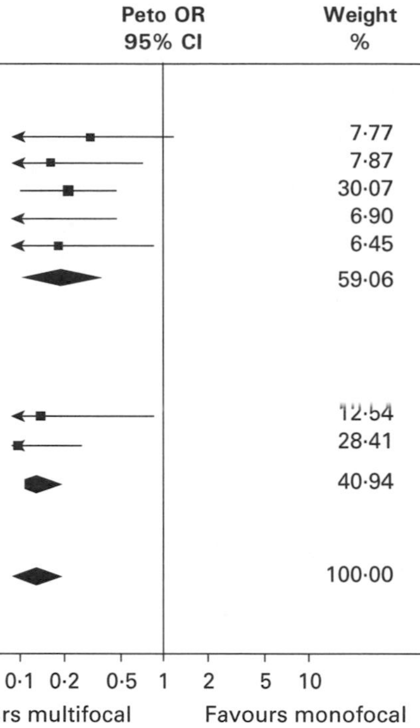

```
        0·1 0·2  0·5  1   2    5   10
        Favours multifocal    Favours monofocal
```

Figure 34.6 Spectacle dependence

However, in no trial did more than half of the participants achieve spectacle independence.

Question

Does the use of multifocal intraocular lenses offer benefits over monofocal intraocular lenses for in terms of depth of field?

The evidence

Four trials measured depth of field (the amount of defocus consistent with retention of useful acuity). Depth of field was improved with the multifocal IOL compared to the monofocal. One trial tested acuity with defocus from emmetropia, and reported the proportion achieving better than or equal to 6/12 acuity at each level of defocus. In the trial, 76% and 57% of multifocal and monofocal patients respectively achieved 6/12 with minus 1·25 D defocus, compared with 96% and 4% at minus 2·5 D defocus. Three trials measured the number of dioptres of defocus through which a 6/12 acuity was achieved, across a range of 3–6 dioptres plus or minus from emmetropia. The data were not presented in such a way as to be combined in a meta-analysis. However, each study reported increased depth of field with the multifocal IOL.

Question

Does the use of multifocal intraocular lenses offer benefits over monofocal intraocular lenses in terms of contrast sensitivity and glare?

The evidence

Contrast is the difference between the brightness of an image and its background divided by the total brightness of image plus background. Contrast sensitivity is the inverse of target contrast threshold. Six trials assessed contrast sensitivity (Table 34.3). All reported lower contrast sensitivity with the multifocal IOL, which is consistent with the expected optical effect of the lens.

Three trials objectively assessed glare using the Brightness Acuity Tester. The differences between lenses was not statistically significant. Seven trials reported subjective results and all describe an increased incidence of adverse visual phenomena with the multifocal IOL (Figure 34.7). In those trials that separated glare from haloes, the latter is the more frequently observed. The TyPE questionnaire quantifies the degree of bother from glare, haloes, and rings around lights on a scale of 0–4, where "not at all" scores 0, "a little bit" scores 1, "moderately" scores 2, "quite a bit" scores 3 and "extremely" scores 4. The mean scores (without glasses on) were 1·57 for the multifocal IOL and 0·43 for the monofocal.[7] Median

Table 34.3 Contrast sensitivity (CS) results

Study	Method	Outcome	Multifocal	Monofocal
El-Magrahby *et al*, 1992[6]	Not tested	–	–	–
Steinert, 1992[10]	Regan contrast acuity charts	Acuity (lines read) at 96%, 50%, 25% and 11% contrast	CS lower at all levels. 2·59 lines (SD 2.01) at 11%	Statistically significant at 11% 4·37 lines (SD 2.05)
Percival and Setty, 1993[8]	Regan contrast acuity charts	Acuity (lines read) at 96%, 50%, 25% and 11% contrast	CS lower at all levels (no analysis)	2·1 lines better acuity at 11% level
Rossetti *et al*, 1994[9]	Pelli–Robson chart	Mean score (log units)	1·70	1·73
Allen *et al*, 1996[5]	VCTS chart (6500 near, 6000 distance)	Mean of CS at 5 spatial frequencies, at 3 light levels (log units)	CS 57·9 to 83·9 lower	CS 57·9 to 83·9 higher
Javitt and Steinert 2000[7]	Not tested	–	–	–
Kamlesh *et al*, 2001[14]	Pelli–Robson chart	Mean CS score (log units)	1·38	1·56
Leyland *et al*, 2002[12]	Pelli–Robson chart	Mean (SD) CS score (log units)	1·66 (0·16)	1·74 (0·15)

scores of 1 (multifocal) and 0 (monofocal) were reported in the other study using the TyPE instrument.[12]

Comment

Contrast sensitivity was lower in participants with the multifocal IOL. The differences were smaller than would be expected, given the division of light between distance and near focus, which may result from post-receptoral visual processing. Whether the reduction in contrast sensitivity induced by the IOL would be clinically significant would depend on the contrast presented by the visual target and the contrast sensitivity of the patient's retina. No significant differences between IOLs with respect to objective glare were reported. Subjective experience of adverse visual phenomena (glare/halo) was more likely with multifocal IOLS.

Question

Does the use of multifocal intraocular lenses offer benefits over monofocal intraocular lenses in terms of quality of life?

The evidence

The overall visual satisfaction results from the monofocal IOL control groups illustrate the high level of satisfaction with these lenses. The non-validated multifocal subjective data are inconclusive. Using the TyPE instrument, one study found a small but statistically significant increase in overall visual satisfaction with the multifocal IOL[7] (8·4/10 with the multifocal compared to 7·9/10 with the monofocal) and, as expected, a larger beneficial effect with respect to near vision (7·4/10 and 5·3/10). Another study found unaided overall visual satisfaction to be the same in the two IOL groups (median 8/10).[12]

Only El-Maghraby *et al.* (1992)[6] did not report any subjective assessment. Of the other seven trials, only Javitt and Steinert (2000)[7] and Leyland *et al.* (2002)[12] used a validated instrument: the TyPE cataract questionnaire. The data could not be combined for meta-analysis, and are instead presented in Table 34.2.

Comment

Subjective outcomes are fundamental to the evaluation of multifocal IOLs but, like near vision, measurements were flawed in most of the trials. There was no consistent effect on visual satisfaction evident.

Adverse subjective visual phenomena, particularly haloes or rings around lights, were more prevalent and more troublesome in participants with the multifocal IOL. The lack of a consistent drop in patient satisfaction despite the prevalence of these phenomena could be interpreted as evidence that patients do not perceive them as severe.

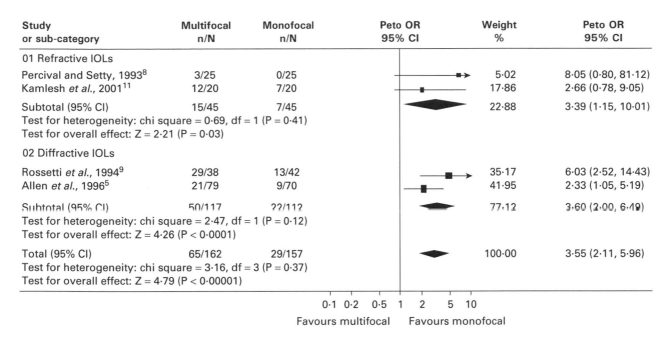

Study or sub-category	Multifocal n/N	Monofocal n/N	Peto OR 95% CI	Weight %	Peto OR 95% CI
01 Refractive IOLs					
Percival and Setty, 1993[8]	3/25	0/25		5·02	8·05 (0·80, 81·12)
Kamlesh *et al.*, 2001[11]	12/20	7/20		17·86	2·66 (0·78, 9·05)
Subtotal (95% CI)	15/45	7/45		22·88	3·39 (1·15, 10·01)
Test for heterogeneity: chi square = 0·69, df = 1 (P = 0·41)					
Test for overall effect: Z = 2·21 (P = 0·03)					
02 Diffractive IOLs					
Rossetti *et al.*, 1994[9]	29/38	13/42		35·17	6·03 (2·52, 14·43)
Allen *et al.*, 1996[5]	21/79	9/70		41·95	2·33 (1·05, 5·19)
Subtotal (95% CI)	50/117	22/112		77·12	3·60 (2·00, 6·49)
Test for heterogeneity: chi square = 2·47, df = 1 (P = 0·12)					
Test for overall effect: Z = 4·26 (P < 0·0001)					
Total (95% CI)	65/162	29/157		100·00	3·55 (2·11, 5·96)
Test for heterogeneity: chi square = 3·16, df = 3 (P = 0·37)					
Test for overall effect: Z = 4·79 (P < 0·00001)					

0·1 0·2 0·5 1 2 5 10

Favours multifocal   Favours monofocal

Figure 34.7 Glare/haloes

Discussion

Six of the eight included trials involved participants who had surgery on only one eye.[5,6,8–12] Unilateral trials allow measurement of uniocular outcomes such as visual acuity, but are of limited use when attempting to measure the effect of the multifocal intraocular lenses on quality of life, especially where the fellow eye has good vision.

Implications for practice

There is good evidence that use of multifocal intraocular lenses improves near vision without any adverse effect on distance acuity. Spectacle independence is considerably more likely with use of these intraocular lenses when compared to the standard practice of monofocal implantation.

Whether the improvement in unaided near vision and increased incidence of spectacle independence are sufficiently high to outweigh the loss of contrast sensitivity and the experience of haloes is a matter for an individual patient to decide. The final choice for a patient is likely to depend on his or her motivation to be free of spectacles, guided by realistic expectations as to the likelihood of achieving this aim and understanding of the compromises involved.

Implications for research

The optical and visual effects of multifocal intraocular lenses are now well known. Future research on these and similar intraocular lenses should use validated subjective outcome criteria and strive for clarity in reporting of objective outcomes, particularly with regard to near vision. The search for alternative strategies to achieve spectacle independence such as monovision and accommodating intraocular lenses should continue.

References

1. Desai P, Reidy A, Minassian D. The National Cataract Surgery Survey 1997/98. A report of the results of the clinical outcomes. *Br J Ophthalmol* 1999;**83**:1336–40.
2. Minassian D, Rosen P, Dart J, Reidy A, Desai P, Sidhu M. Extracapsular cataract extraction compared with small incision surgery by phacoemulsification: a randomised trial. *Br J Ophthalmol* 2001;**85**(7): 822–9.
3. Javitt J, Wang F, Trentacost D, Rowe M, Tarantino N. Outcomes of cataract extraction with multifocal intraocular lens implantation. *Ophthalmology* 1997;**104**:589–99.
4. Holladay J, van Dijk H, Lang A, Portney V, Willis T, Sun R, Oksman H. Optical performance of multifocal intraocular lenses. *J Cataract Refract Surg* 1990;**16**:413–22.
5. Allen E, Burton R, Webber S *et al.* Comparison of a diffractive bifocal and a monofocal intraocular lens. *J Cataract Refract Surg* 1996;**22**:446–51.
6. El-Maghraby A, Marzouky A, Gazayerli E *et al.* Multifocal versus monofocal intraocular lenses. Visual and refractive comparisons. *J Cataract Refract Surg* 1992;**18**:147–52.

7. Javitt JC, Steinert RF. Cataract extraction with multifocal intraocular lens implantation. A multinational clinical trial evaluating clinical, functional, and quality-of-life outcomes. *Ophthalmology* 2000;**107**: 2040–8.

8. Percival SP, Setty SS. Prospectively randomized trial comparing the pseudoaccommodation of the AMO ARRAY multifocal lens and a monofocal lens. *J Cataract Refract Surg* 1993;**19**:26–31.

9. Rossetti L, Carraro F, Rovati M, Orzalesi N. Performance of diffractive multifocal intraocular lenses in extracapsular cataract surgery. *J Cataract Refract Surg* 1994; **20**:124–8.

10. Steinert RF, Post CT Jr, Brint SF *et al.* A prospective, randomized, double-masked comparison of a zonal-progressive multifocal intraocular lens and a monofocal intraocular lens. *Ophthalmology* 1992;**99**:853–60.

11. Kamlesh M, Dadeya S, Kaushik S. Contrast sensitivity and depth of focus with aspheric multifocal versus conventional monofocal intraocular lens. *Can J Ophthalmol* 2001;**36**:197–201.

12. Leyland M, Langan L, Goolfee F, Lee N, Bloom P. Prospective randomised double-masked trial of bilateral multifocal, bifocal or monofocal intraocular lenses. *Eye* 2002;**16**:481–90.

13. Jadad AR, Moore RA, Carroll D. Assessing the quality of reports of randomized clinical trials: is blinding necessary? *Control Clin Trials* 1996;**17**:1–12.

35 Perioperative management of cataract surgery

Vincenzo Maurino

Background

Modern cataract surgery is effective, fast and safe and its complication rate has decreased enormously in recent years. However there are some conditions, such as cystoid macular oedema, endophthalmitis and postoperative inflammation, which continue to have an adverse effect on the clinical outcome. A number of different techniques have been proposed for the management of these rare complications of cataract surgery.

This chapter sets out the evidence available in the following areas of perioperative management for cataract surgery:

- prevention and treatment of cystoid macular oedema
- prevention and treatment of endophthalmitis
- postoperative anti-inflammatory treatment.

Prevention and treatment of cystoid macular oedema

Background

Cystoid macular oedema (CMO) remains one of the most common causes of decreased vision after cataract surgery. Strategies for preventing and treating CMO are based largely on the proposed mechanism of its pathogenesis. Prostaglandins are involved in human intraocular inflammation and in triggering CMO formation following cataract surgery. Corticosteroids and non-steroidal anti-inflammatory drugs (NSAIDs) are inhibitors of the cyclo-oxygenase pathway of prostaglandin biosynthesis and they have been tested clinically to prevent and to treat CMO.

Question

Is it possible to prevent the onset of cystoid macular oedema after uneventful cataract surgery?

The evidence

Fifteen randomised controlled trials (RCTs) have looked at the prevention of CMO following cataract surgery (Table 35.1). In fourteen of those studies, NSAIDs have been compared either with placebos or steroids.[1–14] The remaining study compared steroid treatment to placebo.[15] In the two studies that tested oral NSAIDs no difference was found in angiographic or clinically significant CMO.[1,2] In the 13 studies that looked at topical NSAID administration, two studies failed to show a difference between placebo and diclofenac in preventing angiographic CMO.[3,4] Two other studies showed a lower incidence of angiographic CMO with diclofenac compared to topical steroid but no difference in visual outcome.[5,6]

Topical indometacin versus placebo was evaluated in four RCTs,[7–10] which showed a lower incidence of angiographic CMO with topical indometacin. However, where final visual acuity was measured no difference was found.

Indometacin was compared with other NSAIDs and with steroids in three further studies.[11–13] No difference in angiographic CMO was found after using indometacin and ketorolac.[11] A significantly lower incidence of angiographic CMO was found with indometacin,[12,13] fluribrofen,[13] ketorolac[14] and dexamethasone[12,15] than placebo. However, a sustained difference in final visual acuity was not found.

Comment

A common problem of these studies is related to the clinical value of the outcomes investigated. Angiographic CMO was used as the main outcome measure. This is not associated with visual acuity impairment and can spontaneously resolve. Therefore its value in clinical practice is unclear. Moreover, clinically significant CMO, which is associated with visual acuity loss, is difficult to define, its natural course in unknown and has not been used as primary outcome measure in the majority of the studies. Comparison between studies is difficult since the procedures and surgical techniques used varied enormously and the incidence of complications including CMO has progressively declined with time.

Overall, the evidence supports the use of topical NSAIDs and steroids to prevent angiographic CMO formation, especially when used in combination. In the majority of

Table 35.1 Cystoid macular oedema prevention

Authors	Methods	Intervention	Participants	Outcomes	Results	Notes
Abelson et al, 1989[1]	RCT FU 12/12 ECCE + IOL	Oral piroxicam v placebo	178 eyes piroxicam – 85 placebo – 93	• Clinically significant CMO (incidence, time of onset, severity, final visual acuity)	• No difference found between treated and untreated groups	Concomitant administration of topical antibiotics and corticosteroids
Sholiton et al, 1979[2]	RCT FU 2/12 ICCE +/–IOL	Oral indometacin v placebo	42 eyes indomethacin – 20 placebo – 22	• Angiographic CMO	• No difference found between the two groups	Concomitant administration of topical antibiotics and corticosteroids
Quentin et al, 1989[3]	RCT FU 6/12 ICCE + AC IOL	Topical diclofenac v placebo	179 eyes diclofenac – 80 placebo – 73	• Angiographic CMO	• Reduced incidence of ang o-CMO in the treated group. • No SSD found	Concomitant administration of topical antibiotics and corticosteroids
Rossetti et al, 1996[4]	RCT FU 6/12 Phaco/ECCE + IOL	Topical diclofenac v placebo	88 eyes diclofenac – 42 placebo – 46	• Angiographic CMO • AC inflammtion • Contrast sensitivity	• Lower angio-CMO in the treated group only at 1/12. No SSD between the two groups thereafter • Better contrast sensitivity in diclofenac group	Concomitant administration of topical antibiotics and corticosteroids Small numbers
Miyake et al, 2000[5]	RCT FU 8/52 phaco + IOL	Topical 0·1% diclofenac v 0·1% fluorometholone	106 eyes diclofenac – 53 fluorometholone – 53	• Angiographic CMO • AC laser-cell phototometry	• CMO incidence: 5·7% diclofenac group 54·7% FML group SSD found • No SSD in final VA	
Italian Diclofenac Study Group, 1997[6]	RCT FU 5/12 ECCE+IOL	Topical diclofenac 0·1% v dexamethasone 0·1%	281 eyes diclofenac – 141 dexamehtasone – 140	• AC inflammation • angiographic CMO	• Incidence of angio-CMO two times higher in the dexamethasone group • No difference in postoperative inflammation prevention	
Urner-Bloch, 1983[7]	RCT FU 4/12 ICCE/ECCE +/– IOL	Topical indometacin v placebo	72 patients indometacin – 35 placebo – 38	• Angiographic CMO	• SSD found at 12/52 from surgery in angio-CMO • No differences in VA	Concomitant administration of topical antibiotics and corticosteroids
Yannuzzi et al, 1981[8]	RCT FU 3–12/12 ECCE	Topical indometacin v placebo	231 eyes indometacin – 100 placebo – 131	• Angiographic CMO	• Only at 5/52 SSD in ang o-CMO between the two groups • No SSD in final VA	Concomitant administration of topical antibiotics and corticosteroids

(Continued)

Table 35.1 (Continued)

Authors	Methods	Intervention	Participants	Outcomes	Results	Notes
Kraft et al, 1982[9]	RCT FU 6–12/12 ECCE or phaco + IOL	Topical indometacin v placebo	500 eyes (78% had FFA) indometacin – 330 placebo – 170	• Angiographic CMO • Final VA	• SSD in angio-CMO • No difference in final VA	Concomitant administration of topical antibiotics and corticosteroids. All patients had PPC
Miyake et al, 1980[10]	RCT FU up to 1 year ICCE	Topical indometacin v placebo	218 eyes indometacin – 112 placebo – 106	• Angiographic CMO	• Angio-CMO higher incidence in the placebo group up to 6/12, thereafter no SSD found	Concomitant administration of topical antibiotics and corticosteroids
Le Rebeller, et al, 1994[11]	RCT FU 1/12 ECCE +/– IOL	Topical ketorolac tromethamine 0·5% v Indocollyre 0·1%	100 eyes ketorolac – 50 Indocollire – 50	• AC tyndall • Angiographic CMO	• No SSD between the two groups	Small in numbers
Ahluwalia et al, 1988[12]	RCT FU 6/52 ICCE	Topical indometacin v dexamethasone v placebo	60 eyes indometacin – 20 dexamethasone – 20 placebo – 20	• Angiographic CMO • Clinically significant CMO	• Lower incidence in indometacin and dexamethasone groups v placebo • Final VA similar in the three groups	
Solomon, 1995[13]	RCT FU 6/52 ECCE+IOL	Topical 0·03% flurbiprofen v 1% indometacin v placebo	681 eyes flurbiprofen – 226 indometacin – 234 placebo – 221	• Angiographic CMO • Clinical CMO • Snellen VA • Contrast sensitivity (Vistech test)	• At 2/12 F-U angio-CMO, clinical CMO, Snellen VA and contrast sensitivity worse in the placebo group (SSD found) • At final FU no SSD found between the 3 groups	Concomitant administration of topical antibiotics and corticosteroids
Flach et al, 1990[14]	RCT FU 2/12 ECCE	Topical ketorolac tromethamine 0·5% v placebo	50 patients undergoing bilateral surgery randomised to placebo treatment or vice versa	• Angiographic CMO at 40th day • AC fluorophotometry and graded SLE observations	• SSD found in angio-CMO	Single surgeon
Krishnan et al, 1985[15]	RCT FU 6/52	Topical dexamethasone v placebo ICCE	56 eyes dexamethasone – 28 placebo – 28	• Angiographic CMO • AC inflammation • Corneal oedema	• No cases of angio-CMO in the steroid group (SSD found) • No SSD in AC inflammation	

RCTs that tested NSAIDs, concomitant steroid eyedrops were administered and therefore it is difficult to separate the effect of the two drugs. The evidence on the efficacy of NSAIDs and steroids in preventing clinically significant CMO and related visual loss is not clear-cut. Where final visual acuity or clinical significant CMO were chosen as study outcomes, no statistical significant difference was found.

Question

What is the evidence for the treatment of clinically significant CMO after cataract surgery?

The evidence

Five RCTs have investigated the treatment of CMO after cataract surgery (Table 35.2). Four studies looked at the treatment of chronic CMO.[16–19] No difference was found between oral indometacin[16] or topical fenoprofen[17] when compared with placebo. Both studies had very small numbers of participants and CMO was well established. Topical ketorolac was effective in improving the visual acuity compared to placebo.[18,19] However, the improvement in visual acuity was not always matched with an angiographic appearance of CMO resolution.

Treatment of acute pseudophakic CMO was investigated in a recent study that compared ketorolac alone and prednisolone alone versus combined ketorolac and prednisolone.[20] The study showed better outcomes in terms of visual acuity and contrast sensitivity in the combined treatment group.

Comment

Direct inter-study comparison is not possible given the different type of CMO (acute and chronic, aphakic and pseudophakic) and the different treatment regimens. Overall, there is some evidence to support the topical treatment of acute and chronic CMO after cataract surgery with topical NSAIDs in combination with topical steroids. However, more rigorous trials are needed to confirm the efficacy of the treatment of CMO, the best method of administration, the long-term visual acuity benefit and whether the treatment influences the severity and chronicity of CMO that may develop at a later stage.

Prevention and treatment of endophthalmitis after cataract surgery

Background

Endophthalmitis is a rare but devastating complication of cataract surgery, with an estimated incidence of between 0·07% and 0·30% in the developed world. The best way to avoid such a serious complication has not yet been determined. Preoperative, postoperative and intraoperative antibiotics and other agents have been variously advocated to reduce the risk of endophthalmitis.

Question

Does preoperative povidone-iodine reduce the risk of postoperative endophthalmitis after cataract surgery?

The evidence

Seven studies evaluated the use of preoperative povidone-iodine to prevent endophthalmitis (Table 35.3).[21–27] Two studies looked at the incidence of postoperative endophthalmitis in eyes treated with prophylactic povidone-iodine compared with controls.[21,22] One found a significantly higher incidence of endophthalmitis in the control group. However, these studies have a number of weaknesses mainly related to the difficulty in designing and conducting a prospective study on such a rare event like endophthalmitis.

Four other studies showed that povidone-iodine reduced the conjuctival bacterial flora intraoperatively and in the immediate postoperative period compared with either controls or preoperative topical antibiotics.[23–26] No toxicity from the administration of povidone-iodine in the conjunctival cul-de-sac was noted.

Comment

Overall, evidence shows that the administration of povidone-iodine is effective in reducing the bacterial flora when it is applied into the conjunctival fornices prior to surgery. This may be helpful in reducing the occurrence of endophthalmitis after cataract surgery.

Question

Do preoperative topical antibiotics help to reduce the occurrence of acute endophthalmitis following cataract surgery?

Table 35.2 Cystoid macular oedema treatment

Authors	Methods	Intervention	Participants	Outcomes	Results	Notes
Yannuzzi et al., 1977[16]	RCT FU 6/52 ICCE	Oral indometacin v placebo	23 eyes indometacin – 10 eyes placebo – 13 eyes	• Angio-CMO • VA	• No differences found	• Oral treatment • Chronic aphakic CMO
Burnett et al., 1983[17]	RCT FU 2/12 ICCE	Topical fenoprofen sodium v placebo	14 patients fenoprofen – 6 placebo – 8	• Angio-CMO • VA	• No differences found	• Topical treatment • Chronic aphakic CMO
Flach et al., 1987[18]	RCT FU 4/12 ECCE +/– IOL	Topical ketorolac v placebo	26 patients ketorolac – 13 eyes placebo – 13 eyes	• Angio-CMO • VA	• Improved VA in the ketorolac group • No differences in angio-CMO appearance	• Small numbers • Chronic aphakic/ pseudophakic CMO
Flach et al., 1991[19]	RCT FU 5/12 ECCE +/– IOL	Topical ketorolac v placebo	120 patients ketorolac – 61 placebo – 59	• VA improvement	• Statistically significant improvement in distance VA at all examination	• Chronic aphakic/ pseudophakic CMO
Heier et al., 2000[20]	RCT FU 4/12 Phaco IOL	Topical ketorolac v prednisolone v combined (k+p)	26 patients ketorolac – 9 prednisolone – 8 combined regimen – 9	• Snellen VA • Leakage on angiogram • Contrast sensitivity	• Better outcome when combined treatment • Faster improvement	• Small sample size • Lack of controls • Acute pseudophakic CMO

Table 35.3 Preoperative povidone-iodine

Authors	Methods	Intervention	Participants	Outcomes	Results	Notes
Mork, 1987[21]	RCT Cataract surgery 5-year study period	PVD-I v nothing	4111 eyes PVD-I – 2550 control – 1561	• Incidence of endophthalmitis diagnosed clinically	• Higher incidence of endophthalmitis in non PVD-I group but lack of SSD	
Speaker and Mekinoff, 1991[22]	CCT FU 12/12 Intraocular eye surgery	PVD-I v silver protein solution	8083 patients PVD-I – 3489 silver protein – 4594	• Incidence of endophthalmitis (culture proven)	• Lower endophthalmitis incidence in the PVD-I group • SSD found	• Uncontrolled use of preop antibiotics
Apt et al., 1984[23]	CCT Intraocular surgery	PVD-I v controls (unoperated fellow eyes)	30 patients	• Bacterial colony and species isolated from pre-postop conj swabs	• PVD-I showed SS reduction in colony and species compared with controls	
Apt et al., 1995[24]	CCT Cataract, strabismus, RD and KP surgery	PVD-I v polimixin B sulfate-neomicin sulfate-gramicidin v controls (fellow unoperated eyes)	40 patients PVD-I – 21 eyes antibiotic – 21 eyes control – 38 eyes	• Bacterial colony and species isolated from pre-postop conj swabs	• PVD-I more effective than Ab • SSD found	• Preop antibiotics to all eyes • PVD-I applied for 10 minutes • Small numbers
Apt et al., 1989[25]	RCT eye surgery	Preop 3-day course of PVD-I v antibiotics	40 patients	• Bacterial colony and species isolated from pre-postop conj swabs	• Better results in the group receiving preoperative antibiotics and perioperative PVD-I	• All cases received perioperative PVD-I
Isenberg et al., 1985[26]	RCT	PVD-I v 3-day course of preoperative antibiotics v combined treatment	35 patients undergoing ocular surgery randomly divided in three groups	• Bacterial colony and species isolated from pre-postop conj swabs	• Marked reduction in conjunctival flora in the PVD-I and preop antibiotics groups, even better in the combined group	• Small numbers
Walters et al., 1993[27]	RCT ECCE	PVD-I v control group	146 patients PVD-I – 73 control – 73	• PVD-I toxicity • Bacterial colony count from AC samples	• Reduced culture positivity in the PVD-I group but no SSD found • No toxicity shown	• Preop Ab drops administered

The evidence

Three studies compared the efficacy of povidone-iodine versus preoperative topical antibiotics in sterilising the conjunctiva[24–26] (Table 35.4). Two showed that preoperative antibiotics were effective in reducing conjunctival bacterial flora[25, 26] and one showed that they were not.[24]

Table 35.4 summarises the studies on the efficacy of preoperative topical antibiotics. Only one study uses the incidence of endophthalmitis as an outcome measure,[28] whilst the others look at bacterial growth from conjunctival swabs or anterior chamber and vitreous aspirates.[29–34] There was no difference in the incidence of endophthalmitis after topical chloramphenicol compared with sub-conjunctival penicillin.[28] Gentamicin and ciprofloxacin were most effective in sterilising the conjunctiva compared to other antibiotics.[29,30] Four further studies compared different topical antibiotics with placebos.[31–34] No difference in bacterial contamination was found with neomycin,[31] norfloxacin[33] or gentamicin[34] when compared with placebo. A significant reduction of positive conjunctival bacterial cultures was found with fusidic acid.[32]

Comment

Overall, there is little evidence regarding the efficacy of preoperative antibiotic before cataract surgery to prevent postoperative acute endophthalmitis.

Question

Are intraoperative antibiotics administered during cataract surgery effective in prevention of acute endophthalmitis?

The evidence

Table 35.5 summarises the studies looking at the use of intraoperative antibiotics added to the infusion fluid during cataract surgery. Only one controlled clinical study used the incidence of acute postoperative endophthalmitis as an outcome measure.[35] This study showed a lower rate of endophthalmitis in the treatment group. The study does have several pitfalls: small numbers of controls, absence of masking, lack of randomisation and no statistical analysis. Five studies commented on the use of aminoglycosides in the infusion fluid during phacoemulsification to reduce the risk of intraocular bacterial contamination.[36–40] A reduction in the rate of positive cultures was shown in the patients

given a combination of vancomycin and gentamicin[38,39] or vancomycin alone[40] compared with placebo. However, in two further studies no difference was found between intraocular gentamicin or vancomycin with placebos.[36,37]

Comment

Overall these studies show conflicting results and the evidence for intraocular antibiotics is not clear-cut. Moreover, a relationship between positive intraocular cultures at the end of the surgery and endophthalmitis has not been proven. Large multi-centre randomised clinical trials are needed if we are to address the question of whether intraocular antibiotics are useful in the prevention of acute endophthalmitis after cataract surgery.

Question

Does the administration of antibiotics in the sub-conjunctival space at the end of the cataract surgery help to prevent acute endophthalmitis?

The evidence

Three RCTs evaluated the administration of antibiotics in the sub-conjunctival space at the end of cataract surgery to prevent acute endophthalmitis (Table 35.6). In two studies the outcome chosen was the occurrence of endophthalmitis.[28,41] One of these studies showed a significant reduction in endophthalmitis incidence with sub-conjunctival antibiotics[28] while the other did not.[41] A significant reduction in preoperative versus postoperative bacterial counts from lid and conjunctival swabs was found with sub-conjuntival antibiotics compared with preoperative antibiotics.[42]

Comment

Overall, there is conflicting evidence for the use of sub-conjunctival antibiotics to reduce the risk of acute endopthalmitis. However, sub-conjunctival antibiotics do reduce the conjunctival bacterial flora.

Question

What is the best evidence-based approach for the treatment of acute endophthalmitis following cataract surgery?

Table 35.4 Preoperative topical antibiotics

Authors	Methods	Intervention	Participants	Outcomes	Results	Notes
Christy and Sommer, 1979[28]	RCT Study period 1973–1977 FU 1/52 ICCE	Sub-conjunctival penicillin v no sub-conj All eyes had preoperative antibiotics	6618 patients 3309 sub-conjunctival 3309 no sub-conj	• Endophthalmitis incidence	• Rate of endophthalmitis 0·15% in sub-conjunctival group, 0·45% in the control group SSD	• Randomisation and masking not described
Fahmy, 1980[29]	RCT	G. chloramphenicol v G. gentamicin v occ.oxytetracycline-polymyxin B v G. sulphamethizole v G. bacitracin-Neomycin v G. ristocetin-polymyxinB	60 patients randomised to 10 per group	• Conjunctival swabs cultures before and after surgery	• Only gentamicin was able to eliminate bacteria	• Small numbers • Lack of placebo group
Lemimg et al., 1994[30]	RCT ECCE + IOL	Ciprofloxacin v norfloxacin	39 patients ciprofloxacin – 18 norfloxacin – 20	• Mean pre-postoperative bacterial counts isolated from lid swabs	• Statistically significant decrease in eyelid flora with ciprofloxacin	• Small numbers • Lack of placebo group
Mistlberger et al., 1997[31]	RCT FU 24/12 Phaco/ECCE + IOL	Neomycin v placebo	700 patients randomly divide	• Pre-postop conjunctival swabs cultures • AC aspirates cultures	• No SSD between study groups • Only finding: reduced bacterial counts on postop conjunctival swabs following antibiotic v control	• No endophthalmitis
Gray et al., 1993[32]	RCT	Fusidic acid v placebo	79 patients fusidic acid – 39 placebo – 40	• Bacterial colony and species isolated from pre-postop conj swabs	• SSD reduction of the bacteria isolated in the treatment group	
Chiktara et al., 1994[33]	RCT ECCE + IOL	Norfloxacin v placebo	80 patients randomly divided	• Bacterial contamination of AC aspirates obtained at the end of surgery	• No difference between norfloxacin and placebo	
Gelfand et al., 1998[34]	RCT PPV	Gentamicin v placebo	40 patients randomly divided	• Bacterial contamination of vitreous sample	• No differences between the two groups	• Intraocular contamination less common after PPV

Table 35.5 Preoperative intraocular antibiotics

Authors	Methods	Intervention	Participants	Outcomes	Results	Notes
Peyman et al., 1977[35]	CCT ICCE	Gentamicin v controls (topical/ systemic Ab)	2026 eyes gentamicin – 1626 control – 400	• Culture proven endophthalmitis incidence	• 0·37% in the study group v 3·6% in the control group	• Small number of eyes in the control group • No masking • No statistical analysis
Gimbel et al., 1996[36]	RCT Phaco IOL	BSS + gentamicin v palcebo	97 eyes gentamicin – 48 placebo – 49	• Intra-op AC aspirates culturing	• No SSD in the positive culture rate	• All cultures were negative but for one in the placebo group • PVD-I administered preop
Feys et al., 1997[37]	CCT Phaco + IOL	Vancomicin v placebo	372 eyes treatment – 182 control – 190	• Bacterial intraocular contamination	• No difference found between the two groups	
Ferro et al., 1997[38]	RCT Phaco IOL	Vancomycin and gentamicin v placebo	125 eyes 60 treated eyes 65 placebo eyes	• Intra-op AC aspirates culturing	• Higher rate of postop positive cultures in the placebo group but no SSD found	• PVD-I administered preop
Beigi et al., 1998[39]	RCT Phaco IOL	Vancomycin and gentamicin v placebo	220 eyes 110 eyes in each group	• Intra-op AC aspirates culturing	• High reduction in microbial contamination of the AC aspirates in the treatment group (SSD found)	• PVD-I administered preop • One case of endophthalmitis in the Ab group
Mendivil and Mendivil, 2001[40]	RCT Phaco IOL FU 2/12	Vancomycin and preop PVD-I Vancomycin Preop PVD-I Placebo	400 eyes randomised 100 eyes per each of the four group	• MIC • Intra-op AC aspirates culturing	• MIC of vancomycin maintained two hours from surgery • Lower rate of positive cultures in the vancomycin groups (SSD) • No SSD between PVD-I groups and placebos • However number of positive cultures greater in the placebo group	• No cases of endophthalmitis

Table 35.6 Perioperative sub-conjunctival antibiotics

Author	Methods	Intervention	Participants	Outcomes	Results	Notes
Chalkley and Schoch 1967[42]	RCT ICCE	Sub-conj penicillin-streptomycin v nothing	852 patients sub-conj – 571 non-sub-conj – 281	• Endophthalmitis incidence	• No SSD found but higher rate of endophthalmitis in the untreated group	
Christy and Sommer 1979[28]	RCT Study period 1973–1977 FU 1/52 ICCE	Sub-conjunctival penicillin v no sub-conj	6618 patients 3309 sub-conjunctival 3309 no sub-conj	• Endophthalmitis incidence	• Rate of endophthalmitis 0.15% in sub-conjunctival group, 0.45% in the control group • SSD	• Preoperative topical Ab to all eyes • Randomisation and masking not described
Dallison et al., 1989[43]	RCT Cataract surgery	Preoperative fucidic acid Preoperative chloramphenicol Sub-conjunctival cephazolin	fusidic – 42 eyes chloramphenicol – 21 sub-conj Ab – 17	• Quantitative bacterial count from conj and lid swabs preop v postop	• Reduction in the sub-conj Ab group compared with the two preop Ab groups	• In the treatment group delayed onset endophthalmitis seen

Table 35.7 Treatment of endophthalmitis after cataract surgery

Author	Methods	Intervention	Participants	Outcomes	Results
EVSG, 1995[43]	Multi-centre RCT: acute endophthal-mitis after cataract and II IOL procedures FU 12/12	• PPV + IV Ab • PPV alone • Vitreal tap + IV Ab • Vitreal tap alone • Pars plana vitrectomy	420 eyes with clinical diagnosed acute endophthalmitis within 6/52 from cataract or II IOL surgery (396 completed the FU)	• Final visual acuity • Ocular media clarity	• No difference found in the main outcomes with or without IV Ab • SSD in the treatment groups found • Better results with PPV only if presenting VA of LP or less

The evidence

One RCT has looked at the treatment of acute endophthalmitis following cataract surgery[43] and especially at the benefit of vitrectomy versus vitreous tap (Table 35.7). The benefit of vitrectomy over vitreous tap was limited to a specific subgroup of eyes with presenting visual acuity of light perception or worse. The study did not find differences in final visual acuity and media clarity with or without intravenous antibiotics administration.

Comment

More studies are needed to identify the best evidence-based approach for the treatment of acute endophthalmitis following cataract surgery.

Treatment of postoperative inflammation after cataract surgery

Background

The surgical trauma induced by the removal of the cataract and IOL implantation, although minimised by the use of modern techniques of phacoemulsification and foldable IOL implantation, causes intraocular inflammation that may complicate the otherwise uneventful postoperative course. Anti-inflammatory drugs and especially topical steroids have been used to minimise the onset of intraocular inflammation after cataract surgery.

Question

Is the administration of sub-conjunctival steroids at the end of the cataract operation useful in reducing the inflammatory response?

The evidence

Six RCTs have assessed the efficacy of sub-conjunctival steroid injections at the end of the cataract procedures (Table 35.8). Five studies found no difference between sub-conjunctival steroid injection and controls.[44–48] One study found a beneficial effect of the sub-conjunctival steroid administration.[49] This was limited to the first postoperative day and was found in the normal and the inflammatory eyes subgroups but not in the diabetic eye subgroup. In all six studies small numbers of eyes were evaluated and thus further large studies may be warranted.

Comment

In summary, there is not enough evidence to support the usefulness of sub-conjunctival steroid injections administered at the end of the cataract procedure to prevent postoperative inflammation and blood aqueous barrier breakdown.

Question

Are collagen shields systems a better way of delivering drugs than sub-conjunctival injection?

Table 35.8 Perioperative sub-conjunctival steroids

Authors	Methods	Intervention	Participants	Outcomes	Results	Notes
Shah et al., 1992[43]	RCT FU 3/12 ECCE	Sub-conjunctival cefuroxime + bethamethasone v cefuroxime alone	10 eyes in each group	• AC inflammation • Laser flare-cell meter evaluation	• No difference in cells and flare at any time between the two groups	• Small numbers • Uncomplicated eyes
Sanders et al., 1992[44]	RCT FU 3/12 ECCE + IOL	Sub-conjunctival cefuroxime + bethamethasone v topical dexamethasone + neomycin	60 patients sub-conjunctival group – 30 topical group – 30	• AC activity • Conjunctival injection	• Worse AC activity and conjunctival injection in the sub-conj group (SSD at 48h only)	• Preop topical chloramphenicol to all eyes • Small numbers
Schmitt and Hessemer, 1995[45]	RCT ECCE + IOL	Sub-conjunctival dexamethasone v topical prednisolone	30 patients 15 in each group	• Laser flare-cell meter • AC activity	• No difference at day 1–2 after surgery	• Small numbers
Nicolas et al., 1995[46]	RCT FU 6/12	Sub-conjunctival methylprednisolone v nothing	50 patients 25 eyes per group	• Laser flare photometry	• No difference found between groups	• Small numbers
Fukushima et al., 2001[47]	RCT FU 2/52 Phaco IOL	Sub-conjunctival dexamethasone + gentamicin v gentamicin alone	104 diabetic patients 52 eyes per group	• Laser flare-cell meter • AC activity	• No difference found between the two groups	• Transient significant blood glucose increase day of surgery
Corbett et al., 1993[48]	RCT FU 3/12 ECCE or phaco + IOL	Sub-conjunctival bethamethasone v placebo	246 eyes 123 eyes in each group (further subdivided in uncomplicated, diabetic and previous inflammation)	• AC activity	• Significantly lower inflammatory score with sub-conj, especially in the uncomplicated group and previous inflammation subgroups at day one postop only	• No effect in the diabetic subgroup

Table 35.9 Perioperative collagen shields drug delivery

Authors	Methods	Intervention	Participants	Outcomes	Results
Menchini *et al*, 1994[49]	RCT ECCE + IOL 1/7 FU	Collagen (Ab + steroids) shields *v* sub-conjunctival inj	50 patients randomised to shields or sub-conj	• AC inflammation • Tolerance • Corneal oedema	• No SSD found between the two groups • SI higher corneal oedema in the shielded group
Renard *et al*, 1994[50]	RCT ECCE + IOL 1/12 FU	Collagen (Ab + steroids) shields *v* sub-conjunctival inj *v* combined treatment	61 patients randomly divided in three groups	• Sub-conjunctival haemorrhage • AC flare • Corneal oedema • Pain level	• Shield better • SSD found
Haaskjold *et al*, 1994[51]	RCT FU 1/52 ECCE phaco + IOL	Collagen (Ab + steroids) shields *v* sub-conjunctival/ peribulbar inj	183 patients shields – 93 sub-conj – 90	• Sub-conjunctival haemorrhage • AC flare • Corneal oedema • Pain level	• Shield better • SSD found for pain, haemorrhage, corneal oedema

The evidence

Three studies comment on collagen shield drug delivery at the end of cataract surgery compared with periocular injections (Table 35.9). In one study there was no difference between the two modalities of drug delivery in postoperative intraocular inflammation, corneal oedema and discomfort.[50] Two other studies showed significantly more discomfort and conjunctival haemorrhage with the injections.[51,52]

Question

Is there any difference in the anti-inflammatory efficacy of steroids and NSAIDs after cataract surgery?

The evidence

Nine studies compared the anti-inflammatory effectiveness of different topical steroids versus various NSAIDs eyedrops[53–62] (Table 35.10).

Comment

Overall, evidence suggests that both steroids and NSAIDs are equally effective in reducing postoperative inflammation following cataract surgery. The advantages of using NSAIDs are related to the lack of ocular side effects such as intraocular pressure rise, impairment of cicatrisation or reduced immune defence response with risk of infection, especially of herpetic disease recurrence. On the other hand, NSAIDs are more likely to cause ocular intolerance. Studies are needed to support the efficacy of topical NSAIDs in the postoperative treatment of inflammation after complicated and complex cataract surgery.

Implications for practice

It is difficult to draw conclusions on the perioperative management of cataract surgery given the paucity of well-designed randomised clinical trials. Overall, there is evidence to support the treatment of CMO and also the possible reduction of endophthalmitis occurrence by preoperative povidone-iodine application. Less clear-cut is the benefit of active treatment to prevent CMO. There is not sufficient evidence that preoperative antibiotics and intraocular antibiotics reduce the risk of endophthalmitis after uneventful cataract surgery. There is conflicting evidence for the use of periocular injections either of steroids or antibiotics at the end of the surgery. In uneventful surgeries and low-risk patients, the anti-inflammatory efficacy of steroids eyedrops is not superior to that of NSAIDs.

Implications for research

In the field of perioperative management there is a need for larger, multi-centre randomised clinical trials to clarify these issues.

Table 35.10 Postoperative topical steroids and non-steroidal anti-inflammatory drugs

Authors	Methods	Intervention	Participants	Outcomes	Results	Notes
Sanders and Kraff, 1984[52]	RCT FU 2/52 ECCE + IOL	Indometacin v dexamethasone v placebo v combined indometacin-dexamethasone	283 patients indometacin/dexa – 60 indometacin/placebo – 78 dexa/placebo – 86 placebo/placebo – 59	• AC fluorophotometry • Unacceptable inflammation • AC inflammation clinical grading	• Unacceptable inflammation worse in the placebo/placebo group (SSD) • Better result in the combined treatment group • Similar results in the indometacin and dexamethasone groups	
Hessemer and Schmitt, 1995[53]	RCT ECCE + IOL	Indometacin v prednisolone v combined treatment	30 eyes divided in three equal groups	• AC fluorophotometry	• Indometacin and prednisolone equally effective • Better results in the combined indometacin-prednisolone group compared with the monotherapy groups (SSD)	
Renard et al, 1996[54]	RCT FU 1/12 ECCE + IOL	Indometacin/gentamicin v dexamethasone/neomycin	220 patients randomised in two groups of 110 eyes	• AC inflammation clinical grading • Eyedrops tolerance	• No difference found	
Suharwardy et al, 1994[55]	RCT FU 6/52 ECCE + IOL	Diclofenac/gentamicin v dexamethasone/neomycin	78 patients diclofenac – 38 dexamethasone – 40	• AC inflammation by clinical grading • Laser cell-flare meter, • Treatment tolerance	• No difference found in AC inflammation • Worse tolerance for the diclofenac (due to gentamicin?)	
Othenin et al, 1994[56]	RCT FU 2/12 ECCE + IOL	Diclofenac v dexamethasone	24 patients 12 in each group	• AC inflammation by clinical grading • Laser cell-flare meter • Tolerance	• No difference found in any outcomes	• Small numbers • One allergic reaction to diclofenac reported
Roberts and Brennan, 1995[57]	RCT FU 1/12 Phaco + IOL	Diclofenac v prednisolone	52 patients randomly divided	• AC inflammation by clinical grading • Laser cell-flare meter • IOP	• No difference found	

(Continued)

Table 35.10 (Continued)

Authors	Methods	Intervention	Participants	Outcomes	Results	Notes
Demco et al., 1997[58]	RCT FU 2/52 Phaco + IOL	Diclofenac v prednisolone	101 patients diclofenac – 57 prednisolone – 59	• AC inflammation • Conjunctival hyperaemia • Local tolerance burning stinging	• Only the burning was statistically significantly more with diclofenac	
Butt et al., 1998[59]	RCT FU 1/12 ECCE + IOL	Diclofenac-gentamicin v dexamethasone-neomycin-polymyxin B	259 patients diclofenac – 131 dexamethasone – 128	• AC inflammation • Conjunctival hyperaemia • Local tolerance	• No SSD found for any variable • More drug-related adverse event in the diclofenac (due to gentamicin?) • No SSD	
Flach et al., 1989[60]	RCT FU 1/12 ECCE + IOL	Ketorolac v dexamethasone	127 patients ketorolac – 63 dexamethasone – 64	• SLE fluorophotometry • AC inflammation • Grading	• No SSD found between the two groups	
Ostrov et al., 1997[61]	RCT FU 6/52 ECCE/phaco + IOL	Ketorolac v prednisolone v dexamethasone	157 patients ketorolac – 57 prednisolone – 59 dexamethasone – 41	• AC inflammation • Clinical grading • Fluorophotometry	• No SSD found between the two groups	• Periocular steroid injection given
Simone et al., 1999[62]	RCT FU 1/12 Phaco/ECCE + IOL	Ketrolac v prednisolone	59 patients ketorolac – 29 prednisolone – 30	• Postop pain • AC inflammation • Clinical grading	• Only at 1/52 prednisolone had fewer • AC activity then ketorolac (SSD found) • Less pain with ketorolac (no SSD)	

283

References

1. Abelson MB, Smith LM, Ormerod LD. Prospective, randomized trial of oral piroxicam in the prophylaxis of postoperative cystoid macular edema. *J Ocul Pharmacol* 1989;**5**:147–53.
2. Sholiton DB, Reinhart WJ, Frank KE. Indomethacin as a means of preventing cystoid macular edema following intracapsular cataract extraction. *Am Intraocul Implant Soc J* 1979;**5**:137–40.
3. Quentin C-D, Behrens-Bauman W, Gaus W. Prevention of cystoid macular edema with diclofenac eyedrops in intracapsular cataract extraction using the Choice Mark IX anterior chamber lens. *Fortschr Ophthalmol* 1989;**86**:546–9.
4. Rossetti L, Bujtar E, Castoldi D, Torrazza C, Orzalesi N. Effectiveness of diclofenac eyedrops in reducing inflammation and the incidence of cystoid macular edema after cataract surgery. *J Cataract Refract Surg* 1996;**22**(Suppl 1):794–9.
5. Miyake K, Masuda B, Shirato S *et al.* Comparison of diclofenac and fluorometholone in preventing cystoid macular edema after small incision cataract surgery: a multicentered prospective trial. *Jpn J Ophthalmol* 2000;**44**:58–67.
6. Italian Diclofenac study Group. Efficacy of diclofenac eyedrops in preventing postoperative inflammation and long-term cystoid macular edema. *J Cataract Refract Surg* 1997;**23**:1183–9.
7. Urner-Bloch U. Prevention of aphakic cystoid macular edema by topical indomethacin. *Klin Monatsbl Augenheilkunde* 1983;**182**: 495–6.
8. Yannuzzi LA, Landau AN, Turtz AI. Incidence of aphakic cystoid macular edema with the use of topical indomethacin. *Ophthalmology* 1981;**88**:947–54.
9. Kraff MC, Sanders DR, Jampol LM, Peyman GA, Lieberman HL. Prophylaxis of pseudophakic cystoid macular edema with topical indomethacin. *Ophthalmology* 1982;**89**:885–90.
10. Miyake K, Sakamura S, Miura H. Long-term follow-up study on prevention of aphakic cystoid macula oedema by topical indomethacin. *Br J Ophthalmology* 1980;**64**:324–8.
11. Le Rebeller MJ, Riss I, Rosier Diallo L, Albinet JL, Merot JL. Etude de la prevention des reactions inflammatoires apres chirurgie de la cataracte par le Ketorolac tromethamine 0·5% versus Indocollire 0·1%. *Opthalmology* 1994;**8**:201–4.
12. Ahluwalia BK, Kalra SC, Parmar IP, Khurana AK. A comparative study of the effect of antiprostaglandins and steroids on aphakic cystoid macular oedema. *Ind J Ophthalmol* 1988;**36**:176–8.
13. Solomon LD. Efficacy of topical flurbiprofen and indomethacin in preventing pseudophakic cystoid macular edema. Flurbiprofen-CME study group I. *J Cataract Refract Surg* 1995;**21**:73–81.
14. Flach AJ, Stegman RC, Graham J, Kruger LP. Prophylaxis of aphakoc cystoid macular edema without corticosteroids. A paired-comparison, placebo controlled double-masked study. *Ophthalmology* 1990;**97**(10): 1253–8.
15. Krishnan MM, Lath NK, Govind A. Aphakic macular edema: some observation on prevention and pathogenesis. *Ann Ophthalmol* 1985;**17**:253–7.
16. Yannuzzi LA, Klein RM, Wallyn RH, Cohrn N, Katiz I. Ineffectiveness of indomethacin in the treatment of chronic cystoid macular edema. *Am J Ophthalmol* 1977;**84**(4):517–19.
17. Burnett J, Tessler H, Isenberg S, Tso MOM. Double-masked trial of fenoprofen sodium: treatment of chronic aphakic cystoid macular edema. *Ophthalmic Surg* 1983;**14**:150–2.
18. Flach AJ, Dolan BJ, Irvine AR. Effectiveness of ketorolac tromethamine 0·5% ophthalmic solution for chronic aphakic and pseudophakic cystoid macular edema. *Am J Ophthalmol* 1987;**103** (4):479–86.
19. Flach AJ, Jampol LM, Weinberg D. Improvement in visual acuity in chronic aphakic and pseudophakic cystoid macular edema after treatment with topical 0·5% ketorolac tromethamine. *Am J Ophthamol* 1991;**112**:514–19.
20. Heier JS, Topping TM, Baumann W, Dirks MS, Chern S, Flach AJ. Ketorolac versus predinisolone versus combination therapy in the treatment of acute pseudophakic cystoid macular edema. *Ophthalmology* 2000;**107**(11):2034–9.
21. Mork P. Polyvinylpyrrolidone-iodine as a disinfectant in eye surgery for five years. *Acta Ophthalmology Copenh* 1987;**65**(6):572–4.
22. Speaker MG, Mekinoff JA. Prophylaxis of endophthalmitis with topical povidone-iodine. *Ophthalmology* 1991;**98**(12):1769–75.
23. Apt L, Isenberg S, Yoshimori R, Paez JH. Chemical preparation of the eye in ophthalmic surgery. III. Effect of povidone-iodine on the conjunctiva. *Arch Ophthalmol* 1984;**102**:728–9.
24. Apt L, Isenberg SJ, Yoshimori R *et al.* The effect of povidone-iodine solution applied at the conclusion of ophthalmic surgery. *Am J Ophthalmol* 1995;**119**(6):701–5.
25. Apt L, Isenberg SJ, Yoshimori R, Spierer A. Outpatient topical use of povidone-iodine in preparing the eye for surgery. *Opthalmology* 1989;**96**(3):289–92.
26. Isenberg SJ, Apt L, Yoshimory R, Khwarg S. Chemical preparation of the eye in ophthalmic surgery. IV. Comparison of povidone-iodine on the conjunctiva with a prophylactic antibiotic. *Arch Ophthalmol* 1985;**103**:1340–2.
27. Walters RF, Boase DL, Cockcroft PM *et al.* Povidone-iodine and the prevention of bacterial contamination of the eye during extracapsular cataract surgery. *Eur J Implant Refract Surg* 1993;**5**(4):242–6.
28. Christy NE, Sommer A. Antibiotic prophylaxis of postoperative endophthalmitis. *Ann Ophthalmol* 1979;**11**(8):1261–5.
29. Fahmy JA. Bacterial flora in relation to cataract extraction. V. effects of topical antibiotics on the preoperative conjunctival flora. *Acta Ophthalmolog Copenh* 1980;**58**(4):567–75.
30. Leeming JP, Diamond JP, Trigg RR, White L, Hoh HB, Easty DL. Ocular penetration of topical ciprofloxacin and norfloxacin drops and their effect upon eyelid flora. *Br J Ophthalmol* 1994;**78**(7):546–8.
31. Mistlberger A, Ruckhofer J, Raithel E *et al.* Anterior chamber contamination during cataract surgery with intraocular lens implantation. *J Cataract Refract Surg* 1997;**23**:1064–9.
32. Gray TB, Keenan JI, Clemett RS, Allardyce RA. Fusidic acid prophylaxis before cataract surgery: patient self-administration. *Aust NZ J Ophthalmol* 1993;**21**:99–103.
33. Chitkara DK, Manners T, Chapman F, Stoddart MG, Hill D, Jenkins D. Lack of effect of preoperative norfloxacin on bacterial contamination of anterior chamber aspirates after cataract surgery. *Br J Ophthalmol* 1994;**78**(10):772–4.
34. Gelfand YA, Mezer E, Linn S, Miller B. Lack of effect of prophylactic gentamicin treatment on intraocular and extraocular fluid culturs after pars plana vitrectomy. *Ophthalmic Surg Lasers* 1998;**29**:497–501.
35. Peyman GA, Sathar ML, May DR. Intraocular gentamicin as intraoperative prophylaxis in South India eye camps. *Br J Ophthalmol* 1977;**61**:260–2.
36. Gimbel HV, Sun R, DeBroff BM, Yang HM. Anterior chamber fluid cultures following phacoemulsification and posterior chamber lens implantation. *Ophthalmic Surg Lasers* 1996;**27**(2):121–6.
37. Feys J, Salvanet-Bouccara A, Emond J, Dublanchet A. Vancomycin prophylaxis and intraocular contamination during cataract surgery. *J Cataract Refract Surg* 1997;**23**:894–7.
38. Ferro JF, de Plablos M, Logrono MJ, Guisasola L, Aizpuru F. Postoperative contamination after using vancomycin and gentamicin during phacoemulsification. *Arch Ophthalmol* 1997;**115**(2):165–70.
39. Beigi B, Westlake W, Chang B, Marsh C, Jacob J, Riordan T. The effect of intracameral, peroperative antibiotics on microbial contamination of anterior chamber aspirates during phacoemulsification. *Eye* 1998;**12**(3A):390–4.
40. Mendivil Soto A, Mendivil MP. The effect of topical povidone-iodine, intraocular vancomycin, or both on aqueous humor cultures at the time of cataract surgery. *Am J Ophthalmol* 2001;**3**:293–300.
41. Chalkley TFH, Schoch D. An evaluation of prophylactic subconjunctival antibiotic injection in cataract surgery. *Am J Ophthalmol* 1967;**64**: 1084–7.
42. Dallison IW, Simpson AJ, Keenan JI, Clemett RS, Allardyce. Topical antiobiotic prophylaxis for cataract surgery: a controlled trial of fucidic acid and chloramphenicol. *Aust NZ J Ophthalmol* 1989;**17**: 289–93.
43. Shah SM, McHugh JD, Spalton DJ. The effects of suconjunctival bethamethasone on the blood aqueous barrier following cataract surgery: a double-blind randomised prospective study. *Br J Ophthalmol* 1992;**76**(8):475–8.

44. Sanders R, MacEwen CJ, Haining WM. A comparison of prophylactic, topical and subconjunctival treatment in cataract surgery. *Eye* 1992;**6**(1):105–10.

45. Schmitt K, Hessemer V. Is subconjunctival steroid injection necessary in addition to topical therapy after cataract surgery? A laser flare-cell meter study. *Ophthalmology* 1995;**92**:303–6.

46. Nicolas T, Benitez del Castillo J M, Diaz D, Castillo A, Garcia Sanchez J.Effects of subconjunctival methylprednisolone on the blood aqueous barrier following cataract surgery. *Int Ophthalmol.*1995;**19**(4):235–8.

47. Fukushima H, Kato S, Kaiya T *et al.* Effect of subconjunctival steroids injection on intraocular inflammation and blood glucose level after cataract surgery in diabetic patients. *J Cataract Refract Surg* 2001;**27**:1386–91.

48. Corbett MC, Hingorani M, Boulton JE, Shilling JS. Subconjunctival bethamethasone is of benefit after cataract surgery. *Eye* 1993;**7**(6):774–8.

49. Menchini U, Lanzetta P, Ferrari E, Soldano F, Vita S. Efficacy of collagen shields after extracapsular cataract extraction. *Eur J Ophthalmol* 1994;**4**:175–80.

50. Renard G, Bennani MD, Lutaj P, Richard C, Triquand C. Comparative study of a collagen corneal shield and a subconjunctival injection at the end of cataract surgery. *J Cataract Refract Surg* 1993;**19**:48–51.

51. Haaskjold E, Ohrstrom A, Uusitalo RJ *et al.* Use of collage shields in cataract surgery. *J Cataract Refr Surg* 1994;**20**:150–3.

52. Sanders DR, Kraff M. Steroidal and nonsteroidal anti-inflammatory agents. Effects on postsurgical inflammation and blood-aqueous humor barrier breakdown. *Arch Ophthalmol* 1984;**102**:1453–6.

53. Hessmer V, Schmitt K. Monotherapy versus combination therapy with topical prednisolone and indomethacin. *Ophthalmology* 1995;**92**: 31–4.

54. Renard G, Adenis JP, Rouland JF *et al.* Efficacy and safety of a combination of indomethacin and gentamicin after cataract surgery. *J Fr Ophthalmol* 1996;**19**(11):689–95.

55. Suharwardy J, Ling C, Bell JA, Munton CG. A comparative trial between diclofenac-gentamicin and betamethasone-neomycin drops in patients undergoing cataract extraction. *Eye* 1994;**8**(5):550–4.

56. Othenin-Girard P, Tritte JJ, Pittet N, Herbort CP. Dexamethasone versus diclofenac sodium eyedrops to treat inflammation after cataract surgery. *J Cataract Refract Surg* 1994;**20**:9–12.

57. Roberts CW, Brennan KM. A comparison of topical diclofenac with prednisolone for postcataract inflammation. *Arch Ophthalmol* 1995;**113**(6):725–7.

58. Demco TA, Sutton H, Demco CJ, Suder Raj P. Topical diclofenac sodium compared with prednisolone acetate after pahcoemulsification-lens implant surgery. *Eur J Ophthalmol* 1997;**7**(3):236–40.

59. Butt Z, Fsadni MG, Sunder Raj P. Diclofenac-gentamicin combination eye drops compared with corticosteroid-antibiotic combination eye drops after cataract surgery. *Clin Drug Inv* 1998;**15**:229–34.

60. Flach AJ, Jaffe NS, Akers WA. The effect of ketorolac tromethamine in reducing postoperative inflammation: double-mask parallel comparison with dexamethasone. *Ann Ophthalmol* 1989;**21**(11): 407–11.

61. Ostrov SC, Sirkin SR, Deutsch WE, Masi RJ, Chandler JW, Lindquist TD. Ketorolac, prednisolone and dexamethasone for postoperative inflammation. *Clin Ther* 1997;**19**(2):259–72.

62. Simone JN, Pendelton RA, Jenkins JE. Comparison of the efficacy and safety of ketorolac tromethamine 0·5% and prednisolone acetate 1% after cataract surgery. *J Cataract Refract Surg* 1999;**25**: 699–704.

Section IX

Retinal diseases

Bill Aylward, Editor

Retina: mission statement

Had this volume been written a hundred years ago, the retina section would have been very short indeed. Some of the conditions featured in this section had not been fully described, and none of them had any treatments that could remotely be described as effective. Since then there have been advances in our understanding of retinal disease, and in combination with significant technological advances, treatments have emerged. One such example was the realisation by Jules Gonin in the 1920s that the key to curing retinal detachment was to close the retinal holes. His initial treatment efforts using thermocautery increased the success rate for treatment from zero to 50% overnight. Subsequent developments have increased this further, so that now the vast majority of detached retinas can be re-attached, albeit sometimes with more than one operation! The introduction of the laser into ophthalmology made treatment of a whole range of retinal disorders possible, and the invention of pars plana vitrectomy in the 1970s enabled hitherto undreamt of treatment possibilities. A classic example is the surgical treatment of macular holes. The interval between Gass' observations on the likely pathology, and macular hole surgery becoming an accepted, widely available, and routine treatment was less than six years.

The rapid advances described above achieved successful treatments for many previously untreatable conditions. As a result, evidence from trials has often lagged behind. For example, given the knowledge of the natural history, it would clearly not be appropriate to test retinal detachment surgery against no treatment in a randomised trial. However, there are many aspects of the variety of treatment methods which have been, and could be, subjected to evidence-based assessment. The aim of this section is to pull together such trials and to highlight those gaps where more evidence is required.

The chapters cover everyday retinal conditions including age related macular degeneration, the commonest cause of visual loss in the western world, retinal detachment, retina vein occlusions, and macular hole.

36 Age-related macular degeneration

Jennifer Evans

Background

Definition

Age-related macular degeneration (AMD) is defined as degeneration of the macula that occurs after 50 years of age and which cannot be attributed to an obvious systemic or ocular cause. There are two types of AMD – geographic atrophy and neovascular AMD. In geographic atrophy the retinal pigment epithelium atrophies with secondary loss of the photoreceptors. In neovascular AMD new vessels grow from the choroidal circulation through Bruchs membrane and into the retinal pigment epithelium. Choroidal new vessels are commonly defined as "classic" or "occult". Classic neovascularisation is seen as well-defined leakage observed early during fluorescein angiography. Occult neovascularisation presents as ill-defined fluorescence. It is thought that these two angiographic patterns reflect the different extent to which the vessels have penetrated the retinal pigment epithelium, occult vessels lying underneath the retinal pigment epithelium.

AMD is associated with "drusen", which are yellow spots clinically observable on the retina. Drusen and pigmentary abnormalities are commonly seen in older people, not all of whom will go on to develop visually impairing age-related macular degeneration. People with large, ill-defined "soft" drusen are more likely to develop age-related macular degeneration. A classification system has been proposed to enable comparison between different studies.[1]

Incidence/prevalence

Age-related macular degeneration is the most important cause of visual loss in most industrialised countries, accounting for approximately half of all registrations for blindness and partial sight.[2] Pooled analysis of the major population-based studies of AMD shows that the prevalence of geographic atrophy in at least one eye increases from 0·7/1000 at ages 55 to 59 to 106/1000 at ages 90 and over.[3] Neovascular AMD increases from 0·3/1000 at ages 55 to 59 to 113/1000 at ages 90 and over.

The Beaver Dam Eye Study estimated that the five-year incidence of AMD increased from 0·4% in the 55–64 age-group to 5·4% in the 75 and over age-group. The overall incidence in the Beaver Dam Study (ages 43 and over) was 0·9%.[4]

Aetiology

Most of the aetiological studies on AMD have been conducted in white populations in North America, Europe and Australia. These studies have been both population based and hospital based. The main risk factor for development of AMD is age. People aged 90 years and above are over 50 times more likely to have AMD causing visual impairment compared to those aged 55–59.[5] Genetic predisposition is the next most important aetiological factor. People with a sibling who has the disease are 20 times more likely to develop the disease compared to those who do not have a sibling with the disease.[6] The only other risk factor that has been demonstrated consistently in observational studies to be associated with AMD is cigarette smoking. People who smoke are two to three times more likely to develop AMD. A variety of other factors have been studied, including cardiovascular disease and its risk factors, dietary levels of antioxidant micronutrients, lifetime light exposure and oestrogens in women. Inconsistent results have been found.

Prognosis

Large drusen and retinal pigment epithelial hyper-pigmentation are significant risk factors for developing neovascular AMD. It has been estimated that approximately 12% of people with bilateral soft drusen will develop either unilateral or bilateral neovascular AMD within 10 years, 4% will develop bilateral disease and 2·5% will become legally blind.[7] In one cohort, 26% of people with neovascular AMD in one eye developed neovascular disease in their fellow eye within five years.[8] Almost half of these were legally blind by five years. Approximately half of eyes with geographic atrophy and good visual acuity will experience significant visual loss (doubling of visual angle) within two years.[9]

Overview of interventions

Treatments for age-related macular degeneration can be divided into the following categories: first, interventions designed to treat choroidal neovascular membranes and, second, interventions designed to slow down the progression of the disease more generally. In addition, there have been attempts to relocate the retina physically in order to restore vision after the retina has been damaged by AMD.

Box 36.1 Approaches to treatment of AMD

Treatment of choroidal neovascular membranes

- Laser treatment

  - thermal laser photocoagulation,* laser treatment combined with photoreactive drugs (photodynamic therapy)*

- Radiation treatment

  - external beam using photon or proton beams*
  - brachytherapy

- Heat treatment (transpupillary thermotherapy)
- Treatments with antiangiogenic drugs

  - interferon*
  - thalidomide
  - steroids

- Physical removal of the new vessels

  - submacular surgery with or without injection of fibrinolytic agent*

Treatments designed to halt the progression of AMD
- Antioxidant vitamin and mineral supplements*
- Laser treatment of drusen at risk of progression to advanced AMD*

Treatments designed to improve the choroidal circulation
- Membrane differential filtration*
- Pentoxifylline*
- Heparin*
- Lipotriad*

Relocation of the retina

Box 36.1 shows the approaches that have been taken to treat AMD. The interventions marked with an asterisk are ones for which randomised controlled trials are available and are therefore considered in this review.

Question

In people with choroidal neovascularisation (CNV) lesions associated with AMD does thermal laser photocoagulation reduce the risk of vision loss?

The evidence

The aim of thermal laser photocoagulation of CNV lesions is to seal off the new vessels and prevent them from leaking and/or growing larger.

We found 11 randomised controlled trials that have evaluated thermal laser photocoagulation – MPS-SMDS,[10] COSG-AMD,[11] MPS-AMDS K,[12] Mestres *et al.* (1993),[13] MMSG,[14] Yassur *et al.* (1982),[15] MPS-subfoveal recurrent,[16] MPS-subfoveal new,[17] Coscas *et al.* (1991),[18] Bressler *et al.* (1996)[19] and Arnold *et al.* (1997).[20] All the trials were parallel group studies. Two trials enrolled two eyes from some of the patients but did not adjust for this in the analysis. However, the number of people with two eyes enrolled was small and this was unlikely to have affected the results. None of the studies were double-blind studies, that is, in all the studies, either the patient or the outcome assessment was unmasked to treatment group. In five of the studies, all other quality parameters were considered to be adequate.[10–12,16,17] In none of the other trials was concealment of the randomisation schedule adequately described.

Participants in these studies were aged 50 years or over and had some visual acuity reduction associated with AMD. Most studies specified a lower limit for visual acuity ranging between 20/320 and 20/100. All studies recruited men and women and nine studies reported the numbers of men and women. The percentage of women ranged from 49% to 76%. Almost all studies excluded people who had had previous laser photocoagulation or other eye/systemic disease incompatible with the study. One study (MPS-subfoveal recurrent) examined treatment of new vessels after previous laser photocoagulation.

Participants were selected into the different studies according to the location of the CNV relative to the foveal avascular zone (FAZ). Extrafoveal CNV was defined where the border of the lesion was more than 200 microns from the centre of the FAZ. Juxtafoveal CNV was defined 1–199 microns from the centre of the FAZ and subfoveal CNV occurred directly under the centre of the FAZ. In most studies, the CNV was classic and generally well defined. Three studies examined poorly demarcated/occult subfoveal CNV.[18–20]

The type of intervention differed according to the location and type of CNV. Argon green or blue-green laser was developed first and evaluated for the treatment of extrafoveal CNV. Krypton red laser was thought to have advantages for treating CNV close to the fovea because the red wavelength was not absorbed by xanthophyll in the inner retina. Two studies used dye red laser or a combination of the krypton/argon/yellow dye as chosen by the treating clinician. Poorly demarcated subfoveal CNV was treated with perifoveal and scatter laser photocoagulation.

Most studies compared laser photocoagulation with no treatment. Two studies compared different types of laser,[11,13] while two studies compared argon and krypton lasers against no treatment.[16,17]

In general, the primary outcome was visual acuity. This was usually presented as change in visual acuity from baseline to a defined follow up time, usually between 12 and 36 months. In most studies, logMAR charts were used (ETDRS or Bailey-Lovie) and the proportion of people experiencing a doubling of the visual angle (three or more lines lost) or quadrupling of the visual angle (six or more lines lost) could be estimated from the report. Secondary outcomes were more variable but included contrast sensitivity, reading speed and progression of the disease.

The results of the studies are presented in Table 36.1. MPS-SMDS found that laser photocoagulation of classic CNV located more than 200 microns from the FAZ was effective with a relative risk of 0·32 (95% CI 0·18–0·57) and number needed to treat (NNT) of 3·3 (2·3–5·7).

The results of studies treating classic CNV closer to the FAZ were more equivocal. In the MPS-AMDS K study,[12] 58% of the no treatment group experienced a loss of six or more lines of visual acuity 36 months after randomisation compared to 49% of the group treated with krypton red laser. This gives a relative risk of 0·85 (CI 0·70–1·04) corresponding to a number needed to treat (NNT) of 11·7. However, this result does not exclude a harmful effect of treatment. The authors concluded that treatment was to be recommended because of a trend in visual acuity improvement in the treated group (P = 0·02) and a subgroup analysis (unclear whether defined *a priori*) showing a larger effect in people without hypertension. A similar effect size was seen in MMSG,[14] which included people with juxtafoveal and extrafoveal CNV. Pooling the results of these two trials using a fixed effects model gives a pooled relative risk of 0·85 (CI 0·72–0·99) for loss of vision (two or more/six or more lines) at 24 or 36 months. Calculating an NNT based on the pooled risk difference gives an estimate of 10 people to be treated (CI 5·3–100) for one person to benefit.

Three studies have examined thermal laser photocoagulation of classic CNV directly below the FAZ. The MPS studies examined subfoveal new vessels and subfoveal vessels developing after previous laser photocoagulation.[16,17] In both studies they demonstrated a benefit of treatment with NNTs of 6·1 (CI 3·6–20·6) and 5·1 (CI 2·8–26·9), respectively for six or more lines of visual acuity lost at 24 months follow up. The pooled relative risk from these trials is 0·47 (CI 0·31–0·71). Yassur *et al*.[15] demonstrated a similar effect size but the length of follow up was unclear.

In two studies of macular scatter (grid) laser photocoagulation of poorly defined subfoveal CNV, little benefit of treatment was detected. Bressler *et al*.[19] found a relative risk of 0·93 (CI 0·48–1·78) and Arnold *et al*.[20] found a relative risk of 1·36 (CI 0·84–2·18) for loss of six or more lines of visual acuity at 24 and 60 months, respectively. In contrast, Coscas *et al*.[18] found that perifoveal treatment of poorly demarcated subfoveal CNV was effective with a relative risk of 0·68 (CI 0·53–0·88) and NNT of 4 (CI 2·4–10·4). However, the study group for this study included participants with well-defined, presumably classic, subfoveal CNV.

There was no evidence to suggest that either argon green or krypton red laser was more effective.[11,16,17]

Comment

Overall, it is likely that laser photocoagulation of classic CNV is an effective treatment when compared to no treatment. However, the size of the treatment effect is not well estimated to date. There has been only one trial randomising 224 people with extrafoveal CNV. It is a little surprising that trials of the treatment of subfoveal CNV (new vessels and recurrent vessels) indicate a more favourable result than trials of juxtafoveal CNV. There is little evidence that laser photocoagulation is effective for occult CNV. Two trials of macular scatter (grid) photocoagulation for occult subfoveal CNV did not demonstrate any benefit. One trial of perifoveal photocoagulation demonstrated an effect for classic and occult subfoveal CNV, but this was a poorer quality study and has not been repeated.

Question

In people with CNV lesions associated with AMD does photodynamic therapy reduce the risk of vision loss?

The evidence

Photodynamic therapy aims to treat the CNV without affecting the retina. Photoreactive chemicals are injected into the blood and irradiated with light as they pass through the CNV. The light activates the chemicals, causing them to emit free radicals that destroy the new vessel.

There has been one Cochrane review of photodynamic therapy.[21] This includes one published parallel group randomised trial (TAP Study – 609 participants).[22] This was a high-quality study with adequate allocation concealment, reasonable attempts to mask participants and outcome assessment and one eye only enrolled for each participant. Rates of follow up were high. The majority of the participants were white (98%) with a mean age of 75 years.

People with vision 20/40 to 20/200 were included and CNV lesions were less than 5400 microns in diameter and had to have a classic component. People with previous treatment or other significant eye or systemic disease were excluded.

Tabel 36.1 Thermal laser photocoagulation

Study	Intervention	Control	No. randomised	Lines visual acuity lost[a]	Follow up (months)	Outcome				
						% Treatment group	% Control group	RR	95% CI	Fisher's exact (2-sided)
Well-demarcated classic extrafoveal CNV (> 200 microns from centre of foveal avascular zone)										
MPS-SMDS	A-BG	No treatment	224	6+	Up to 24	15	45	0·32	0·18–0·57	<0·001
COSG-AMD	K-RED	A-G	191	6+	12	30	39	0·77	0·52–1·15	0·221
Well-demarcated classic juxtafoveal CNV (1–199 microns from centre of foveal avascular zone)										
MPS-AMDSUK	K-RED	No treatment	496	6+	36	49	58	0·85	0·70–1·04	0·13
Well-demarcated classic juxta/extrafoveal CNV										
Mestres et al, 1993[13]	A-G	Dye red	41	–	12	No significant differences in visual field indices				
MMSG,1982[14b]	A	No treatment	128	2+	24	67	80	0·83	0·66–1·06	0·178
Well-demarcated classic subfoveal CNV (directly under centre of foveal avascular zone)										
Yassur et al., 1982[15]	K-RED	No treatment	123[c]	*	Unclear	32	67	0·48	0·33–0·71	<0·001
MPS-subfoveal Recurrent	A-G v K-RED	No treatment	206	6+	24	9	28	0·3	0·09–0·98	0·028
MPS-subfoveal new	A-G v K-RED	No treatment	373[c]	6+	24	20	37	0·55	0·36–0·85	0·008
Poorly demarcated subfoveal CNV (directly under centre of foveal avascular zone)										
Coscas et al., 1991[18d]	Perifoveal K-RED/A G/yellow dye	No treatment	127	3+	42	54	80	0·68	0·53–0·88	0·003
Bressler et al, 1996[19]	K-RED scatter	No treatment	103	6+	24	38	41	0·93	0·48–1·78	1
Arnold et al., 1997[20]	K-RED scatter	No treatment	57	6+	60	68	50	1·36	0·84–2·18	0·259

K-RED, krypton red; A, Argon; A-G, Argon green; A-BG, argon blue-green; RR, relative risk

[a]In most studies logMAR charts (Bailey-Lovie/EDTRS) were used: MMSG and Arnold et al. (1997) used Snellen; Coscas et al. (1991) chart was not stated

[b]100–1500 microns from centre of foveal avascular zone

[c]These trials enrolled more than one eye per person in the trial; in none of the trials was this taken into account

[d]Includes well-demarcated as well

*Deterioration: moving to a worse visual acuity group: three groups defined at beginning of study: 6/9–6/18; 6/21–6/60; <6/60

Verteporfin 6 mg/m² of body surface area) was compared to placebo (5% dextrose in water) administered via intravenous infusion of 30 ml over 10 minutes. This was followed after 15 minutes by application of 83 seconds of laser light at 689 nm delivered as 50 joules/cm² at an intensity of 600 mW/cm² using a spot size with a diameter 1000 microns larger than the greatest linear dimension of the CNV lesion.

Visual acuity was the main outcome. It was measured using the ETDRS chart, and two outcomes – loss of three or more lines of visual acuity and loss of six or more lines of visual acuity – were examined at 12 and 24 months.

The trial found that photodynamic therapy was effective in preventing visual loss. At 24 months, the relative risk of losing six or more lines of visual acuity was 0·61 (CI 0·45–0·81) with an NNT of 8·3 (CI 5·3–20). Subgroup analyses, specified *a priori*, suggested that the benefits of treatment may be confined to people with no signs of occult CNV.

The VIP study from the same group (not yet incorporated into the Cochrane review) enrolled patients with subfoveal occult CNV. The study was of a similar design to the TAP Study. At two years, 55% of the treatment group compared with 68% of the control group lost at least three lines of visual acuity ($P = 0·032$). Twenty-nine per cent of the treated group compared to 47% of the control group lost at least six lines of acuity ($P = 0·004$).

Photodynamic therapy in people with classic and occult choroidal neovascularisation due to AMD is effective in reducing the risk of visual loss.

Comment

Trials to date have been funded by the manufacturer. Further independent evidence is required.

Question

In people with CNV lesions associated with AMD does radiation therapy reduce the risk of vision loss?

The evidence

Ionising radiation inhibits vascular endothelial cell proliferation *in vitro*. It is thought that the retina can withstand cumulative doses up to 25 Gy without significant harm. The aim of radiation therapy is to slow down or prevent the progression of CNV without damaging the retina. The biological effect of radiation therapy depends on the dose per fraction, the number of fractions and the time between fractions. There have been two methods proposed for delivering the dose – external beam radiotherapy and brachytherapy. There are no reported trials for the latter, but the trials of external beam radiotherapy are summarised below.

Table 36.2 shows out details of the five randomised controlled trials that have evaluated external beam radiotherapy – Bergink *et al.* (1998),[23] Kobayashi and Kobayashi (2002),[24] RAD Study (1999),[25] Marcus *et al.* (2001)[26] and Char *et al.* 1999.[27] All the trials were parallel group studies. In one trial[23] it was not clear if one or both eyes had been enrolled in the trial. Two of the studies made efforts to mask patients and outcome assessors to treatment group using "sham irradiation".[25,26] The role of sham treatment in keeping the patients unaware of their treatment was demonstrated by Marcus *et al.*[26]

The average age of participants in these studies ranged between 72 and 76 years. The proportion of women ranged from 48% to 64%. Some studies specified an upper limit for visual acuity of 20/40,[27] 20/50[24] or 20/200[23]; the others specified a lower limit of 20/320[26] or 20/400.[25] There was little consistency on exclusions, although eligibility for laser photocoagulation, previous treatment for CNV, other eye disease and other systemic disease were considered in some studies. All studies enrolled participants with subfoveal CNV. In Bergink *et al.*[23] and RAD Study[25] this was further described as classic or occult. It must be assumed that in the absence of any clear statement, patients with classic or occult CNV were enrolled in the other studies.

The dose of radiation used differed in all the studies. Bergink *et al.*[23] used the highest dose with 24 Gy delivered in four fractions. Char *et al.*[27] delivered the lowest dose with one fraction of 7·5 Gy. Follow up ranged from 12 to 24 months. In Char[27] follow up ranged from seven to 32 months. The results of the studies are presented in Table 36.2.

The RAD Study,[25] which was the highest quality study, found little evidence of an effect of 16 Gy of radiation delivered in eight fractions on visual acuity loss to due CNV (relative risk 0·97, CI 0·73–1·28). Similarly Marcus *et al.*,[26] which was the only other study to use sham irradiation in the control group, found little effect of 14 Gy delivered in seven fractions (relative risk 1·23, CI 0·56–2·68). Bergink *et al.*[23] and Kobayashi and Kobayashi[24] used higher doses of radiation and found more evidence of a protective effect of radiation. In Kobayashi and Kobayashi,[24] results of analysis of mean logMAR scores were highly statistically significant in favour of treatment. However, these studies were not double masked. The study using the lowest dose[27] found the strongest effect, but this was not statistically significant and may be subject to several biases due to the study design.

Comment

Overall there is little evidence that low-dose radiation therapy (less than 20 Gy) is effective in preventing visual

Tabel 36.2 External beam radiotherapy

Study	Intervention			Outcome					
	Total dose (Gy)	No. of fractions	Fraction size (Gy)	Control	No. randomised	Lines visual acuity lost	Follow up (months)	% Treatment group	% Control group	RR	95% CI	Fisher's exact (2-sided)

Study	Total dose (Gy)	No. of fractions	Fraction size (Gy)	Control	No. randomised	Lines visual acuity lost	Follow up (months)	% Treatment group	% Control group	RR	95% CI	Fisher's exact (2-sided)
Subfoveal CNV												
*Bergink et al., 1998[23]	24	4	6	No treatment	68	3+	12	32	52	0·63	0·36–1·10	0·141
Kobayashi and Kobayashi, 2000[24]	20	10	2	No treatment	101	6+	24	22	43	0·52	0·27–1·01	0·062
RAD Study, 1999[25]	16	8	2	Sham irradiation	205	3+	12	51	53	0·97	0·73–1·28	0·883
Marcus et al., 2001[26]	14	7	2	Sham irradiation	83	6+	12	30	24	1·23	0·56–2·68	0·788
Char et al., 1999[27]	7·5	1	–	No treatment	27	3+	7–32	29	62	0·46	0·18–1·18	0·128

*Visual acuity measured using Snellen chart (all other studies used logMAR chart)

loss due to subfoveal CNV. Of the published studies to date, higher quality studies have been less likely to demonstrate treatment effects. High-quality trials of higher doses of radiation (20 to less than 25 Gy) need to be undertaken using sham irradiation as a control group.

Question

In people with CNV lesions associated with AMD does interferon alfa-2a reduce the risk of vision loss?

The evidence

Interferon alfa-2a has antiangiogenic properties, which is why it has been proposed as a treatment for CNV associated with AMD.

Table 36.3 sets out details of the three randomised controlled trials that have evaluated subcutaneous interferon alfa-2a – Engler *et al.* (1994),[28] Poliner *et al.* (1993)[29] and PTMDSG (1997).[30] All the trials were parallel group studies. In two of the trials[28,29] it was not clear whether one or two eyes were enrolled in the trial and/or whether the analysis of the eyes was conducted appropriately.

The average age of participants in these studies was 73 years[28,30] and 77 years.[29] The proportion of women ranged from 40% to 61%. All three studies specified a lower limit of visual acuity for inclusion in the study of 20/200,[29] 20/320[30] or 20/400.[28] Exclusion criteria included other eye disease, other systemic disease and previous treatment. PTMDSG specified that the lesion should be less than 12 disc areas (Macular Photocoagulation Study definitions).[30]

All three studies used a dose of 3 million international units (IU) of interferon injected subcutaneously. PTMDSG also examined doses of 1·5 million IU and 6 million IU.[30] Dose frequencies were similar in the three studies with Engler *et al.*[28] and PTMDSG[30] using a schedule of three injections per week and Poliner *et al.*[29] using a schedule of alternate days. The length of treatment varied, with PTMDSG treating for 12 months and the other studies for two months.

PTMDSG, which was the highest quality study, found little evidence that 12-month treatment with interferon alfa-2a is effective in preventing visual loss due to CNV associated with AMD.[30] Follow up at 12 months showed that 50% of the treatment group compared with 38% of the control group had lost three or more lines of visual acuity (relative risk 1·30, CI 0·99–1·71). This result is approaching statistical significance in the direction of harm of treatment with one person harmed for every nine persons treated (NNH = 8·7). There was no apparent dose–response effect.

The other two studies were small. Engler *et al.*[28] enrolled 43 patients and treated them with 3 million IU of

interferon. They found a highly beneficial effect of treatment with a relative risk of 0·22 (CI 0·06–0·88). It is difficult to explain why this finding should be so different from that of PTMDSG – there are no obvious differences between the studies other than the duration of treatment (2 months *v* 12 months). PTMDSG was a better quality and considerably larger study.

Comment

Overall there is little evidence that interferon alfa-2a (3 million IU subcutaneously) is effective in preventing visual loss due to subfoveal CNV when used over a 12-month period. Different doses and different treatment schedules could usefully be studied.

Question

In people with CNV lesions associated with AMD does submacular surgery reduce the risk of vision loss?

The evidence

"Submacular surgery" refers to the surgical removal of CNV lesions along with associated scar tissue and blood.

We found no trials reporting a comparison of submacular surgery versus no treatment. One trial[31] did not find a difference when a fibrinolytic agent (tissue plasminogen activator) was used during submacular surgery and compared to balanced salt solution. Although this was a high-quality study it was small (80 patients randomised) and therefore modest differences in effect cannot be ruled out.

A large multi-centre trial, SSTS, is ongoing in the USA. Submacular surgery is being compared to thermal laser photocoagulation. The results of the pilot study have been published.[32] Until the results of SSTS are available there is not enough evidence on the effects of submacular surgery to recommend its use.

Question

In people with early AMD or AMD, does supplementation with antioxidant vitamin and/or mineral supplements reduce the risk of vision loss?

The evidence

The retina is subject to the combined effects of light and oxygen leading to the development of harmful free radicals. Antioxidant vitamin and mineral supplementation aims to protect the retina from the effects of free radicals,

Table 36.3 Subcutaneous interferon alfa-2a

Study	Intervention Dose (million IU)	Frequency	Duration of treatment (months)	Control	No. randomised	Lines visual acuity lost	Follow up (months)	Outcome % Treatment group	% Control group	RR	95% CI	Fisher's exact (2-sided)
Subfoveal CNV												
*Engler et al., 1994[28]	3	3 per week	2	Placebo	43	2+	2	11	50	0·22	0·06–0·88	0·008
**Poliner et al., 1993[29]	3/m²	Alternate days	2	No treatment	20	Final acuity <20/200	6	50	50	1·00	0·42–2·40	1·000
PTMDSG, 1997[30]	1,5,3,6	3 per week	12	Placebo	481	3+	12	50	38	1·30	0·99–1·71	0·062

RR, relative risk; PTSG, Pharmacological Therapy Study Group

*Includes juxtafoveal

**Eyes, not people

thereby slowing down the progression of AMD and vision loss.

There has been one Cochrane review of the effects of antioxidant vitamin and mineral supplementation in people with AMD.[33] Seven trials that randomised 4119 people were included in the review. The majority of people (88%) were enrolled in one trial (AREDS).[34] This was a high-quality study that had an average of six years of supplementation and follow up. There were three intervention groups: antioxidants (vitamin C 500 mg, vitamin E 400 IU, beta-carotene 15 mg), zinc (80 mg zinc oxide) and antioxidants plus zinc. People supplemented daily with antioxidants and/or zinc were less likely to lose 15 or more letters of visual acuity (equivalent to a doubling of the visual angle) (odds ratio 0·79, 99% CI 0·60–1·04), when compared to people taking placebo. This effect was seen more strongly in people with moderate to severe disease (OR 0·73, 99% CI 0·54–0·99). The other trials included in the review were small and their results inconsistent.

Comment

AREDS was a large high-quality study. It is likely that its results are relevant to people similar to those enrolled in the study, that is a relatively well-nourished subgroup of the American population. Further trials in populations with different nutritional status are required.

Question

In people with drusen likely to progress to advanced AMD, does thermal laser photocoagulation reduce the risk of vision loss?

The evidence

Thermal laser photocoagulation can induce drusen to disappear, even if the drusen are not treated directly. The exact mechanism behind this is unknown. The rationale behind laser treatment of drusen is that reducing the burden of drusen may decrease the likelihood of progression to AMD.

Table 36.4 sets out details of the trials that have evaluated laser treatment of drusen – CNVPT,[35] Olk *et al.* (1999),[36] Figueroa and Regeuras (1997),[37] Little *et al.* (1997)[38] and Frenneson and Nilsson (1995).[39] Two types of studies have been done. Where people with both eyes affected by drusen at risk of developing into AMD have been enrolled these studies are called "bilateral drusen studies". People with exudative AMD in one eye and drusen in the other have been enrolled in "fellow eye studies". The usual study design in bilateral drusen studies is to enrol both eyes in the study and then randomly assign one eye to treatment. In the

fellow eye studies, only the eye with drusen and not exudative AMD is enrolled in the study and participants randomly assigned to treatment or no treatment. CNVPT[35] and Olk *et al.*[36] reported bilateral drusen and fellow eye studies. Figueroa and Regeuras[37] enrolled both bilateral drusen and fellow eye patients. The latter were not randomised but all treated with laser. They are not included in Table 36.4. Frennesson enrolled both types of patient but did not present the results separately.

Bilateral drusen studies present particular problems in analysis. They are essentially matched pair studies. The matching has to be taken into account in the analysis. Although trialists may use appropriate statistical tests, reporting of these data in a form that enables the reader to calculate relevant effect measures, such as relative risk and NNT, is very rarely done. Figueroa and Regeuras[37] and Olk *et al.*[36] did not analyse eyes appropriately. None of the trials were "double masked" and none described generation of the allocation sequence.

The average age of participants in these studies ranged from 69 to 75 years and the proportion of women ranged from 59% to 67%. Most studies specified a lower limit for visual acuity in the study eye. This limit ranged from 20/25 to 20/63. Olk *et al.*[36] CNVPT[35] and Little *et al.*[38] specified a minimum number of large drusen for inclusion in the study (5, 10 and 20, respectively). Exclusion criteria were not consistently applied but included previous eye treatment and other systemic and ocular diseases.

Two types of laser photocoagulation were used. CNVPT[35] and Olk *et al.*[36] applied the laser in a scatter or grid pattern. Figueroa and Regeuras[37] and Little *et al.*[38] applied the laser directly at the drusen. Frennesson[39] used a mixture of these techniques. The number of laser burns used ranged from 20 in CNVPT[35] to 132 (range 23 to 516) in Little *et al.*[38] Olk *et al.*[36] compared visible and invisible (subthreshold) burns.

Although all the studies reported a significant reduction in the number of drusen, prevention of visual loss was not demonstrated convincingly in any of the studies. In a post-hoc subgroup analysis in the CNVPT study, it was found that laser-treated eyes with 50% or more drusen reduction at one year were less likely to lose vision.[35] However, the overall results for the trial did not indicate any overall benefit of scatter/grid laser photocoagulation of eyes with drusen in preventing vision loss.

Olk *et al.*'s[36] was a pilot study for planning a larger multi-centre randomised controlled trial. In an analysis that ignored the matched pairs they found a significant improvement in vision in treated eyes. However, this was not statistically significant when the bilateral drusen and fellow eye studies were separated and analysed appropriately.

Figueroa and Regeuras,[37] Little *et al.*[38] and Frennesson and Nilsson[39] were small studies that would be unlikely to detect anything other than large treatment effects.

Tabel 36.4   Laser treatment of drusen

Study	Intervention							Outcome				
	Type of laser	Wavelength	Spot diameter (microns)	No. of laser burns	No. randomised	***Lines visual acuity lost	Follow up (months)	% Treatment group	% Control group	RR	95% CI	Fisher's exact (2-sided)
Bilateral drusen studies – scatter/grid laser photocoagulation												
CNVPT, 1998[35]	Not specified		100	20	156	3+	12	6	1	Not enough data to calculate		
**Olk et al, 1999[36]	Infrared	810 nm	125	48	154	2+	24	No available data		0·44****	0·17–1·07	0·076
Bilateral drusen studies – laser photocoagulation applied to drusen directly												
Figueroa and Regeuras , 1997[37]	Argon green	Not specified	100	Agerage 39 (range 18–47)	30		1·5–5	Not available data		–	–	–
Little et al, 1997[38]	Rhodamine dye	577–620 nm	100–200	Average 132 (range 23–516)	27		12–72	No available date		–	–	–
Fellow eye studies – scatter/grid laser photocoagulation												
*CNVPT, 1998[35]	Not specified		100	20	120	3+	12	3	4	0·820·05–12·48		1
**Olk et al, 1999[36]	Infrared	810 nm	125	48	75	2+	24	54	40	1·35	0·77–2·36	0·315
Mixture bilateral drusen/fellow eye – scatter/grid laser photocoagulation and laser applied to drusen directly												
Frennesson and Nilsson, 1995[39]	Argon green	Not specified	200	51–154	39	Mean Snellen visual acuity	12	0·91 (0·2)	0·89 (0·1)	–	–	0·699*****

All interventions were compared to no treatment
*CNVPT, applied laser burns avoiding drusen
**Macular grid: visible compared with subthreshold
***Figueroa and Regeuras, 1997; Frennesson, 1995 Snellen acuity
****Matched pair data: relative risk is approximated by odds ratio
*****T-test

Comment

There is little evidence to support the use of prophylactic laser treatment of drusen in the prevention of AMD. Published studies to date do not answer this question adequately – in general, they have been small and at risk of bias. In addition, specific issues as to the analysis of matched pair data have not always been addressed. The results of ongoing trials are awaited.

Question

In people with AMD do treatments aiming to improve the choroidal circulation reduce the risk of vision loss?

The evidence

A number of treatments have been studied whose overall aim is to improve some (often undetermined) aspects of the microcirculation with the aim of halting the progression of AMD. The studies are listed below in chronological order.

- Brunner *et al.* (2000)[40] – membrane differential filtration
- Kruger (1998)[41] – oral pentoxifylline
- Lebuisson *et al.* (1986)[42] – ginkgo biloba extract
- Brown (1974)[43] – lipotriad
- Zahn (1968)[44] – heparin
- Havener and Sheets (1958)[45] – heparin.

The trials of heparin[44,45] and lipotriad[43] were done before trial methodology was well established in ophthalmology. They were small, at risk of bias and, as the treatments considered are not currently debated, they are not considered further here.

The trial on *Ginkgo biloba* extract[42] has been included in a Cochrane review.[46] However, it was the only trial available and, as only 20 patients were randomised and it was not masked, it does not contribute to the evidence and is not considered further.

The trial on pentoxifylline[41] demonstrated that a 3-month course of oral pentoxifylline treatment increased choroidal but not retinal blood flow. Further trials are needed to establish whether it prevents visual loss over a longer period.

Brunner *et al.*[40] randomised 40 patients in a trial of membrane differential filtration, which aims to improve the microcirculation by removing high molecular weight proteins and lipoproteins from the blood. The treatment group was treated five times over a period of 21 weeks. The study was small and did not follow up the participants for a long enough period. There was a marginal improvement in visual acuity in the treated group compared to the control group but this was small and, as the study was unmasked, could well be attributable to bias.

Comment

None of the treatments aimed to improve the microcirculation have been demonstrated to be effective in preventing visual loss in AMD. Studies have been small and poor quality. Some of these treatments suffer from lack of a credible biological hypothesis, and some of them may involve considerable inconvenience and potential risk to patients (membrane differential filtration).

Implications for research

Although many different interventions have been proposed for the treatment of AMD, few have been evaluated sufficiently thoroughly to provide meaningful estimates of risks and benefits either for people with AMD or for ophthalmologists. Large, well-designed randomised controlled trials of interventions for AMD are required. Small trials are to be discouraged. The research community needs to focus on using common outcome measures that are relevant to patients.

Implications for practice

Treatment of neovascular AMD with photodynamic therapy and laser photocoagulation will slow down the progression of the disease, provided treatment is started early enough. The implications of photodynamic therapy for screening, healthcare provision and costs have not been explored fully. Other treatments should not be provided outside the remit of randomised controlled trials to evaluate their effectiveness.

References

1. Bird AC, Bressler NM, Bressler SB *et al.* An international classification and grading system for age-related maculopathy and age-related macular degeneration. The International ARM Epidemiological Study Group. *Surv Ophthalmol* 1995;**39**:367–74.
2. Evans JR. Causes of blindness and partial sight in England and Wales 1990–1991. *Studies on Medical and Population Subjects* 57. London: HMSO, 1995.
3. Owen CG, Fletcher AE, Donoghue M, Rudnicka AR. How big is the burden of visual loss caused by age-related macular degeneration in the UK? *Br J Ophthalmol* 2003;**87**:312–17.
4. Klein R, Klein BE, Jensen SC, Meuer SM. The five-year incidence and progression of age-related maculopathy: the Beaver Dam Eye Study. *Ophthalmology* 1997;**104**:7–21.
5. Evans JR. Risk Factors for age-related macular degeneration. *Prog Ret Eye Res* 2001;**20**:227–53.
6. Silvestri G, Johnston PB, Hughes AE. Is genetic predisposition an important risk factor in age-related macular degeneration? *Eye* 1994;**8**: 564–8.
7. Lanchoney DM, Maguire MG, Fine SL. A model of the incidence and consequences of choroidal neovascularization secondary to age-related macular degeneration. Comparative effects of current treatment and potential prophylaxis on visual outcomes in high-risk patients. *Arch Ophthalmol* 1998;**116**:1045–52.

8. Macular Photocoagulation Study Group. Five year follow-up of fellow eyes of patients with age-related macular degeneration and unilateral extrafoveal choroidal neovascularization. *Arch Ophthalmol.* 1993; **111**:1189–99.

9. Sunness JS. The natural history of geographic atrophy, the advanced atrophic form of age-related macular degeneration. *Mol Vis* 1999; **5**:25.

10. MPSG. Argon laser photocoagulation for senile macular degeneration. Results of a randomized clinical trial. *Arch Ophthalmol* 1982;**100**:912–18.

11. Willan AR, Cruess AF, Ballantyne M. Argon green *v.* krypton red laser photocoagulation for extrafoveal choroidal neovascularization secondary to age-related macular degeneration: 3-year results of a multicentre randomized trial. *Can J Ophthalmol* 1996;**31**:11–97.

12. MPSG. Krypton laser photocoagulation for neovascular lesions of age-related macular degeneration. Results of a randomized clinical trial. Macular Photocoagulation Study Group. *Arch Ophthalmol* 1990; **108**:816–24.

13. Duch Mestres F, Vilaplana D, Rutllan Civit J, Torres F, Barraquer J. Static perimetry evaluation of argon green and dye red laser treatment for choroidal nevovascular membranes. *Lasers Light Ophthalmol* 1993;**6**:27–32.

14. The Moorfields Macular Study Group. Treatment of senile disciform macular degeneration: a single-blind randomised trial by argon laser photocoagulation. The Moorfields Macular Study Group. *Br J Ophthalmol* 1982;**66**:745–53.

15. Yassur Y, Axer-Siegel R, Cohen S, Svetliza E, Ben-Sira I. Treatment of neovascular senile maculopathy at the foveal capillary free zone with red krypton laser. *Retina* 1982;**2**:127–33.

16. MPSG. Laser photocoagulation of subfoveal recurrent neovascular lesions in age-related macular degeneration. Results of a randomized clinical trial. Macular Photocoagulation Study Group. *Arch Ophthalmol* 1991;**109**:1232–41.

17. MPSG. Laser photocoagulation of subfoveal neovascular lesions in age-related macular degeneration. Results of a randomized clinical trial. Macular Photocoagulation Study Group. *Arch Ophthalmol* 1991;**109**:1220–31.

18. Coscas G, Soubrane G, Ramahefasolo C, Fardeau C. Perifoveal laser treatment for subfoveal choroidal new vessels in age-related macular degeneration: results of a randomized clinical trial. *Arch Ophthalmol* 1991;**109**:1258–65.

19. Bressler NM, Maguire MG, Murphy PL *et al.* Macular scatter ("grid") laser treatment of poorly demarcated subfoveal choroidal neovascularization in age-related macular degeneration: results of a randomized pilot trial. *Arch Ophthalmol* 1996;**114**:1456–64.

20. Arnold J, Algan M, Soubrane G, Coscas G, Barreau E. Indirect scatter laser photocoagulation to subfoveal choroidal neovascularization in age-related macular degeneration. *Graefe's Arch Clin Exp Ophthalmol* 1997;**235**:208–16.

21. Wormald R, Evans J, Smeeth L, Henshaw K. Photodynamic therapy for neovascular age-related macular degeneration (Cochrane review). In: Cochrane Collaboration: *Cochrane Library.* Issue 1. Oxford: Update software, 2003.

22. Treatment of Age-Related Macular Degeneration with Photodynamic Therapy (TAP) Study Group. Photodynamic therapy of subfoveal choroidal neovascularization in age-related macular degeneration with verteporfin: two-year results of 2 randomized clinical trials – TAP report 2. *Arch Ophthalmol* 2001;**119**:198–207.

23. Bergink G-J, Hoyng CB, van der Maazen RWM, Vingerling JR, van Daal WAJ, Deutman AF. A randomized controlled clinical trial on the efficacy of radiation therapy in the control of subfoveal choroidal neovascularization in age-related macular degeneration: radiation versus observation. *Graefe's Arch Clin Exp Ophthalmol* 1998;**236**: 321–5.

24. Kobayashi H, Kobayashi K. Age-related macular degeneration: long-term results of radiotherapy for subfoveal neovascular membranes. *Am J Ophthalmol* 2000;**130**:617–35.

25. The Radiation for Age-related Macular Degeneration (RAD) Study Group. A prospective, randomized, double-masked trial on radiation therapy for neovascular age-related macular degeneration (RAD Study). *Ophthalmology* 1999;**106**:2239–47.

26. Marcus DM, Sheils WC, Johnson MH *et al.* External beam irradiation of subfoveal choroidal neovascularization complicating age-related macular degeneration. *Arch Ophthalmol* 2001;**119**:171–80.

27. Char DH, Irvine AI, Posner MD, Quivey J, Phillips TL, Kroll S. Randomized trial of radiation for age-related macular degeneration. *Am J Ophthalmol* 1999;**127**:574–8.

28. Engler C, Sander B, Villumsen J, Lund-Andersen H. Interferon alfa-2a modifies the course of subfoveal and juxtafoveal choroidal neovascularisation. *Br J Ophthalmology* 1994;**78**:749–53.

29. Poliner LS, Tornambe PE, Michelson PE, Heitzmann JG. Interferon alpha-2a for subfoveal neovascularization in age-related macular degeneration. *Ophthalmol* 1993;**100**:1417–24.

30. PTMDSG. Interferon alfa-2a is ineffective for patients with choroidal neovascularization secondary to age-related macular degeneration. Results of a prospective randomized placebo-controlled clinical trial. Pharmacological Therapy for Macular Degeneration Study Group. *Arch Ophthalmol* 1997;**115**:865–72.

31. Lewis H, Medendorp SV. Tissue plasminogen activator-assisted surgical excision of subfoveal choroidal neovascularization in age-related macular degeneration: a randomized, double-masked trial. *Ophthalmology* 1997; **104**:1847–52.

32. Submacular Surgery Trials Pilot Study Investigators. Submacular surgery trials randomized pilot trial of laser photocoagulation versus surgery for recurrent choroidal neovascularization secondary to age-related macular degeneration: 1. Ophthalmic outcomes. *Am J Ophthalmol* 2000;**130**:387–407.

33. Evans JR. Antioxidant vitamin and mineral supplements for age-related macular degeneration (Cochrane review). In: Cochrane Collaboration: *Cochrane Library.* Issue 1. Oxford: Update Software, 2003.

34. Age-Related Eye Disease Study Research Group. A randomized, placebo-controlled, clinical trial of high-dose supplementation with vitamins C and E, beta carotene, and zinc for age-related macular degeneration and vision loss: AREDS report no. 8. *Arch Ophthalmol* 2001;**119**:1417–36.

35. The Choroidal Neovascularization Prevention Trial Research Group. Laser treatment in eyes with large drusen. Short-term effects seen in a pilot randomized clinical trial. Choroidal Neovascularization Prevention Trial Research Group. *Ophthalmology* 1998;**105**:11–23.

36. Olk RJ, Friberg TR, Stickney KL *et al.* Therapeutic benefits of infrared (810-nm) diode laser macular grid photocoagulation in prophylactic treatment of nonexudative age-related macular degeneration: two-year results of a randomized pilot study. *Ophthalmology* 1999;**106**: 2082–90.

37. Figueroa MS, Regeuras A. Laser photocoagulation for macular soft drusen. Updated results. *Retina* 1997;**17**:378–84.

38. Little HL, Showman JM, Brown BW. A pilot randomized controlled study on the effect of laser photocoagulation of confluent soft macular drusen. *Ophthalmology* 1997;**104**:623–31.

39. Frennesson IC, Nilsson SE. Effects of argon (green) laser treatment of soft drusen in early age-related maculopathy: a 6 month prospective study. *Br J Ophthalmol* 1995;**79**:905–9.

40. Brunner R, Widder RA, Walter P *et al.* Influence of membrane differential filtration on the natural course of age-related macular degeneration: a randomized trial. *Retina* 2000;**20**:483–91.

41. Kruger A, Matulla B, Wolzt M *et al.* Short-term oral pentoxifylline use increases choroidal blood flow in patients with age-related macular degeneration. *Arch Ophthalmol* 1998;**116**:27–30.

42. Lebuisson DA, Leroy L, Rigal G. Traitement des degenerescences "maculaires seniles" par l'extrait de Ginkgo biloba. *Presse Medicale* 1986;**15**:1556–8.

43. Brown CA. Lipotriad. A double-blind clinical trial. *Trans Ophthalmol Soc UK* 1974;**94**:578–82.

44. Zahn K. Heparin treatment of senile macular degeneration. *Gerontolog Clin* 1968;**10**:288–92.

45. Havener WH, Sheets J, Cook MJ. Evaluation of heparin therapy of senile macular degeneration. *Arch Ophthalmol* 1959;**61**:76–87.

46. Evans JR. Ginkgo biloba extract for age-related macular degeneration (Cochrane review). In: Cochrane Collaboration: *Cochrane Library.* Issue 1. Oxford: Update Software, 2003.

37 Treatment of lattice degeneration and asymptomatic retinal breaks to prevent rhegmatogenous retinal detachment

Charles P Wilkinson

Background

Lattice degeneration and retinal breaks are visible lesions that are risk factors for later retinal detachment. Lattice degeneration exists in 6–8% of the general population, and asymptomatic retinal breaks are almost as common, although a substantial number of these occur within lattice lesions.[1] Retinal detachments occur when fluid in the vitreous cavity passes through tears or holes in the retina and separates the retina from the underlying retinal pigment epithelium. Non-traumatic retinal detachments occur in approximately 1/10 000 persons/year,[2,3] and they are significantly more common in eyes with significant myopia[4] and following cataract surgery.[5,6] Phakic retinal detachments are associated with lattice degeneration in approximately 30% of cases.[1] Patients with non-traumatic retinal detachments in their first eye are at significantly greater risk for a similar event in their second eye.

Prevention of retinal detachment has been a major goal for many decades, and this has been of particular interest in patients in whom a detachment has occurred in their first eye and the surgical outcome has been less than desirable. Based upon the traditional mechanisms that lead to retinal detachment, theoretical manoeuvres that might reduce the incidence of detachment would include measures that retard vitreous liquification, reduce vitreoretinal traction, prevent focal lesions that predispose an eye to the development of a retinal break from doing so, and seal existing retinal breaks so that fluid cannot pass through them. Of these options, only the latter two are widely practised at this time.

Thus, creation of an adhesion around lattice degeneration and or retinal breaks, with laser photocoagulation or cryotherapy, has been recommended as an effective contemporary means of preventing retinal detachment. This therapy is of value in the management of retinal tears associated with the symptoms of flashes and floaters and persistent vitreous traction upon the retina, because such symptomatic retinal tears are associated with a high progression to retinal detachment.[7] Lattice degeneration and retinal breaks not associated with acute symptoms are significantly less likely to be the sites of retinal tears that are responsible for later retinal detachment. Nevertheless, treatment of these problems is also frequently recommended, in spite of the fact that the effectiveness of this therapy is unproven.[8]

Enthusiasm for treating asymptomatic retinal breaks and their precursors such as lattice degeneration was probably most popular before the time that the high frequency of these lesions in the general population and the low risk of retinal detachment, with or without therapy, were appreciated.[8] Creation of an adhesion around the retinal break(s) or lattice lesion(s) was originally performed with diathermy, which was replaced by xenon photocoagulation, which in turn was supplanted by trans-scleral cryotherapy or laser photocoagulation. Improved methods of delivering laser energy have resulted in this being most commonly employed modality at the present time. The primary problem in treating focal lesions is not that treatment does not prevent retinal detachment from a break at the treated site, but rather that later breaks will occur elsewhere, in regions of the retina that appeared "normal" prior to detachment. For this reason, some authors have recommended 360 degrees of peripheral laser burns in an effort to treat the regions in which the vast majority of retinal breaks arise. However, such extensive treatment is not without risks, is not always effective, and has not been subjected to prospective randomised trials comparing therapy with observation.[8]

Question

What is the effectiveness of treating lattice degeneration and asymptomatic retinal breaks to prevent retinal detachment?

The evidence

A systematic search for randomised controlled trials of therapy to prevent retinal detachment is included in a 2001 edition of the *Cochrane Library*.[9] The review attempted to identify any and all trials in which one treatment of lattice degeneration and asymptomatic retinal breaks was compared to control or to another form of therapy.

The review documented a lack of any studies that met the inclusion criteria, because no prospective randomised trials were identified. An additional more recent literature search was unproductive in discovering such trials.

Implications for practice and research

There are no randomised controlled trials to support conclusions regarding the value of treating lattice degeneration or asymptomatic retinal breaks to prevent retinal detachment. Although lattice degeneration and asymptomatic holes are genuine risk factors for rhegmatogenous retinal detachment, the value of treating these lesions is not supported by available evidence in the literature. Prospective randomised trials of treatment of eyes with these lesions and with additional risk factors should offer the best opportunity to provide outcome data that are statistically meaningful.

References

1. Byer NE. Long-term natural history of lattice degeneration of the retina. *Ophthalmology* 1989;**96**:1396–402.
2. Haimann MH, Burton TC, Brown CK. Epidemiology of retinal detachment. *Arch Ophthalmol* 1982;**100**:289–92.
3. Wilkes SR, Beard CM, Kurland LT, Robertson DM, O'Fallon WM. The incidence of retinal detachment in Rochester, Minnesota, 1970–1978. *Am J Ophthalmol* 1982;**94**:670–3.
4. The Eye Disease Case–Control Study Group. Risk factors for idiopathic rhegmatogenous retinal detachment. *Am J Epidemiol* 1993;**137**:749–57.
5. Tielsch JM, Legro MW, Cassard SD *et al.* Risk factors for retinal detachment after cataract surgery. A population-based case–control study. *Ophthalmology* 1996;**103**:1537–45.
6. Rowe JA, Erie JC, Baratz KH *et al.* Retinal detachment in Olmsted County, Minnesota, 1976–1995. *Ophthalmology* 1999;**106**:154–9.
7. Shea, M, Davis, MD, Kamel, I. Retinal breaks without detachment, treated and untreated. *Mod Probl Ophthalmol* 1974;**12**:97–102.
8. Wilkinson, CP. Evidence-based analysis of prophylactic treatment of asymptomatic retinal breaks and lattice degeneration. *Ophthalmology* 2000;**107**:12–18.
9. Wilkinson, C. Interventions for asymptomatic retinal breaks and lattice degeneration for preventing retinal detachment retinal detachment (Cochrane Review). In: Cochrane Collaboration: *Cochrane Library.* Issue 4. Oxford: Update Software, 2001.

38 Surgery for proliferative vitreoretinopathy

David G Charteris

Background

Proliferative vitreoretinopathy (PVR) is a condition of cellular proliferation and migration resulting in the formation of contractile periretinal membranes. PVR may complicate rhegmatogenous retinal detachment and variants of the process can occur in other situations, for example, following penetrating ocular trauma. Series of surgical repair of rhegmatogenous retinal detachments report incidences of PVR of between 5% and 12%.[1–8] Higher incidences are seen in more complex forms of vitreoretinal disease:16–41% of giant retinal tears[9–13] and 10–45% of eyes with penetrating trauma[14,15] are complicated by PVR.

Retinal breaks and neural retinal separation result in blood–retinal barrier breakdown, increased concentrations of fibrogenic growth factors and the formation of complex epi- and sub-retinal membranes. These consist of mixed retinal pigment epithelial, glial, fibroblastic and inflammatory cells in a collagenous extracellular matrix.[16–18] Membranes cause retinal distortion and shortening, which can potentially result in re-opening of retinal breaks and recurrent detachment. Re-detachment is normally considered the defining event in PVR development. However, degrees of membrane formation may take place without detaching the retina where the combination of retinopexy and surgical release of vitreoretinal traction are sufficient to counteract the re-detaching force produced by PVR membrane formation. Analysis of the results of PVR clinical trials should take account of the possibility of such subclinical disease. It can also be argued that post-detachment macular pucker reflects a lesser degree of the proliferative process where the retina remains attached.

Once PVR is established and the retina re-detaches, progression to extensive retinal detachment and profound visual loss is inevitable. Anatomic (defined as total retinal reattachment) success rates of 90% and 73% have been reported for initial and repeat PVR surgery in uncontrolled series.[19,20] Visual results are often poor with 19% and 11% respectively achieving 20/100.[19,20] It has been noted that the vision of the fellow eye in PVR cases is frequently threatened. In a retrospective series, 53% had sight-threatening pathology in the fellow eye and 26% of these had final visual acuity of 20/250 or less.[21]

Question

What is the optimal intraocular tamponade agent in the surgical management of PVR?

The evidence

The Silicone Study analysed the efficacy and complications of intraocular gas and silicone oil tamponade for severe PVR and reported its results in a series of publications.[22–33] The Silicone Study was a prospective, randomised, multi-centre surgical trial which evaluated 1000 centistoke (measure of viscosity) silicone oil against (i) sulphur hexafluoride (SF6) and (ii) perfluoropropane (C3F8) gases in eyes undergoing vitrectomy surgery for severe (grade C3[1] or worse) PVR. The study protocol was revised after two years: SF6 gas was replaced by C3F8 to preserve the clinical relevance of the trial, which ran for a further three years. Cases were divided into those which had (group 1) and those which had not (group 2) undergone previous vitrectomy surgery. Primary outcome measures were anatomical reattachment of the posterior retina (macula) and visual acuity of 5/200 or better. Secondary outcome measures were lens opacification, intraocular pressure abnormalities and corneal damage. The trial recruited a total of 404 patients.

Silicone oil was demonstrated to be a superior tamponade agent to SF6 both in terms of visual acuity ($P <0·05$) and macular attachment ($P<0·05$, Chi square analysis). Hypotony was more common in the SF6 group ($P <0·05$) as was keratopathy ($P <0·05$ at 6 and 18 months, $P <0·01$ at 24 months). Silicone oil and C3F8 gas were similar in visual acuity and anatomical outcomes. There was a borderline advantage of C3F8 gas in achieving complete posterior retinal reattachment in group 1 eyes ($P= 0·045$). No difference was found in keratopathy rates and persistent hypotony was more common in C3F8 treated eyes ($P <0·05$). The authors concluded that silicone oil and C3F8 gas produced similar outcomes in PVR surgery and both were superior to SF6 gas.

A further prospective randomised controlled trial has analysed the use of silicone oil and C3F8 gas in the management of giant retinal tears complicated by PVR (grade C2 or worse).[34] There were no significant differences in rates of anatomical success, visual acuity or complications. The total number of patients recruited is relatively small (47 cases) and no details of the method of sample size calculation are given.

Comment

The Silicone Study has provided valuable information on the use of tamponade agents in established PVR. However, the relative efficacy of these agents in other areas of vitreoretinal surgery remains uninvestigated. For example, individual surgeons may have strong preferences for intraocular gas or silicone oil in the management of giant retinal tears or complex primary retinal detachments but as yet there is no evidence base to inform surgical decision making. Likewise in the area of posterior segment trauma there is a lack of good information on the optimal tamponading agent.

> ### Question
>
> Can adjunctive agents prevent the occurrence or recurrence of PVR?

The evidence

One large-scale, multi-centre, randomised controlled trial has investigated the potential of an intraocular infusion of the antiproliferative agent daunorubicin to improve the prognosis in surgery for established PVR.[35] A total of 286 patients with established PVR grade C2 or greater were recruited and randomised to a 10 minute intraoperative infusion of daunorubicin (7·5 micrograms/ml) or placebo. Patients underwent vitrectomy surgery with silicone oil tamponade. The primary outcome measure, retinal attachment without additional vitreoretinal surgery at six months, showed a trend towards a benefit in the treatment group, which marginally failed to reach significance: 62·7% success in the treatment group, 54·1% in the placebo group (odds ratio 1·43, 95% CI 0·88–2·30). Of the two secondary outcome measures the number of vitreoretinal re-operations within one year was significantly reduced in the treatment group (50 patients *v* 65 in the control group, $P = 0·005$, Cochran-Mantel-Haenszel test) and there was no significant difference in visual acuity change between the groups. The authors concluded that there was some benefit of the adjunctive medication and that PVR was amenable to pharmacological treatment.

A prospective, randomised, controlled trial analysed the effect of postoperative irradiation in preventing reproliferation in eyes with established (grade D1–D3) PVR.[36] The numbers recruited are relatively small (30 in each group) and the sample size calculation is not documented. A total dose of 3000 cGy was given in 8–10 applications postoperatively. No significant difference was seen in retinal reattachment rates at six or 14 months. It was concluded that irradiation does not influence the course of PVR, but the study was probably underpowered.

A prospective, randomised pilot study investigated the potential of combined heparin and dexamethasone in the vitrectomy infusion fluid to reduce reproliferation in established PVR.[37] The pilot study randomised 62 patients with PVR grade C3 or worse to heparin 100 units/ml and dexamethasone 4 micrograms/ml in balanced salt solution (BSS) infusion fluid or placebo control. The treatment group had a higher anatomical success rate and a lower rate of reproliferation but these results were not statistically significant. There was significantly more postoperative haemorrhage (hyphaema, vitreous haemorrhage) in the treatment group ($P = 0·02$, Fisher's exact test).

The potential of adjunctive medication to improve the outcome in patients with retinal detachment at high risk of developing PVR was investigated in a randomised, controlled study of intraoperative infusion of 5-fluorouracil (5FU) and low molecular weight heparin (LMWH) against placebo.[38] Patients were selected as high risk on the basis of a previous prospective analysis of known risk factors for PVR.[39] The study medications were infused for one hour during vitrectomy at concentrations of 200 micrograms/ml (5FU) and 5 IU/ml (LMWH) in Hartmann's solution. A total of 174 patients were recruited. The primary outcome measure, development of postoperative PVR, was significantly improved in the treatment group (12·6% *v* 26·4%, $P = 0·02$, Wilcoxon rank sum analysis). Secondary outcome measures did not show significant differences between treatment and control groups and there was no difference in complication rates. It was concluded that this treatment regime should be used routinely in patients at risk of PVR.

Implications for practice

The use of a combination of 5-fluorouracil and low molecular weight heparin in patients at high risk of PVR would now appear to have reasonable justification although the use in other situations remains unproven.

Implications for research

Adjunctive treatments have been proposed to improve the success rates of vitreoretinal procedures for over 20 years, particularly to control intraocular proliferation. It is only recently that prospective randomised studies have been published on the use of adjuncts in PVR.[35,38] Various questions are unanswered – other adjunctive agents may be more effective and the range of vitreoretinal conditions that would benefit is uncertain. Improved control of the biological response following vitreoretinal intervention remains a major target of vitreoretinal research.

References

1. The Retina Society Terminology Committee. The classification of retinal detachment with proliferative vitreoretinopathy. *Ophthalmology* 1983;**90**:121–5.

2. Speicher MA, Fu AD, Martin JP, von Fricken MA. Primary vitrectomy alone for repair of retinal detachments following cataract surgery. *Retina* 2000;**20**(5):459–64.

3. Duquesne N, Bonnet M, Adeleine P. Preoperative vitreous haemorrhage associated with rhegmatogenous retinal detachment: a risk factor for postoperative proliferative vitreoretinopathy? *Graefe's Arch Clin Exp Ophthalmol* 1996;**234**(11):677–82.

4. Greven CM, Sanders RJ, Brown GC *et al.* Pseudophakic retinal detachments. Anatomic and visual results. *Ophthalmology* 1992;**76**(2): 257–62.

5. Girard P, Mimoun G, Karpouzas I, Montefiore G. Clinical risk factors for proliferative vitreoretinopathy after retinal detachment surgery. *Retina* 1994;**14**(5):417–24.

6. Gartry DS, Chignell AH, Franks WA, Wong D. Pars plana vitrectomy for the treatment of rhegmatogenous retinal detachment uncomplicated by advanced proliferative vitreoretinopathy. *Br J Ophthalmol* 1993; **77**(4):199–203.

7. Bonnet M, Fleury J, Guenoun S, Yaniali A, Dumas C, Hajjar C. Cryopexy in primary rhegmatogenous retinal detachment: a risk factor for postoperative proliferative vitreoretinopathy? *Graefe's Arch Clin Exp Ophthalmol* 1996;**234**(12):739–43.

8. Heimann H, Bornfeld N, Friedrichs W *et al.* Primary vitrectomy without scleral buckling for rhegmatogenous retinal detachment. *Graefe's Arch Clin Exp Ophthalmol* 1996;**234**(9):561–8.

9. Chang S. Giant retinal tears: surgical management with perfluorocarbon liquids. In: Lewis H, Ryan SJ (eds). *Medical and Surgical Retina: advances, controversies and management.* St Louis: Mosby, 1994, pp. 199–207.

10. Chang S, Lincoff H, Zimmerman NJ, Fuchs W. Giant retinal tears. Surgical techniques and results using perfluorocarbon liquids. *Arch Ophthalmol* 1989;**107**(5):761–6.

11. Kertes PJ, Wafapoor H, Peyman GA, Calixto N Jr, Thompson H. The management of giant retinal tears using perfluoroperhydrophenanthrene. A multicenter case series. Vitreon Collaborative Study Group. *Ophthalmology* 1997;**104**(7):1159–65.

12. Kreiger AE, Lewis H. Management of giant retinal tears without scleral buckling. Use of radical dissection of the vitreous base and perfluoro-octane and intraocular tamponade. *Ophthalmology* 1992;**99**(4):491–7.

13. Verstraeten T, Williams GA, Chang S *et al.* Lens-sparing vitrectomy with perfluorocarbon liquid for the primary treatment of giant retinal tears. *Ophthalmology* 1995;**102**(1):17–20.

14. Cardillo JA, Stout T, LaBree L *et al.* Post-traumatic proliferative vitreoretinopathy: the epidemiologic profile, onset, risk factors, and visual outcome. *Ophthalmology* 1997;**104**:1166–73.

15. Mittra RA, Mieler WF. Controversies in the management of open-globe injuries involving the posterior segment. *Surv Ophthalmol* 1999;**3**:215–25.

16. Charteris DG. Proliferative vitreoretinopathy: pathobiology, surgical management and adjunctive treatment. *Br J Ophthalmol* 1995;**79**: 953–60.

17. Pastor JC. Proliferative vitreoretinopathy: an overview. *Surv Ophthalmol* 1998;**43**(1):3–18.

18. Campochiaro PA. Pathogenic mechanisms in proliferative vitreoretinopathy. *Arch Ophthalmol* 1997;**115**(2):237–41.

19. Lewis H, Aaberg TM, Abrams GW. Causes of failure after initial vitreoretinal surgery for severe proliferative vitreoretinopathy. *Am J Ophthalmol* 1991;**111**:8–14.

20. Lewis H, Aaberg TM. Causes of failure after repeat vitreoretinal surgery for recurrent proliferative vitreoretinopathy. *Am J Ophthalmol* 1991;**111**:15–19.

21. Schwartz SD, Kreiger AE. Proliferative vitreoretinopathy: a natural history of the fellow eye. *Ophthalmology* 1998;**105**:785–8.

22. Azen SP, Boone DC, Barlow W *et al.* and The Silicone Study Group. Methods, statistical features, and baseline results of a standardized, multicentered ophthalmologic surgical trial: The Silicone Study. *Control Clin Trials* 1991;**12**:438–55.

23. The Silicone Study Group. Vitrectomy with silicone oil or sulfur hexafluoride gas in eyes with severe proliferative vitreoretinopathy: results of a randomized clinical trial. Silicone Study Report 1. *Arch Ophthalmol* 1992;**110**:770–9.

24. The Silicone Study Group. Vitrectomy with silicone oil or perfluoropropane gas in eyes with severe proliferative vitreoretinopathy: results of a randomized clinical trial. Silicone Study Report 2. *Arch Ophthalmol* 1992;**110**:780–92.

25. McCuen BW, Azen SP, Stern W *et al.* and The Silicone Study Group. Vitrectomy with silicone oil or perfluoropropane gas in eyes with severe proliferative vitreoretinopathy. Silicone Study Report 3. *Retina* 1993;**13**:279–84.

26. Barr CC, Lai MY, Lean JS *et al.* and The Silicone Study Group. Postoperative intraocular pressure abnormalities in the Silicone Study. Silicone Study Report 4. *Ophthalmology* 1993;**100**:1629–35.

27. Blumenkranz MS, Azen SP, Aaberg T *et al.* and The Silicone Study Group. Relaxing retinotomy with silicone oil or long-acting gas in eyes with severe proliferative vitreoretinopathy. Silicone Study Report 5. *Am J Ophthalmol* 1993;**116**:557–64.

28. Hutton WL, Azen SP, Blumenkranz MS *et al.* for The Silicone Study Group. The effects of silicone oil removal. Silicone Study Report 6. *Arch Ophthalmol* 1994;**112**:778–85.

29. Abrams GW, Azen SP, Barr CC *et al.* and The Silicone Study Group. The incidence of corneal abnormalities in the Silicone Study. Silicone Study Report 7. *Arch Ophthalmol* 1995;**113**:764–9.

30. Cox MS, Azen SP, Barr CC *et al.* for The Silicone Study Group. Macular pucker after successful surgery for proliferative vitreoretinopathy. Silicone Study Report 8. *Ophthalmology* 1995;**102**:1884–91.

31. Lean J, Azen SP, Lopez PF, Qian D, Lai MY, McCuen B for The Silicone Study Group. The prognostic utility of the Silicone Study classification system. Silicone Study Report 9. *Arch Ophthalmol* 1996;**114**:286–92.

32. Diddie KR, Azen SP, Freeman HM *et al.* for The Silicone Study Group. Anterior proliferative vitreoretinopathy in the Silicone Study. Silicone Study Report 10. *Ophthalmology* 1996;**103**:1092–9.

33. Abrams GW, Azen SP, McCuen BW, Flynn HW, Lai MY, Ryan SJ for The Silicone Study Group. Vitrectomy with silicone oil or long-acting gas in eyes with severe proliferative vitreoretinopathy: results of additional and long-term follow-up. Silicone Study Report 11. *Arch Ophthalmol* 1997;**115**:335–44.

34. Batman C, Çekiç O. Vitrectomy with silicone oil or long-acting gas in eyes with giant retinal tears: long-term follow-up of a randomized clinical trial. *Retina* 1999;**19**:188–92.

35. Wiedemann P, Hilgers RD, Bauer P, Heimann K. Adjunctive daunorubicin in the treatment of proliferative vitreoretinopathy: results of a multicenter clinical trial. *Am J Ophthalmol* 1998;**126**:550–9.

36. Binder S, Bonnet M, Velikay M *et al.* Radiation therapy in proliferative vitreoretinopathy: a prospective randomized study. *Graefe's Arch Clin Exp Ophthalmol* 1994;**232**:211–14.

37. Williams RG, Chang S, Comaratta MR, Simoni G. Does the presence of heparin and dexamethasone in the vitrectomy infusate reduce reproliferation in proliferative vitreoretinopathy? *Graefe's Arch Clin Exp Ophthalmol* 1996;**234**:496–503.

38. Asaria RHY, Kon CH, Bunce C *et al.* Adjuvant 5-fluorouracil and heparin prevents proliferative vitreoretinopathy: results from a randomized, double-blind, controlled clinical trial. *Ophthalmology* 2001;**108**:1179–83.

39. Kon CH, Asaria RH, Occleston NL, Khaw PT, Aylward GW. Risk factors for proliferative vitreoretinopathy after primary vitrectomy: a prospective study. *Br J Ophthalmol* 2000;**84**:506–11.

39 Rhegmatogenous retinal detachment

Graham Duguid, Sarit Lesnik-Oberstein

Background

Retinal detachment is a relatively rare condition but comprises a significant proportion of the workload of vitreo-retinal surgeons. As opposed to tractional or exudative retinal detachment, the pathognomonic feature of rhegmatogenous (Greek *rhegma*, "tear") retinal detachment is the presence of a full-thickness break or hole in the retina through which fluid from the vitreous cavity can pass and accumulate in the subretinal space. Central vision is impaired if this fluid accumulates under the fovea, and left untreated the retina may become totally detached, scarred and irreparable. A potentially blinding condition, considered untreatable until the 1920s, its prognosis has significantly improved in recent decades with advances in surgical techniques.

Aetiology

For a primary or secondary rhegmatogenous retinal detachment to occur, three factors must coexist: a full-thickness retinal break, liquefied vitreous and, arguably, traction on the adjacent retina.

In primary detachments, full-thickness retinal breaks occur spontaneously. These may be either as atrophic round holes often found in areas of lattice degeneration, as U-shaped tears in the retinal periphery complicating posterior vitreous detachment formation, or as retinal dialyses (disinsertions) at the ora serrata.

Posterior vitreous detachment (PVD) is considered a normal process and is age-related: vitreous lacunae have been reported in 90% of the population over the age of 40, and posterior vitreous detachment is found in 27% of individuals aged 60 to 69, and in 63% aged 70 or over.[1] In comparison to the high incidence of normal syneresis and PVD formation, progression to retinal U-tear formation is rare. Tears may form either as a result of unusually strong vitreo-retinal adhesion or at an area of relatively thin or weak retina, often in the region of lattice degeneration or a retinal blood vessel, resulting in vitreous haemorrhage. Round holes and operculated breaks rarely progress to retinal detachment, in contrast to retinal U-tears, giant tears or dialyses, in which the risk of detachment is high. The latter three conditions all have associated vitreal traction on the edge of the full-thickness tear. Once started, the retinal detachment usually progresses with the accumulation of further subretinal fluid until the entire retina including the macula is detached and floating freely, constrained by its attachments to the ora serrata and the optic nerve.

Prognosis

The natural history of total retinal detachment is for the retina to become ischaemic and to lose function. Usually proliferative retinopathy ensues as a typical scarring response, but this results in stiffening and contraction of the retina. Once the contraction involves the ciliary body, ocular hypotony and, later, phthisis follows. Sometimes the retinal detachment becomes stable and remains localised, usually inferiorly, the long-standing nature reflected by the development of a pigmented tide-mark at the edge of the detachment. Rarely the ischaemic retina develops surface neovascularisation and rubeosis iridis.

With surgical repair, approximately 95% of retinal detachments will be reattached. Visual acuity is usually maintained if the macula is not involved. However, if the acuity has fallen due to macular involvement the recovery of acuity is less predictable and usually partial.

Treatment of retinal detachment is surgical and has been evaluated in some prospective randomised controlled trials. Easily measured end-points in most studies are the first-time and final reattachment rates, final visual acuity and the incidence of complications.

Question

Which is the best method of retinopexy?

The evidence

In vitro[2] and *in vivo* experiments[3] have studied retinal adhesion and methods of retinopexy. There is little to choose between laser and cryotherapy as methods of retinopexy. Cryotherapy is quicker, in that a larger area can be treated with one application, and indentation with the cryotherapy probe may allow holes to be treated in the presence of subretinal fluid. Laser is more precise, less inflammatory and perhaps better if extensive areas require treatment. The ultimate adhesive strength of both laser and cryotherapy scars is twice normal by two to three weeks, but laser adhesion takes one day compared with five for cryotherapy. Cryotherapy also disperses pigment epithelial cells, which theoretically may increase the risk of proliferative vitreoretinopathy (PVR) formation, but this has not been proven. Cryotherapy and laser have not been formally compared in a prospective randomised controlled trial (RCT).

Comment

Thus, all forms of retinopexy appear to be effective in the long run, presumably by inducing scar formation; however, if a rapid bond is required, laser photocoagulation or diathermy are probably preferable.

Question

Is there a need for drainage of subretinal fluid?

The evidence

The need for drainage was addressed convincingly by Hilton *et al.*[4] in a randomised controlled trial of 120 consecutive patients undergoing scleral buckling procedures. The study excluded cases in which drainage was either impossible (due to the shallow nature of the subretinal fluid) or essential (for example, for very bullous detachments) and matched the two populations very accurately. Surgery was carried out by a single surgeon, and the decision on whether to drain subretinal fluid was assigned at random preoperatively, and there was no significant difference in the first time rate of flattening (87% in the drainage group *v* 82% in the non-drainage group), final flattening rate (97% in both groups) or visual acuity outcome.

Comment

It can be concluded that drainage of subretinal fluid is only indicated in specific situations, many of which (for example, giant retinal tears, detachments due to macular breaks and proliferative vitreoretinopathy) have since been managed by vitrectomy.

Current practice for drainage in scleral buckling surgery is to allow closure of the retinal breaks during cryotherapy, in order to make space within the eye to allow a large scleral indent and to allow better visualisation of breaks in bullous detachments. Drainage is not free from potential complications, which include choroidal haemorrhage, retinal incarceration and intraocular infection.

Question

Which is the best method of drainage?

The evidence

Several methods of drainage have been described: scleral cut-down and choroidal puncture with diathermy, needle drain where the sclera and choroid are punctured in one stab with a 3 mm suture needle, and the laser drain where a scleral cut-down is performed and the choroid punctured by argon laser via an indirect ophthalmoscope or endoprobe.

Three trials have prospectively compared needle and laser drainage. Das and Jalali[5] showed an increased complication rate in the needle drainage group (4/25) than in the lasered group but provided no statistical analysis. Ibanez *et al.*[6] similarly randomised 175 patients to either laser drainage choroidotomy using an endoprobe, or needle drainage. No significant difference was found in the complication rate between the two groups (13% *v* 16%). Aylward *et al.*[7] performed a randomised prospective, controlled trial comparing suture needle drainage with argon laser drainage in 1995. Argon laser drainage was associated with a higher rate (98%) of complete or partial but adequate drainage, compared with suture needle drainage (85%), and a lower rate of clinically significant subretinal haemorrhage (4·3% *v* 28·3.%, respectively). The larger sclerostomy created by the argon laser drain was not associated with any increase in the rate of retinal incarceration between the two groups.

Comment

Subretinal haemorrhage is problematic if it tracks back under the macula. Therefore, current practice favours the expediency of a needle drain when the macula is attached and the submacular space is closed, while the safer laser drain is preferred when the macula is off.

Question

When should cryotherapy be carried out if drainage is necessary?

The evidence

Cryotherapy is thought to dilate the choroidal vasculature. Traditionally the sequence of surgical steps was to carry out cryotherapy after drainage in order to decrease the risk of choroidal haemorrhage. Pearce *et al.*[8] randomised 80 cases undergoing scleral buckle procedures either to the surgical sequence of drain, air, cryotherapy, explant or cryotherapy, drain, air, explant. The incidence of subretinal haemorrhage in each of the groups was low and not significantly different.

Comment

Current opinion is that providing needle drainage is technically well performed with elevation of the intraocular pressure at the time of drainage, the sequence of steps is less important.

Question
Is it necessary to soak silicone sponge explants pre-operatively?

The evidence

The two commonly used types of scleral explant are silicone sponges or the harder solid silicone bands. A higher infection rate has been associated with silicone sponges compared with the solid elements, probably due to their porous nature, which means the sponge can harbour bacteria if it is contaminated preoperatively. Arribas *et al.* carried out a prospective trial to determine whether preoperative soaking of the sponge would reduce the rate of infection and extrusion. In 921 consecutive cases in which a sponge was used, for every alternate case the sponge was soaked in a 2 ml aqueous solution of penicillin (500 000 units) and gentamicin (40 mg). Peroperative soaking was associated with a seven-fold reduction of infection and extrusion of the explant.[9]

Comment

Although this trial was not a properly randomised study, it suggests that soaking sponge explants in antibiotic reduces the rate of infection.

Question
Is encirclement necessary in aphakic patients?

The evidence

An explant may be either a localised buckle placed over the break or an encircling band placed around the region of the vitreous base. Which should be used in aphakic patients: this was the subject of a randomised trial by Singh.[10] Eighty-four patients with aphakic retinal detachments were randomised either to local scleral buckling or one combined with scleral encirclement. Both techniques had similar first time anatomical reattachment rates (90% and 91%, respectively).

Comment

Encirclement offers no advantage over local buckling, except that the indent is permanent. Aphakic retinal detachment is less common though still an issue in developing countries where intracapsular extraction is still performed.

Question
Does pneumatic retinopexy have a role in retinal detachment repair?

The evidence

Pneumatic retinopexy was described by Rosengren in 1938[11] but did not become popular until the 1980s in United States.[12] The technique involves treating the retinal break with cryotherapy and then injecting a gas bubble into the vitreous cavity to tamponade the break. The patient is required to posture in order to allow the gas bubble to press against the break and flatten the retina allowing adhesion to occur. It is a relatively quick procedure that can be carried out under local anaesthetic with the patient as an out-patient. Several controlled trials have evaluated the results.

Injecting gas and applying cryotherapy, without performing a vitrectomy (pneumatic retinopexy), was found to have a comparable success rate to vitrectomy with cryotherapy and gas in a prospective randomised controlled trial of 120 cases in 1987.[13] The Retinal Detachment Study Group conducted a multi-centre trial comparing pneumatic retinopexy with scleral buckling, and reported results in 198 patients at six months[14] and in 179 patients at two years follow up.[15] At six months, there was no significant difference in either first time (82% *v* 73%) or final (98% *v* 99%) reattachment rate for scleral buckling and pneumatic retinopexy, respectively. Pneumatic retinopexy, however, had less morbidity and better visual acuity. Importantly, this study showed that aphakic or pseudophakic eyes had lower reattachment rates with pneumatic retinopexy. At two years follow up, the retinal detachment recurrence rate was small (1%) in each group, but the incidence of cataract was significantly greater in the scleral buckling group. Better visual outcome in the pneumatic retinopexy group persisted.

Mulverhill *et al.*[16] randomised 20 consecutive patients, who met inclusion criteria, to be treated either by scleral buckling or pneumatic retinopexy. Retinal flattening was achieved in one operation in 90% of the pneumatic retinopexies and 100% of the scleral buckles. Visual outcome was comparable between the two groups.

However, in a meta-analysis of pneumatic retinopexy compared to primary scleral buckling procedures, scleral buckling was found to have a higher primary success rate than pneumatic retinopexy.[17]

Comment

Pneumatic retinopexy is an effective procedure and has found its strongest advocates in the United States where office-based procedures are more common. Since the success rate is only marginally less than scleral buckling, it is a viable alternative and is often used in patients unfit for general anaesthetic or when access to an operating theatre is difficult.

Question

Is an internal approach the best method?

The evidence

There have been no randomised controlled trials comparing an external and internal approach, although one multi-centre trial is currently under way in Europe.

Comment

Internal approach by vitrectomy, internal search, retinopexy and internal tamponade is increasing in popularity as the primary approach for retinal detachment repair. It offers the advantages of easier visualisation with internal illumination, magnification from the microscope and scleral indentation, arguably reducing the risk of failure from a missed retinal break. The disadvantages of vitrectomy are that cataract is very common postoperatively, there is a risk of endophthalmitis (not present in an external approach not requiring drainage), and there is a higher risk of inflammation and proliferative vitreoretinopathy. The internal approach is thought to be specifically indicated if the retinal break is large and/or posteriorly placed, for giant retinal tears (since it allows the tear to be unfolded and the vitreous cleared from behind the tear), and in any retinal detachments that require internal manipulation, such as clearance of vitreous haemorrhage, removal of PVR membranes or retinectomy. Retinal detachments in pseudophakic eyes are also more easily managed by

vitrectomy, since the breaks are usually small and close to the ora serrata, and hence difficult to visualise externally. Vitrectomy may also be combined with scleral indentation, either segmentally or by encirclement.

Question

Is silicone oil superior to long-acting gas in retinal detachment repair by vitrectomy?

The evidence

The choice of intraocular tamponade in vitrectomy depends on the duration of tamponade required and the size and location of the tear. Agents currently available are sulphahexafluoride (SF6), hexafluoroethane (C2F6), perfluoropropane (C3F8) and silicone oil.

When using intraocular gas as a tamponading agent, the use of nitrous oxide as an anaesthetic agent is generally considered contraindicated as this can adversely affect the size of the gas bubble. In a small prospective randomised trial comparing patients given nitrous oxide or propofol as an anaesthetic agent the postoperative volumes of intraocular gas were found to be similar.[18]

Peyman *et al.*[19] carried out a randomised trial comparing the use of gas (20% C3F8 or 30% C3F8) and silicone oil in a group of 50 patients with complex retinal detachments or vitreous haemorrhage. Unfortunately, the patients were of mixed diagnoses, including proliferative diabetic retinopathy (PDR) with or without retinal detachment and with or without vitreous haemorrhage, proliferative vitreoretinopathy (PVR), and traumatic retinal detachment. Both groups achieved a high anatomical success rate (82% in the oil-treated and 83% in the gas-treated groups), and there was no significant difference in the visual outcome. However, the gas-treated group was associated with a greater incidence of late elevation of intraocular pressure and with postoperative vitreous haemorrhage.

The Silicone Oil Study Group conducted a large multi-centre randomised controlled trial in the United States between 1 September 1985 and 31 October 1990 in 11 centres. The main objective of the study was to compare silicone oil with intraocular gas in the treatment of retinal detachment in eyes with severe proliferative vitreoretinopathy. The primary outcome measures were macular reattachment and postoperative visual acuity. The secondary outcome measures were to assess the potential complications of the two forms of intraocular tamponade.[20] A total of 404 patients were recruited and 101 were in the initial randomisation for silicone oil or SF6 as the intraocular tamponade. The superiority of silicone oil over SF6 in retinal detachment associated with severe PVR, in terms of visual outcome and incidence of complications, was apparent within two years of the study.[21] However, at this point C3F8 was shown to have longer and more effective intraocular tamponade than SF6. It was therefore introduced to begin a second phase in the study[22] in which 265 eyes were recruited. The most important conclusion was that C3F8 and silicone oil showed no difference in posterior pole reattachment rate or visual acuity at the last follow up examination.[23] No differences were found between patients who had previous vitrectomy at randomisation and those who had not. However, if multiple surgeries were necessary to reattach the macula, the final visual acuity was likely to be worse.[24]

After these main outcome measures of anatomic and functional success had been analysed, various secondary outcome measures, mainly the occurrence of complications, were assessed. Chronically raised intraocular pressure was found to be more in eyes with silicone oil. This could be reduced by the presence of an inferior peripheral iridectomy and oil removal. A relatively high incidence of hypotony was an unexpected finding. This was more likely to occur in C3F8 eyes and eyes in which the retina was still detached. Risk factors for hypotony are preoperative hypotony, anterior diffuse contraction of the retina, rubeosis and large retinal breaks. Hypotony was also correlated with poor postoperative vision.[25]

Almost a third of the study patients had a relaxing retinotomy at the time of surgery. Most of these patients were found to have had a worse PVR grading before surgery with more diffuse anterior traction and subretinal fibrosis. For patients who had had a previous vitrectomy, the retinotomy did not affect their outcome. However, patients who had not had a prior vitrectomy did less well after retinotomy, especially if C3F8 was used for the tamponade.[26]

Anterior proliferative vitreoretinopathy was redefined during the Silicone Study, as anterior vitreous traction seemed to have an important prognostic value for surgical outcome. Patients with posterior traction only had better postoperative visual acuity and better reattachment rates. For anterior PVR (>D1) there was a poorer visual prognosis and more hypotony, especially in the C3F8 eyes.[27]

The removal of the silicone oil from eyes during the study was at the surgeon's discretion, which introduced selection bias, as eyes having oil removed were more likely to have an attached retina. A matched pair analysis was performed to control for this bias, which showed that oil-removed eyes tended to have a greater improvement in visual acuity compared to oil-retained eyes. Oil-removed eyes also had a lower incidence of keratopathy.[28] Risk factors for keratopathy after vitrectomy were aphakia or pseudophakia and rubeosis preoperatively. Postoperatively high aqueous flare, number of reoperations and silicone oil-corneal touch were risk factors.[29] The preoperative risk factors for

postoperative macular pucker in an attached retina were pseudophakia or aphakia, large (inferior) retinal breaks and iris new vessels.[30]

In the final Silicone Study Report with long-term follow up, the main findings were that success at the first surgery was most important for attaining a good visual result and if the macula was still attached at three years it was likely to stay attached.[31]

Comment

Although there was little benefit in retinal reattachment rate with silicone oil over C3F8 gas, silicone oil does offer an indefinitely longer tamponade, which can be useful. Whilst both techniques will work if all the breaks are adequately sealed, silicone oil does have the advantage of offering a period of stability as a result of its indefinite tamponade. The longer term complications need to be considered.

Question

What is the best intraocular tamponade for treating giant retinal tears?

The evidence

Whilst giant retinal tears have been shown to be successfully repaired using vitrectomy and silicone oil, a prospective trial by Batman and Cekic[32] involving 47 patients with giant tears associated with PVR equally randomised between the two groups, demonstrated that C3F8 and silicone oil have similar outcomes (attachment rates, visual acuity 5/200 or better and complication rates) at five years follow up.

Question

Does removing the corneal epithelium peroperatively in order to improve visibility of the retina have any long-term effects?

The evidence

Removing oedematous corneal epithelium provides a straightforward solution to poor preoperative retinal visibility but it has been questioned whether this has any effect on the corneal epithelium postoperatively. Hung[33] measured corneal sensation using an esthesiometer preoperatively and at several time internals postoperatively in a group of 26 patients randomised to have the epithelium either removed or left intact peroperatively. In the non-removal group, five of 14 patients had slightly reduced sensation and this had returned to normal in all patients by one week postoperatively. This was compared with 10 of 12 patients having reduced sensation postoperatively in the removal group, and this took one month to recover in seven patients and three months to recover in the remaining three patients. This should be borne in mind when allowing patients to return to contact lens wear postoperatively.

Comment

Usually the corneal epithelium is left intact unless the surgeon is forced to remove it due to the poor operative visibility.

Question

Do postoperative steroids affect clinical outcome?

The evidence

Postoperatively, many surgeons advocate the use of sub-conjunctival steroids with or without antibiotics, a course of topical antibiotics and steroids, and a period of posturing in an appropriate position to tamponade the breaks if necessary. The use of antibiotic and steroid makes good clinical sense, but the evidence for their benefit has never been subjected to a clinical trial. In the early 1970s, choroidal detachment was a common postoperative problem, and Burton *et al.* conducted a prospective trial to evaluate the effect of sub-conjunctival depot steroid on its incidence.[34] They reported no significant difference in the incidence of choroidal detachment between the groups treated (44%) and untreated (38%) with depot steroid and also found no difference in the incidence of postoperative infection.

Comment

There is no evidence of either benefit or harm from depot steroid injections. In current practice, their use is not widespread.

Question

Should physical activity be restricted following detachment surgery?

The evidence

The lack of need for restriction in physical activity was demonstrated by a randomised controlled trial by Bovino and Marcus in 1984.[35] Following scleral buckling surgery, 108 patients were divided into two groups, one advised to avoid bending, lifting, straining at stool, driving, sexual activity, lawn-mowing, gardening, athletics and returning to work for six weeks postoperatively, and the other allowed to resume normal activity immediately. No difference in the redetachment, reoperation and final reattachment rates was found at six months or in final visual acuity at one year.

Comment

This study confirms that physical activity need not be avoided postoperatively. This seems logical since in rapid eye movement sleep, unavoidable forces are applied to the eye.

Question

Are there proven methods to control postoperative pain?

The evidence

The use of analgesics postoperatively is both essential and commonplace. Non-steroidal anti-inflammatory drugs (NSAIDs) are likely to be beneficial in scleral buckling surgery due to their already proven effect on scleritis. A randomised placebo controlled trial of the use of oral indometacin by Sadiq *et al.*[36] studied 28 patients undergoing scleral buckling surgery. Patients receiving indometacin 100 mg by suppository and 50 mg orally twice daily for 10 days had significantly lower pain scores measured at both three and 10 days postoperatively.

For postoperative analgesia the use of a regional block in addition to general anaesthesia has been shown to be beneficial and is gaining popularity. Duker *et al.*[37] studied the effect of retrobulbar bupivacaine injection in a prospective, randomised, double-masked trial of 50 patients. Only 12% of the group who received bupivacaine required parenteral analgesic in the first 24 hours following surgery, compared with 72% of those who received placebo. This effect was significant up to 48 hours postoperatively in a similar study by Gottfredsdottir *et al.*[38] Bourke *et al.*[39] found a similar benefit with bupivacaine administered in a peribulbar/subtenon injection in scleral buckling surgery. Chung *et al.*[40] reported 28 patients undergoing general anaesthesia for retinal detachment, who were randomly assigned to receive a retrobulbar block or nothing. The operative procedure was not reported but was presumably a cryotherapy and scleral explant procedure. Postoperative pain score and speed of recovery of anaesthesia were both significantly better in those who received a retrobulbar block.

Comment

Indometacin is not much used in current practice, having been replaced by more modern NSAIDS. Use of subtenon bupivacaine 0·5% administered at the start of all vitrectomy and scleral buckling procedures is common practice.

Question

Can entry-site breaks be prevented in vitrectomy surgery?

The evidence

Entry-site breaks in the retina are reported to occur in 5–10% of vitrectomy operations. Territo et al.[41] showed that use of a cannulated sclerostomy system can reduce this from 7·7% in the non-cannulated group to 1% in the cannulated group.

Question

Can the incidence of postoperative cystoid macular oedema be reduced?

The evidence

Cystoid macular oedema has been reported to occur in 30–43% of patients following retinal detachment surgery. It may result from a number of factors theoretically, including vitreomacular traction, inflammation and hypotony, although no one factor has been proven. However, the randomised trial of Miyake et al.[42] involving 124 patients randomised to receive topical indometacin or placebo following retinal detachment surgery suggests inflammation is causative. Topical indometacin, which reduces inflammation, reduced the incidence and severity of cystoid macular oedema in patients treated in the early (four to six weeks) but not the late (12 weeks) postoperative period. The presence of cystoid macular oedema was associated with reduced visual acuity.

Comment

Cystoid macular degeneration is perhaps an under-reported complication, but this trial does show that there is further benefit to the use of NSAIDs in addition to their analgesic properties.

Question

Can ocular motility problems be avoided after retinal detachment surgery?

The evidence

After scleral buckling surgery, diplopia is a common complaint. It was thought to be caused either by the presence of an explant or the manipulation of the rectus muscles during the procedure. A trial by Mester et al.[43] compared 60 patients undergoing scleral buckling surgery, randomised to receive either a permanent silicone sponge explant or a temporary, removable balloon buckle. Orthoptic evaluation revealed no difference between the ocular motility findings between the groups at one week postoperatively (i.e. immediately after the balloon was removed), but significantly better ocular motility in the balloon-treated group at four weeks and 26 weeks postoperatively.

Comment

This study supports the view that permanent explants cause ocular motility problems, and this is further borne out by the common experience that the ocular motility symptoms improve when an explant is removed.

Implications for research

Over the past 80 years, rhegmatogenous retinal detachment has evolved from being an untreatable condition to being one with an excellent prognosis for surgical outcome. Randomised clinical trials have been crucial in evaluation of the various components of possible treatment and has helped to refine techniques. The major questions remaining to be answered are those of how to preserve visual function following macular retinal detachment and how to improve the outcome of retinal detachments complicated by PVR.

Implications for practice

The large proportion of rhegmatogenous retinal detachments require surgical repair. However, a conservative approach may be indicated if the detachment is inferior and long standing (implied by a pigmented tide-mark at the demarcation of detached and attached retina), or conversely if a successful surgical outcome is considered unlikely due to advanced PVR. However, this rationale is based on common practice and experience rather than any scientific evidence.

An external approach with cryotherapy or laser retinopexy and scleral explant is indicated when the retinal breaks are anteriorly placed, can be clearly visualised, and/or there is no posterior vitreous detachment. The subretinal fluid may be drained transclerally. Other surgical approaches are pars plana vitrectomy or pneumatic retinopexy.

Drainage of subretinal fluid is indicated if there is excessive subretinal fluid to allow retinopexy, to create intraocular space if a large explant or encirclement is required, and tends to be associated with increased success in the treatment of inferior breaks.

References

1. Foos RY, Wheeler NC. Vitreoretinal juncture: Synchysis senilis and posterior vitreous detachment. *Ophthalmology* 1982;**89**:1502–12.
2. Yoon YH, Marmor MF. Rapid enhancement of retinal adhesion by laser photocoagulation. *Ophthalmology* 1988;**95**:1385–8.
3. Kita M, Negi A, Honda Y, Marmor MF. The recovery of retinal adhesion and subretinal fluid absorption after experimental retinal detachment.
4. Hilton GF, Grizzard WS, Avins L *et al*. The drainage of subretinal fluid. A randomized controlled clinincal trial. *Retina* 1981;**1**:271–80.
5. Das TP, Jalali S. Laser-aided external drainage of subretinal fluid: prospective randomized comparison with needle drainage. *Ophthalmic Surg* 1994;**25**:236–9.
6. Ibanez HE, Bloom SM, Olk RJ *et al*. External argon laser choroidotomy versus needle drainage technique in primary scleral buckle procedures. A prospective randomised study. *Ophthalmology* 1994;**14**:348–50.
7. Aylward GW, Orr G, Scwhartz SD, Leaver PK. Prospective, randomised, controlled trial comparing suture needle drainage and argon laser drainage of subretinal fluid. *Br J Ophthalmol* 1995;**79**: 724–7.
8. Pearce IA, Wong D, McGalliard J, Groenewald C. Does cryotherapy before drainage increase the risk of intraocular haemorrhage and affect outcome? *Br J Ophthalmol* 1997;**81**:563–7.
9. Arribas NP, Olk RJ, Schertzer M *et al*. Preoperative antibiotic soaking of silicone sponges. Does it make a difference? *Ophthalmology* 1984;**91**:1684–9.
10. Singh M. Surgery of aphakic retinal detachment. *Br J Ophthalmol* 1988;**72**:820–2.
11. Rosengren B. Cases of retinal detachment treated with diathermy and the injection of air into the vitreous body. *Acta Ophthalmol* 1938;**15**:573–9.
12. Hilton GF, Kelly NE, Salzano TC, Tornambe PE, Wells JW, Wendel RT. Pneumatic retinopexy: a collaborative report of the first 100 cases. *Ophthalmology* 1987;**94**:307–14.
13. Van Effenterre G, Haut J, Larricart P, Abi-Rached J, Vachet JM. Gas tamponade as a single technique in the treatment of retinal detachment: is vitrectomy needed? *Graefe's Arch Clin Exp Ophthalmol* 1987;**225**:254–8.
14. Tornambe PE, Hilton GF, The Retinal Detachment Study Group. Pneumatic retinopexy. A multicenter randomized controlled trial comparing pneumatic retinopexy with scleral buckling. *Ophthalmology* 1989;**96**:772–84.
15. Tornambe PE, Hilton GF, Brinton DA *et al*. Pneumatic retinopexy. A two-year follow-up study of the multi-center clinical trial comparing pneumatic retinopexy with scleral buckling. *Ophthalmology* 1991;**98**:1115–23.
16. Mulverhill A, Fulcher T, Datta V, Acheson R. Pneumatic retinopexy versus scleral buckling: a randomised controlled trial. *Ir J Med Sci* 1996;**165**:274–7.
17. Sharma S. Meta-analysis of clinical trials comparing scleral buckling surgery to pneumatic retinopex. *Evidence-based Eye Care* 2002; **3**:125–8.
18. Briggs M, Wong D, Groenewald C, McGalliard J, Kelly J, Harper J. The effect of anaesthesia on the intraocular volume of the C3F8 gas bubble. *Eye* 1997;**11**:47–52.
19. Peyman GA, Kao GW, de Corral LR. Randomized clinical trial of intraocular silicone *v*. gas in the management of complicated retinal detachment and vitreous hemorrhage. *Int Ophthalmol* 1987;**10**: 221–34.
20. Azen SP, Boone DC, Barlow W *et al*. Methods, statistical features and baseline results of a standardised, multicentered ophthalmic surgical trial: the silicone study. *Control Clin Trials* 1991;**12**:438–55.
21. The Silicone Study Group. Vitrectomy with silicone oil or sulphahexafluoride gas in eyes with severe proliferative vitreoretinopathy: results of a randomised trial: Silicone Study Report 1. *Arch Ophthalmol* 1992;**110**:770–9.
22. Lincoff H, Mardirossian J, Lincoff A, Liggett P, Iwamoto T, Jakobiec F. Intravitreal longevity of three perfluorocarbon gases. *Arch Ophthalmol* 1980;**98**:1610–11.
23. The Silicone Study Group. Vitrectomy with silicone oil or perfluoropropane gas in eyes with sever proliferative vitreoretinopathy: results of a randomised clinical trial: Silicone Study Report 2. *Arch Ophthalmol* 1992;**110**:780–92.
24. McCuen BW, Azen SP, Stern W *et al*. Vitrectomy with silicone oil or perfluoropropane gas in eyes with severe proliferative vitreoretinopathy: results in group 1 versus group 2. Silicone Study Report 3. *Retina* 1993;**13**:279–84.
25. Barr CC, Lai MY, Lean JS *et al*. Postoperative intraocular pressure abnormalities in the Silicone Study. Silicone Study Report 4. *Ophthalmology* 1993;**100**:1629–35.
26. Blumenkranz MS, Azen SP, Aaberg TM *et al*. Relaxing retinotomy with silicone oil or long-acting gas in eyes with severe proliferative vitreoretinopathy. Silicone Study Report 5. *Am J Ophthalmol* 1993;**116**:557–64.
27. Diddie KR, Azen SP, Freeman HM *et al*. Anterior proliferative vitreoretinopathy in the Silicone Study. Silicone Study Report 10. *Ophthalmology* 1996;**107**:1092–9.
28. Hutton WL, Lee MBF, Blumenkranz MS *et al*. The effects of silicone oil removal in the Silicone Study. Silicone Study Report 6. *Arch Ophthalmol* 1994;**112**:778–85.
29. Abrams GW, Azen SP, Barr CC *et al*. The incidence of corneal abnormalities in the Silicone study. *Arch Ophthalmol* 1995;**113**: 764–9.
30. Cox MS, Azen SP, Barr CC *et al*. Macular pucker after successful surgery for proliferative vitreoretinopathy. Silicone Study Report 8. *Ophthalmology* 1995;**102**:1884–91.
31. Abrams GW, Azen SP, McCuen BW *et al*. Vitrectomy with silicone oil or long-acting gas in eyes with severe proliferative vitreoretinopathy: results of additional long-term follow-up. Silicone Study Report 11. *Arch Ophthalmol* 1997;**115**:335–44.
32. Batman C, Cekic O. Vitrectomy with silicone oil or long-acting gas in eye with giant retinal tears. Long-term follow-up of a randomised clinical trial. *Retina* 1999;**19**:188–92.
33. Hung JY. Corneal sensation in retinal detachment surgery. *Ann Ophthalmol* 1987;**19**:313–18.
34. Burton TC, Stevens TS, Harrison TJ. The influence of subconjunctival depot corticosteroid on choroidal detachment following retinal detachment surgery. *Trans Am Acad Ophthalmol Otolaryngol* 1975;**79**:845–9.
35. Bovino JA, Marcus DF. Physical activity after retinal detachment surgery. *Am J Ophthalmol* 1984;**98**:171–9.
36. Sadiq SA, Stevenson L, Gorman C, Orr GM. Use of indomethacin for pain relief following scleral buckling surgery. *Br J Ophthalmol* 1998;**82**:429–31.

37. Duker J, Neilsen J, Vandeer JF *et al*. Retrobulbar bupivcaine irrigation for post-operative pain after scleral buckling surgery. A prospective study. *Ophthalmology* 1991;**98**:514–18.

38. Gottfredsdottir MS, Gislason I, Stefansson E *et al*. Effects of retrobulbar bupivcaine on post-operative pain and nausea in retinal detachment surgery. *Acta Ophthalmol* 1993;**71**:544–7.

39. Bourke RD, Dowler JG, Heyworth P, Cooling RJ, Moore C. Extraconal bupivacaine in scleral buckling procedures. *Retina* 1996;**16**:240–5.

40. Chung F, Westerling, Chisholm LDJ, Squires GW. Postoperative recovery after general anaesthesia with and without retrobulbar block in retinal detachment surgery. *Anaesthesia* 1988;**43**:943–6.

41. Territo C, Gieser JP, Wilson CA, Anand R. Influence of the cannulated vitrectomy system on the recurrence of sclerotomy retinal tears. *Retina* 1997;**17**:430–3.

42. Miyake K, Miyake Y, Maekubo K, Asakura M, Manabe R. Incidence of cystoid macular oedema after retinal detachment surgery and the use of topical indomethacin. *Am J Ophthalmol* 1983;**95**:451–6.

43. Mester U, Volker B, Pefferman U. A comparison of the influence of temporary balloon buckles and permanent episcleral sponges on postoperative ocular motility in retinal detachment surgery. *Graefe's Arch Clin Exp Ophthalmol* 1986;**224**:76–7.

40 Surgical management of full-thickness macular hole

Eric Ezra

Background

Epidemiology

Idiopathic full-thickness macular hole (FTMH) occurs in approximately 1/3300 and predominantly affects patients in their sixth to eighth decades of life. A significant number (15–20%) of patients with a unilateral FTMH will develop fellow-eye involvement over the first five years.[1]

Aetiology and natural history

In 1988 and subsequently in 1995, Gass proposed that FTMH arise from tangential vitreofoveal traction as the posterior vitreous cortex contracts with progressive ageing.[2,3] This results in centrifugal traction on the fovea, leading to a localised foveal detachment and loss of the foveal reflex and depression on biomicroscopy. This configuration is termed stage 1a or an impending hole and is associated with a yellow spot biomicroscopically. With progressive traction, a small foveal dehiscence occurs and is associated with the development of a preretinal glial membrane (probably an attempted reparative response). The dehiscence is usually not visible beneath the membrane and is termed "occult". This stage 1b lesion is characterised by the appearance of a yellow ring at the fovea, which is thought to represent displaced xanthophyll at the edges of the occult hole. Recent data from optical coherence tomography have shown that some stage 1a lesions may actually represent a foveal cyst rather than a full thickness foveal detachment.

Subsequently, a dehiscence occurs in the membrane itself and this extends either in a centric or pericentric ("can-opener") fashion, termed stage 2. Only about 50% of stage 1 lesions progress to stage 2, with the remainder either arresting or resolving, usually due to the release of traction as a result of localised vitreofoveal separation. In 80% of stage 2 lesions, localised vitreofoveal separation occurs with the formation of an operculum (visible in about 80% of lesions), which remains attached to the separated posterior vitreous cortex at the fovea (stage 3), while the remainder (20%) may arrest or resolve spontaneously. Approximately 20% of stage 3 lesions subsequently develop a full posterior vitreous detachment (stage 4). Although spontaneous closure occurs in approximately 20% of stage 2 lesions, it is much rarer for this to happen in stage 3 (7%) and 4 (<1%) lesions.[4]

The description of the pathophysiology of macular hole formation has led to the evolution of surgical treatments for the condition using modern vitrectomy and posterior segment techniques. The evidence for the effectiveness of these techniques is summarised below.

Question

Is surgical treatment effective in preventing progression of stage 1 (impending) lesions?

The evidence

In the late 1980s and early 1990s, a number of investigators evaluated the benefit of vitrectomy and posterior vitreous cortex (PVC) removal in stage 1 lesions in an attempt to prevent FTMH formation by removing vitreous traction. The procedure consisted of a three-port pars plana vitrectomy and PVC separation without the use of intraocular gas tamponade. Initial results from uncontrolled pilot studies appeared favourable, with a rate of progression to stage 2 of 20% in operated eyes.[5,6] However, a randomised trial that included a no-treatment group, revealed a progression rate of 37% in the surgical group compared to 40% in the observation group and showed no statistical benefit in terms of vision.[7–9] Full recruitment to the study could not be completed and no definitive recommendations could be offered. In the light of these data and in view of the favourable surgical results achieved for FTMH, impending holes are rarely treated.

Question

Is surgery effective in achieving anatomical closure and vision improvement in stage 2, 3 and 4 FTMH?

The evidence

Kelly and Wendel were the first to report successful surgical closure of FTMH.[10,11] In their initial report,[6] using vitrectomy, PVC separation, epiretinal membrane (ERM) dissection and intraocular gas tamponade, anatomical closure was achieved in 58% of eyes, with visual improvement in 42%. A number of subsequent case-control series[11–13] demonstrated improved outcomes, which led to a prospective randomised controlled trial conducted by the Vitrectomy for Treatment of Macular Hole Study Group.[15–17] The results were difficult to interpret and showed only a marginal benefit in vision and a relatively high rate of sight-threatening complications in the treated group compared to the observation eyes. A number of confounding factors, in terms of study design, are thought to account for these results. First, the surgery was performed by a large number of surgeons, with different levels of expertise, in a wide range of centres. Second, patients undergoing vitrectomy were precluded from having cataract surgery afterwards, and with visual results being reported at only six months after macular hole surgery, it is highly likely that the visual benefit was masked. It is generally agreed that further trials are required to evaluate the exact visual benefit of macular hole surgery.[18,19]

Question

Does the use of intraoperative adjunctive substances improve the results of FTMH surgery?

The evidence

The demonstration by histological studies that successfully sealed holes are closed or "bridged" by glial cells led a number of investigators to examine the possibility of encouraging postoperative healing with the use of substances that stimulate glial activation and migration. The rationale and potential advantages of such substances appear attractive for a number of reasons. First, they might enhance the closure rate in less favourable cases, such as stage 3 and 4 holes. Second, they might obviate the need to perform intraoperative ERM dissection, which can prove difficult in some cases where the membranes are very nebulous. Third, they might obviate the need for patients to posture in the postoperative period. Potential disadvantages include cost, prolongation of the procedure risking intra-ocular infection, and stimulation of an over-aggressive glial response postoperatively, leading to ERM formation and traction around the edges of the hole.

In 1992, Glaser reported the use of bovine transforming growth factor-β2 (TGF-β2),[20–22] with or without epiretinal membrane dissection, which produced impressive results in uncontrolled case series but which were less successful with recombinant TGF-β.[23,24]

Liggett *et al.* reported the use of autologous serum as an adjunct in a small pilot study, achieving a closure rate comparable to that achieved with bovine TGF-β2.[25] This substance has also been shown to stimulate proliferation and migration of glia, retinal pigment epithelial (RPE) cells and fibroblasts, and to facilitate chorioretinal adhesion in animal models.[26] Initial reports from uncontrolled studies using autologous serum have proved encouraging with closure rates of about 70%.[27] More recently, the Vitrectomy for Treatment of Macular Hole Study Group reported non-randomised data on vitrectomy plus autologous serum versus vitrectomy alone and found no difference in results between the two groups.[28]

Autologous platelet concentrates, which are also potent stimulants of cellular migration and proliferation,[29,30] have been shown to be promising[31–33] with closure rates of 95%.[31,32] Other substances that have been evaluated as adjuncts include autologous plasma–thrombin mixture,[34] autologous fibrin,[35] Tissucol[36] and bovine thrombin.[37] Although all these substances have shown encouraging early results, they await further evaluation in properly designed trials.

Question

Is reoperation effective in eyes with persistent FTMH after primary surgery?

The evidence

There are no randomised controlled trials addressing this issue, but given that the failure rate may be as high as 20%, reoperation is often considered. Three case series have specifically reported the outcome of reoperation after unsuccessful primary surgery with anatomical success rates of 80–90%[38–40] with significant visual improvement of two Snellen lines in over 60% of eyes,[39] but this effect may be exaggerated and better quality trial data are required.

Question

What are the complications of FTMH surgery?

The evidence

Although patients undergoing FTMH surgery may develop general complications related to closed intraocular surgery, a number of complications specific to macular hole surgery have been reported although generally these are rarely sight-threatening.[2–73] Early postoperative complications include problems related to posturing, such as neck and back discomfort. These should be anticipated pre-operatively, particularly in the elderly, who may have osteoarthritis of the neck. Some patients have developed ulnar nerve compression syndromes due to prolonged pressure on the elbows during posturing.[41] For these reasons, a number of investigators have examined whether surgery with less rigorous or no posturing is feasible and have reported case series with good surgical results.[42,43]

Another early complication is intraocular pressure elevation. This is usually secondary to postoperative gas expansion and is usually transient,[24] responding rapidly to medical treatment. Gas overfill and angle closure can occur. Postoperative sterile hypopyon has also been noted in some cases, particularly with the use of adjuncts.[37] The possibility of infection needs to be excluded in these cases.

Other complications include retinal tears (3%)[44] and detachments (1·8–14%),[44–46] RPE damage or phototoxicity (1–3%)[44,45,47,48] and glaucoma.[49] A number of reports have described the occurrence of non-progressive peripheral, absolute, wedge-shaped field defects after apparently uncomplicated surgery.[50–59] Nerve fibre layer damage during separation of the PVC and/or air drying have been postulated as possible mechanisms.

Longer term complications have also been reported. Hole persistence, after failed surgery (in 5–30% of cases), is associated with enlargement of the hole diameter and further decline in acuity.[60] For these cases, reoperation should be considered.[61–63] Late reopening of the hole after successful surgery has also been reported (<10% of cases)[64–68] and these are also amenable to reoperation. The mechanism of reopening may be related to foveal stress due either to ERM contraction or cystoid oedema, particularly after cataract extraction, although in the majority of cases no specific cause can be identified.

The most common long-term complication is nuclear cataract after surgery, and like nucleosclerosis after vitrectomy for ERM peeling,[69] it may occur in up to 80% of patients at two years[70] with 25% requiring extraction.[10,14] Simultaneous macular hole and cataract surgery, particularly with modern phacoemulsification, may be considered in some cases.[42,71,72] Combining these procedures may be associated with increased risk of postoperative pseudophakic cystoid macular oedema[72] and late reopening.

In view of the frequency of nuclear cataract progression, hole persistence or reopening and other complications, patients should be warned of the possibility of requiring reoperation and/or cataract surgery after macular hole surgery and other complications. Further clinical data from ongoing prospective trials will provide greater understanding of the benefits and risks of macular hole surgery. Future developments such as enzyme-assisted vitrectomy[73] may allow atraumatic separation of the PVC and reduce the incidence of complications.

New developments in macular hole surgery

Despite the plethora of adjunctive substances that have undergone only preliminary evaluation, researchers continue to report ever-increasing surgical success rates using vitrectomy without adjuncts, emphasising the importance of patient selection (hole size and shorter duration). Some have questioned the absolute necessity of using longer acting gases and prone posturing although further randomised data evaluating these variables is required. In addition, a number of surgical refinements have been introduced, including internal limiting membrane (ILM) peeling[74–77] with or without the use of dyes such as indocyanine green,[78] to enhance visualisation of the ILM. Although initial non-randomised studies have demonstrated encouraging results,[74,75,77,79] prompting many clinicians to adopt ILM peeling, others have failed to show any improvement in success rates.[80,81] Clearly, further data from randomised studies are required.

Conclusions and recommendations

Over the past decade, macular hole surgery has continued to develop rapidly. Although intraoperative adjuncts showed early promise, clinical data have failed to demonstrate significant positive statistical effects for the majority of agents. The improvement in surgical success rates in recent years has been attributable predominantly to improved surgical techniques and preoperative case selection rather than the use of adjuncts. The use of ILM peeling ensures complete removal of the scaffold and glial elements from around the hole, and although its precise role remains to be determined some anecdotal data suggest that it may be useful for larger or more chronic lesions. Further prospective randomised clinical studies are required to evaluate its role, although given the rapid evolution of surgical techniques and the already high (>90%) anatomical success rates in most studies, these will be difficult to carry out.

References

1. Ezra E, Wells JA, Gray RH *et al.* Incidence of idiopathic full-thickness macular holes in fellow eyes. A 5-year prospective natural history study. *Ophthalmology* 1998;**105**:353–9.
2. Gass JDM. Idiopathic senile macular hole its early stages and development. *Arch Ophthalmol* 1988;**106**:629–39.

3. Johnson RN, Gass JDM. Idiopathic macular holes. Observations, stages of formation and implications for surgical intervention. *Ophthalmology* 1988;**95**:917–24.

4. Ezra E, Gregor ZJ. Moorfields Macular Hole Study Group. Surgery for idiopathic full-thickness macular hole: 2-year results of a prospective randomised clinical trial comparing natural history, vitrectomy and vitrectomy plus autologous serum. Moorfields Macular Hole Study Group (MMHSG). Report No 1. *Arch Ophthalmol* 2003. (In press).

5. Smiddy WE, Michels RG, Glaser BM, de Bustros S. Vitrectomy for impending macular holes. *Am J Ophthalmol* 1988;**105**:371–6.

6. Jost BF, Hutton WL, Fullet DG *et al.* Vitrectomy in eyes at risk of macular hole formation. *Ophthalmology* 1990;**97**:843–7.

7. de Bustros S. Early stages of macular holes: to treat or not to treat. *Arch Ophthalmol* 1990;**108**:979–82.

8. de Bustros S. Vitrectomy for prevention of macular hole study. *Arch Ophthalmol* 1991;**109**:1057.

9. de Bustros S, The Vitrectomy for Prevention of Macular Hole Study Group. Vitrectomy for the prevention of macular holes: results of a randomized clinical trial. *Ophthalmology* 1994;**101**:1055–60.

10. Kelly NE, Wendel RT. Vitreous surgery for idiopathic macular holes: results of a pilot study. *Arch Ophthalmol* 1991;**190**:654–9.

11. Wendel RT, Patel AC, Kelly NE, Salzano TC, Wells JW, Novack GD. Vitreous surgery for macular holes. *Ophthalmology* 1993;**100**:1671–6.

12. Orrellana J, Lieberman RM. Stage III macular hole surgery. *Br J Ophthalmol* 1993;**77**:555–8.

13. Ryan EH, Gilbert HD. Results of surgical treatment of recent onset full-thickness idiopathic macular holes. *Arch Ophthalmol* 1994;**112**:1545–53.

14. Ruby AJ, Williams DF, Grand MG *et al.* Pars plana vitrectomy for treatment of Stage 2 macular holes. *Arch Ophthalmol* 1994;**112**:359–64.

15. Kim JW, Freeman WR, Azen SP *et al.* Prospective randomised trial of vitrectomy for stage 2 macular holes. *Am J Ophthalmol* 1996;**121**:605–14.

16. Freeman WR, Azen SP, Kim JW *et al.* Vitrectomy for the treatment of full-thickness stage 3 or 4 macular holes. Results of a multicentre randomised controlled trial. *Arch Ophthalmol* 1997;**115**:11–22.

17. Kim JW, Freeman WR, El-Haig W, Maguire AM, Arevalo JF, Azen SP. Baseline characteristics, natural history, and risk factors to progression in eyes with Stage 2 macular holes. Results from a prospective randomized clinical trial. *Ophthalmology* 1995;**102**:1818–29.

18. Fine SL. Macular hole: a continuing saga. *Arch Ophthalmol* 1999;**117**:248–9.

19. Ho AC, Guyer DR, Fine SL. Macular hole (review). *Surv Ophthalmol* 1998;**42**:393–416.

20. Smiddy WE, Glaser BM, Green WR *et al.* Transforming growth factor beta: a biological chorioretinal glue. *Arch Ophthalmol* 1989;**107**:577–80.

21. Glaser BM, Michels RG, Kupperman BD *et al.* The effects of pars plana vitrectomy and transforming growth factor-beta 2 for the treatment of full-thickness macular holes: a prospective randomized study. *Ophthalmology* 1992;**99**:1162–73.

22. Lansing MB, Glaser BM, Liss H *et al.* The effect of pars plana vitrectomy and transforming growth factor-beta 2 without epiretinal membrane peeling on full-thickness macular holes. *Ophthalmology* 1993;**100**:868–71.

23. Thompson JT, Smiddy WE, Williams GA *et al.* Comparison of recombinant transforming growth factor beta-2 and placebo as an adjunctive agent for macular hole surgery. *Ophthalmology* 1998;**105**:700–6.

24. Thompson JT, Sjaarda RN, Glaser BM, Murphy RP. Increased intraocular pressure after macular hole surgery. *Am J Ophthalmol* 1996;**121**:615–22.

25. Liggett PE, Skolik S, Horio B *et al.* Human autologous serum for the treatment of full thickness macular holes: a preliminary study. *Ophthalmology* 1995;**102**:1071–6.

26. Christmas NJ, Skolik SA, Howard MA, Saito Y, Barnstable CJ, Liggett PE. Treatment of retinal breaks with autologous serum in an experimental model. *Ophthalmology* 1995;**102**:263–71.

27. Wells JA, Gregor ZJ. Surgical treatment of full-thickness macular holes using autologous serum. *Eye* 1996;**10**:593–9.

28. Banker AS, Freeman WR, Azen SP, Lai MY. A multicentred clinical study of serum as adjunctive therapy for surgical treatment of macular holes. Vitrectomy for Macular Hole Study Group. *Arch Ophthalmol* 1999;**117**:1499–1502.

29. Hitaizumi Y, Transfeldt EE, Kwahara N, Sung JH, Knighton D, Fiegel VD. In vitro angiogenesis by platelet-derived wound-healing formula in injured spinal cord. *Brain Res Bull* 1993;**30**:353–7.

30. Ksander GA, Swamura S, Ohawa Y, Sundsumo J, McPherson J. The effect of platelet release on wound healing in animal models. *J Am Acad Dermatol* 1990;**22**:781–91.

31. Gaudric A, Massin P, Paques M *et al.* Autologous platelet concentrate for the treatment of full thickness macular holes. *Graefe's Arch Clin Exp Ophthalmol* 1995;**233**:549–54.

32. Paques M, Chastang C, Mathis A *et al.* Effect of autologous platelet concentrate in surgery for idiopathic macular hole: results of a multicentre, double-masked, randomised trial. *Ophthalmology* 1999;**106**:932–8.

33. Korobelnik JF, Hannouche D, Belayachi N *et al.* Autologous platelet concentrate as an adjunct in macular hole surgery: a pilot study. *Ophthalmology* 1996;**103**:590–4.

34. Blumenkranz MS, Coll GE, Chang S, Morse LS. Use of autologous plasma–thrombin mixture as adjuvant therapy for macular hole. *Ophthalmology* 1994;**101**(Suppl):769.

35. Iwasaki T, Sanda A, Yamamoto K, Okade A, Usui NM. The use of fibrin tissue adhesive in the treatment of macular holes. *Invest Ophthalmol Vis Sci* 1995;**36**:1050–6.

36. Tilanus MA, Deutman AF. Full-thickness macular holes treated with vitrectomy and tissue glue. *Int Ophthalmol* 1994–95;**18**:355–8.

37. Olsen TW, Sternber P, Martin DF *et al.* Postoperative hypopyon after intravitreal bovine thrombin for macular hole surgery. *Am J Ophthalmol* 1996;**121**:575–7.

38. Ie D, Glaser BM, Thompson JT, Sjaarda RN, Gordon LW. Retreatment of full-thickness macular holes persisting after prior vitrectomy: a pilot study. *Ophthalmology* 1993;**100**:1787–93.

39. Smiddy WE, Sjaarda RN, Glaser BM *et al.* Reoperation after failed macular hole surgery. *Retina* 1996;**16**:13–18.

40. Ezra E, Aylward WG, Gregor ZJ. Membranectomy and autologous serum for the retreatment of full-thickness macular holes. *Arch Ophthalmol* 1997;**115**:1276–80.

41. Holekamp NM, Meredith TA, Landers MB *et al.* Ulnar neuropathy as a complication of macular hole surgery. *Arch Ophthalmol* 1999;**117**:1607–10.

42. Tornambe PE, Poliner LS, Grote KD. Macular hole surgery without face-down positioning. A pilot study. *Retina* 1997;**17**:179–85.

43. Mulhern MG, Cullinane A, Cleary PE. Visual and anatomical success with short-term macular tamponade and autologous platelet concentrate. *Graefe's Arch Clin Exp Ophthalmol* 2000;**238**:577–83.

44. Park SS, Marcus DM, Duker JS *et al.* Posterior segment complications after vitrectomy for macular hole. *Ophthalmology* 1995;**102**:775–81.

45. Banker AS, Freeman WR, Kim JW *et al.* Vision threatening complications of surgery for full-thickness macular holes. Vitrectomy for Macular Hole Study Group. *Ophthalmology* 1997;**104**:1442–52.

46. Tabandeh H, Chaudhry NA, Smiddy WE. Retinal detachments associated with macular hole surgery: characteristics, mechanisms and outcomes. *Retina* 1999;**19**:281–6.

47. Charles S. Retinal pigment epithelial abnormalities after macular hole surgery. *Retina* 1993;**13**:176.

48. Poliner LS, Tornambe PE. Retinal pigment epitheliopathy after macular hole surgery. *Ophthalmology* 1992;**99**:1671–7.

49. Chen C. Glaucoma after macular hole surgery. *Ophthalmology* 1996;**103**(Suppl):124.

50. Melberg NS, Thomas MA. Field loss after pars plana vitrectomy with air/fluid exchange. *Am J Ophthalmol* 1995;**120**:386–8.

51. Boldt HC, Munden PM, Folk JC, Mehaffey MG. Visual field defects after macular hole surgery. *Am J Ophthalmol* 1996;**122**:371–81.

52. Kerison JB, Haller JA, Elman M, Miller NR. Visual fields loss following vitreous surgery. *Arch Ophthalmol* 1996;**114**:564–9.

53. Pendergast SD, McCuen BW. Visual field loss after macular hole surgery. *Ophthalmology* 1996;**103**:1069–77.

54. Bopp S, Lucke K, Hille U. Peripheral visual field loss after vitreous surgery for macular hole. *Graefe's Arch Clin Exp Ophthalmol* 1997;**235**:362–71.

55. Paques M, Massin P, Santiago PY *et al*. Visual field loss after vitrectomy for full-thickness macular holes. *Am J Ophthalmol* 1997;**124**:88–94.

56. Ohji M, Nao-I N, Saito Y, Hayashi A, Tano Y. Prevention of visual field defect after macular hole surgery by passing air used for fluid–air exchange through water. *Am J Ophthalmol* 1999;**127**:62–6.

57. Groenewald CP, Wong D, Pearce I, Hiscott P, Grierson I. Nasal epipapillary membrane causing visual field loss following macular hole surgery. *Eye* 1998;**12**:328–30.

58. Cullinane AB, Cleary PE. Prevention of visual field defects after macular hole surgery. *Br J Ophthalmol* 2000;**84**:372–7.

59. Evaluation of patients with visual field defects following macular hole surgery using multifocal electroretinography. *Retina* 2000;**20**:238–43.

60. Leonard RE, Smiddy WE, Flynn HW. Visual acuity and macular hole size after unsuccessful macular hole surgery. *Am J Ophthalmol* 1997;**123**:84–9.

61. Ie D, Glaser BM, Thompson JT, Sjaarda RN, Gordon LW. Retreatment of full-thickness macular holes persisting after prior vitrectomy: a pilot study. *Ophthalmology* 1993;**100**:1787–93.

62. Smiddy WE, SjaardaRN, Glaser BM *et al*. Reoperation after failed macular hole surgery. *Retina* 1996;**16**:13–18.

63. Thompson JT, Sjaarda RN. Surgical treatment of macular holes with multiple recurrences. *Ophthalmology* 2000;**107**:1073–7.

64. Duker JS, Wendel RT, Patel AC, Puliafito CA. Late reopening of macular holes following initially successful vitreous surgery. *Ophthalmology* 1994;**101**:1373–8.

65. Del Priore LV, Kaplan HJ, Bonham FD. Laser photocoagulation and fluid–gas exchange for recurrent macular hole. *Retina* 1994;**14**:381–2.

66. Paques M, Massin P, Santiago PY *et al*. Late reopening of successfully treated macular holes. *Br J Ophthalmol* 1997;**81**:658–62.

67. Christmas NJ, Smiddy WE, Flynn HW. Reopening of macular holes after initially successful repair. *Ophthalmology* 1998;**105**:1835–8.

68. Paques M, Massin P, Blain P, Duquesnoy AS, Gaudric A. Long-term incidence of reopening of macular holes. *Ophthalmology* 2000;**107**:760–5.

69. de Bustros S, Thompson JT, Michels RG, Enger C, Rice TA, Glaser BM. Nuclear sclerosis after vitrectomy for idiopathic epiretinal membrane. *Am J Ophthalmol* 1988;**105**:160–4.

70. Thompson JT, Glaser BM, Sjaarda RN, Murphy RP. Progression of nuclear sclerosis and long-term visual results after vitrectomy with transforming growth factor beta-2 for macular holes. *Am J Ophthalmol* 1995;**119**:48–54.

71. Miller JH, Googe JM, Hoskins JC. Combined macular hole and cataract surgery. *Am J Ophthalmol* 1997;**123**:705–7.

72. Sheidow TG, Gonder JR. Cystoid macular oedema following combined phacoemulsification and vitrectomy for macular hole. *Retina* 1998;**18**:510–14.

73. Trese MT, Williams GA, Hartzer MK. A new approach to stage 3 macular holes. *Ophthalmology* 2000;**107**:1607–11.

74. Olsen TW, Sternberg P, Capone A *et al*. Macular hole surgery using thrombin activated fibrinogen and selective removal of the internal limiting membrane. *Retina* 1998;**18**:322–9.

75. Park DW, Sipperly JO, Sneed SR, Dugel PU, Jacobsen J. Macular hole surgery with internal limiting membrane peeling and intravitreous air. *Ophthalmology* 1999;**106**:1392–0.

76. Freeman WR, Azen SP. Evaluation of new techniques in macular surgery. *Ophthalmology* 1999;**106**:861–2.

77. Mester V, Kuhn F. Internal limiting membrane removal in the management of full-thickness macular hole. *Am J Ophthalmol* 2000;**129**:769–77.

78. Kadonosono K, Itoh N, Uchio E, Nakamura S, Ohno S. Staining of the internal limiting membrane in macular hole surgery. *Arch Ophthalmol* 2000;**118**:1116–18.

79. Brooks HL. Macular hole surgery with and without internal limiting membrane peeling. *Ophthalmology* 2000;**107**:1939–48.

80. Margherio RR, Margherio AR, Williams GA, Chow DR, Banach MJ. Effect of perifoveal tissue dissection in the management of acute full-thickness macular holes. *Arch Ophthalmol* 2000;**118**:495–8.

81. Smiddy WE, Feuer W, Cordahi G. Internal limiting membrane peeling in macular hole surgery. *Ophthalmology* 2001;**108**:1471–6.

41 Retinal vein occlusion

Heather Baldwin

Background

Retinal vein occlusion is a common clinical condition that forms a serious threat to visual acuity, particularly in older people.

Aetiology and risk factors

There is an increasing incidence of retinal vein occlusion (RVO) with age, with greater than 50% of patients being over 65.[1] There is an approximately equal sex distribution.[2] Established cardiovascular risk factors are the predominant medical associations for both central (CRVO) and branch (BRVO) vein occlusions. The main risk factor for both types of vein occlusion is hypertension, and is more prevalent in BRVO.[2–4] Inadequately controlled hypertension is associated with recurrence of RVO in the same or fellow eye. Hyperlipidaemia (cholesterol ≥6·5 mmol/l) is the predominant association in the younger age group of RVO patients, and is associated in up to 50% of older patients.[3,5,6] Diabetes mellitus is associated with RVO, which may be due to an increase of other cardiovascular risk factors.[4,5,7] Interestingly, there is no direct evidence linking smoking to retinal vein occlusion.[2,8] Primary open angle glaucoma has been implicated in the aetiology of CRVO, but not of BRVO.[5] Myeloproliferative disorders are an important association, occurring in 1% of patients presenting with retinal vein occlusion. Thrombophilic abnormalities have been implicated but their significance in the aetiology is unclear. The subject is thoroughly reviewed by Fegan.[9] Kirwan *et al.*[10] looked at a case series of 588 retinal vein occlusion patients including women on the combined oral contraceptive pill and on hormone replacement therapy (HRT), and suggested that RVO is a contraindication to the use of the contraceptive pill, but also that HRT was not a major risk factor for retinal vein occlusion. In patients less than 50 years of age with BRVO, there are usually underlying systemic conditions such as hypertension or hyperlipidaemia.[11] Patients in the younger age group with CRVO, however, present a particular problem in investigation and management, and other rare associations may need to be investigated, such as use of the oral contraceptive pill, optic disc vasculitis, and thrombophilic factors.

Prognosis

Some 65–80% of CRVO is non-ischaemic, with 7–20% of these converting to the ischaemic type.[12] The visual prognosis is unpredictable, and mainly depends on the degree of involvement of the macula and on the length of time that macula oedema is present. In one study, two-fifths retained good visual acuity but two-fifths fared very badly.[13] A greater proportion of younger people (less than 50 years old) with CRVO are thought to have a benign outcome, with spontaneous regression of the occlusive event being more common. However, at least 20% of patients have poor visual outcome with severe neovascular complications.

Question

Do patients with retinal vein occlusion experience a better visual outcome and/or less neovascular glaucoma when treated with anticoagulants, fibrinolytic agents, antiplatelet drugs or steroids?

The evidence

We found four randomised controlled trials investigating the use of these agents for retinal vein occlusion.[14–17]

The first study, published in 1973, described results in 12 patients (three women, nine men) ranging from 33 to 69 years old, who were assigned to either fibrinolysis (intravenous streptokinase) or fibrinolysis with anticoagulants (intravenous heparin) using Horbach's randomising model.[14] Five patients had branch vein occlusions and seven had central vein occlusions. Outcome measures were visual acuity, macular morphology and fluorescein angiographic features. The results were not presented with statistical analysis as the numbers were small. The authors reported an improvement in central visual function in the streptokinase group after eight days, which was sustained until the final follow up reported at 90 days, with most of the anticoagulant alone group showing no improvement in vision.

In the following year another randomised controlled trial investigated the role of streptokinase in the treatment of central retinal vein occlusion.[15] Forty patients were randomised (details not given) to receive intravenous streptokinase or no therapy. There was no statistically significant difference in visual acuity between the groups at the outset of the trial, and no significant difference between the treated and control groups in the final visual acuity at 12 months. Three of the control group developed thrombotic glaucoma, compared with none in the treatment group, although the authors comment on the low rate of the complication even in the untreated group compared with data from other studies. The authors concluded that the hazards of the treatment, including vitreous haemorrhage, and the lack of evidence for a definite benefit for visual outcome, meant that streptokinase has no useful role to play in the management of central vein occlusion.

Hyperaggregation of platelets has been implicated in the aetiology of retinal vein occlusion, suggesting the possible role of inhibitors of platelet aggregation in the management of this condition. A double-blind randomised controlled trial investigating the use of ticlopidine was published in 1984.[16] Eighty-nine patients (46 men and 43 women, from "less than 40" to "over 80" years of age) were assigned to oral treatment or placebo (randomisation methods are not described). Thirty-five patients had central vein occlusion and 54 had branch vein occlusion. In the BRVO group, a statistical significant improvement in visual acuity was achieved in the treatment group at six months, with the same trend in the CRVO group, but this did not reach statistical significance. The main complication of treatment was gastric irritation.

Abnormal blood viscosity has also been implicated in the aetiology of retinal vein occlusion, leading to investigation into the role of troxerutin, an inhibitor of platelet and red cell aggregation.[17] Fifty-three patients were included in a prospective, randomised double-masked controlled trial, of whom 27 had central vein occlusion and 26 had branch vein occlusion. A total of 20 women and 33 men were included, ranging in age from 36 to 85 years. Methods for randomisation were not specified. At two years, a significant improvement was seen in the treatment group, both in terms of visual acuity and decrease in macular oedema. No complications of the treatment were described.

Comment

Anticoagulants (such as heparin), fibrinolytic agents (such as streptokinase and tissue plasminogen activator) and antiplatelet drugs (such as aspirin, prostacyclin, and ticlopidine) would seem to be logical treatments, but results from trials have been disappointing, with limited evidence of benefit owing to adverse effects of retinal and vitreous haemorrhage. To date these trials have been small, and have used a variety of follow up periods and outcome measures. Some authorities advocate the use of steroids in CRVO in the younger age group, but there is no published evidence to support this.

Question

Do patients with BRVO or CRVO experience a better visual outcome and/or less neovascular glaucoma when treated with haemodilution?

The evidence

Isovolaemic haemodilution is used to reduce blood viscosity, with the intention of improving retinal circulation. We found eight papers describing five randomised controlled trials of haemodilution in the management of retinal vein occlusion.[12,18–23] The main features of each trial are listed in Table 41.1.

The first of these randomised controlled trials, published in 1985,[18] compared the effect of isovolaemic haemodilution with and without prior xenon-arc panretinal photocoagulation on visual acuity following central retinal vein occlusion. Seven of the 17 patients who had haemodilution retained a better visual acuity at one year, compared with only one of 17 in the control group. The authors commented that the haemodilution seemed to be more effective in patients with ischaemic than with non-ischaemic CRVO.

The same group published another study[19] omitting the panretinal photocoagulation. Only non-ischaemic patients were investigated, so that the effect of haemodilution could be compared with no treatment. At one year, six out of 13 haemodiluted patients retained better visual acuity, compared with none of 11 control group patients.

Wolf *et al.* published a series of papers looking at the short-term,[20] intermediate-term[21] and long-term results[22] of haemodilution in 40 patients with central retinal vein occlusion. They performed a single-blind randomised prospective investigation, and found a statistically significant improvement in visual acuity at one year for the treated group compared with the control group.[21] This improvement was sustained after three years.[22] There was no statistically significant difference between the two groups in the progression to ischaemic central vein occlusion.

However, in 1996, Luckie *et al.*[12] published the results of a randomised controlled trial investigating the effect of haemodilution on 59 patients with central retinal vein occlusion, stating that the incidence rates for improvement in visual acuity and iris neovascularisation were not different between the treated and control groups. Moreover, this trial found that the incidence rate of deterioration in visual acuity was 5·3 times higher in the treated group.

Finally, the role of haemodilution in patients with reduced visual acuity secondary to branch retinal vein occlusion was investigated by Chen *et al.*,[23] who found a statistically significant difference in visual acuity at one year, with the treated group having a better outcome.

Table 41.1 Main features of RCTs of haemodilution in the management of RVO

Reference	No. of patients	Men/ Women	BRVO/ CRVO	Method of allocation	Interventions	Outcome measures
Hansen *et al.*, 1985[18]	38	Not specified	CRVO	Lottery system	Haemodilution Photocoagulation	Visual acuity
Hansen *et al.*, 1989[19]	25	12/13	CRVO	Lottery system	Haemodilution	Visual acuity
Wolf *et al.*, 1991[20], 1994[21], 1996[22]	40	Not specified	CRVO	Not specified	Haemodilution Placebo	Visual acuity
Luckie *et al.*, 1996[12]	59	37/22	CRVO	Sealed envelopes	Haemodilution	Visual acuity Rubeosis iridis
Chen *et al.*, 1998[23]	34	Not specified	BRVO	Consecutively numbered envelopes, lottery system	Haemodilution	Visual acuity Retinal appearance

Comment

Analysis of the available randomised trials shows the effects of haemodilution to be inconsistent, although results from further trials are awaited. Double-masked studies are not possible as "placebo haemodilution" cannot be performed. The procedure is not without complications, particularly in the elderly, and those with respiratory problems or ischaemic heart disease.

Question

Is it possible to ameliorate morbidity and mortality associated with retinal vein occlusion?

The evidence

Retinal vein occlusions are associated with an increase in vascular causes of death (both cerebral and cardiovascular) in large prospective follow up studies.[8,24] It is now proven that drug treatment of hypertension reduces the severity of its complications, and additional therapy of aspirin reduces the cardiovascular event rate.[8,24] Recent trials of reducing cholesterol levels using statins have shown reduction of cardiovascular morbidity and mortality.[8] The risk of future cardiovascular disease in retinal vein occlusion patients may be calculated using the Framingham algorithm, and this risk estimate may be used to guide decisions about preventive treatment for cardiovascular disease in these patients.[25] There is evidence for the roles of treatment of hypertension, lipid lowering and the regular use of aspirin in reducing morbidity from cardiovascular disease.

Question

Do patients with retinal vein occlusion experience a better visual outcome and/or less neovascular glaucoma with medical management of underlying systemic risk factors?

The evidence

This question is pertinent in cases of "pre-occlusive" retinal vein occlusion, sometimes referred to as "venous stasis". These patients should undergo medical investigation for underlying systemic risk factors and should be treated urgently, as it is potentially possible to prevent progression or to reverse the existing occlusion.[8] Antiplatelet agents may be of benefit. In exceptional circumstances other measures may be considered, but there is only anecdotal evidence of their benefit, and they may be potentially harmful.

Comment

In all cases of retinal vein occlusion, involvement of the fellow eye is a concern. Several studies have demonstrated that recurrence of retinal vein occlusion may occur in the affected eye or in the fellow eye in 9–15% of patients over a five-year follow up period.[1,8] In view of the poor potential visual outcome for patients with recurrent retinal vein occlusion, this aspect has been studied, but not in controlled trials. The available data support the concept that recurrence of retinal vein occlusion may be reduced by medical treatments of underlying cardiovascular risk factors with the addition of aspirin/persantin.

The evidence

Disc or retinal neovascularisation following BRVO is an indication for photocoagulation to the ischaemic retina (sector photocoagulation). The available evidence suggests that waiting until vitreous haemorrhage occurs before using laser treatment does not adversely affect the visual prognosis.

The two principal papers that provide this evidence come from the Branch Vein Occlusion Study Group[26] and Hayreh *et al.*[27] The Branch Vein Occlusion Study Group set up a randomised controlled trial to investigate the effect of argon laser scatter photocoagulation in branch vein occlusions in 316 patients. One hundred and seventy-three men and 146 women patients were randomised either to a treated group or an untreated control group by a computer-generated random allocation schedule issued by the study coordinator. Results from this study showed that there was significantly less neovascularisation and less vitreous haemorrhage in the treated eyes compared with the untreated group. This study suggested that peripheral scatter treatment should be applied after rather than before the development of neovascularisation.

These findings were confirmed in a second randomised controlled trial from Hayreh's group, who also looked at the effect of scatter photocoagulation on peripheral visual fields. Two hundred and seventy-one patients were allocated to treatment or no treatment using a random number table, and a follow up of five years was provided. This paper echoed the recommendations of treatment only following development of neovascularisation, particularly in view of their demonstration of the detrimental effects of photocoagulation on peripheral visual fields in this study.

Evidence supports the use of argon laser panretinal photocoagulation (PRP) when iris new vessels or angle new vessels are visible following central retinal vein occlusion.

The largest study investigating this treatment is from the Central Vein Occlusion Study group.[28] This was a multi-centre, randomised controlled clinical trial. Of a total of 725 patients recruited in the entire Central Vein Occlusion Study, 90 were assigned to receive immediate PRP and 91 to close observation with PRP only administered at the first sign of iris or angle neovascularisation. The patients ranged from 20 to 92 years with a mean age of 65, and were assigned using computer-generated random allocation. The results showed that prophylactic PRP did not totally prevent iris or angle neovascularisation, and that prompt regression of such neovascularisation was more likely to occur in eyes

that had not been treated previously. The study advised "frequent" follow up in the early months in all untreated patients with features of retinal ischaemia, including undilated iris examination and detailed examination of the angle by gonioscopy. In circumstances where regular follow up is impractical, prophylactic treatment may be appropriate.

The evidence

In the Branch Vein Occlusion Study Group publication,[29] 139 eyes were randomly assigned to laser treatment or no treatment using computer-generated random allocation. At three years treated patients had a gain of at least two lines of visual acuity from baseline. This led the group to recommend argon laser photocoagulation for macular oedema as described in the study.

In the same year, Shilling and Jones[30] found that treatment of macular oedema by laser in some patients did not significantly alter their visual prognosis. They investigated 90 patients in two groups (methods not specified); the first with macular oedema and a broken perifoveal capillary ring on fluorescein angiography, and the second with macular oedema and intact or broken perifoveal capillary rings. The research showed that treatment with argon laser photocoagulation to areas of retina with incompetent capillaries did not significantly improve the visual prognosis at one year, and that patients with an intact perifoveal arcade have a better visual prognosis than those with a broken arcade.

Patients with severe visual loss (less than 6/60 vision) are unlikely to benefit from laser treatment and those in whom symptoms have been present for more than a year are likely to have a limited benefit from photocoagulation.

A paper by Battaglia *et al.*[31] looked at grid pattern argon laser treatment specifically in macular branch vein occlusion, using 99 patients randomly assigned to control group, early grid at three months or delayed grid at six to 18 months. The mean age of the patients was 70 years, but no other population data were provided. Results showed that neither early nor delayed grid laser treatment reduced macular oedema more than the natural evolution, and visual acuity was not improved.

Macular oedema following CRVO causes visual loss but randomised controlled trials have failed to indicate benefit from grid treatment. The most important of these is the

Central Vein Occlusion Study Group M Report,[32] which looked at laser treatment for macular oedema in a subset of the 725 patients recruited to the main study. Computer-generated random assignment of 155 patients to grid treatment (77 patients) or to observation (78 patients) was used to examine the role of grid laser for macular oedema in perfused central vein occlusion. Visual acuity had to be 20/50 or worse, and macular oedema was judged using fluorescein angiography. Patients with non-perfusion were excluded. Interestingly, although the treatment reduced the angiographic evidence of macular oedema, there was no difference in visual acuity between the treated and untreated groups at any point during the three-year follow up period, and the study group therefore did not support macular grid photocoagulation for this population.

Chorioretinal anastomosis is an experimental treatment for improving retinal blood flow following CRVO. This technique shows promise but the results of randomised clinical trials are not yet available. Trials of other treatments such as optic nerve sheathotomy to improve retinal circulation and pars plana vitrectomy in the management of macular oedema are underway.

Implications for research

The literature search performed for this chapter reveals several areas requiring further evaluation. First, the role of rheologic factors in the aetiology of retinal vein occlusion, and their manipulation in management and prophylaxis needs further investigation. The role of steroids in young patients with central vein occlusion requires scientific evaluation. However, small numbers of patients, and favourable prognosis in a subset of these, will provide a challenge in study design. Surgical techniques of chorioretinal anastomosis, optic nerve sheathotomy and pars plana vitrectomy for macular oedema have all provided some preliminary results that show promise, and require larger randomised controlled trials to complete their evaluation.

Implications for practice

The evidence presented in this chapter may have some impact on current management of retinal vein occlusions. In the first instance, the available data on the effect of haemodilution suggest that this treatment may be suitable for some patients in some cases. Patients who are medically fit, with vein occlusion affecting only one eye could be considered, and experienced advice may need to be sought. Secondly, the timing and indications for scatter treatment both in branch and central vein occlusions vary in different units around the country. This also applies to the frequency of follow up of newly diagnosed cases. The evidence base provides guidelines for practice in these situations.

Acknowledgements

This chapter was written with the help of the Royal College of Ophthalmologists Vein Occlusion Study Group, in particular Mr John Shilling (Consultant, St Thomas' Hospital) and Dr Paul Dodson (Consultant, Birmingham Heartlands Hospital).

References

1. Hayreh SS, Zimmerman MB, Podhajsky P. Incidence of various types of retinal vein occlusion and their recurrence and demographic characteristics. *Am J Ophthalmol* 1994;**117**:429–41.
2. Mitchell P Smith W, Chang A. Prevalence and associations of retinal vein occlusion in Australia. *Arch Ophthalmol* 1996;**114**(10):1243–7.
3. The Eye Disease Case-control study group. Risk factors for branch retinal vein occlusion. *Am J Ophthalmol* 1993;**116**(3):286–96.
4. Elman MJ, Bhatt AK, Quinlan PM, Enger C. The risk for systemic vascular diseases and mortality in patients with central retinal vein occlusion. *Ophthalmology* 1990;**97**(11):1543–8.
5. The Eye Disease Case-control study group. Risk factors for central retinal vein occlusion. *Arch Ophthalmol* 1996;**114**(5):545–54.
6. Dodson PM, Galton DJ, Hamilton AM, Blach RK. Retinal vein occlusion and the prevalence of lipoprotein abnormalities. *Br J Ophthalmol* 1982;**66**(3):161–4.
7. Dodson PM, Kritzinger EE, Clough CG. Diabetes mellitus and retinal vein occlusion in patents of Asian, West Indian and white European origin. *Eye* 1992;**6**:66–8.
8. Dodson PM, Kritzinger EE. Medical cardiovascular treatment trials: relevant to medical ophthalmology in 1997? *Eye* 1997;**11**:3–11.
9. Fegan CD. Central retinal vein occlusion and thrombophilia. *Eye* 2002;**11**:98–106.
10. Kirwan JF, Tsaloumas MD, Vinall H, Prior P, Kritzinger EE, Dodson PM. Sex hormone preparations and retinal vein occlusion. *Eye* 1997;**11**:53–6.
11. Dodson PM, Kritzinger EE. Underlying medical conditions in young patients and ethnic differences in retinal vein occlusion. *Trans Ophthalmol Soc UK* 1985;**104**(2):114–19.
12. Luckie AP, Wroblewski JJ, Hamilton P *et al.* A randomised prospective study of outpatient haemodilution for central retinal vein obstruction. *Aust NZ J Ophthalmol* 1996;**24**(3):223–32.
13. Rubenstein K, Jones EB. Retinal vein occlusion: long term prospects. *Br J Ophthalmol* 1976;**60**:148–50.
14. Hohmann R, Martin M, Weigelin E. Fibrinolysis in retinal vein occlusions. A preliminary report. *Graefe's Arch Clin Exp Ophthalmol* 1973;**187**(4):327–40.
15. Kohner EM, Hamilton AM, Bulpitt CJ, Dollery CT. Streptokinase in the treatment of central retinal vein occlusion. A controlled trial. *Trans Ophthalmol Soc UK* 1974;**94**(2):599–603.
16. Houtsmuller AJ, Vermeulen JA, Klompe M *et al.* The influence of ticlopidine on the natural course of retinal vein occlusion. *Agents Actions Suppl* 1984;**15**:219–29.
17. Glacet Bernard A, Coscas G, Chabanel A, Zourdani A, Lelong F, Samama MM. A randomised, double-masked study on the treatment of retinal vein occlusion with troxerutin. *Am J Ophthalmol* 1994;**118**(4):421–9.
18. Hansen LL, Danisevskis P, Arntz HR, Hovener G, Wiederholt M. A randomised prospective study on treatment of central retinal vein occlusion by isovolaemic haemodilution and photocoagulation. *Br J Ophthalmol* 1985;**69**(2):108–16.

19. Hansen LL, Weik J, Wiederholt M. A randomised prospective study of treatment of non-ischaemic central retinal vein occlusion by isovolaemic haemodilution. *Br J Ophthalmol* 1989;**73**(11):895–9.

20. Wolf S, Arend O, Bertram B *et al.* [Haemodilution in patients with central retinal vein thrombosis. A placebo-controlled randomised study]. *Fortschr Ophthalmol* 1991;**88**(1):35–43.

21. Wolf S, Arend O, Bertram B, Remky A, Schulte K, Wald KJ, Reim M. Haemodilution therapy in central retinal vein occlusion. One year results of a prospective randomised study. *Graefe's Arch Clin Exp Ophthalmol* 1994;**232**(1):33–9.

22. Wolf S, Arend O, Bertram B, Knabben H, Reim M. Long term results after haemodilution therapy in central retinal vein occlusion. *Clin Hemorheol* 1996;**16**(3):357–65.

23. Chen HC, Wiek J, Gupta A, Luckie A, Kohner EM. Effect of isovolaemic haemodilution on visual outcome in branch retinal vein occlusion. *Br J Ophthalmol* 1998;**82**(2):162–7.

24. Tsaloumas MD, Kirwan J, Vinall H *et al.* Nine year follow-up study of morbidity and mortality in retinal vein occlusion. *Eye* 2000;**14**: 821–7.

25. Martin SC, Butcher A, Martin N *et al.* Cardiovascular risk assessment in patients with retinal vein occlusion. *Br J Ophthalmol* 2002;**86**: 774–6.

26. Branch Vein Occlusion Study Group. Argon laser scatter photocoagulation for prevention of neovascularisation and vitreous haemorrhage in branch vein occlusion. A randomised clinical trial. *Arch Ophthalmol* 1986;**104**(1):34–41.

27. Hayreh SS, Rubenstein L, Podhajsky P. Argon laser scatter photocoagulation in treatment of branch retinal vein occlusion. A prospective clinical trial. *Ophthalmology* 1993;**206**(1):1–14.

28. Central Vein Occlusion Study Group. A randomised clinical trial of early panretinal photocoagulation for ischaemic central vein occlusion. The Central Vein Occlusion Study Group N report. *Ophthalmology* 1995;**102**(10):1434–44.

29. Branch Vein Occlusion Study Group. Argon laser photocoagulation for macular edema in branch vein occlusion. *Am J Ophthalmol* 1984;**98**(3):271–82.

30. Shilling JS, Jones CA. Retinal branch vein occlusion: A study of argon laser photocoagulation in the treatment of macular oedema. *Br J Ophthalmol* 1984;**68**(3):196–8.

31. Battaglia Parodi M, Saviano SD, Ravalico G. Grid laser treatment in macular branch retinal vein occlusion. *Graefe's Arch Clin Exp Ophthalmol* 1999;**237**(12):1024–7.

32. Central Vein Occlusion Study Group. Evaluation of grid pattern photocoagulation for macular oedema in central vein occlusion. The Central Vein Occlusion Study Group M report. *Ophthalmology* 1995;**102**(10):1425–33.

Section X

Diabetic retinopathy

Bernd Richter, Editor

Diabetic retinopathy: mission statement

Diabetic retinopathy is the most frequent cause of visual loss in the working age population, even though laser treatment has been available for almost three decades. The risk of retinopathy is directly related to the degree and duration of hyperglycaemia.

For both type 1 and type 2 diabetic patients, strict metabolic control has been shown to reduce the incidence and progression of early retinopathy. Intensive therapy of elevated blood pressure, using atenolol or captopril, reduces diabetic retinopathy progression and decreases diabetes-related death and stroke in type 2 diabetes.

Laser treatment is effective in treating high risk proliferative diabetic retinopathy and clinical significant macular oedema.

Diabetic patients with vitreous haemorrhage and active fibrovascular proliferation profit from early vitrectomy.

Retinal photography with mydriasis appears to be the most effective strategy for screening for diabetic retinopathy. Though annual screening is proposed in guidelines, data for screening intervals are conflicting, suggesting individualised approaches especially in high risk patients.

With the exception of antiplatelet agents which are not contraindicated in people with retinopathy when used to prevent macrovascular disease, no other pharmacotherapy slows progression of retinopathy. Several clinical trials in progress may find newer more effective therapies to prevent visual loss.

42 Medical interventions for diabetic retinopathy

Bernd Richter, Eva Kohner

Background

Diabetic retinopathy is a highly specific vascular complication of both type 1 and type 2 diabetes mellitus. Overall, diabetic retinopathy is estimated to be the most frequent cause of new blindness among adults aged 20–74 years, especially in the young-onset, type 1 group.[1] The risk of retinopathy is directly related to the degree and duration of hyperglycaemia.[2]

Definition/classification

Patients whose eyes have microaneurysms only, with or without associated retinal oedema, are classified as having mild, non-proliferative diabetic retinopathy. A patient is classified as having moderate or severe non-proliferative diabetic retinopathy, depending mostly on the extent and severity of intraretinal microvascular abnormalities, intraretinal haemorrhage and venous beading.[3]

Proliferative diabetic retinopathy is defined as the presence of new vessels on the surface of the retina or optic disc. Patients with neovascularisation of the disc progress more rapidly and therefore have a worse prognosis.[3–5]

Prevalence/incidence

In the Wisconsin Epidemiologic Study of Diabetic Retinopathy (WESDR) the frequency of any visual impairment in people with diabetes was 7·8%.[6] In the clinic-based Insulin-Dependent Diabetes Mellitus Patients in Europe (EURODIAB IDDM) Complications Study, 2·3% of patients aged 15 to 50 years were blind. In a sample of African Americans with type 1 diabetes obtained from hospital admissions in New Jersey, 11% were visually impaired and 3·1% of patients were legally blind.[7–9]

The prevalence of blindness due to diabetic retinopathy was similar for African Americans (5%) and Caucasians (6%) with type 2 diabetes in the population-based Baltimore Eye Study, although the rate of visual impairment was higher in African Americans.[10]

In the WESDR, the estimated annual incidence rate of blindness due to diabetes was 3·3 per 100 000 population. In all groups, the frequency of macular oedema increased with increasing duration of diabetes.[11]

Aetiology/predictors/risk factors

Loss of vision due to retinopathy is more likely to be associated with proliferative retinopathy in type 1 diabetes and with macular oedema in type 2 diabetes.

In the main randomised controlled trial, the United Kingdom Prospective Diabetes Study (UKPDS), risk factors were assessed after three months' diet from the time of diagnosis of diabetes.[12] By six years 22% of 1919 patients with no retinopathy had developed retinopathy – that is, microaneurysms in both eyes or worse.

Development of retinopathy (incidence) was strongly associated with baseline glycaemia, glycaemic exposure over six years, higher blood pressure and with not smoking.

Microaneurysms are important predictive lesions for progression of diabetic retinopathy. Six years after diagnosis, 5·6% of type 2 diabetes patients with five or more microaneurysms had photocoagulation or vitreous haemorrhage.[13–15]

Data from epidemiologic studies suggest the following important predictors of progression of retinopathy.

- **Metabolic control**: elevated glycated haemoglobin and the glycaemic exposure over time are strongly related to the incidence and progression of diabetic retinopathy in people with type 1 and type 2 diabetes.[16–18]
- **Ethnicity**: data from several studies are conflicting but a nationwide US population-based study revealed greater prevalences of diabetic retinopathy in non-Hispanic African Americans (27%) and Mexican Americans (33%) than in non-Hispanic Caucasians (18%).[19]
- **Duration of diabetes and age**: diabetic retinopathy is rare before the age of 10 years, regardless of the duration of diabetes. Vision-threatening retinopathy is not observed under age 15 and affects 2·5% of people aged 15–19.[20]
- **Elevated blood pressure**: elevated blood pressure is an independent risk factor for any retinopathy, macular oedema and loss of vision in both type 1 and type 2 diabetes.[21–24]

- **Lipids:** lipid deposits, especially when they are beneath the centre of the macula, are associated with retinal damage and permanent loss of vision.[25] The extent of these lipid deposits is correlated with serum lipid concentrations.[26,27] In the Diabetes Control and Complications Trial (DCCT) and the Early Treatment Diabetic Retinopathy Research Study (ETDRS) elevated serum cholesterol was related to the development and severity of retinal hard exudates in the macula or the risk of visual loss (50% increase of relative risk (RR) when comparing serum cholesterol of less and more than 6·3 mmol/l at baseline).[28,29] Interestingly, in the UKPDS there was no relationship between hard exudates, macular oedema and serum cholesterol (personal communication).
- **Pregnancy:** pregnancy is an independent risk factor for retinopathy progression with patients at greatest risk who have the poorest control at baseline, the largest improvement in glycaemic control during early pregnancy, hypertension and pre-eclampsia.[30–32] Adverse outcomes in delivery are especially predicted by the severity of diabetic retinopathy in the first trimester.[33]
- **Cigarette smoking/alcohol:** neither cigarette smoking nor alcohol consumption appear to be independent risk factors for retinopathy.[34,35] The UKPDS established an association of reduced incidence of retinopathy with current smoker status (odds ratio (OR) for retinopathy 0·63, 95% CI 0·48–0·82).[36]

Prognosis

The baseline severity of retinopathy strongly predicts the prognosis. Untreated eyes with high-risk proliferative retinopathy are at very high risk of blindness.[37,38]

The natural history of the development of sight-threatening retinopathy is approximately constant from discovery of any retinopathy[36]: one third of those with retinopathy of more than microaneurysms progress to photocoagulation by 12 years.

Question

What is the effect of diabetes control in preventing/treating diabetic retinopathy?

The evidence

In the DCCT, 1441 patients with type 1 diabetes (726 with no retinopathy, 715 with mild-to-moderate non-proliferative retinopathy at baseline) were randomly assigned to receive either intensive or conventional insulin

therapy. The mean follow up was 6·5 years. There was a reduction in the rate of the development or progression of retinopathy, diabetic nephropathy and neuropathy among patients assigned to intensive treatment.[39] For development of serious retinopathy the number needed to treat (NNT) 5 years was 4 (95% CI 2–20).

In the UKPDS, of 3867 newly diagnosed type 2 diabetes patients, 2729 patient were randomly assigned to intensive treatment aiming for fasting plasma glucose levels less than 6 mmol/l and 1138 patients were allocated to conventional dietary treatment aiming at fasting plasma glucose levels less than 15 mmol/l without hyperglycaemic symptoms. Most of the relative risk reduction in the main outcome "any diabetes-related aggregate end-point" ($NNT_{10years}$ 20, 95% CI 10–500) was due to a 25% relative risk reduction (RR 7–40, P = 0·0099) in microvascular end-points, including the need for retinal photocoagulation.

Comment

Improved glycaemic control is associated with fewer microvascular end-points. This is in concordance with observational studies, implicating hyperglycaemia in the development of chronic microvascular complications of diabetes.

Question

Is there an association between rapid improvement of glycaemic control and progression of diabetic retinopathy?

The evidence

When intensive treatment is to be instituted in patients who have proliferative or severe non-proliferative retinopathy, ophthalmological consultation is desirable because photocoagulation may be indicated. Better control of hyperglycaemia lowers but does not eliminate the risk of retinopathy and other complications of diabetes. The DCCT[39] and other investigators[40] have shown that early deterioration of retinopathy at the time of normoglycaemic re-entry is possible. This deterioration was most marked in those with more advanced retinopathy.[29,41]

Comment

It appears that patients with proliferative retinopathy should be treated simultaneously with photocoagulation and intensified insulin therapy and have to be followed up carefully.[42]

The evidence

In the UKPDS, all patients had their blood pressure checked at three-monthly intervals, and 22% were part of the blood pressure control study, two thirds of whom had tight control of their blood pressure.[24] A total of 1148 patients with type 2 diabetes and hypertension were stratified for presence or absence of previous hypertensive treatment, while 758 patients were allocated to tight blood pressure control aiming for a blood pressure of less than 150/85 mmHg by first-line use of captopril or atenolol. Tight blood pressure control reduced the risk for diabetes-related complications or death, stroke and microvascular disease. The $NNT_{10years}$ for any complication was six (95% CI 3–10) and a 35% relative reduction of risk of retinal photocoagulation was observed ($P = 0.023$).

Comment

Type 2 diabetes patients with hypertension and tight blood pressure control have a reduced risk of developing a diabetes-related clinical end-point, diabetes-related death, stroke and microvascular disease. This treatment is also cost-effective.

The evidence

A directive to reduce visual loss and blindness as a result of diabetes was embodied in the St Vincent Declaration of 1989.[43] Diabetic retinopathy screening appears to offer a chance to reduce this major cause of blindness and partial sightedness in the working age group. A systematic review of the English language literature on screening and monitoring tests for diabetic retinopathy identified 22 prospective cohort studies comparing the screening method with a reference standard in a masked fashion.[44] No randomised controlled trial could be identified and no formal meta-analysis was carried out.

Comment

The British Diabetic Association has proposed levels of at least 80% sensitivity and 95% specificity for screening tests

for diabetic retinopathy,[45] which was used as the basis for assessing the effectiveness of the screening/monitoring tests in the systematic review. The authors concluded that retinal photography with mydriasis is the most effective strategy for screening. This is supported by an older systematic review/meta-analysis and other investigators.[46–48]

Direct ophthalmoscopy alone is inadequate with a sensitivity below 80% in most of the studies across all professional groups. Non-mydriatic polaroid prints achieved a poor detection rate of 56% even for sight-threatening diabetic retinopathy. The reviewers could not adequately address the question of the value of undertaking an examination of visual acuity in screening, who should perform the screening and where the screening should be carried out.

The evidence

A recent consensus document advised that diabetic patients should have annual screening for retinopathy.[49] In the UKPDS cohort any patient with type 2 diabetes and little or no retinopathy was unlikely to progress to the need for photocoagulation for several years.[36] If eyes were clear of retinopathy (or had only minimal lesions) the risk of progression to photocoagulation was slight (2/1000 patients in three years), provided blood pressure and glycaemia are under control. Such patients could be re-screened after three years.[50,51] Moreover, on the basis of cost-effectiveness Vijan *et al.* suggested that screening should be tailored to the patients needs, rather than screening everybody annually.[50,51]

Comment

Retinal photography with mydriases is the preferred screening modality with less reliance on the status of the observer. There are conflicting data for screening intervals, which should probably be individualised, especially in high-risk patients.

Several systematic reviews/meta-analyses were performed on screening modalities indicating that retinal photography with mydriasis should form the basis of any formal screening programme. No study has clearly shown a decrease in blindness incidence directly attributable to a retinopathy screening programme. There are no adequate data to reach a definite conclusion either on screening intervals or the effects of screening itself, both of which currently have to be estimated by reliance on competing models. Since critical factors for any screening programme's effectiveness are prevalence of treatable disease among screened patients, test validity and treatment effectiveness, efficiency may be increased by tailoring screening to the patients' needs and risk profile.

Question

What are the effects of pharmacological interventions for diabetic retinopathy?

The evidence

No systematic review on the effects of pharmacological treatments for diabetic retinopathy could be found. A number of randomised controlled trials investigating various drugs were found. At present, there is no firm evidence for the value of any drug, mainly because the studies have been too small, of poor quality and the assessments have often been subjective and not independent from the observers. These trials are summarised in Tables 42.1 and 42.2. Only the calcium dobesilate, aldose reductase inhibitors (ARIs) and lisinopril trials had more than 100 participants.

Pharmacological interventions

Aldose reductase inhibitors (sorbinil, tolrestat and ponalrestat)

In seven randomised controlled trials (six of double-blind design) 56 patients were treated with aldolase reductase inhibitors (ARIs). Aldose reductase facilitates the conversion of glucose to sorbitol, which accumulates in cells during hyperglycaemia and may result in cell death.[52–58] Only one study provided a power calculation. One trial with a topical ARI reported significant differences in reversion of reduced corneal sensitivity and abnormal morphological characteristics of corneal epithelial cells.

Angiotensin converting enzyme inhibitors (lisinopril)

A randomised double-blind trial of lisinopril suggested that inhibition of this enzyme or blood pressure lowering, even in non-hypertensive patients, may slow the progression of diabetic retinopathy.[59] The primary end-point was the urinary albumin excretion rate. The authors also provided a power calculation for the secondary end-point – retinopathy (80% power to detect a reduction in

retinopathy progression from 24% on placebo to 10% on lisinopril).

The HbA_{1c} adjusted odds ratio for progression to proliferative retinopathy was 0·20 (95% CI 0·04–0·91) in favour of lisinopril versus placebo (calculated $NNT_{2years} = 19$). The Diabetic Retinopathy Candesartan Trials (DIRECT) large scale study is now in progress to confirm these findings. DIRECT consists of three randomised, double-masked, parallel, placebo controlled to determine the impact of treatment with candesartan on diabetic retinopathy. It is anticipated that it will be completed in 2004.

Data from the UKPDS suggest that the blood pressure lowering rather than a specific retinal vascular response to the inhibition of angiotensin-converting enzyme may be responsible for slowing the progression of retinopathy, as both captopril and atenolol (a beta-adrenergic antagonist) slowed the progression of retinopathy equally well.[60,61]

Antioxidants

In one controlled clinical trial the effects of buckwheat herbs, ruscus extract and troxerutin were compared with each other.[62] The study had no power calculation and did not supply relevant statistics. Vitamin E was given to 36 patients in one randomised double-blind trial and resulted in improved retinal haemodynamics.[63] The study provided a power calculation.

Antiplatelet agents

A systematic review of randomised controlled trials of aspirin therapy in people with diabetic retinopathy concluded that the treatment with aspirin did not affect the progression of retinopathy, the risk of visual loss or the risk of vitreous haemorrhage among patients with proliferative retinopathy.[64] It concluded that there are no ocular contraindications to taking aspirin if required as part of a treatment for cardiovascular diseases[65] or other medical indications.

Ticlopidine was investigated in two randomised double-blind studies administering 500 mg ticlopidine per day for three years to 269 patients.[66,67] The larger trial[67] reported a significant decrease in the number of definite microaneurysms, weighted for angiographic quality (0·48 ± 5·79 microaneurysms per year in the ticlopidine versus 1·44 ± 4·67 in the placebo group, $P = 0·03$). Thirteen per cent of patients receiving ticlopidine had to discontinue treatment due to adverse effects. Neither study provided a power calculation.

Calcium dobesilate

In eight randomised or controlled clinical trials (seven of double-blind design) around 280 patients received calcium

Table 42.1 Key features of randomised controlled trials with less than 100 patients investigating the treatment of diabetic retinopathy in type 1 or type 2 diabetes patients

Drug	No. of studies	No. of patients*	Dose**	Duration	Drop-out rate*	Efficacy	Adverse reaction rate*
Clofibrate	1	15	2000 mg	24 months	20%	No significant effect	?
Cyclandelate	2	25	1600 mg	3–12 months	8%***	No significant effect	0–17%
Danaparoid sodium	2	21	750 anti-Xa units s.c.	1·5–2 months	0–8%	No significant effect	Up to 42%[1]
Factor VIII derivative	1	15	1 mg	6 months	10%	No significant effect	Nil
Gingko biloba	1	14	160 mg	6 months	24%	Significant ($P=0.046$) improvement of colour vision in patients without retinal ischaemia	?
Methandienone	1	44	10 mg	12 months	21%	No significant effect	27%
Naftidrofuryl	1	23	600 mg	6 months	30%	Significant differences ($P<0.05$) no. of microaneurysms/ retinal bleeding	4%
Octreotide	2	21	400–5000 micrograms s.c	12–15 months	4–36%	No significant effect	Up to 29%***
Pentoxifylline	1	5	2000 mg	3 months	?	No significant effect	?
Sulindac	1	12	400 mg	6 months	?	Improvements in the blood–retina barrier	?
Troxerutin, ruscus extract, buckwheat	1	20 in all groups	?	3 months	0%	No significant effect	?
Vitamin E	1	36	1800 IU	4 months	31%	Significant ($P<0.001$) increase in retinal blood flow	11%

*Data are shown for active compound only.
** Total daily dose.
***Only one study provided data.

dobesilate (an "angioprotective" agent, thought to reduce microvascular hyperpermeability)[68–74] No study provided a power calculation. Two studies reported "significant" differences, for example, in microaneurysms, haemorrhages or capillary hyperpermeability, but did not supply the relevant statistics.

Clofibrate

One randomised double-blind trial in 15 patients investigated clofibrate (a blood lipid reducing agent).[75] The study did not provide a power calculation.

Cyclandelate

Two randomised double-blind trials investigated the effects of cyclandelate (a compound thought to have stabilising effects on the blood–retinal barrier; its metabolites could also have ARI-inhibiting activities) in 25 patients.[76,77] Neither study reported a power calculation.

Table 42.2 Key features of randomised controlled trials with more than 100 patients investigating the treatment of diabetic retinopathy in type 1 or type 2 diabetes patients

Drug	No. of studies	No. of patients*	Dose**	Duration	Drop-out rate*	Efficacy	Adverse reaction rate*
Aldose reductase enzyme inhibitors (ARIs)							
Ponalrestat	2	45	600 mg	6–18 months	0–16%	No significant effect	?
Sorbinil	3	268	250 mg	1–30 months	0–33%	No significant effect	Up to 14%
Tolrestat	1	14	200 mg	6 months	Nil	No significant effect	?
Topical AR	1	20	4×/die 0·5% suspension	6 months	?	Significant effects on surrogate outcomes	?
Angiotensin converting enzyme (ACE) inhibitors							
Lisinopril	1	202	10–20 mg	24 months	23%	Significant ($P=0·04$) difference in progression to proliferative retinopathy	?
Calcium dobesilate							
Calcium dobesilate	8	approx. 280	750–1500 mg	6–24 months	8–41%	No significant effect	up to 27%[†]

*Data are shown for active compound only.
**Total daily dose.
[†]Only one study provided data.

Danaparoid sodium

Two trials investigated the effects of danaparoid sodium (a mixture of glycosaminoglycans consisting mainly of heparan sulfate, thought to induce a regression of retinal hard exudates) in 21 patients.[78,79] Both studies had a randomised double-blind design, and one early report provided a retrospective analysis of the trial. One study supplied a power calculation.

Factor VIII

Bovine factor VIII derivative (thought to have positive effects on capillary basement membranes and on vascular endothelium) was given to 15 patients in one randomised double-blind trial.[80] The study had no power calculation.

Gingko biloba

In one randomised double-blind trial 14 patients were treated with gingko biloba (a medicine thought to protect cell membranes in retinopathy and have oedema-reducing efficacy).[81] The study had no power calculation. Due to multiple comparisons in a small group of patients the partly significant study results have to be interpreted with caution.

Methandienone

In one randomised single-blind study 44 patients received methandienone (an anabolic steroid that can be given by mouth).[82] The study had no power calculation.

Naftidrofuryl

In one randomised double-blind trial 23 patients were treated with naftidrofuryl (a compound thought to reduce platelet aggregation as well as influence plasticity of erythrocytes).[83] The authors reported a low *post hoc* power estimation of 50%.

Pentoxifylline

One randomised double-blind trial in five patients investigated pentoxifylline (a methylxanthine thought to improve blood flow velocity and blood viscosity).[84] No power calculation was reported. Some significant differences for retinal capillary blood velocity were shown.

Somatostatin analogues

In two randomised controlled pilot trials the use of octreotide (a growth hormone inhibiting somatostatin analogue with antiproliferative effects) was explored in 21 patients.[85,86] No study reported a power calculation. Large-scale studies on the efficacy of somatostatin analogues are in progress.

Sulindac

One randomised double-blind trial examined the use of sulindac in 12 patients.[87] No power calculation was performed.

Comment

At the moment, pharmacological therapy of diabetic retinopathy does not appear to be useful with regard to relevant end-points, such as progression of retinopathy. Better therapeutic principles have to be discovered (for example, trials investigating inhibition of protein kinase $C_{\beta 2}$[88] are in progress) and well assessed in adequately powered trials.

Summary

Thirty-six studies investigated 20 different compounds thought to influence the course of diabetic retinopathy. Approximately half of the trials was performed with calcium dobesilate or aldose reductase inhibitors. With the exception of antiplatelet agents around 1100 patients were investigated for a maximum of two and a half years showing no significant effects of pharmacotherapy for diabetic retinopathy.

Implications for practice

Improved glycaemic control is associated with fewer microvascular end-points. Tight blood pressure control in type 2 diabetes patients reduces several diabetes-related end-points as well as microvascular disease. There are no ocular contraindications to aspirin if required for medical indications. At the moment, any other pharmacological therapy of diabetic retinopathy does not appear useful with regard to relevant clinical end-points.

Implications for research

Randomised controlled, high-quality long-term trials of adequate power investigating new therapeutic principles should focus on patient-oriented outcomes, such as prevention or progression of retinopathy, and health-related quality of life and costs.

References

1. Klein R, Klein BEK. Vision disorders in diabetes. In: *Diabetes in America. 2nd edn.* Washington: National Diabetes Data Group, National Institute of Diabetes and Digestive and Kidney Diseases, National Institutes of Health, 1995, pp. 293–338.
2. Klein R, Klein BE, Moss SE. The Wisconsin epidemiological study of diabetic retinopathy: a review. *Diabetes Metab Rev* 1989;**5**:559–70.
3. Early Treatment Diabetic Retinopathy Study Research Group. Fundus photographic risk factors for progression of diabetic retinopathy. ETDRS report number 12. *Ophthalmology* 1991;**98**:823–33.
4. Early Treatment Diabetic Retinopathy Study Research Group. Grading diabetic retinopathy from stereoscopic color fundus photographs – an extension of the modified Airlie House classification. ETDRS report number 10. *Ophthalmology* 1991;**98**: 786–806.
5. Rand LI, Prud'homme GJ, Ederer F, Canner PL. Factors influencing the development of visual loss in advanced diabetic retinopathy. Diabetic Retinopathy Study (DRS) Report No. 10. *Invest Ophthalmol Vis Sci* 1985;**26**:983–91.
6. Klein R, Klein BE, Moss SE. Visual impairment in diabetes. *Ophthalmology* 1984;**91**:1–9.
7. Roy MS. Diabetic retinopathy in African Americans with type 1 diabetes: The New Jersey 725: II. Risk factors. *Arch Ophthalmol* 2000;**118**:105–15.
8. Sjolie AK, Stephenson J, Aldington S *et al.* Retinopathy and vision loss in insulin-dependent diabetes in Europe. The EURODIAB IDDM Complications Study. *Ophthalmology* 1997;**104**:252–60.
9. Klein R, Klein BE, Moss SE, Davis MD, DeMets DL. The Wisconsin epidemiologic study of diabetic retinopathy. III. Prevalence and risk of diabetic retinopathy when age at diagnosis is 30 or more years. *Arch Ophthalmol* 1984;**102**:527–32.
10. Tielsch JM, Sommer A, Witt K, Katz J, Royall RM. Blindness and visual impairment in an American urban population. The Baltimore Eye Survey. *Arch Ophthalmol* 1990;**108**:286–90.
11. Klein R, Klein BE, Moss SE, Davis MD, DeMets DL. The Wisconsin epidemiologic study of diabetic retinopathy. IV. Diabetic macular edema. *Ophthalmology* 1984;**91**:1464–74.
12. Stratton IM, Kohner EM, Aldington SJ *et al.* UKPDS 50: risk factors for incidence and progression of retinopathy in Type II diabetes over 6 years from diagnosis. *Diabetologia* 2001;**44**:156–63.
13. Kohner EM, Stratton IM, Aldington SJ, Turner RC, Matthews DR. Microaneurysms in the development of diabetic retinopathy (UKPDS 42). UK Prospective Diabetes Study Group. *Diabetologia* 1999;**42**: 1107–12.
14. Klein R, Meuer SM, Moss SE, Klein BE. The relationship of retinal microaneurysm counts to the 4-year progression of diabetic retinopathy. *Arch Ophthalmol* 1989;**107**:1780–5.
15. Klein R, Meuer SM, Moss SE, Klein BE. Retinal microaneurysm counts and 10-year progression of diabetic retinopathy. *Arch Ophthalmol* 1995;**113**:1386–91.
16. Reichard P. Risk factors for progression of microvascular complications in the Stockholm Diabetes Intervention Study (SDIS). *Diabetes Res Clin Pract* 1992;**16**:151–6.
17. UK Prospective Diabetes Study (UKPDS) Group. Intensive blood-glucose control with sulphonylureas or insulin compared with conventional treatment and risk of complications in patients with type 2 diabetes (UKPDS 33). *Lancet* 1998;**352**:837–53.
18. Anonymous. The relationship of glycemic exposure (HbA1c) to the risk of development and progression of retinopathy in the diabetes control and complications trial. *Diabetes* 1995;**44**:968–83.
19. Harris MI, Klein R, Cowie CC, Rowland M, Byrd-Holt DD. Is the risk of diabetic retinopathy greater in non-Hispanic blacks and Mexican Americans than in non-Hispanic whites with type 2 diabetes? A U.S. population study. *Diabetes Care* 1998;**21**:1230–5.
20. Klein R, Klein BEK, Moss SE. Severe retinopathy in insulin-taking children and young adults. *Pediatr Adolesc Endocrinol* 1988;**17**: 146–52.
21. Klein R, Moss SE, Klein BE, Davis MD, DeMets DL. The Wisconsin epidemiologic study of diabetic retinopathy. XI. The incidence of macular edema. *Ophthalmology* 1989;**96**:1501–10.

22. Klein R, Klein BE, Moss SE, Davis MD, DeMets DL. Is blood pressure a predictor of the incidence or progression of diabetic retinopathy? *Arch Intern Med* 1989;**149**:2427–32.

23. Stephenson JM, Fuller JH, Viberti GC, Sjolie AK, Navalesi R. Blood pressure, retinopathy and urinary albumin excretion in IDDM: the EURODIAB IDDM Complications Study. *Diabetologia* 1995;**38**: 599–603.

24. UK Prospective Diabetes Study Group. Tight blood pressure control and risk of macrovascular and microvascular complications in type 2 diabetes: UKPDS 38. *BMJ* 1998;**317**:703–13.

25. Sigurdsson R, Begg IS. Organised macular plaques in exudative diabetic maculopathy. *Br J Ophthalmol* 1980;**64**:392–7.

26. Chew EY, Klein ML, Ferris FL *et al.* Association of elevated serum lipid levels with retinal hard exudate in diabetic retinopathy. Early Treatment Diabetic Retinopathy Study (ETDRS) Report 22. *Arch Ophthalmol* 1996;**114**:1079–84.

27. Klein BE, Moss SE, Klein R, Surawicz TS. The Wisconsin Epidemiologic Study of Diabetic Retinopathy. XIII. Relationship of serum cholesterol to retinopathy and hard exudate. *Ophthalmology* 1991;**98**:1261–5.

28. Ferris FL, III, Chew EY, Hoogwerf BJ. Serum lipids and diabetic retinopathy. Early Treatment Diabetic Retinopathy Study Research Group. *Diabetes Care* 1996;**19**:1291–3.

29. Diabetes Control and Complications Trial Research Group. Progression of retinopathy with intensive versus conventional treatment in the Diabetes Control and Complications Trial. *Ophthalmology* 1995;**102**:647–61.

30. Klein BE, Moss SE, Klein R. Effect of pregnancy on progression of diabetic retinopathy. *Diabetes Care* 1990;**13**:34–40.

31. Rosenn B, Miodovnik M, Kranias G *et al.* Progression of diabetic retinopathy in pregnancy: association with hypertension in pregnancy. *Am J Obstet Gynecol* 1992;**166**:1214–18.

32. Lovestam-Adrian M, Agardh CD, Aberg A, Agardh E. Pre-eclampsia is a potent risk factor for deterioration of retinopathy during pregnancy in Type 1 diabetic patients. *Diabet Med* 1997;**14**:1059–65.

33. Klein BE, Klein R, Meuer SM, Moss SE, Dalton DD. Does the severity of diabetic retinopathy predict pregnancy outcome? *J Diabetes Complications* 1988;**2**:179–84.

34. Moss SE, Klein R, Klein BE. The association of alcohol consumption with the incidence and progression of diabetic retinopathy. *Ophthalmology* 1994;**101**:1962–8.

35. Moss SE, Klein R, Klein BE. Cigarette smoking and ten-year progression of diabetic retinopathy. *Ophthalmology* 1996;**103**:1438–42.

36. Kohner EM, Stratton IM, Aldington SJ, Holman RR, Matthews DR. Relationship between the severity of retinopathy and progression to photocoagulation in patients with Type 2 diabetes mellitus in the UKPDS (UKPDS 52). *Diabet Med* 2001;**18**:178–84.

37. Early Treatment Diabetic Retinopathy Study Research Group. Fundus photographic risk factors for progression of diabetic retinopathy. ETDRS report number 12. *Ophthalmology* 1991;**98**:823–33.

38. Davis MD, Fisher MR, Gangnon RE *et al.* Risk factors for high-risk proliferative diabetic retinopathy and severe visual loss: Early Treatment Diabetic Retinopathy Study Report 18. *Invest Ophthalmol Vis Sci* 1998;**39**:233–52.

39. The Diabetes Control and Complications Trial Research Group. The effect of intensive treatment of diabetes on the development and progression of long-term complications in insulin-dependent diabetes mellitus. *New Engl J Med* 1993;**329**:977–86.

40. Lauritzen T, Frost-Larsen K, Larsen HW, Deckert T. Effect of 1 year of near-normal blood glucose levels on retinopathy in insulin-dependent diabetics. *Lancet* 1983;**1**:200-4.

41. Anonymous. The effect of intensive diabetes treatment on the progression of diabetic retinopathy in insulin-dependent diabetes mellitus. The Diabetes Control and Complications Trial. *Arch Ophthalmol* 1995;**113**:36–51.

42. Chantelau E, Kohner EM. Why some cases of retinopathy worsen when diabetic control improves. *BMJ* 1997;**315**:1105–6.

43. Diabetes care and research in Europe: the Saint Vincent declaration. *Diabet Med* 1990;**7**:360.

44. Hutchinson A, McIntosh A, Peters J *et al.* Effectiveness of screening and monitoring tests for diabetic retinopathy – a systematic review. *Diabet Med* 2000;**17**:495–506.

45. British Diabetic Association. *Retinal photography screening for diabetic eye disease. A British Diabetic Association Report.* London: British Diabetic Association, 1997.

46. Bachmann MO, Nelson SJ. Impact of diabetic retinopathy screening on a British district population: case detection and blindness prevention in an evidence-based model. *J Epidemiol Community Health* 1998;**52**:45–52.

47. Harding SP, Broadbent DM, Neoh C, White MC, Vora J. Sensitivity and specificity of photography and direct ophthalmoscopy in screening for sight threatening eye disease: the Liverpool Diabetic Eye Study. *BMJ* 1995;**311**:1131–5.

48. Taylor R, Lovelock L, Tunbridge WM *et al.* Comparison of non-mydriatic retinal photography with ophthalmoscopy in 2159 patients: mobile retinal camera study. *BMJ* 1990;**301**:1243–7.

49. Porta M, Kohner E. Screening for diabetic retinopathy in Europe. *Diabet Med* 1991;**8**:197–8.

50. Vijan S, Kent DM, Hayward RA. Are randomized controlled trials sufficient evidence to guide clinical practice in type II (non-insulin-dependent) diabetes mellitus? *Diabetologia* 2000;**43**:125–30.

51. Vijan S, Hofer TP, Hayward RA. Cost-utility analysis of screening intervals for diabetic retinopathy in patients with type 2 diabetes mellitus. *JAMA* 2000;**283**:889–96.

52. Anonymous. A Randomized Trial of Sorbinil, an Aldose Reductase Inhibitor, in Diabetic Retinopathy. Sorbinil Retinopathy Trial Research Group. *Arch Ophthalmol* 1990;**108**:1234–44.

53. Arauz-Pacheco C, Ramirez LC, Pruneda L, Sanborn GE, Rosenstock J, Raskin P. The effect of the aldose reductase inhibitor, ponalrestat, on the progression of diabetic retinopathy. *J Diabetes Complications* 1992;**6**:131–7.

54. Biersdorf WR, Malone JI, Pavan PR, Lowitt S. Cone electroretinograms and visual acuities of diabetic patients on sorbinil treatment. *Doc Ophthalmol* 1988;**69**:247–54.

55. Cunha-Vaz JG, Mota CC, Leite EC, Abreu JR, Ruas MA. Effect of sorbinil on blood-retinal barrier in early diabetic retinopathy. *Diabetes* 1986;**35**:574–8.

56. Hosotani H, Ohashi Y, Yamada M, Tsubota K. Reversal of abnormal corneal epithelial cell morphologic characteristics and reduced corneal sensitivity in diabetic patients by aldose reductase inhibitor, CT-112. *Am J Ophthalmol* 1995;**119**:288–94.

57. Tromp A, Hooymans JM, Barendsen BC, van Doormaal JJ. The effects of an aldose reductase inhibitor on the progression of diabetic retinopathy. *Doc Ophthalmol* 1991;**78**:153–9.

58. van Gerven JM, Boot JP, Lemkes HH, van Best JA. Effects of aldose reductase inhibition with tolrestat on diabetic retinopathy in a six months double blind trial. *Doc Ophthalmol* 1994;**87**:355–65.

59. Chaturvedi N, Sjolie AK, Stephenson JM *et al.* Effect of lisinopril on progression of retinopathy in normotensive people with type 1 diabetes. The EUCLID Study Group. EURODIAB Controlled Trial of Lisinopril in Insulin-Dependent Diabetes Mellitus. *Lancet* 1998;**351**: 28–31.

60. UK Prospective Diabetes Study Group. Tight blood pressure control and risk of macrovascular and microvascular complications in type 2 diabetes: UKPDS 38. *BMJ* 1998;**317**:703–13.

61. UK Prospective Diabetes Study Group. Efficacy of atenolol and captopril in reducing risk of macrovascular and microvascular complications in type 2 diabetes: UKPDS 39. *BMJ* 1998;**317**:713–20.

62. Archimowicz CB. Clinical effect of buckwheat herb, Ruscus extract and troxerutin on retinopathy and lipids in diabetic patients. *Phytother Res* 1996;**10**:659–62.

63. Bursell SE, Clermont AC, Aiello LP *et al.* High-dose vitamin E supplementation normalizes retinal blood flow and creatinine clearance in patients with type 1 diabetes. *Diabetes Care* 1999;**22**: 1245–51.

64. Bergerhoff K, Clar C, Richter B. Aspirin in diabetic retinopathy – a systematic review. *Endocrinol Metab Clin North Am* 2002;**31**: 779–93.

65. ETDRS Investigators. Aspirin effects on mortality and morbidity in patients with diabetes mellitus. Early Treatment Diabetic Retinopathy Study report 14. *JAMA* 1992;**268**:1292–300.

66. Belgian Ticlopidine Retinopathy Study Group (BTRS). Clinical study of ticlopidine in diabetic retinopathy. *Ophthalmology* 1992;**204**:4–12.

67. The TIMAD Study Group. Ticlopidine treatment reduces the progression of nonproliferative diabetic retinopathy. *Arch Ophthalmol* 1990;**108**:1577–83.

68. Haas A. Effect of calcium dobesilate on progression of diabetic retinopathy. *Klin Monatsbl Augenheilkunde* 1995;**207**:17–21.

69. Vojnikovic B. Doxium (calcium dobesilate) reduces blood hyperviscosity and lowers elevated intraocular pressure in patients with diabetic retinopathy and glaucoma. *Ophthalmic Res* 1991;**23**: 12–20.

70. Salama Benarroch I, Nano H, Perez H, Elizalde F, Bisceglia H, Salama A. Assessment of calcium dobesilate in diabetic retinopathy. A double-blind clinical investigation. *Ophthalmology* 1977;**174**:47–51.

71. Daubresse JC, Meunier R, Dumont P. A controlled clinical trial of calcium dobesylate in the treatment of diabetic retinopathy. *Diabetes Metabol* 1977;**3**:27–30.

72. Freyler H. Microvascular protection with calcium dobesilate (Doxium) in diabetic retinopathy. *Ophthalmology* 1974;**168**:400–16.

73. Larsen HW, Sander E, Hoppe R. The value of calcium dobesilate in the treatment of diabetic retinopathy. A controlled clinical trial. *Diabetologia* 1977;**13**:105–9.

74. Stamper RL, Smith ME, Aronson SB *et al.* The effect of calcium dobesilate on nonproliferative diabetic retinopathy: a controlled study. *Ophthalmology* 1978;**85**:594–606.

75. Cullen JF, Town SM, Campbell CJ. Double-blind trial of Atromid-S in exudative diabetic retinopathy. *Trans Ophthalmol Soc UK* 1974;**94**:554–62.

76. Cunha-Vaz JG, Reis Fonseca J, Hagenouw JR. Treatment of early diabetic retinopathy with cyclandelate. *Br J Ophthalmol* 1977;**61**: 399–404.

77. Mota MC, Leite E, Ruas MA, Verjans HL, Blakemore CB, Cunha-Vaz JG. Effect of cyclospasmol on early diabetic retinopathy. *Int Ophthalmol* 1987;**10**:3–9.

78. van der Pijl JW, van der Woude FJ, Swart W, Van Es LA, Lemkes HH. Effect of danaparoid sodium on hard exudates in diabetic retinopathy. *Lancet* 1997;**350**:1743–5.

79. van der Pijl JW, Lemkes HH, Frolich M, van der Woude FJ, van der Meer FJ, Van Es LA. Effect of danaparoid sodium on proteinuria, von Willebrand factor, and hard exudates in patients with diabetes mellitus type 2. *J Am Soc Nephrol* 1999;**10**:1331–6.

80. Bandello F, Lattanzio R, Maestranzi G, Brancato R. Bovine factor VIII derivative in the treatment of non-proliferative diabetic retinopathy. *Ophthalmologica* 1995;**209**:149–54.

81. Lanthony P, Cosson JP. The course of color vision in early diabetic retinopathy treated with Ginkgo biloba extract. A preliminary double-blind versus placebo study. *J Fr Ophtalmol* 1988;**11**:671–4.

82. Hunter PR, Cotton SG, Kelsey JH, Bloom A. Controlled trial of methandienone in treatment of diabetic retinopathy. *BMJ* 1967;**3**: 651–3.

83. Klein M, Hirche H. Naftidrofuryl in the treatment of simple diabetic retinopathy. A double-blind study. *Klin Monatbl Augenheilkunde* 1985;**187**:195–201.

84. Sonkin PL, Kelly LW, Sinclair SH, Hatchell DL. Pentoxifylline increases retinal capillary blood flow velocity in patients with diabetes. *Arch Ophthalmol* 1993;**111**:1647–52.

85. Grant MB, Mames RN, Fitzgerald C *et al.* The efficacy of octreotide in the therapy of severe nonproliferative and early proliferative diabetic retinopathy: a randomized controlled study. *Diabetes Care* 2000;**23**:504–9.

86. Kirkegaard C, Norgaard K, Snorgaard O, Bek T, Larsen M, Lund-Andersen H. Effect of one year continuous subcutaneous infusion of a somatostatin analogue, octreotide, on early retinopathy, metabolic control and thyroid function in Type I (insulin-dependent) diabetes mellitus. *Acta Endocrinol* 1990;**122**:766–72.

87. Cunha-Vaz JG, Mota CC, Leite EC, Abreu JR, Ruas MA. Effect of sulindac on the permeability of the blood–retinal barrier in early diabetic retinopathy. *Arch Ophthalmol* 1985;**103**:1307–11.

88. Frank RN. Potential new medical therapies for diabetic retinopathy: protein kinase C inhibitors. *Am J Ophthalmol* 2002;**133**:693–8.

43 Photocoagulation for sight threatening diabetic retinopathy

Jonathan GF Dowler

Background

Definition

Sight threatening diabetic retinopathy takes two forms (see Box 43.1). Diabetic macular oedema involves thickening of the central retina (macula) associated with microvascular abnormalities caused by diabetes. There may be related deposition of lipid exudates, or cystic change at the centre of the macula. Proliferative diabetic retinopathy involves new blood vessels arising from the optic disc (new vessels disc, NVD), or from retinal vessels (new vessels elsewhere, NVE). These may give rise to haemorrhage into the vitreous gel, or retinal detachment.

Incidence/prevalence

In a probability sample of a Wisconsin population, the ten-year incidence of diabetic macular oedema was 14–25%,[1] and that of proliferative retinopathy 10–30%.[2] (See Table 43.1.)

Aetiology

In diabetic macular oedema hyperglycaemia causes injury to retinal microvasculature. Resulting leakage through or between retinal capillary endothelial cells results in extracellular fluid accumulation, retinal thickening and impaired function. Intracellular fluid accumulation and leakage through the retinal pigment epithelium may also contribute.

In proliferative diabetic retinopathy hyperglycaemia-induced changes to blood elements, vessel walls and flow causes occlusion of retinal capillaries. Enhanced production of growth factors by ischaemic retina appears to cause retinal capillary endothelial cell proliferation and new vessel formation.

Risk factors

Risk factors for more rapid retinopathy progression include longer duration of diabetes, type 1 and insulin treated type 2 diabetes, certain ethnicities, male sex, poor glycaemic or tightened glycaemic control, hypertension, renal dysfunction, pregnancy, and possibly cataract surgery, as well as specific ophthalmoscopic signs (see Box 43.2).

Prognosis

Diabetic retinopathy is the commonest cause of blindness in the working population of the western world and the commonest cause of preventable blindness in the UK. Prior to the advent of photocoagulation, the prognosis for vision was very poor.

Questions

1 In patients with proliferative diabetic retinopathy, does photocoagulation reduce the risk of visual loss?
2 In patients with diabetic macular oedema, does photocoagulation reduce the risk of visual loss?
3 In patients with diabetic retinopathy that has not reached the high risk proliferative stage, does photocoagulation (early treatment) reduce the risk of visual loss?
4 Does photocoagulation technique affect treatment outcome?

All randomised controlled trials found have been included. Smaller trials superseded by larger, better controlled trials were excluded.[3,4]

Question

In patients with proliferative diabetic retinopathy, does photocoagulation reduce the risk of visual loss?

The evidence

One large (n = 1758) multi-centre RCT of high quality, the Diabetic Retinopathy Study (DRS), was identified.[5] Patients with severe non-proliferative (NPDR) or proliferative diabetic retinopathy (PDR) in both eyes were included. Patients with visual acuity 6/30, those who had undergone

Box 43.1 Definitions

Clinically significant macular oedema: the clinical level at which macular/focal laser should be applied, being one of the following:

- Thickening of the retina at or within 500 microns of the fovea
- Hard exudates at or within 500 microns of the fovea if associated with retinal thickening
- A zone of retinal thickening 1 disc area or larger any part of which is within 1 disc diameter of fovea

High risk proliferative diabetic retinopathy: the clinical level at which panretinal/scatter laser should be applied for proliferative diabetic retinopathy, being one of the following:

- Moderate to severe optic disc new vessels
- Any grade of optic disc new vessels associated with preretinal or vitreous haemorrhage
- Moderate to severe new vessels elsewhere associated with preretinal or vitreous haemorrhage
- Non-proliferative diabetic retinopathy: retinopathy prior to the development of optic disc or retinal new vessels
- Focal/macular laser: laser treatment appropriate for macular oedema
- Scatter/panretinal laser: laser treatment appropriate for proliferative retinopathy

TABLE 43.1   Ten-year incidence of macular oedema and proliferative retinopathy in diabetes

Age diagnosed	Macular oedema (%)	Proliferative retinopathy (%)
Diagnosed at age less than 30 years	20	30
Diagnosed at age greater than 30 years, patient uses insulin	25	24
Diagnosed at age greater than 30 years, patient does not use insulin	14	10

Box 43.2 Risk factors for retinopathy progression

Patient attributes
- longer duration of diabetes
- diabetes type: type 1 > insulin treated type 2 > non-insulin treated type 2
- ethnicity
- male sex

Systemic status
- poor glycaemic control
- hypertension
- renal dysfunction

Specific risk factors
- tightening of glycaemic control
- pregnancy
- cataract surgery

Retinal signs
- extensive haemorrhage
- irregularity of venous calibre (venous beading)
- irregularly branching vascular structures (intraretinal microvascular abnormalities, IRMA)
- cotton wool spots

prior photocoagulation, and those in which photocoagulation was not possible, were excluded. One eye of each patient was assigned randomly to scatter (panretinal) photocoagulation, and the other to indefinite deferral of photocoagulation. The principal outcome variable was development of severe visual loss (visual acuity ≤1·5/60 on two successive visits). Severe visual loss occurred in 26% of untreated versus 12% of treated eyes with "high risk proliferative retinopathy" in two years (number needed to treat (NNT) 8, 95% CI 5–18).

Comment

This study established the benefit of panretinal photocoagulation for proliferative diabetic retinopathy. Quantum treatments were applied to eyes at specific high risk disease thresholds. Titrating the amount of treatment to the risk of visual loss might be equally valid.

Questions

In patients with diabetic macular oedema, does photocoagulation reduce the risk of visual loss?

In patients with diabetic retinopathy that has not reached the high risk proliferative stage, does photocoagulation (early treatment) reduce the risk of visual loss?

The evidence

One large (n = 3711) high quality multi-centre RCT, the Early Treatment Diabetic Retinopathy Study (ETDRS) was identified.[6] Patients with diabetic retinopathy in both eyes having either no macular oedema and more severe non-proliferative or early proliferative retinopathy and visual acuity 6/12 or macular oedema and mild, moderate or severe non-proliferative retinopathy or early proliferative retinopathy, and visual acuity 6/60 were included. Patients with high risk proliferative retinopathy or other significant ocular disease were excluded. One eye of each patient was assigned randomly to early photocoagulation and the other to deferral of photocoagulation until high risk proliferative retinopathy developed. Eyes selected for photocoagulation received one of four combinations of focal (macular) laser therapy or mild/full scatter (panretinal) laser therapy. The principal outcome variables were the development of severe visual loss (visual acuity ≤1·5/60 on two successive visits) and moderate visual loss (loss of ≥ three lines of visual acuity). Moderate visual loss occurred in 12% of treated eyes with clinically significant diabetic macular oedema versus 24% of untreated eyes in three years (NNT 9, 95% CI 6–16).

The five-year risk of severe visual loss was 2·6% in the early treatment group versus 3·7% in the deferred treatment group; a difference of borderline significance ($P = 0·035$ versus the chosen significance level of 0·01; NNT 86, 95% CI 51–275). Early treatment was also associated with a higher incidence of adverse effects. Subgroup analysis suggests, however, that early treatment may be more beneficial in patients with type 2 diabetes.[7]

Comment

This study established the benefits of macular laser therapy for diabetic macular oedema. Clinical examination does, however, underestimate the incidence of retinal thickening. Better recognition of thickening, for example, using optical coherence tomography, might improve the effectiveness of laser therapy, and less destructive treatment, for example, using micropulse laser, might reduce adverse effects.

"Early treatment" photocoagulation of eyes with retinopathy that has not yet reached the high risk proliferative stage cannot be unequivocally recommended on the basis of the ETDRS findings. In addition, randomisation categories did not include eyes with high risk proliferative retinopathy and clinically significant macular oedema. A non-randomised study suggested that results comparable to the ETDRS can be achieved by immediate application of focal and one fraction of scatter, followed two to four weeks later by the second fraction of scatter.[8]

Question

Does photocoagulation technique affect treatment outcome?

The evidence

Xenon-arc versus argon laser photocoagulation

One large (n = 1758) multi-centre RCT of high quality, the Diabetic Retinopathy Study (DRS),[5] and three small (n = 15–63) RCTs were identified.[9–11] Eyes were randomised to treatment in the DRS and were further randomised to xenon arc or argon laser photocoagulation; in the other studies, eyes with proliferative diabetic retinopathy were randomised to argon or xenon treatment. There was no significant difference in therapeutic benefit between xenon and argon treatment in any of the studies. In the DRS, a persistent treatment-related loss of one to four lines of visual acuity was encountered in 9·3% of argon treated eyes and 19·1% of xenon treated eyes, and severe visual field loss in 7% and 41% of eyes, respectively (number needed to harm (NNH) 11 and 3, respectively).

Comment

Xenon treatment is now rarely used.

Laser wavelength

One large (n = 696) high quality multi-centre RCT, the Krypton Argon Regression Neovascularisation Study (KARNS),[12] and 11 other smaller RCTs (n = 8–210) were identified.[13-23] Eyes with proliferative retinopathy (10 studies) or macular oedema (two studies) and clear media were included. People with significant vitreous haemorrhage in eyes with proliferative retinopathy were excluded. In the KARNS and three other studies[14,21,23] eyes were randomised to argon blue-green or krypton red panretinal photocoagulation. Other comparisons included argon blue-green versus diode infrared[15,19] dye orange[20] and dye orange or dye yellow[17]; argon green versus krypton red[23]; argon green versus diode infrared[22]; dye yellow versus dye red[13]; and frequency-doubled Nd:YAG yellow-green versus argon green.[16] The principal outcome variables included regression of neovascularisation/macular oedema, visual acuity, visual fields. No difference in therapeutic effect, visual acuity or adverse effect was encountered in any study.

Comment

Wavelength appears not to be a critical treatment parameter for either macular or panretinal laser.

Laser delivery parameters

Pattern of laser application

Two small RCTs (n = 40, 42) were identified.[24,25] The inclusion criterion was proliferative diabetic retinopathy. Interventions studied were peripheral versus more central panretinal photocoagulation. Neither study showed a difference between techniques in regression of neovascularisation or visual acuity. One study[26] showed greater field loss with more central photocoagulation, the other did not. One study[27] showed more tendency for macular oedema with more central photocoagulation, the other study did not examine this.

Burn characteristics

Two small RCTs were identified (n = 12,34).[26,28] The inclusion criterion was proliferative diabetic retinopathy. Intervention was long duration versus short duration burns, intense versus light. No difference between techniques in therapeutic effect was demonstrated. Intense laser had more adverse effect on visual field than light.

Comment

The practice of applying intense laser has grown less common, which limits the relevance of the older studies on pattern of laser delivery to current practice.

Temporal distribution of laser application

Two small (n = 35, 50) but well-controlled RCTs were identified.[27,29] One study divided laser application over several visits (fractionation), the other applied early retreatment to eyes in which high risk retinopathy did not regress within three weeks. Principal outcome variables were regression of neovascularisation and visual acuity. Neither treatment strategy affected regression of neovascularisation or visual acuity.

Comment

The ETDRS data show a higher rate of early visual loss in eyes randomised to immediate panretinal photocoagulation when compared to the deferral group, especially in eyes randomised to full compared to mild panretinal photocoagulation. Although the ETDRS study cohort did not include eyes with high risk proliferative retinopathy, its data are used by some to justify fractionation of the treatment of high risk eyes.

Summary

Panretinal photocoagulation for high risk proliferative diabetic retinopathy and macular laser therapy for diabetic macular oedema reduce visual loss, and the technique of photocoagulation appears to have relatively little effect on these benefits. Early photocoagulation, before the development of high risk proliferative retinopathy reduces slightly the rate of visual loss, but rates are in any case low and there are significant adverse effects of treatment.

Implications for practice

To reduce the risk of visual loss, laser therapy is indicated for macular oedema when it meets the definition of clinical significance and for proliferative disease when it meets the definition of high risk retinopathy.

Implications for research

Any trial of novel therapy for treating diabetic retinopathy should involve comparison of its risks and benefits with laser treatment applied according to the recommendations of the Diabetic Retinopathy and Early Treatment retinopathy study.

Reference

1. Klein R, Klein BE, Moss SE, Cruickshanks KJ. The Wisconsin Epidemiologic Study of Diabetic Retinopathy. XV. The long-term incidence of macular edema. *Ophthalmology* 1995;**102**:7–16.
2. Klein R, Klein BE, Moss SE, Cruickshanks KJ. The Wisconsin Epidemiologic Study of diabetic retinopathy. XIV. Ten-year incidence and progression of diabetic retinopathy. *Arch Ophthalmol* 1994;**112**:1217–28.

3. Olk RJ. Modified grid argon blue green laser photocoagulation for diffuse diabetic macular oedema. *Ophthalmology* 1986;**93**:938–50.
4. Uehara M, Tamura N, Kinjo M, Shinzato K, Fukuda M. A prospective study on necessary and sufficient retinal photocoagulation for diabetic retinopathy. *J Japan Ophthalmol Soc* 1993;**1993**:83–9.
5. Diabetic Retinopathy Study Research Group. Photocoagulation treatment of proliferative diabetic retinopathy. The second report of diabetic retinopathy study findings. *Ophthalmology* 1978;**85**:82–106.
6. Early Treatment Diabetic Retinopathy Study Research Group. Early photocoagulation for diabetic retinopathy. ETDRS report 9. *Ophthalmology* 1991;**98**:766–85.
7. Ferris F. Early photocoagulation in patient with either type 1 or type 2 diabetes. *Trans Am Ophthalmolog Soc* 1996;**94**:505–37.
8. Olk RJ, Lee CM, Akduman L. Combined modified grid and panretinal photocoagulation for diffuse diabetic macular edema and proliferative diabetic retinopathy. *Ophthalmic Surg Lasers* 2000;**31**:292–300.
9. Plumb AP, Swan AV, Chignell AH, Shilling JS. A comparative trial of xenon arc and argon laser photocoagulation in the treatment of proliferative diabetic retinopathy. *Br J Ophthalmol* 1982;**66**:213–18.
10. Hamilton AM, Townsend C, Khoury D, Gould E, Blach RK. Xenon arc and argon laser photocoagulation of diabetic disc neovascularisation. Part 1. Effect on disc vessels, visual fields and visual acuity. *Trans Ophthalmolog Soc UK* 1981;**101**:87–92.
11. Crick MDP, Chignell AH, Shilling JS. Argon laser versus xenon arc photocoagulation in proliferative diabetic retinopathy. *Trans Ophthalmolog Soc UK* 1978;**98**:170–1.
12. Krypton Argon Regression Neovascularization Study Research Group. Randomized comparison of Krypton versus Argon scatter photocoagulation for diabetic disc neovascularization. *Ophthalmology* 1993;**100**:1655–64.
13. Atmaca LS, Idil A, Gunduz K. Dye laser treatment in proliferative diabetic retinopathy and maculopathy. *Acta Ophthalmol Scand* 1995;**73**:303–7.
14. Blankenship GW, Gerke E, Batlle JF. Red krypton and blue green argon laser diabetic panretinal photocoagulation. *Graefe's Arch Clin Exp Ophthalmol* 1989;**227**:364–8.
15. Bandello F, Brancato R, Trabucchi G, Lattanzio R, Malegori A. Diode versus argon-green laser panretinal photocoagulation in proliferative diabetic retinopathy: a randomized study in 44 eyes with a long follow-up time. *Graefe's Arch Clin Exp Ophthalmol* 1993;**231**:491–4.
16. Bandello F, Brancato R, Lattanzio R, Trabucchi G, Azzolini C, Malegori A. Double-frequency Nd:YAG laser *v* argon-green laser in the treatment of proliferative diabetic retinopathy: randomized study with long-term follow-up. *Lasers Surg Med* 1996;**19**:173–6.
17. Canning C, Polkinghorne P, Ariffing A, Gregor Z. Panretinal laser photocoagulation for proliferative diabetic retinopathy: the effect of laser wavelength on macular function. *Br J Ophthalmol* 1991;**75**:608–10.
18. Capoferri C, Bagini M, Chizzoli A, Pece A, Brancato R. Electroretinographic findings in panretinal photocoagulation for diabetic retinopathy. A randomized study with blue-green argon and red krypton lasers. *Graefe's Arch Clin Exp Ophthalmol* 1990;**228**:232–6.
19. Buckley S, Jenkins L, Benjamin L. Field loss after panretinal photocoagulation with diode and argon lasers. *Doc Ophthalmol* 1992;**82**:317–22.
20. Seiberth V, Schatanek S, Alexandridis E. Panretinal photocoagulation in diabetic retinopathy: argon versus dye laser coagulation. *Graefe's Arch Clin Exp Ophthalmol* 1993;**231**:318–22.
21. Schulenburg WE, Hamilton AM, Blach RK. A comparative study of argon laser and krypton laser in the treatment of diabetic optic disc neovascularisation. *Br J Ophthalmol* 1979;**63**:412–17.
22. Akduman L, Olk RJ. Diode laser (810 nm) versus argon green (514 nm) modified grid photocoagulation for diffuse diabetic macular edema. *Ophthalmology* 1997;**104**:1433–41.
23. Olk RJ. Argon green (514 nm) *v* krypton red (647 nm) modified grid laser photocoagulation for diffuse diabetic macular edema. *Ophthalmology* 1990;**97**:1101–13.
24. Theodossiadis GW, Boudouri A, Georgopoulos G, Kousandrea Ch. Central field changes after panretinal photocoagulation in proliferative diabetic retinopathy. *Ophthalmologia* 1990;**201**:71–8.
25. Blankenship GW. A clinical comparison of central and peripheral argon laser panretinal photocoagulation for proliferative diabetic retinopathy. *Ophthalmology* 1988;**95**:170–7.
26. Wade EC, Blankenship GW. The effect of short versus long exposure times of argon laser panretinal photocoagulation on proliferative diabetic retinopathy. *Graefe's Arch Clin Exp Ophthalmol* 1990;**228**:226–31.
27. Doft BH, Metz DJ, Kelsey SF. Augmentation laser for proliferative diabetic retinopathy that fails to respond to initial panretinal photocoagulation. *Ophthalmology* 1992;**99**:1728–35.
28. Seiberth V, Alexandridis E. Function of the diabetic retina after panretinal argon laser photocoagulation. Influence of the intensity of the coagulation spots. *Ophthalmologia* 1991;**202**:10–17.
29. Doft BH, Blankenship GW. Single versus multiple treatment sessions of argon laser panretinal photocoagulation for proliferative diabetic retinopathy. *Ophthalmology* 1982;**89**:772–9.

44 Vitrectomy for diabetic retinopathy

Paul Sullivan, Alistair Laidlaw

Background

Diabetic retinopathy is the commonest cause of blind registration in working age in the western world. Blindness in diabetic patients generally occurs by one of two pathological mechanisms.

Proliferative diabetic retinopathy is characterised by the growth of extraretinal new blood vessels. These vessels are prone to rupture (causing vitreous haemorrhage) or act as foci for traction on the retina, leading to retinal detachment. These pathological processes may render photocoagulation ineffective or impossible (advanced diabetic eye disease). Blindness may also occur due to diabetic maculopathy, which is characterised by a microangiopathy affecting the macula with visual loss due the effects of leakage and ischaemia. The exact proportion of patients progressing to sight-threatening retinopathy is dependent on type of diabetes and duration of disease.[1,2]

Vitrectomy for proliferative diabetic retinopathy was proposed in 1971.[3] The rationale of the treatment was to improve vision by clearing the visual axis of blood and removing membranes from the surface of the retina that might distort or detach it. One problem with approaching the evidence in support of vitrectomy is the rapid rate of technical advance. Vitreoretinal instruments and surgical techniques have been constantly refined since Machemer first advocated vitrectomy,[3] so that the common surgical practice now is not that of 30 years ago. Particularly important in this respect is the development of fluid–gas exchange techniques to reattach the retina hydraulically, the advent of endolaser probes allowing peroperative laser and the development of special instruments for the excision of fibrovascular scars.

Four questions will be addressed by this review of the evidence:

- Does early vitrectomy reduce the chance of visual loss in eyes with advanced diabetic eye disease with poor vision due to vitreous haemorrhage?
- Does early vitrectomy reduce the chance of visual loss in eyes with advanced diabetic eye disease and useful vision?
- Is vitrectomy beneficial in eyes with diabetic maculopathy?
- Can any adjunctive treatment reduce the risk of surgical complications?

> ## Question
>
> Does early vitrectomy reduce the chance of visual loss in eyes with advanced diabetic eye disease with poor vision due to vitreous haemorrhage?

The evidence

Untreated, advanced diabetic eye disease has a high risk of severe visual loss.[4] We found one multi-centre randomised control trial with a total of 600 eyes.[5] The Diabetic Retinopathy Vitrectomy Study (DRVS) was a multi-centre randomised control trial that studied three groups of patients. Group H consisted of eyes with severe vitreous haemorrhage of less than six months' duration reducing visual acuity to 5/200 or less. Principal exclusion criteria included photocoagulation in the three months prior to randomisation, severe iris neovascularisation and retinal detachment affecting the macula. Patients with age of onset of diabetes prior to age 20 were classified as type I while those with onset after age 40 were classified as being type II (those with intermediate age of onset being assigned to an intermediate group). Patients were randomly assigned to immediate vitrectomy or deferral for one year. Patients in the deferral group received further photocoagulation at the discretion of the clinician, while patients in the immediate vitrectomy group did not receive photocoagulation during surgery and only received postoperative photocoagulation for rubeosis or for severe and progressive retinal neovascularisation after discussion with the trial coordinators.

The principal outcomes were best corrected visual acuity at two and four years after randomisation. Visual acuity of 10/20 at two years was found in 62 of 253 eyes with early vitrectomy and 37 of 244 eyes in the deferral group (relative risk (RR) of achieving 10/20 1·61, 95% CI 1·1–2·3; number needed to treat (NNT) for benefit 11, 95% CI 7–43). This beneficial effect was more apparent in type I patients (RR of achieving 10/20 3, 95% CI 1·7–5·5); than type II (RR of achieving 10/20 0·87, 95% CI 0·4–1·74). There was no significant difference in the numbers of patients with no perception of light between the two groups at two years (RR 1·3, 95% CI 0·9–1·8).

Comment

There have been significant technical advances since the DRVS study was carried out. These are likely to have reduced the complication rate of vitrectomy for diabetic retinopathy and increased the benefit from early surgery. The benefits were confined to type I patients who were more likely to have adhesions between the retina and vitreous. A relatively high proportion of eyes in both groups lost perception of light. Rubeotic glaucoma was a significant cause of visual loss after vitrectomy in this study but is seldom seen since the advent of retinal endolaser, so it is possible that the beneficial effect of early vitrectomy would be more marked if the trial were repeated today.

Question

Does early vitrectomy reduce the chance of visual loss in eyes with advanced diabetic eye disease and useful vision?

The evidence

We found one multi-centre randomised control trial with a total of 370 patients: group P in the DRVS study.[6] Patients with advanced preretinal fibrovascular proliferation and best corrected visual acuity of 10/200 or better were eligible – significant exclusion criteria were as for group H of the study (see above). Patients were randomly allocated to early vitrectomy with removal of preretinal membranes or deferral of vitrectomy until retinal detachment or severe vitreous haemorrhage developed. The protocol for photocoagulation was similar to that in the vitreous haemorrhage arm of the study (see above).

The principal outcomes were best corrected visual acuity at four years after randomisation. Visual acuity of 10/20 was found in 64 of 145 eyes with early vitrectomy and 39 of 138 eyes in the deferral group ($P = 0.008$; RR of achieving 10/20 1·56, 95% CI 1·13–2·1; NNT for benefit 7, 95% CI 4 harm–22 benefit). The investigators state that the type of diabetes did not seem to exert an independent effect on visual outcome. There was no significant difference in the numbers of patients with no perception of light between the two groups at two years (RR 1·2, 95% CI 0·76–1.9, $P = 0.51$).

Comment

Most of the comments relating to the evidence for early vitrectomy for severe vitreous haemorrhage can equally be applied to eyes with useful vision undergoing vitrectomy.

Question

Is vitrectomy beneficial for diabetic maculopathy?

The evidence

We found no published randomised controlled trials regarding the efficacy of vitrectomy for diabetic macular oedema.[7,8]

Comment

The current clinical understanding regarding vitrectomy for diabetic macular oedema is that patients fall into four groups. This classification may not, however, stand the test of time. The aim of this review is to identify potentially pertinent subgroups of patients with diabetic macular oedema and to provide a framework against which future publications might be assessed.

Group 1: Patients with clinically identifiable vitreo-retinal traction

This group includes patients with epiretinal membranes, fibrovascular tissue resulting from proliferative diabetic retinopathy in the absence of a tractional detachment, vitreous haemorrhage and those with frank tractional detachments. There are only scant uncontrolled data relating to 36 patients on this very diverse group.[9,10] A potential treatment effect has been reported. The dearth of data means that it is not possible to draw even preliminary conclusions regarding the role of vitrectomy in this group. The heterogeneous nature of this group of patients also makes it difficult to envisage randomised trials.

Group 2: Patients with a taut thickened posterior hyaloid

Patients in this group demonstrate an exaggerated glistening premacular hyaloid membrane, which is occasionally thick enough to preclude laser.[11] The premacular vitreous has a hammered appearance but there are no signs of retinal striae or tractional detachment. Angiography may demonstrate a deep diffuse leak with prominent cystoid oedema.[12] Uncontrolled data regarding vitrectomy on 112 eyes fulfilling this definition have been reported.[10,11,13–17] Overall, oedema resolved in 61% and acuity improved in 75%. Recent investigations using Optical Coherence Tomography (OCT), suggest that vitreo-retinal microtraction may be important in patients with a taut thickened posterior hyaloid (TTPH).[12,18] OCT also provides a reliable objective quantification of macular thickness.[19] Accordingly, any randomised controlled trials (RCTs) of this subject should include OCT quantification of macular thickness as well as qualitative assessment of the vitreo-retinal interface.

Group 3: Patients with no retinal traction and no clinically apparent posterior vitreous detachment

These patients may well constitute the most commonly encountered group in clinical practice. The literature contains uncontrolled reports of surgery on 114 patients.[20–23] The studied populations have also been ethnically diverse and a variety of different outcome measures and follow up durations have been employed in a non-systematic fashion. The reported data suggest an acuity benefit from vitrectomy. Rates of oedema resolution were, however, highly variable and recurrence has been observed.[21] Randomised trials are clearly required in this area and OCT is likely to form an important part of patient assessment.[20,21,24]

Group 4: Eyes with a posterior vitreous detachment

There are published uncontrolled data regarding the results of vitrectomy in 20 patients.[10,25] These data are insufficient to allow even preliminary conclusions to be drawn.

Summary

Carefully planned and systematically reported randomised trials, which incorporate technical measures of outcome such as acuity and macular thickness as well as qualitative assessments such as OCT vitreo-retinal interface assessment, are required. The costs and inherent risk of vitrectomy might be expected to be greater than those of macular laser. Accordingly, both economic and quality of life assessments will be important.

Question

Can any adjunctive treatment reduce the risk of surgical complications?

The evidence

A number of measures have been proposed to make vitrectomy in diabetic patients easier to perform and to reduce the risk of iatrogenic complications, and some of these have been the subjects of small clinical trials.

Insertion of a gas tamponade at the end of surgery has been the subject of two clinical trials,[26,27] the rationale being that the presence of air at the bleeding site may promote haemostasis. Koutsandrea *et al.*[26] investigated the effect of an intravitreal bubble of sulphur hexafluoride (SF6)

gas in an RCT of 33 patients undergoing vitrectomy for diabetic eye disease. The major outcome measure was the incidence of postoperative vitreous haemorrhage. The authors reported no reduction in the incidence of postoperative vitreous haemorrhage (RR of haemorrhage with SF6 1·41, 95% CI 0·31–6·49). Joondeph *et al.*[27] performed a similar study using air, which is resorbed more quickly, with similar findings (RR of haemorrhage with air 1·41, 95% CI 0·87–2·2). Both of these studies noted some evidence of harm in the form of a greater incidence of lens opacity with gas (RR of cataract with SF6 1·64, 95% CI 0·62–4·57; RR of cataract with air 1·95, 95% CI 0·86–4·5).

Two trials have studied the effect of procoagulants to reduce bleeding. Packer *et al.*[28] performed an RCT on 26 patients undergoing vitrectomy for diabetic eye disease. These eyes were randomly allocated to receiving intravitreal injections of sodium hyaluronate or saline at the end of surgery. There was a significant difference between the two groups (RR of opaque media 0·54, 95% CI 0·28–0·9 with sodium hyaluronate, $P = 0·016$; NNT 3 for benefit). This benefit had disappeared at two weeks. Thompson *et al.*[29] performed a prospective double-blind study on the effect of the addition of thrombin to the infusate on the bleeding time of severed neovascular stalks. Twenty-eight patients undergoing vitrectomy for diabetic eye disease were studied. The authors reported a significantly reduced bleeding time (12 seconds compared to 111 seconds) in patients receiving thrombin. This study included some non-randomised patients in its analysis, the report includes few raw data and a significant proportion of the thrombin-treated patients developed intraocular inflammation.

There has been much interest in the possibility of chemically removing the vitreous. Tissue plasminogen activator (TPA) converts plasminogen to plasmin which, in addition to its fibrinolytic role, is thought to dissolve the structural proteins at the vitreoretinal interface, thereby facilitating surgical dissection. Le Mer *et al.*[30] randomised 56 patients undergoing vitrectomy for diabetic eye disease to adjunctive TPA or placebo. There was no significant difference between the two groups in either of the two main outcomes studied: retinal breaks (RR 0·93, 95% CI 0·41– 2·1) and retinal detachment (RR 0·93, 95% CI 0·41–2·1). The authors felt that the TPA might not have had enough time to work and considerable interest remains in this area.

Implications for practice

There is a good evidence base for consideration of early vitrectomy in diabetic patients with vitreous haemorrhage and with active fibrovascular proliferation. The procedure still has a significant complication rate, but development of new surgical approaches and treatment adjuncts are likely in the future. Vitrectomy for diabetic maculopathy is an attractive treatment option because maculopathy is a significant cause of visual loss in diabetic patients and existing treatment has limited therapeutic effect. Clinical trials are underway but to date there is no evidence base supporting this intervention.

Implications for research

There has been a recent explosion in interest in the potential for vitrectomy in diabetic retinopathy and in particular in its use as an alternative to laser in the management of diabetic maculopathy. Carefully planned and systematically reported randomised trials, which incorporate technical measures of outcome such as acuity and macular thickness as well as qualitative assessments such as OCT vitreo-retinal interface assessment, are required. Surgery should also be compared to other emerging treatments such as intravitreal triamcinolone injection or sustained release steroid implants. The financial costs and inherent risk of vitrectomy might be expected to be greater than those of macular laser or drug injection. Accordingly, both economic and quality of life assessments will be important.

References

1. Klein R, Klein BE, Moss SE, Davis MD, DeMets DL. The Wisconsin Epidemiologic Study of diabetic retinopathy III. Prevalence and risk of diabetic retinopathy when age at diagnosis is 30 or more years. *Arch Ophthalmol* 1984;**102**:527–32.
2. Klein R, Klein BE, Moss SE, Davis MD, DeMets DL. The Wisconsin Epidemiologic Study of diabetic retinopathy II. Prevalence and risk of diabetic retinopathy when age at diagnosis is less than 30 years. *Arch Ophthalmol* 1984;**102**:520–6.
3. Machemer R, Buettner H, Norton EW, Parel JM. Vitrectomy: a pars plana approach. *Trans Am Acad Ophthalmol Otolaryngol* 1971;**75**:813–20.
4. The Diabetic Retinopathy Vitrectomy Study Research Group. Two year course of visual acuity in severe proliferative diabetic retinopathy with conventional management. *Ophthalmology* 1985;**92**:492–502.
5. The Diabetic Retinopathy Vitrectomy Study Research Group. Early vitrectomy for severe vitreous hemorrhage in diabetic retinopathy. Two-year results of a randomized trial. Diabetic Retinopathy Vitrectomy Study Report 2. *Arch Ophthalmol* 1985;**103**:1644–52.
6. The Diabetic Retinopathy Vitrectomy Study Research Group. Early Vitrectomy for Severe Proliferative Diabetic Retinopathy in Eyes with Useful Vision. Results of a Randomised Trial – Diabetic Retinopathy Study Report 3. *Ophthalmology* 1988;**5**:1307–20.
7. Lewis H. The role of vitrectomy in the treatment of diabetic macular edema. *Am J Ophthalmol* 2001;**131**:123–5.
8. Capone A, Jr, Panozzo G. Vitrectomy for refractory diabetic macular edema. *Semin Ophthalmol* 2000;**15**:78–80.
9. Hoerle S, Poestgens H, Schmidt J, Kroll P. Effect of pars plana vitrectomy for proliferative diabetic vitreoretinopathy on preexisting diabetic maculopathy. *Graefe's Arch Clin Exp Ophthalmol* 2002;**240**:197–201.
10. Yamamoto T, Akabane N, Takeuchi S. Vitrectomy for diabetic macular edema: the role of posterior vitreous detachment and epimacular membrane. *Am J Ophthalmol* 2001;**132**:369–77.
11. Pendergast SD, Hassan TS, Williams GA *et al.* Vitrectomy for diffuse diabetic macular edema associated with a taut premacular posterior hyaloid. *Am J Ophthalmol* 2000;**130**:178–86.
12. Kaiser PK, Riemann CD, Sears JE, Lewis H. Macular traction detachment and diabetic macular edema associated with posterior hyaloidal traction. *Am J Ophthalmol* 2001;**131**:44–9.
13. Harbour JW, Smiddy WE, Flynn HW, Jr, Rubsamen PE. Vitrectomy for diabetic macular edema associated with a thickened and taut posterior hyaloid membrane. *Am J Ophthalmol* 1996;**121**:405–13.
14. Gandorfer A, Messmer EM, Ulbig MW, Kampik A. Resolution of diabetic macular edema after surgical removal of the posterior hyaloid and the inner limiting membrane. *Retina* 2000;**20**:126–33.
15. Abrams GW, Blumenkranz MS, Campo RV. Vitrectomy for diabetic macular traction and edema associated with posterior hyaloidal traction. *Ophthalmology* 1992;**99**:753–9.
16. Pendergast SD. Vitrectomy for diabetic macular edema associated with a taut premacular posterior hyaloid. *Curr Opin Ophthalmol* 1998;**9**:71–5.
17. van Effenterre G, Guyot-Argenton C, Guiberteau B, Hany I, Lacotte JL. [Macular edema caused by contraction of the posterior hyaloid in diabetic retinopathy. Surgical treatment of a series of 22 cases]. *J Fr Ophtalmol* 1993;**16**:602–10.
18. Giovannini A, Amato GP, Mariotti C, Ripa E. Diabetic maculopathy induced by vitreo-macular traction: evaluation by optical coherence tomography (OCT). *Doc Ophthalmol* 1999;**97**:361–6.
19. Massin P, Vicaut E, Haouchine B, Erginay A, Paques M, Gaudric A. Reproducibility of retinal mapping using optical coherence tomography. *Arch Ophthalmol* 2001;**119**:1135–42.
20. Otani T, Kishi S. Tomographic assessment of vitreous surgery for diabetic macular edema. *Am J Ophthalmol* 2000;**129**:487–94.
21. Duguid G, Massin P, Haouchine B, Erginay A, Gaudric A. Vitrectomy for Diabetic Macular Oedema: the effect on visual acuity and optical coherence tomography appearances. *Assoc Res Vis Ophthalmol Abstracts* 2000:Abstract no. 585.
22. Ikeda T, Sato K, Katano T, Hayashi Y. Vitrectomy for cystoid macular oedema with attached posterior hyaloid membrane in patients with diabetes. *Br J Ophthalmol* 1999;**83**:12–14.
23. La Heij EC, Hendrikse F, Kessels AG, Derhaag PJ. Vitrectomy results in diabetic macular oedema without evident vitreomacular traction. *Graefe's Arch Clin Exp Ophthalmol* 2001;**239**:264–70.
24. Patel JI, Cree IA, Gregor ZJ, Boulton ME, Hykin PG. Vascular Endothelial Growth Factor and diabetic macular edema. *Assoc Res Vis Ophthalmol Abstracts* 2001:Abstract no. 3974.
25. Ikeda T, Sato K, Katano T, Hayashi Y. Improved visual acuity following pars plana vitrectomy for diabetic cystoid macular edema and detached posterior hyaloid. *Retina* 2000;**20**:220–2.
26. Koutsandrea CN, Apostolopoulos MN, Chatzoulis DZ, Parikakis EA, Theodossiadis GP. Hemostatic effects of SF6 after diabetic vitrectomy for vitreous hemorrhage. *Acta Ophthalmol Scand* 2001;**79**:34–8.
27. Joondeph BC, Blankenship GW. Hemostatic effects of air versus fluid in diabetic vitrectomy. *Ophthalmology* 1989;**96**:1701–6.
28. Packer AJ, McCuen BW 2nd, Hutton WL, Ramsay RC. Procoagulant effects of intraocular sodium hyaluronate (Healon) after phakic diabetic vitrectomy. A prospective, randomized study. *Ophthalmology* 1989;**96**:1491–4.
29. Thompson JT, Glaser BM, Michels RG *et al.* The use of intravitreal thrombin to control hemorrhage during vitrectomy. *Ophthalmology* 1986;**93**:279–82.
30. Le Mer Y, Korobelnik JF, Morel C, Ullern M, Berrod JP. TPA-assisted vitrectomy for proliferative diabetic retinopathy: results of a double-masked, multicenter trial. *Retina* 1999;**19**:378–82.

Section XI

Neuro-ophthalmology

James Acheson, Editor

Neuro-ophthalmology: mission statement

This section on evidence-based neuro-ophthalmology focuses on acquired optic neuropathies. These diseases are important, firstly from the standpoint of accurate diagnosis of more generalised neurological conditions, and secondly from the point of view of the ophthalmologist's duty to try to optimise management to prevent avoidable and devastating neural blindness. All the topics which have been selected have attracted some controversy in recent years. Some are surgical (CSF diversion surgery for visual failure complicating papilloedema and traumatic optic neuropathy). Others are medical (optic neuritis, ischaemic optic neuropathy and toxic optic neuropathies). However, they share the emphasis on the need for well informed and well timed interventions to try to improve visual outcomes in these disorders.

45 Optic neuritis

Simon J Hickman

Background

Definition

Optic neuritis usually presents as acute unilateral loss of vision with retro-ocular pain and pain on eye movement. Bilateral cases and painless presentations are possible. The degree of visual loss varies from minor blurring to no perception of light in the affected eye. Decreased colour vision, a central or paracentral scotoma and a relative afferent pupillary defect are also usually seen on examination. The optic disc may appear swollen but is often normal in appearance, hence the term retrobulbar optic neuritis.[1,2]

Incidence/prevalence

The age- and sex-adjusted incidence is 1–5 per 100 000/year.[3–5] It principally affects young adults and is more common in females. Childhood cases are seen, a higher proportion of which are bilateral.[6]

Aetiology

Most cases of optic neuritis are due to idiopathic inflammatory demyelinating disease. It may occur in isolation or as a manifestation of multiple sclerosis (MS).[7]

Prognosis

The natural history of acute optic neuritis is for spontaneous improvement in vision to occur with most patients showing a good functional recovery. The mean visual acuity one year following entry into the Optic Neuritis Treatment Trial (ONTT) was better than 6/5, although approximately 7% had a visual acuity of worse than 6/12.[8]

The cumulative probability of having recurrent optic neuritis after five-years' follow-up in the ONTT was 19% for the affected eye, 17% for the unaffected eye and 30% for either eye. The risk of recurrence was twice as high in patients who had developed clinically definite MS (CDMS).[9]

The cumulative risk of developing MS increases with time. In one series the 10-year risk was 39% rising to 60% for the 40-year risk.[5] The strongest predictor for the subsequent development of MS is the presence of asymptomatic white matter lesions on brain magnetic resonance imaging (MRI) on presentation with acute optic neuritis. The five-year risk of CDMS was 16% in 202 patients with no brain lesions, but was 51% in the 89 patients with three or more lesions on entry to the ONTT.[7]

Question

Do corticosteroids improve visual recovery after acute optic neuritis?

The evidence

I found one meta-analysis which included four randomised controlled trials (RCTs) with a total of 556 participants[10] and one systematic review by the Quality Standards Subcommittee of the American Academy of Neurology, which included the RCTs analysed in the above meta-analysis and other studies.[11] A Cochrane review was in progress at the time of writing.

The meta-analysis showed that corticosteroids reduced the number of patients without clinical improvement at 30 days (odds ratio 0·60, range 0·42–0·85) but did not find long-term improvement in disability (odds ratio 0·96, range 0·71–1·31).[10]

The largest reported trial was the ONTT, in which patients with acute optic neuritis were randomised into three groups.[12] People in the first group (n = 151) were admitted to hospital and received intravenous methylprednisolone (IVMP), 250 mg every six hours for three days, followed by 1 mg/kg oral prednisolone for 11 days and a short period thereafter of tapered withdrawal. The second group (n = 156) received 1 mg/kg oral prednisolone for 14 days followed again by dose tapering. The third group (n = 150) received oral placebo according to the oral prednisolone schedule. The estimated treatment effect was 30% with an α error of 0·02 and a power of 90%. The rate of return of vision to normal was higher in the IVMP group compared to the placebo group ($P = 0·0001$ for visual field, $P = 0·02$ for contrast sensitivity, and $P = 0·09$ for visual acuity). The differences were greatest on day four and day 15 and then declined such that by one year no treatment benefit was seen for any of the visual parameters tested.[8] When the presenting visual acuity was 6/12 or better then IVMP conferred no benefit, even during the initial stages of recovery.[12] Oral prednisolone produced no significant improvements in the rate of recovery for any of the visual measures tested and was associated with a persistent two-fold increased risk of recurrence of optic neuritis compared with the other two groups.[9] The cumulative probability of recurrence at five years was 41% in the prednisolone group, 25% in the IVMP group ($P = 0.003$) and 25% in the placebo group ($P = 0.004$).

The systematic review concluded that 1 mg/kg/day of oral prednisolone did not affect visual recovery. Higher dose oral or parenteral methylprednisolone or adrenocorticotrophic hormone may speed up visual recovery without affecting long-term outcome. The decision to use these medications should therefore be based on other non-evidence-based factors such as quality of life, risk to the patient and visual function in the fellow eye.[11]

Harms

Common minor side effects reported from the use of corticosteroids in optic neuritis include insomnia, mild mood changes, stomach upsets, facial flushing, acneiform eruptions, oedema and weight gain.[12,13] More serious side effects seen in the IVMP arm of the ONTT include one patient developing psychotic depression and another developing pancreatitis.[12]

Comment

High-dose corticosteroids speed up visual recovery in acute optic neuritis but do not affect long-term outcome.

Question

Does intravenous immunoglobulin (IVIG) improve vision in patients with chronic visual impairment after optic neuritis?

The evidence

I found one RCT that studied 55 MS patients with persistent visual acuity worse than 6/12 (logMAR 0·3) after optic neuritis.[14] Participants were randomised to receive either 0·4 g/kg IVIG daily for five days followed by three single infusions monthly for three months, or placebo. The sample size calculated to detect a change of two lines on the logMAR acuity chart with a power of 0·80 was 30 subjects in each arm. Recruitment was terminated early due to negative results following an interim analysis. Visual acuity was unchanged after six months' follow up ($P = 0.766$),

although there was a trend for improvement after 12 months ($P = 0.132$). The improvement was, however, modest, amounting to a mean difference of two letters on the logMAR acuity chart. Exploratory secondary analysis suggested that patients with clinically stable MS benefited more than those with unstable disease.

Harms

Reported adverse effects were rashes, including urticaria, and headache.

Comment

The only RCT did not find a significant beneficial effect for IVIG on chronic visual impairment after optic neuritis.

Question

Do corticosteroids delay the onset of MS after monosymptomatic optic neuritis?

The evidence

Secondary analysis from the ONTT showed that there was a decreased risk for the development of CDMS, which was reduced to 7·5% in the IVMP group compared to the other two groups (14·7% in the prednisolone group, 16·7% in the placebo group) after a follow up period of two years in patients with clinically isolated optic neuritis on entry to the study (n = 389).[15] The adjusted rate ratio for the development of CDMS in IVMP group was 0·34 (95% CI 0·16–0·74) compared with the placebo group. Most of the treatment effect was seen in patients with an abnormal brain MRI on entry to the trial. The beneficial effect was lost by three years with a cumulative incidence of CDMS of 17·3% in the IVMP group, 24·7% in the prednisolone group and 21·3% in the placebo group.[16]

Harms

Harms in the ONTT are reported above.

Comment

These findings were based on a retrospective analysis with an open-label treatment (there was no intravenous placebo arm). The absolute numbers were also small with only 10 in the IVMP group, 21 in the placebo group and 19 in the prednisolone group developing MS at two years. Data were not available for 50 of the participants, which may have introduced bias if there was differential loss to follow up in the treatment arms.

IVMP may delay the onset of MS but this remains controversial. The benefit is short-lived and does not affect either the eventual risk for the development of MS or the development of disability.[7]

Question

Do beta-interferons delay the onset of MS after monosymptomatic optic neuritis?

The evidence

I found no systematic reviews, and two RCTs that addressed this question.[17,18] The CHAMPS study recruited 383 patients following their first demyelinating event (192 with optic neuritis) who, in addition, had two or more clinically silent brain lesions on MRI and were therefore were at greater risk of early development of MS.[17] Half the patients received once weekly 30 micrograms intramuscular interferon beta-1a and half placebo injections. The trial was stopped early after an interim analysis revealed that the cumulative probability of the development of CDMS during the three-year follow-up period was significantly lower in the interferon group than in the placebo group (rate ratio 0·56, 95% CI 0·38–0·81, $P = 0·002$).

The ETOMS study looked at a similar group of patients (n = 309, 98 with optic neuritis) with four asymptomatic white matter lesions (or three if one was enhancing after administration of gadolinium) at entry.[18] The patients were randomised to receive once weekly subcutaneous 22 micrograms interferon beta-1a or placebo injections. After two years the odds ratio for conversion to CDMS was 0·61 (95% CI 0·37–0·99, $P = 0·045$) for the treatment group compared to the placebo group.

Harms

There were no excess major adverse effects in the treatment groups compared to the placebo groups. Significant minor adverse events included influenza-like symptoms (both trials), depression (CHAMPS) and injection-site inflammation (ETOMS).

Comment

Beta-interferons can delay the development of CDMS in patients after an isolated demyelinating event (including optic neuritis) with asymptomatic brain lesions on MRI. These results are consistent with previously reported trials of the beta-interferons in relapsing–remitting MS suggesting that, in patients at high risk of developing CDMS, the beta-interferons have in effect reduced the relapse rate, but not necessarily the eventual occurrence of CDMS. Longer studies are needed to ascertain whether the development of persistent disability is delayed by early introduction of a interferon beta.

Summary

Optic neuritis usually causes acute painful unilateral visual disturbance with most patients making good spontaneous recovery, although poor outcome is possible. Patients with monosymptomatic optic neuritis are at risk of developing MS.

Implications for practice

High dose corticosteroids can speed up the visual recovery but without affecting long-term visual prognosis, and IVMP may delay the onset of MS but this remains to be confirmed. There is also a risk of significant adverse events occurring with their use therefore the decision to use corticosteroids should be based on other factors, the most significant of which is whether the fellow eye is involved or has reduced vision for some other reason. The use of high dose corticosteroids in these cases will shorten the period of functional impairment.

At present there are no treatments that will reverse chronic visual impairment following optic neuritis.

Beta-interferons are generally well tolerated and can delay the development of CDMS in patients after an isolated demyelinating event (including optic neuritis) with asymptomatic brain lesions on MRI. The effects on long-term development of disability are not known.

Implications for research

The lack of benefit of corticosteroids on visual recovery has been postulated on their being given too late to influence outcome.[19] Clinical trials in the hyperacute phase are required to address this issue.

Novel treatments to reverse chronic visual impairment following optic neuritis are needed. Potential therapies could include strategies to induce remyelination[19] and optic nerve transplantation.[20]

Longer term clinical trials of beta-interferons following optic neuritis or targeted trials at those patients at greatest risk for the development of MS[21] are required to address whether the use of beta-interferons in this group can affect the development of disability.

Acknowledgements

Simon J Hickman is supported by The Wellcome Trust.

References

1. Perkin GD, Rose FC. *Optic Neuritis and its Differential Diagnosis.* Oxford: Oxford University Press, 1979.
2. Optic Neuritis Study Group. The clinical profile of optic neuritis: experience of the Optic Neuritis Treatment Trial. *Arch Ophthalmol* 1991;**109**:1673–8.
3. MacDonald BK, Cockerell OC, Sander JWAS, Shorvon SD. The incidence and lifetime prevalence of neurological disorders in a prospective community-based study in the UK. *Brain* 2000;**123**:665–76.
4. Jin Y-P, de Pedro-Cuesta J, Söderström M, Stawiarz L, Link H. Incidence of optic neuritis in Stockholm, Sweden 1990–1995: I. Age, sex, birth and ethnic-group related patterns. *J Neurol Sci* 1998;**159**:107–14.
5. Rodriguez M, Siva A, Cross SA, O'Brien PC, Kurkland LT. Optic neuritis: A population-based study in Olmsted County, Minnesota. *Neurology* 1995;**45**:244–50.
6. Kriss A, Francis DA, Cuendet F *et al.* Recovery after optic neuritis in childhood. *J Neurol Neurosurg Psychiatry* 1988;**51**:1253–8.
7. Optic Neuritis Study Group. The 5-year risk of MS after optic neuritis: Experience of the Optic Neuritis Study Group. *Neurology* 1997;**49**:1404–13.
8. Beck RW, Cleary PA, The Optic Neuritis Study Group. Optic Neuritis Treatment Trial: One-year follow-up results. *Arch Ophthalmol* 1993;**111**:773–5.
9. The Optic Neuritis Study Group. Visual function 5 years after optic neuritis: Experience of the Optic Neuritis Treatment Trial. *Arch Ophthalmol* 1997;**115**:1545–52.
10. Brusaferri F, Candelise L. Steroids for multiple sclerosis and optic neuritis: a meta-analysis of randomised controlled clinical trials. *J Neurol* 2000;**247**:435–42.
11. Kaufman DI, Trobe JD, Eggenberger ER, Whitacker JN. Practice parameter: The role of corticosteroids in the management of acute monosymptomatic optic neuritis. *Neurology* 2000;**54**:2039–44.
12. Beck RW, Cleary PA, Anderson MM Jr *et al.*, The Optic Neuritis Study Group. A randomized, controlled trial of corticosteroids in the treatment of acute optic neuritis. *N Engl J Med* 1992;**326**:581–8.
13. Sellebjerg F, Schaldemose Nielson H, Fredericksen JL, Oleson J. A randomized, controlled trial of oral high-dose methylprednisolone in acute optic neuritis. *Neurology* 1999;**52**:1479–84.
14. Noseworthy JH, O'Brien PC, Petterson TM *et al.* A randomized trial of intravenous immunoglobulin in inflammatory demyelinating optic neuritis. *Neurology* 2001;**56**:1514–22.
15. Beck RW, Cleary PA, Trobe JD *et al.*, The Optic Neuritis Study Group. The effect of corticosteroids for acute optic neuritis on the subsequent development of multiple sclerosis. *N Engl J Med* 1993;**329**:1764–9.
16. Beck RW. The Optic Neuritis Treatment Trial: three-year follow-up results. *Arch Ophthalmol* 1995;**113**:136.
17. Jacobs LD, Beck RW, Simon JH *et al.*, CHAMPS Study Group. Intramuscular interferon beta-1a therapy initiated during a first demyelinating event in multiple sclerosis. *N Engl J Med* 2000;**343**:898–904.
18. Comi G, Filippi M, Barkhof F *et al.*, Early Treatment of Multiple Sclerosis Study Group. Effect of early interferon treatment on conversion to definite multiple sclerosis: a randomised study. *Lancet* 2001;**357**:1576–82.
19. Compston A, Coles A. Multiple sclerosis. *Lancet* 2002;**359**:1221–31.
20. Adachi-Usami E. Optic neuritis: from diagnosis to optic nerve transplantation. *Jpn J Ophthalmol* 2001;**45**:320–1.
21. McDonald WI, Compston A, Edan G *et al.* Recommended diagnostic criteria for multiple sclerosis: guidelines from the International Panel on the diagnosis of multiple sclerosis. *Ann Neurol* 2001;**50**:121–7.

46 Arteritic and non-arteritic anterior ischaemic optic neuropathy

Ahmed Toosy

Background

Definition

Anterior ischaemic optic neuropathy (AION) is acute infarction of the optic nerve head and may be divided into non-arteritic and arteritic (most commonly caused by giant cell arteritis/temporal arteritis) forms. It is the most common acute optic neuropathy in people over the age of 50 years.

Pathogenesis

Anterior ischaemic optic neuropathy is caused by occlusion of the short posterior ciliary arteries (which arise from the ophthalmic artery). These supply the optic nerve head and divide into medial and lateral groups that form a watershed area where their territories overlap. This is thought to be vulnerable to local vascular insufficiency, which consequently may lead to optic nerve head ischaemia or infarction.[1]

In this chapter I consider arteritic and non-arteritic anterior ischaemic optic neuropathy separately.

Arteritic anterior ischaemic optic neuropathy

Introduction

Arteritic anterior ischaemic neuropathy (A-AION) can be caused by a variety of vasculitides but the most common one is giant cell arteritis (GCA, temporal arteritis), which is discussed in this chapter.

Epidemiology

In a community-based population study in the United States, the age and sex adjusted annual incidence for people above 50 years was reported as 17·0 per 100 000 population.[2] The incidence per 100,000 of GCA increased with increasing age (from 2·3 in the sixth decade of life to 44·7 in the ninth decade of life). The mean age of onset is 70 years. There is a female to male preponderance of 2–3:1 and predilection for Caucasians. "Occult GCA" is quite common – 21·2% of patients with proven GCA and visual loss had no systemic symptoms of the disease.[3]

Aetiology/risk factors

Giant cell arteritis is considered to be a severe variant of polymyalgia rheumatica and is caused by T cell mediated inflammation of medium to large sized arteries.[4,5] A combination of genetic and environmental factors is thought to play a role in the aetiology.[6]

Prognosis

The natural history is progressive visual loss and involvement of the second eye in most patients within a few weeks if left untreated.[7] Early and massive visual loss is common – visual acuity of counting fingers or worse was noted in 54% patients in a prospective study.[8] Permanent visual loss is more frequent with transient visual loss, thrombocytosis and cerebrovascular accidents.[9–11] Permanent visual loss or ischaemic complications are less likely with the presence of systemic symptoms (fever, weight loss, myalgia, anorexia), polymyalgia rheumatica and a biochemical inflammatory response (raised C reactive protein or erythrocyte sedimentation rate).[11,12] Survival in patients with GCA is thought to be similar to that of the general population[13]; a retrospective subgroup analysis demonstrated a reduced long-term survival rate in patients with permanent visual loss and in patients who required more than 10 mg/day glucocorticoid at six months after onset.[14] Patients with GCA also have an increased risk of developing thoracic aortic aneurysms.[15] Optic disc cupping usually occurs as a long-term consequence of GCA (in up to 92%) whereas it is hardly seen in non-arteritic ischaemic optic neuropathy (2%).[16]

Treatment options

There is a lack of prospective data regarding steroid treatment in GCA and as a result there is no standardised protocol for its use. Despite this, systemic corticosteroid treatment instituted immediately once GCA is suspected has been shown to suppress the inflammatory process and may help to restore some vision or prevent progression in the affected eye as well as reduce the risk of fellow eye involvement.[17,18]

The following issues will be addressed in this section.

● Is intravenous steroid treatment more effective than oral steroid treatment for GCA?
● What is the role of immunosuppressive steroid-sparing agents in the treatment of GCA?
● Can the long-term complications of osteoporosis with steroid treatment be reduced for patients with GCA?

Question

Is intravenous steroid treatment more effective than oral steroid treatment for GCA?

The evidence

One randomised controlled study was found which prospectively evaluated the steroid sparing effect of an initial pulse of methylprednisolone.[19] A total of 164 patients with GCA were followed up over one year after they were assigned to three treatment arms: 240 mg intravenous (IV) methylprednisolone followed by 0·7 mg/kg/day oral prednisone, 240 mg IV methylprednisolone followed by 0·5 mg/kg/day oral prednisone, or 0·7 mg/kg/day oral prednisone. The cumulative doses of steroids were similar in all three groups ($P = 0.39$) as were steroid resistance and steroid side effects ($P = 0.37$). Pulsed methylprednisolone had no significant steroid sparing effects.

Comment

Randomised, controlled prospective trials with large numbers of participants are required to evaluate fully the differences between oral only and IV (followed by oral) steroid treatments.

Question

What is the role of immunosuppressive steroid-sparing agents (methotrexate, azathioprine, ciclosporin and dapsone) in the treatment of GCA?

The evidence

Methotrexate

A recent randomised, double-blind, placebo controlled trial investigated the efficacy of combined therapy with methotrexate and steroids for GCA.[20] Forty-two patients with biopsy-proven GCA were randomised to one of two arms and followed up for two years: oral prednisone (starting 60 mg/day and tapering gradually) plus oral methotrexate (10 mg/week for two years), or oral prednisone plus placebo. Calcium, vitamin D and folate supplements were given to all patients. Treatment with prednisone and methotrexate was associated with a reduced proportion of patients with at least one relapse compare to the placebo group (45% v 84·2%, $P = 0.02$). Although the frequency and severity of adverse events were similar in the two groups, the prednisone/methotrexate group received a lower cumulative dose of steroids than the placebo group (mean cumulative doses 4187 mg versus 5489·5 mg (mean difference 1302 mg, 95% CI 350–2253, $P = 0.009$).

Azathioprine

The ability of azathioprine to reduce the steroid maintenance dose was investigated in a small, controlled clinical trial in 31 patients with GCA and or polymyalgia rheumatica over one year.[21] A significant difference in mean prednisolone dose was noted in the azathioprine treated group.

Ciclosporin A

Ciclosporin A has been studied in an open, controlled, randomised study.[22] Twenty-two patients with long-standing GCA (mean 39 months' duration) and requiring more than 5 mg/day prednisolone were randomised either to prednisolone or prednisolone plus ciclosporin A and studied for six months. No significant differences were found between the two groups in terms of steroid requirements at six months.

Dapsone

Dapsone has been studied in several small studies and may have a beneficial effect but it is limited by adverse effects. Large, controlled trials are needed.

Comment

Methotrexate has shown some promise in a good quality controlled trial[20] but larger, controlled clinical trials are required to fully evaluate the potential of steroid-sparing immunosuppressants.

Question

Can the long-term complications of osteoporosis with steroid treatment be reduced for patients with GCA?

The evidence

Steroid therapy for GCA is long term (usually six to 24 months and sometimes life-long). Systemic complications include osteoporosis, peptic ulcer, diabetes, hypertension, hypokalaemia, immunosuppression, weight gain, psychiatric disturbances and ocular complications such as cataract and glaucoma. Osteoporosis (characterised by low bone mineral density (BMD)), and subsequent fracture are a major cause of morbidity and mortality, especially in elderly patients. The main treatments for steroid-induced osteoporosis are bisphosphonates, calcium and vitamin D, and calcitonin.

Three systematic reviews[23–25] were found which assessed the evidence for each of these three treatments in chronic inflammatory conditions (including GCA).

Bisphosphonates for steroid-induced osteoporosis[24]

All controlled clinical trials dealing with prevention or treatment of steroid-induced osteoporosis with bisphosphonates were assessed. Participants had to be taking a mean steroid dose of 7·5 mg/day. Thirteen trials (842 patients) were included. At the lumbar spine, the mean weighted difference in BMD between treatment and placebo groups at six to 12 months was 4·3% (95% CI 2·7–5·9). BMD was higher in the treatment group, indicating a beneficial effect. At the femoral neck it was 2·1% (95% CI 0·01–3·8). There was a 24% reduction in odds of spinal fracture, which was not significant (odds ratio (OR) 0·76, 95% CI 0·37–1·53). The reviewers concluded that bisphosphonates are effective at reducing steroid-induced osteoporosis of the lumbar spine and femoral neck. The effect on fracture prevention could not be concluded from the analysis.

Since this review a further randomised controlled trial was published, looking at 83 patients with polymyalgia rheumatica, rheumatoid arthritis and GCA.[26] Etidronate was compared to placebo after one year in patients taking 7·5 mg prednisolone. Lumbar spine BMD was found to be 2·8% higher in the etidronate group ($P = 0.002$). BMD at the femoral neck was also higher in the treatment group compared with placebo, but not significantly so (1·11% ± 1·13).

Calcium and vitamin D for steroid-induced osteoporosis[23]

Randomised controlled trials comparing calcium and vitamin D to calcium alone or placebo in patients on systemic corticosteroids were reviewed. Five trials (274 patients) were included. Analysis was performed at two years after commencement of calcium and vitamin D. There was a significant weighted mean difference in lumber spine (2·6%, 95% CI 0·7–4·5) and radius (2·5%, 95% CI 0·6–4·4),

BMD being higher in the treatment groups compared with the control groups. Other outcome measures (for example, femoral neck bone mass, fracture incidence) were not significantly different. The low toxicity and cost of calcium and vitamin D therapy prompted the reviewers to recommend their use with all patients started on systemic corticosteroids.

Calcitonin for steroid-induced osteoporosis[25]

This review included nine trials (221 patients treated with calcitonin and 220 with placebo). Calcitonin was more effective than placebo at preserving bone mass at the lumbar spine after six and 12 months of therapy with a weighted mean BMD difference of 2·8% (95% CI, 0·3–6·1) at 12 months. This effect was 4·5% (95% CI, −0·6–9·5) at 24 months and was not significant. BMD was also significantly higher in the treatment group after six months for the distal radius (2·9%, 95%CI 1·4–4·4) but not at 12 or 24 months. There was no difference at 6, 12 or 24 months for the femoral neck. The fracture risk was not significantly different between calcitonin and placebo (RR 0·71, 95% CI 0·26–1·89 for vertebral fractures, RR 0·52, 95% CI 0·14–1·96 for non-vertebral fractures). The reviewers concluded that calcitonin appears to preserve bone mass in the first year of steroid therapy and that its efficacy for fracture prevention remains to be established.

Comment

There is evidence that bisphosphonates and calcium with vitamin D retard the development of osteoporosis at two years after commencement of steroids. Their effect on the risk of sustaining fractures requires further investigation.

Non-arteritic anterior ischaemic optic neuropathy (NA-AION)

Epidemiology

The annual incidence of non-arteritic anterior ischaemic optic neuropathy (NA-AION) in the United States is 2·3 to 10·2 per 100 000 persons over 50 years and 0·54 per 100,000 for all ages.[27–29] Men and women are equally affected. The average age of onset is around 60 years.

Aetiology/risk factors

Various vascular risk factors are associated with NA-AION. These include hypertension, diabetes mellitus and cigarette use.[29,30] A retrospective case-control study found no evidence for prothrombotic parameters as risk factors. It did, however, confirm significant associations between NA-AION and vascular risk factors such as ischaemic heart disease (OR 2·9, CI 95% 1·3–6·4), hypercholesterolaemia (OR 2·6 CI 95% 1·6–5·5) and diabetes mellitus (OR 2·3 CI 95% 1·1–4·8).[31] A small cup-to-disc ratio is also associated (disc at risk) with developing NA-AION.[32] Other conditions that are thought to reduce the perfusion pressure of the optic nerve head have also been suggested as risk factors, for example, hypovolaemia secondary to spontaneous or surgical blood loss[33,34] and arterial nocturnal hypotension.[35]

Prognosis

The Ischemic Optic Neuropathy Decompression Trial (IONDT) has provided important data on the natural history of NA-AION. A 24-month update has shown that 31% of 87 patients in the untreated careful follow up group had visual acuities three or more Snellen acuity lines better than baseline and that 21·8% had visual acuities three or more lines worse than baseline.[36] Recurrent NA-AION is very rare in the same eye after two months of onset.[37] NA-AION in the contralateral eye is more common and has been reported in 10·5–73% of patients.[7] Most studies have reported a contralateral recurrence rate of 10–40% after 2–5 years.[37–39] A retrospective natural history study showed patients with NA-AION have an increased risk of dying from vascular related disease (myocardial infarction and stroke).[40]

Question

Is surgery beneficial for patients with acute NA-AION?

The evidence

A systematic review of surgical treatment for NA-AION is in the *Cochrane Library*.[41] The review included one randomised trial – the IONDT – which randomised 258 patients.[42] Results from the 244 participants who achieved six months' follow up showed that participants assigned to surgery did no better than participants assigned to careful follow up with improved visual acuity of three or more Snellen acuity lines at six months as the outcome: 32·6% of the surgery group improved compared with 42·7% of the careful follow up group (OR, adjusted for baseline visual acuity and diabetes, was 0·74 95% CI 0·39–1·38). In addition, participants receiving surgery had a greater risk of losing three or more lines at six months: 23·9% in the surgery group worsened compared with 12·4% in the careful follow up group (adjusted OR 1·96, 95% CI 0·87–4·41).

Since this review was published a 24-month follow up of 174 patients of the IONDT has been published.[36] This confirmed that there is no benefit for surgery compared with careful follow up as 31·0% of patients in the careful follow up group and 29·4% of patients in the surgery group had improved visual acuity of three or more lines (relative risk (RR) 0·95, $P = 0·87$). In comparison, 21·8% of the careful follow up patient group and 20·0% of the surgery group suffered a deterioration in visual acuity (RR 0·92, $P = 0·85$). At three months significantly fewer patients in the careful follow up group had suffered a deterioration in vision compared to the surgery group (9·1% for follow up versus 18·3% for surgery, RR 2·02, $P = 0·04$). A gradual decline in overall mean visual acuity was noted over time in both treatment groups although it was always better than baseline.

Comment

Optic nerve decompression is not effective in acute NA-AION. The IONDT also provided evidence that patients can experience improvement in vision. In addition, while NA-AION may be characterised by initial improvement for many patients, a gradual decline in visual function may occur during subsequent follow-up.

Question

What is the role of aspirin in the treatment of NA-AION?

The evidence

No systematic reviews or randomised controlled trials were found.

Comment

Four retrospective studies were found which compared the effect of aspirin treatment with no treatment on the development of contralateral NA-AION.[39,43–45] These studies suggest that aspirin may prevent the recurrence of NA-AION in the second eye in the short term (over two years). Prospective randomised controlled trials are required to confirm this effect. There is no evidence for the effect of aspirin on the visual outcome of the affected eye following NA-AION.

Question

What other treatment options have been studied for NA-AION?

The evidence

Various medical treatments have been reported including anticoagulants,[46] diphenylhydantoin,[47,48] vasodilators,[49] vasopressors (norepinephrine)[50,51] and corticosteroids,[52,53] hyperbaric oxygen[54] and HELP (heparin induced extracorporeal LDL/fibrinogen precipitation).[55] None of these has been proven effective.

A possible beneficial effect for levodopa has been reported.[56] In a small prospective, randomised, double-masked, placebo-controlled trial 20 patients with NA-AION of 30 months' mean duration received Sinomot (levodopa and carbidopa) or placebo and were followed up for 24 weeks. The levodopa group experienced a significant ($P = 0.016$) mean improvement of visual acuity over the placebo group at 12 weeks, which was still present at 24 weeks ($P = 0.036$). No improvement was observed for mean deviation of visual field loss ($P = 0.82$). Further prospective studies with larger cohorts are required to investigate these findings.

Comment

Levodopa may have a beneficial role in acute and chronic NA-AION but larger, prospective studies are required.

Implications for research

Research that investigates factors involved in the aetiology and pathogenesis of arteritic and non-arteritic anterior ischaemic optic neuropathy is required for effective treatments to be developed. For arteritic anterior ischaemic optic neuropathy, although steroids are known to improve outcome, further research is necessary to optimise their usage with regard to, for example, route of delivery, timing and dosage. There is also the need to investigate other potentially effective immunosuppressant therapies and strategies to minimise side effects of long-term steroid therapy. For non-arteritic ischaemic optic neuropathy, in terms of management, further prospective studies are required in order to investigate potentially beneficial treatments.

Implications for practice

For arteritic anterior ischaemic optic neuropathy, systemic corticosteroid treatment has been shown to suppress the inflammatory process and may help to restore some vision or prevent progression in the affected eye as well as reduce the risk of fellow eye involvement. Steroid therapy is often long term and consideration must be given to minimising side effects such as osteoporosis. Presently a few steroid-sparing agents have shown some promise but further studies are required to assess their efficacy comprehensively.

For non-arteritic anterior ischaemic optic neuropathy, optic nerve decompression is not considered helpful in influencing visual outcome. Some vascular risk factors are known to be important in its aetiology. Aspirin may reduce the frequency of involvement of the fellow eye although its effect on visual prognosis of the affected eye is not known. Levodopa may have some benefit but its role needs to be assessed in greater detail. About 30% of patients may improve their visual acuity over two years.

References

1. Hayreh SS. Anterior ischaemic optic neuropathy. I. Terminology and pathogenesis. *Br J Ophthalmol* 1974;**58**(12):955–63.
2. Machado EB, Michet CJ, Ballard DJ *et al.* Trends in incidence and clinical presentation of temporal arteritis in Olmsted County, Minnesota, 1950–1985. *Arthritis Rheum* 1988;**31**(6):745–9.
3. Hayreh SS, Podhajsky PA, Zimmerman B. Occult giant cell arteritis: ocular manifestations. *Am J Ophthalmol* 1998;**125**(4):521–6.
4. Weyand CM, Goronzy JJ. Pathogenic principles in giant cell arteritis. *Int J Cardiol* 2000;**75**(Suppl 1):S9–15.
5. Evans JM, Hunder GG. Polymyalgia rheumatica and giant cell arteritis. *Rheum Dis Clin North Am* 2000;**26**(3):493–515.
6. Huang D, Zhou Y, Hoffman GS. Pathogenesis: immunogenetic factors. *Best Pract Res Clin Rheumatol* 2001;**15**(2):239–58.
7. Beri M, Klugman MR, Kohler JA, Hayreh SS. Anterior ischemic optic neuropathy. VII. Incidence of bilaterality and various influencing factors. *Ophthalmology* 1987;**94**(8):1020–8.
8. Hayreh SS, Podhajsky PA, Zimmerman B. Ocular manifestations of giant cell arteritis. *Am J Ophthalmol* 1998;**125**(4):509–20.
9. Gonzalez-Gay MA, Blanco R, Rodriguez-Valverde V *et al.* Permanent visual loss and cerebrovascular accidents in giant cell arteritis: predictors and response to treatment. *Arthritis Rheum* 1998;**41**(8): 1497–1504.
10. Gonzalez-Gay MA, Garcia-Porrua C, Llorca J *et al.* Visual manifestations of giant cell arteritis. Trends and clinical spectrum in 161 patients. *Med (Baltimore)* 2000;**79**(5):283–92.
11. Liozon E, Herrmann F, Ly K *et al.* Risk factors for visual loss in giant cell (temporal) arteritis: a prospective study of 174 patients. *Am J Med* 2001;**111**(3):211–17.
12. Cid MC, Font C, Oristrell J *et al.* Association between strong inflammatory response and low risk of developing visual loss and other cranial ischemic complications in giant cell (temporal) arteritis. *Arthritis Rheum* 1998;**41**(1):26–32.
13. Matteson EL, Gold KN, Bloch DA, Hunder GG. Long-term survival of patients with giant cell arteritis in the American College of Rheumatology giant cell arteritis classification criteria cohort. *Am J Med* 1996;**100**(2):193–6.
14. Hachulla E, Boivin V, Pasturel-Michon U *et al.* Prognostic factors and long-term evolution in a cohort of 133 patients with giant cell arteritis. *Clin Exp Rheumatol* 2001;**19**(2):171–6.
15. Evans J, Hunder GG. The implications of recognizing large-vessel involvement in elderly patients with giant cell arteritis. *Curr Opin Rheumatol* 1997;**9**(1):37–40.
16. Danesh-Meyer HV, Savino PJ, Sergott RC. The prevalence of cupping in end-stage arteritic and nonarteritic anterior ischemic optic neuropathy. *Ophthalmology* 2001;**108**(3):593–8.
17. Liu GT. Visual loss: optic neuropathies. In: Liu GT, Volpe NJ, Galetta SL, eds. *Neuro-Ophthalmology: Diagnosis and Management.* Philadelphia: WB Saunders, 2000, pp. 103–87.
18. Chan CC, Paine M, O'Day J. Steroid management in giant cell arteritis. *Br J Ophthalmol* 2001;**85**(9):1061–4.

19. Chevalet P, Barrier JH, Pottier P et al. A randomized, multicenter, controlled trial using intravenous pulses of methylprednisolone in the initial treatment of simple forms of giant cell arteritis: a one year follow up study of 164 patients. J Rheumatol 2000;27(6):1484–91.

20. Jover JA, Hernandez-Garcia C, Morado IC, Vargas E, Banares A, Fernandez-Gutierrez B. Combined treatment of giant-cell arteritis with methotrexate and prednisone, a randomized, double-blind, placebo-controlled trial. Ann Intern Med 2001;134(2):106–14.

21. de Silva M, Hazleman BL. Azathioprine in giant cell arteritis/polymyalgia rheumatica: a double- blind study. Ann Rheum Dis 1986;45(2):136–8.

22. Schaufelberger C, Andersson R, Nordborg E. No additive effect of cyclosporin A compared with glucocorticoid treatment alone in giant cell arteritis: results of an open, controlled, randomized study. Br J Rheumatol 1998;37(4):464–5.

23. Homik J, Suarez-Almazor ME, Shea B, Cranney A, Wells G, Tugwell P. Calcium and vitamin D for corticosteroid-induced osteoporosis. In: Cochrane Collaboration: Cochrane Library. Issue 4. Oxford: Update Software, 2000.

24. Homik J, Cranney A, Shea B et al. Bisphosphonates for steroid-induced osteoporosis. In: Cochrane Collaboration: Cochrane Library. Issue 2. Oxford: Update Software, 2000.

25. Cranney A, Welch V, Adachi JD et al. Calcitonin for the treatment and prevention of corticosteroid-induced osteoporosis. In: Cochrane Collaboration: Cochrane Library. Issue 2. Oxford: Update Software, 2000.

26. Cortet B, Hachulla E, Barton I, Bonvoisin B, Roux C. Evaluation of the efficacy of etidronate therapy in preventing glucocorticoid-induced bone loss in patients with inflammatory rheumatic diseases. A randomized study. Rev Rheum Engl Ed 1999;66(4):214–19.

27. Johnson LN, Arnold AC. Incidence of nonarteritic and arteritic anterior ischemic optic neuropathy. Population-based study in the state of Missouri and Los Angeles County, California. J Neuroophthalmol 1994;14(1):38–44.

28. Hattenhauer MG, Leavitt JA, Hodge DO, Grill R, Gray DT. Incidence of nonarteritic anterior ischemic optic neuropathy. Am J Ophthalmol 1997;123(1):103–7.

29. Anonymous. Characteristics of patients with nonarteritic anterior ischemic optic neuropathy eligible for the Ischemic Optic Neuropathy Decompression Trial. Arch Ophthalmol 1996;114(11):1366–74.

30. Hayreh SS, Joos KM, Podhajsky PA, Long CR. Systemic diseases associated with nonarteritic anterior ischemic optic neuropathy. Am J Ophthalmol 1994;118(6):766–80.

31. Salomon O, Huna-Baron R, Kurtz S et al. Analysis of prothrombotic and vascular risk factors in patients with nonarteritic anterior ischemic optic neuropathy. Ophthalmology 1999;106(4):739–42.

32. Beck RW, Savino PJ, Repka MX, Schatz NJ, Sergott RC. Optic disc structure in anterior ischemic optic neuropathy. Ophthalmology 1984;91(11):1334–7.

33. Johnson MW, Kincaid MC, Trobe JD. Bilateral retrobulbar optic nerve infarctions after blood loss and hypotension. A clinicopathologic case study. Ophthalmology 1987;94(12):1577–84.

34. Williams EL, Hart WM, Jr, Tempelhoff R. Postoperative ischemic optic neuropathy. Anesth Analg 1995;80(5):1018–29.

35. Hayreh SS, Zimmerman MB, Podhajsky P, Alward WL. Nonarteritic anterior ischemic optic neuropathy: role of nocturnal arterial hypotension. Arch Ophthalmol 1997;115(7):942–5.

36. Ischemic Optic Neuropathy Decompression Trial: twenty-four-month update. Arch Ophthalmol 2000;118(6):793–8.

37. Repka MX, Savino PJ, Schatz NJ, Sergott RC. Clinical profile and long-term implications of anterior ischemic optic neuropathy. Am J Ophthalmol 1983;96(4):478–83.

38. Boghen DR, Glaser JS. Ischaemic optic neuropathy. The clinical profile and history. Brain 1975;98(4):689–708.

39. Beck RW, Hayreh SS, Podhajsky PA, Tan ES, Moke PS. Aspirin therapy in nonarteritic anterior ischemic optic neuropathy. Am J Ophthalmol 1997;123(2):212–17.

40. Sawle GV, James CB, Russell RW. The natural history of non-arteritic anterior ischaemic optic neuropathy. J Neurol Neurosurg Psychiatry 1990;53(10):830–3.

41. Dickersin K, Manheimer E. Surgery for nonarteritic anterior ischemic optic neuropathy (Cochrane Review). In: Cochrane Collaboration: Cochrane Library. Issue 2. Oxford: Update Software, 2002.

42. Optic nerve decompression surgery for nonarteritic anterior ischemic optic neuropathy (NAION) is not effective and may be harmful. The Ischemic Optic Neuropathy Decompression Trial Research Group. JAMA 1995;273(8):625–32.

43. Salomon O, Huna-Baron R, Steinberg DM, Kurtz S, Seligsohn U. Role of aspirin in reducing the frequency of second eye involvement in patients with non-arteritic anterior ischaemic optic neuropathy. Eye 1999;13(Pt 3a):357–9.

44. Kupersmith MJ, Frohman L, Sanderson M et al. Aspirin reduces the incidence of second eye NAION: a retrospective study. J Neuroophthalmol 1997;17(4):250–3.

45. Botelho PJ, Johnson LN, Arnold AC. The effect of aspirin on the visual outcome of nonarteritic anterior ischemic optic neuropathy. Am J Ophthalmol 1996;121(4):450–1.

46. Saraux H, Murat JP. [Pseudopapillitis of vascular origin]. Ann Ocul (Paris) 1967;200(1):1–19.

47. Keltner JL, Becker B, Gay AJ, Podos SM. Effect of diphenylhydantoin in ischemic optic neuritis. Trans Am Ophthalmol Soc 1972;70:113–30.

48. Ellenberger C, Jr, Burde RM, Keltner JL. Acute optic neuropathy. Treatment with diphenylhydantoin. Arch Ophthalmol 1974;91(6): 435–8.

49. Bonamour MG. [Apropos of "vascular pseudo-papillitis"]. Bull Soc Ophtalmol Fr 1966;66(9):846–50.

50. Kollarits CR, McCarthy RW, Corrie WS, Swann ER. Norepinephrine therapy of ischemic optic neuropathy. J Clin Neuroophthalmol 1981; 1(4):283–8.

51. Smith JL. Norepinephrine therapy of ischemic optic neuropathy. J Clin Neuroophthalmol 1981;1(4):289–90.

52. Sanders MD. Ischaemic papillopathy. Trans Ophthalmol Soc UK 1971;91:369–86.

53. Hayreh SS. Anterior ischaemic optic neuropathy. III. Treatment, prophylaxis, and differential diagnosis. Br J Ophthalmol 1974;58(12): 981–9.

54. Arnold AC, Hepler RS, Lieber M, Alexander JM. Hyperbaric oxygen therapy for nonarteritic anterior ischemic optic neuropathy. Am J Ophthalmol 1996;122(4):535–41.

55. Haas A, Walzl M, Jesenik F et al. Application of HELP in nonarteritic anterior ischemic optic neuropathy: a prospective, randomized, controlled study. Graefe's Arch Clin Exp Ophthalmol 1997;235(1):14–19.

56. Johnson LN, Gould TJ, Krohel GB. Effect of levodopa and carbidopa on recovery of visual function in patients with nonarteritic anterior ischemic optic neuropathy of longer than six months' duration. Am J Ophthalmol 1996;121(1):77–83.

47 Idiopathic intracranial hypertension

Christian J Lueck, Gawn G McIlwaine

Background

Definition

Idiopathic intracranial hypertension (IIH, also known as benign intracranial hypertension or pseudotumour cerebri) is defined as the presence of raised intracranial pressure without obvious abnormality on CT or MRI imaging of the head (in particular, no space-occupying lesion or enlargement of the ventricles), with no abnormality on examination of the cerebrospinal fluid constituents.[1] It represents a significant cause of visual loss of varying degrees, including complete blindness.

Epidemiology

There have been few epidemiological studies of IIH,[2–4] but these give fairly consistent figures for the incidence of the disease as 1–3 per 100 000 per year in those countries where it has been studied. IIH is much more common in women,[2–5] particularly obese women, when the incidence is as high as 21 per 100,000 per year.[4] It also occurs in children, in whom it is not more common in females[6] and in whom the incidence is reported to be 0·4–2·2 per 100 000 per year.[7]

Presentation

IIH usually presents with headaches and/or visual disturbance. The majority of patients have bilateral papilloedema, but there are reports of patients with unilateral papilloedema[8] and of patients without papilloedema.[9,10] A number of other physical signs may occur occasionally, but the only other physical sign that typically occurs is sixth nerve palsy. Though headache is a major source of morbidity,[11] the only major complication of the condition is visual loss. Blindness has been reported to occur in 10% of cases,[12] but varying degrees of visual loss occur in up to 87% if patients are carefully monitored.[13] The major aim of therapy is thus to prevent visual loss, but other management issues include treatment of headache, and treatment of visual loss once it has occurred.

Aetiology

The cause of IIH remains unknown. Various theories have been proposed relating to the possibility of increased brain, blood or cerebrospinal fluid (CSF) volumes, or the possiblity of increased secretion of CSF. However, the most generally accepted theory is that there is some form of resistance to CSF outflow, possibly at the level of the arachnoid villi. Support for this theory derives from the fact that cortical venous sinus thrombosis (CVST) gives rise to a similar clinical picture (and for many years has been confused with IIH). Modern imaging techniques are now able to detect venous sinus thrombosis relatively easily, and such patients are now not included in the definition of IIH. Accordingly, CVST is not discussed further in this chapter, and the reader is referred to other work for further information.[14]

Risk factors

There have been countless reports in the literature of a potential association between IIH and many different medical conditions or treatments, most notably obesity, vitamin A or its analogues (for example, isoretinoin), tetracyclines, renal disease and the oral contraceptive pill.[15,16] Only two major case-control studies have been performed,[11,17] and these have only shown a statistically significant relationship between IIH and female sex, being of reproductive age, obesity and recent weight gain. However, it should be borne in mind that the numbers involved in these studies were relatively small, and so other possible significant associations cannot be excluded.

Prognosis

The prognosis is variable. In some patients, the disease is relatively self-limiting, but it can continue for many years. It is also possible that patients may relapse following previous resolution of symptoms and signs.

Treatment options

Various different forms of management have been suggested in the literature. These include:

- weight loss either by dieting or aided by gastric (bariatric) surgery[18,19]
- repeated lumbar puncture[20]
- continuous negative abdominal pressure[21]
- pharmacological treatment with diuretics, for example, (most notably acetazolamide), glycerol or corticosteroids[22]
- surgical treament, usually optic nerve sheath fenestration (ONSF)[23–26] or lumboperitoneal shunting (LPS)[27]
- other techniques such as subtemporal decompression,[20] cisternoperitoneal or ventriculoperitoneal shunts.

There are many non-systematic reviews of IIH in the literature,[6,15,16,28–33] and a Cochrane systematic review.[34] Details of the various treatments can be obtained from non-systematic reviews elsewhere.[15,16,33]

Question

What is the best way to manage IIH in order to prevent visual loss?

The evidence

All management techniques have their proponents (and, in some cases, strong opponents).[35] However, a systematic review[34] has found that none of these procedures has yet been subjected to a controlled trial, let alone a randomised controlled trial.

Question

What is the best way to manage the headache that occurs in IIH?

The evidence

None of these treatments has been subjected to RCTs in the context of IIH.

Comment

The various treatments listed have all been reported to reduce headache in some, but not all patients (including, interestingly, ONSF).[23–25] It is often possible to treat the headache with standard headache therapies such as physiotherapy, non-steroidal anti-inflammatory drugs, anti-migraine therapy or tricyclic antidepressants.

Question

What is the best treatment for a patient with IIH who has evidence of visual loss?

The evidence

As above, possible management options for dealing with acute or subacute visual loss include lumbar puncture, surgical procedures, usually ONSF or LPS, but ventriculoperitoneal shunting has also been advocated. Again, no relevant RCTs exist.

Discussion

IIH is a significant cause of visual loss. Because of its numerous symptoms, it is possible for patients to present to various different specialities, including ophthalmology, neurology, neurosurgery, ENT or general medicine. Each discipline is likely to have their own preferred treatment option(s), and the management of individual patients is therefore largely dependent upon which medical speciality they were first referred to, for example, LPS is often easier if patients are being seen by neurosurgeons, ONSF if they are being seen by ophthalmologists. The condition is not rare: because it may go on for many years, the prevalence is considerably higher than the incidence, and patients need to be seen regularly for follow up to make sure they are not losing vision. Consequently, patients with IIH consume a large amount of healthcare resource that might be reduced if only the answers to the above questions were known.

Implications for practice

For the moment, management of patients with IIH has to be done without adequate evidence for or against the various treatment options. In the circumstances, it would seem reasonable to continue to do whatever is felt to be safe and effective until more formal evidence is available. In the absence of adequate information, a guide to "how we do it" has been published elsewhere.[36]

Implications for research

It is clear that there is a desperate need for RCTs in the management of this condition. In particular, there is a need to compare the two major invasive procedures of lumboperitoneal shunting and optic nerve sheath fenestration in a head-to-head trial. In addition, randomised controlled studies of the more non-invasive treatments including diuretics, weight loss and lumbar puncture are needed to work out which of these treatments is most appropriate and in what situation(s) they should be used.

References

1. Miller NR. Papilledema. In: Miller NR, Newman NJ eds. *Walsh & Hoyt's Clinical Neuro-Ophthalmology, 5th edn.* Baltimore: Williams & Wilkins, 1998, pp. 487–548.
2. Durcan FJ, Corbett JJ, Wall M. The incidence of pseudotumor cerebri: population studies in Iowa and Louisiana. *Arch Neurol* 1988;**45**:875–7.
3. Radhakrishnan K, Ahlskog JE, Cross SA, Kurland LT, O'Fallon WM. Idiopathic intracranial hypertension (pseudotumor cerebri). Descriptive epidemiology in Rochester, Minn, 1976 to 1990. *Arch Neurol* 1993; **50**:78–80.
4. Radhakrishnan K, Thacker AK, Bohlaga NH, Maloo JC, Gerryo SE. Epidemiology of idiopathic intracranial hypertension: a prospective and case-control study. *J Neurol Sci* 1993;**116**:18–28.
5. Wall M, George D. Idiopathic intracranial hypertension. A prospective study of 50 patients. *Brain* 1991;**114**:155–80.
6. Warman R. Management of pseudotumor cerebri in children. *Int Pediatr* 2000;**1**:147–50.
7. Gordon K. Pediatric pseudotumor cerebri: descriptive epidemiology. *Can J Neurol Sci* 1997;**24**:219–21.
8. Wall M, White WM. Asymmetric papilledema in idiopathic intracranial hypertension: prospective interocular comparison of sensory visual function. *Invest Ophthalmol Vis Sci* 1998;**39**:134–42.
9. Wang SJ, Silberstein SD, Patterson S, Young WB. Idiopathic intracranial hypertension without papilledema: a case-control study in a headache center. *Neurol* 1998;**51**:245–9.
10. Mathew NT, Ravishankar K, Sanin LC. Coexistence of migraine and idiopathic intracranial hypertension without papilledema. *Neurol* 1996;**46**:1226–30.
11. Giuseffi V, Wall M, Siegel PZ, Rojas PB. Symptoms and disease associations in idiopathic intracranial hypertension (pseudotumor cerebri): a case-control study. *Neurology* 1991;**41**:239–44.
12. Corbett JJ, Savino PJ, Thompson HS. Visual loss in pseudotumor cerebri. Follow-up of 57 patients from five to 41 years and a profile of 14 patients with permanent severe visual loss. *Arch Neurol* 1982;**39**:461–74.
13. Rowe FJ, Sarkies NJ. Assessment of visual function in idiopathic intracranial hypertension. A prospective study. *Eye* 1998;**12**:111–18.
14. de Bruijn SFTM, Deveber G, Stam J. Anticoagulants for cerebral sinus thrombosis (protocol for a Cochrane review). In: Cochrane Collaboration: *Cochrane Library.* Issue 4. Oxford: Update Software, 2001.
15. Digre KB, Corbett JJ. Idiopathic intracranial hypertension (Pseudotumor cerebri): a reappraisal. *Neurologist* 2001;**7**:2–67.
16. Friedman DI. Papilledema and pseudotumor cerebri. *Ophthalmol Clin North Am* 2001;**14**:129–47.
17. Ireland B, Corbett JJ, Wallace RB. The search for causes of idiopathic intracranial hypertension: a preliminary case-control study. *Arch Neurol* 1990;**47**:315–20.
18. Johnson LN, Krohel GB, Madsen RW, March GA. The role of weight loss and acetazolamide in the treatment of idiopathic intracranial hypertension (pseudotumor cerebri). *Ophthalmology* 1998;**105**:2313–17.
19. Sugerman HJ, Felton WL, Sismanis A, Kellum JM, DeMaria EJ, Sugerman EL. Gastric surgery for pseudotumor cerebri associated with severe obesity. *Ann Surg* 1999;**229**:634–40.
20. Johnston I, Paterson A, Besser M. The treatment of benign intracranial hypertension: a review of 134 cases. *Surg Neurol* 1981;**16**:218–24.
21. Sugerman HJ, Felton III WL, Sismanis A *et al.* Continuous negative abdominal pressure device to treat pseudotumor cerebri. *Int J Obes* 2001;**25**:486–90.
22. Go KG. Pseudotumour cerebri: incidence, management and prevention. *CNS Drugs* 2000;**14**:33–49.
23. Brourman ND, Spoor TC, Ramocki JM. Optic nerve sheath decompression for pseudotumor cerebri. *Arch Ophthalmol* 1988; **106**:1378–83.
24. Sergott RC, Savino PJ, Bosley TM. Modified optic nerve sheath decompression provides long-term visual improvement for pseudotumor cerebri. *Arch Ophthalmol* 1988;**106**:1384–90.
25. Corbett JJ, Nerad JA, Tse DT *et al.* Results of optic nerve sheath fenestration for pseudotumor cerebri: the lateral orbitotomy approach. *Arch Ophthalmol* 1988;**106**:1391–7.
26. Herzau V, Baykal HE. Long-term results of optic nerve sheath fenestration in pseudotumor cerebri. *Klin Monatsbl Augenheilkd* 1998;**213**:154–60.
27. Eggenberger ER, Miller NR, Vitale S. Lumboperitoneal shunt for the treatment of pseudotumor cerebri. *Neurology* 1996;**46**:1524–30.
28. Radhakrishnan K, Ahlskog JE, Garrity JA, Kurland LT. Idiopathic intracranial hypertension. *Mayo Clin Proc* 1994;**69**:169–80.
29. Scott IU, Siatkowski RM, Eneyni M, Brodsky MC, Lam BL. Idiopathic intracranial hypertension in children and adolescents. *Am J Ophthalmol* 1997;**124**:253–5.
30. Liu GT, Volpe NJ, Galetta SL. Pseudotumor cerebri and its medical treatment. *Drugs Today* 1998;**34**:563–74.
31. Soler D, Cox T, Bullock P, Calver DM, Robinson RO. Diagnosis and management of benign intracranial hypertension. *Arch Dis Child* 1998;**78**:89–94.
32. Sussman JD, Sarkies N, Pickard JD. Benign intracranial hypertension. Pseudotumour cerebri: idiopathic intracranial hypertension. *Adv Tech Stand Neurosurg* 1998;**24**:261–305.
33. Biousse V, Bousser MG. Benign intracranial hypertension. *Rev Neurol* 2001;**157**:21–34.
34. Lueck C, McIlwaine G. Interventions for idiopathic intracranial hypertension (Cochrane Review). In: Cochrane Collaboration: *Cochrane Library.* Issue 3. Oxford: Update Software, 2002.
35. Rosenberg ML, Corbett JJ, Smith C *et al.* Cerebrospinal fluid diversion procedures in pseudotumor cerebri. *Neurology* 1993;**43**: 1071–2.
36. Lueck CJ, McIlwaine GG. Idiopathic intracranial hypertension. *Practical Neurol* 2002;**2**:262–71.

48 Toxic and nutritional optic neuropathies

Fion Bremner

Background

It has been known for a long time that the optic nerve may be damaged by exposure to toxic substances or through nutritional deprivation. The clinical picture is similar regardless of aetiology, patients typically presenting with painless symmetrical caeco-central scotomata, often with rapid onset. The visual loss is associated in some cases with sensorineural hearing loss or a small fibre sensory peripheral neuropathy. The differential diagnosis includes the hereditary, compressive or inflammatory optic neuropathies, maculopathies and malingering. The clinical challenge is diagnostic (exclude all other causes and identify the toxin or nutritional defect) rather than therapeutic, but in individual cases it is often not possible to ascribe the visual loss to a single toxin or nutrient and the diagnosis remains presumptive.

> ### Question
>
> What is the evidence that exposure to or deficiency of any given substance causes an optic neuropathy?

The evidence

The first level of evidence is to prove that there has been exposure to or deficiency of the substance. In the literature on toxic optic neuropathies, exposure to a putative toxin has most commonly been established from the history (for example, tobacco smoking[1]), occasionally from systemic signs of acute intoxication (for example, ethylene glycol[2]), but rarely from measurement of blood levels (for example, methanol[3]). In the literature on sporadic cases of nutritional optic neuropathy, only vitamins B_{12} and folic acid have been routinely measured in the blood.[4] Other vitamin levels have rarely been assayed (for example, niacin[5]), and in most cases malnutrition has been inferred on clinical grounds (history, general examination and stigmata of specific avitaminoses) when multiple deficiencies are likely to have been present.

Two epidemics of optic neuropathy (Allied prisoners-of-war in the 1940s and Cuba in the 1990s) have afforded epidemiologists the opportunity to assess toxic, dietary and lifestyle risk factors for visual loss at a population level. In the former epidemic gross malnutrition, deficiencies of B vitamins, hard physical labour, male sex and smoking were common to all affected individuals,[6–8] but no case-control studies were performed nor were specific toxins or micronutrients measured. In the more recent epidemic, the Cuba Neuropathy Field Investigation Team conducted a matched-pair case-control study (n = 123) comparing diet, toxin exposure and serum concentrations of vitamin A and carotenoids.[9] Factors identified with an increased risk of visual loss included smoking (consumption of four or more cigars a day was associated with an odds ratio of 22·8) and high cassava intake. Factors associated with a reduced risk of visual loss included high dietary intakes of vitamins B_2, B_{12}, niacin and methionine, and high serum levels of the anti-oxidant carotenoids found in red fruits. In another case-control study mitochondrial DNA analysis showed no genetic predisposition for visual loss in affected cases.[10]

The second level of evidence is to demonstrate a relationship between the substance and the visual loss. Dose-dependence has been demonstrated for some toxins (for example, ethambutol,[11] halogenated hydroxyquinolines[12] and tobacco[9]) but not for any specific nutrients (in man). Improvement in visual function after removing a putative toxin or replacing a specific nutrient has been reported both in individual case reports[1,13–15] and in epidemiological studies[16] but does not occur in all cases.[17] In many studies the reported visual recovery or prevention of visual loss followed much more general measures of nutritional supplementation or toxin avoidance.[18] Visual deterioration on re-challenge with the toxin or nutrient deficiency would be unethical in man, and no reports exist in the literature when this has occurred inadvertently.

Tobacco and alcohol have long been implicated as epigenetic triggers for visual loss in patients harbouring pathogenic mutations for Leber's hereditary optic neuropathy (LHON). Affected patients often smoke or drink excessively[19–21] and mitochondrial DNA analysis occasionally reveals primary LHON mutations in singleton cases diagnosed clinically as tobacco–alcohol amblyopia.[22] Three case-control studies have examined this association, with differing results (see Table 48.1). The first study[23]

Table 48.1   Case–control studies examining the association with alcohol and tobacco

Study	Controls	Cases	Mutation	Alcohol	Tobacco
				Association with:	
Chalmers and Harding, 1996[23]	50	35	11778	NS	NS
		15	14484 or 3460	$P = 0.05$	$P = 0.009$
Tsao, *et al.*, 1999[24]	55	10	11778	–	$P = 0.0009$
Kerrison *et al.*, 2000[25]	158	103	All	$P = 0.0011$	NS

found weak associations between tobacco and alcohol consumption and visual loss for patients with the 14484 or 3460 mutations, but since half of their unaffected "controls" were unrelated (and presumably did not have LHON mutations) it is hard to interpret these data. The second study[24] suggested smoking was a risk factor in one large pedigree with the 11778 mutation. The third and largest study[25] considered only exposure prior to visual loss and found no evidence of risk from smoking and, if anything, a protective role for alcohol consumption.

The third level of evidence is to demonstrate histological damage to optic nerve fibres in patients exposed to or deficient in the substance. There are several postmortem studies in patients who have died of methanol intoxication showing retrobulbar demyelination,[26] central necrosis[27] or atrophy with secondary astrocytic hyperplasia[28] of the distal optic nerves; however most other putative toxins are not fatal and postmortem material has not been available to study. There are a few anecdotal reports of lesions in the optic nerves of patients with pernicious anaemia[29] and in malnourished Allied prisoners-of-war,[30] but patients with specific micronutrient deficiencies usually survive, so autopsy material is rarely available.

The final level of evidence is the establishment of an experimental model proving a causal relationship between the toxin or nutrient and optic neuropathy. Despite the obvious ethical objections there were a number of attempts prior to the second world war to observe the effects of imposing vitamin deficiency on human volunteers[31–33]: systemic disturbances such as anorexia, nausea/vomiting, fatigue and depression were observed at levels known to be found in patients with beriberi or pellagra, but in no case was vision affected. Good animal models have been established for some toxic (methanol[34,35] and ethambutol[36–38]) and nutritional (B_{12}[39,40]) optic neuropathies, but other substances have failed to produce optic nerve damage in animal experiments (for example, cyanide[41] and vitamin B_1[42]).

Discussion

Obtaining evidence to prove a substance caused an optic neuropathy is confounded by the rarity of these cases, the lack of laboratory tests to confirm exposure or deficiency, and the complicated medical backgrounds of this group of patients. There are only a few cases where optic nerve damage can confidently be ascribed to a toxin (methanol, ethambutol) or micronutrient deficiency (vitamin B_{12}); in most cases the association is anecdotal and presumptive. Multiple risk factors usually coexist in these patients, including genetic predisposition, sex, complex nutritional requirements and exposure to toxins many of which have not yet been identified, and it is possible that their combined effect is of more relevance than any individual substance. Despite these diverse risk factors the clinical presentation is impressively stereotyped. This raises the intriguing possibility that in all of these patients there is a final common pathway for damage to optic nerve fibres, perhaps through impairment of mitochondrial ATP production.

Implications for research

Accuracy and specificity when diagnosing toxic or nutritional optic neuropathy needs to be improved by the development of comprehensive, generally available laboratory blood tests to measure exposure or deficiency of different substances. These would enable detailed case-control studies to be conducted examining the role of different toxins and nutrients. Animal models are then important because they allow the investigator to study the pathogenetic mechanisms of damage: discovery of a final common pathway might lead to a range of possible therapeutic interventions that are independent of the underlying aetiology.

References

1. Rizzo JF, Lessell S. Tobacco amblyopia. *Am J Ophthalmol* 1993;**116**:84–7.
2. Friedman EA, Greenberg JB, Merrill JP *et al.* Consequences of ethylene glycol poisoning. *Am J Med* 1962;**32**:891–902.
3. McMartin KE, Amber JJ, Tephly TR. Methanol poisoning in human subjects: role for formic acid accumulation in the metabolic acidosis. *Am J Med* 1980;**68**:414–18.
4. Montgomery RD, Cruickshank EK, Robertson WB *et al.* Clinical and pathological observations on Jamaican neuropathy. *Brain* 1964;**87**:425–62.
5. Knox DL, Chen MF, Guilarte TR *et al.* Nutritional amblyopia. *Retina* 1982;**2**:288–93.
6. Beam AD. Amblyopia due to dietary deficiency: report of eight cases. *Arch Ophthalmol* 1946;**36**:113–19.
7. Bloom SM, Merz EH, Taylor WW. Nutritional amblyopia in American prisoners of war liberated from the Japanese. *Am J Ophthalmol* 1946;**29**:1248–57.
8. Dekking HM: Tropical nutritional amblyopia ("camp eyes"). *Ophthalmologica* 1947;**113**:65–92.
9. Cuba Neuropathy Field Investigation Team. Epidemic optic neuropathy in Cuba: clinical characterization and risk factors. *N Eng J Med* 1995;**333**:1176–82.
10. Newman NJ, Torroni A, Brown MD *et al.* Epidemic neuropathy in Cuba not associated with mitochondrial DNA mutations found in Leber's hereditary optic neuropathy patients. *Am J Ophthalmol* 1994;**118**:158–68.
11. Liebold JE. The ocular toxicity of ethambutol and its relation to dose. *Ann NY Acad Sci* 1966;**135**:904–9.
12. Oakley GP. The neurotoxicity of the halogenated hydroxyquinolines. *JAMA* 1973;**225**:395–7.
13. Greiner JV, Pillai S, Limaye SR *et al.* Sterno-induced methanol toxicity and visual recovery after prompt dialysis. *Arch Ophthalmol* 1989;**107**:643.
14. Golnik KC, Schaible ER. Folate-responsive optic neuropathy. *J Clin Neuro-ophthalmol* 1994;**14**:163–9.
15. Sadun AA, Martone JF, Muci-Mendoza R *et al.* Epidemic optic neuropathy in Cuba: eye findings. *Arch Ophthalmol* 1994;**112**:691–9.
16. Nakae K, Yamamoto S, Shigematsu K *et al.* Relation between subacute myelo-optic neuropathy (SMON) and clioquinol: nationwide survey. *Lancet* 1973;**1**:171–3.
17. Kumar A, Sandramouli S, Verma L *et al.* Ocular ethambutol toxicity: is it reversible? *J Clin Neuro-ophthalmol* 1993;**13**:15–17.
18. Centers for disease control: epidemic neuropathy – Cuba, 1991–1994. *MMWR* 1994;**43**:183–92.
19. Wilson J. Leber's hereditary optic atrophy: some clinical and aetiological considerations. *Brain* 1963;**86**:347–62.
20. Adams JH, Blackwood W, Wilson J. Further clinical and pathological observations on Leber's optic atrophy. *Brain* 1966;**89**:15–26.
21. Riordan-Eva P, Sanders MD, Govan GG *et al.* The clinical features of Leber's hereditary optic neuropathy defined by the presence of a pathogenic mitochondrial DNA mutation. *Brain* 1995;**118**:319–37.
22. Cullom ME, Heher KL, Miller NR *et al.* Leber's hereditary optic neuropathy masquerading as tobacco–alcohol amblyopia. *Arch Ophthalmol* 1993;**111**:1482–5.
23. Chalmers RM, Harding AE. A case-control study of Leber's hereditary optic neuropathy. *Brain* 1996;**119**:1481–6.
24. Tsao K, Aitken PA, Johns DR. Smoking as an aetiological factor in a pedigree with Leber's hereditary optic neuropathy. *Br J Ophthalmol* 1999;**83**:577–81.
25. Kerrison JB, Miller NR, Hsu FC *et al.* A case-control study of tobacco and alcohol consumption in Leber hereditary optic neuropathy. *Am J Ophthalmol* 2000;**130**:803–12.
26. Sharpe JA, Hostovsky M, Bilbao JM *et al.* Methanol optic neuropathy: a histopathological study. *Neurology* 1982;**32**:1093–100.
27. Naeser P. Optic nerve involvement in a case of methanol poisoning. *Br J Ophthalmol* 1988;**72**:778–81.
28. McLean DR, Jacobs H, Mielke BW. Methanol poisoning: a clinical and pathological study. *Ann Neurol* 1980;**8**:161–7.
29. Adams RD, Kubik CS. Subacute combined degeneration of the brain in pernicious anaemia. *N Engl J Med* 1944;**231**:1–9.
30. Fisher CM. Residual neuropathological changes in Canadians held prisoners of war by the Japanese (Strachan's disease). *Can Serv Med J* 1955;**11**:157–99.
31. Elsom KO. Experimental study of vitamin B deficiency. *J Clin Invest* 1940;**14**:40–51.
32. Williams RD, Nason HL, Wilder RM *et al.* Observations on induced thiamine deficiency in man. *Arch Intern Med* 1940;**66**:785–99.
33. Williams RD, Nason HL, Power MH *et al.* Induced thiamine (vitamin B1) deficiency in man. *Arch Intern Med* 1943;**71**:38–53.
34. Baumbach GL, Cancilla PA, Martin-Amat G *et al.* Methyl alcohol poisoning: IV. Alterations of the morphological findings of the retina and optic nerve. *Arch Ophthalmol* 1977;**95**:1859–65.
35. Hayreh MS, Hayreh SS, Baumbach GL *et al.* Methyl alcohol poisoning: III. Ocular toxicity. *Arch Ophthalmol* 1977;**95**:1851–8.
36. Schmidt IG, Schmidt LH. Studies of the neurotoxicity of ethambutol and its racemate for the rhesus monkey. *J Neuropath Exp Neurol* 1966;**25**:40–67.
37. Matsuoka Y, Mukyama M, Sobue I. Histopathological study of experimental ethambutol neuropathy. *Clin Neurol* 1972;**12**:453–9.
38. Lessell S. Histopathology of experimental ethambutol intoxication. *Invest Ophthalmol* 1976;**15**:765–9.
39. Hind VMD. Degeneration in the peripheral visual pathway of vitamin B12-deficient monkeys. *Trans Ophthalmol Soc UK* 1970;**90**:839–46.
40. Agamanolis DP, Chester EM, Victor M *et al.* Neuropathology of experimental vitamin B12 deficiency in monkeys. *Neurology* 1976;**26**:905–14.
41. Foulds WS, Pettigrew AR. Tobacco–alcohol amblyopia. In: Brockhurst RJ, Boruchoff SA, Hutchinson BT *et al.*, eds. *Controversy in Ophthalmology*. Philadelphia: WB Saunders, 1977, pp. 851–65.
42. Cogan DG, Witt ED, Goldman-Rakic PS. Ocular signs in thiamine-deficient monkeys and in Wernicke's disease in humans. *Arch Ophthalmol* 1985;**103**:1212–20.

49 Traumatic optic neuropathy

Andrew S Jacks

Background

Definition

Traumatic optic neuropathy is an injury to the optic nerve following an episode of trauma, which may be direct or indirect.[1,2] Traumatic optic neuropathy is a clinical diagnosis based on reduced vision (not explicable by other ophthalmic problems), presence of a relative afferent pupil defect (RAPD),[3] reduced colour vision, and an associated visual field defect.[4–6] The clinical examination can be complicated by the level of the patient's consciousness and other problems associated with the trauma.

Incidence

The incidence of traumatic optic neuropathy is estimated to be between 0·7% and 2% of all cases with head trauma,[4,7,8] and the population affected is young and predominantly male. The international optic nerve trauma study showed an average age of 34 ± 18 years, of whom 85% were male.[9] Similar results have been seen in other studies.[10–12] These studies used patients who presented to the emergency department with head trauma who were subsequently identified to have an ophthalmic injury.

Aetiology

Motor vehicle or bicycle accidents are the most common cause of trauma.[9–12] Direct optic nerve trauma results from a penetration of the orbit that involves the optic nerve, such as a stab to the orbit. These produce severe and immediate visual loss.[2,13] Indirect optic nerve trauma is caused by forces transmitted from a distant injury to the optic nerve.[1,14] These may be associated with visual recovery and delayed visual loss. The degree of visual loss can be severe or mild.[14]

Prognosis

Visual improvement in untreated cases of indirect traumatic optic neuropathy has been reported in 25% to 45% of patients.[9,10,12,15] The prognosis is less good if the injury is direct and if the initial visual loss is more severe.[10] This leaves a large percentage of indirect traumatic optic neuropathy patients who make no post-trauma improvement and who have visual loss.

Treatment options

The treatment options are no treatment, medical treatment with the use of systemic steroids in high or very high doses, and surgical treatment with decompression of the optic canal.

> **Question**
>
> What is the best form of treatment for visual loss from indirect traumatic optic neuropathy that does not improve spontaneously?

The evidence

No randomised controlled trials were found.

Comment

Only one prospective study of indirect traumatic optic neuropathy has been performed.[9] The study was a non-randomised, non-masked comparative interventional study with concurrent treatment groups. The aim of this study was to compare corticosteroids, optic canal decompression, and no treatment. The study was performed over a three-year period on 206 patients by 76 investigators in 16 countries. The patients were treated as deemed appropriate by the individual investigators according to their customary practice. The results are summarised in Table 49.1. The results show that there is no significant difference in the improvement of vision between the three groups. The confounding features that might have influenced the results were that the surgical group included more severe cases and cases that did not respond to steroid treatment. The study was underpowered because of the relative rarity of the cases.

All other reports are those of retrospective studies,[10,11,12,15] and these have not been randomised, controlled or masked studies. They all produced similar results showing no difference between the three treatment options.

Table 49.1   Results of prospective, non-randomised study[9]

	At least one month follow up			At least three months follow up		
	No treatment	Steroids	Surgery	No treatment	Steroids	Surgery
Overall 3 or more lines improvement	n = 7 4 (57%)	n = 64 33 (52%)	n = 25 8 (32%)	n = 4 2 (50%)	n = 54 29 (54%)	n = 21 8 (38%)
Baseline NLP, LP, HM 3 or more lines improvement	n = 3 1 (33%)	n = 34 15 (44%)	n = 23 6 (26%)	n = 2 1 (50%)	n = 26 12 (46%)	n = 19 6 (32%)
Baseline CF or better 3 or more lines improvement	n = 4 3 (75%)	n = 30 18 (60%)	n = 2 2 (100%)	n = 2 1 (50%)	n = 28 17 (61%)	n = 2 2 (100%)
Unadjusted (adjusted) *P* for comparison with untreated group*	–	1·0 (1·0)	0·38 (1·0)	–	1·0 (1·0)	1·0 (1·0)
Unadjusted (adjusted) *P* for comparison with steroid group*	1·0 (1·0)	–	0·11 (0·52)	1·0 (1·0)	–	0·31 (0·83)

*Fisher's exact test used for unadjusted comparison of proportion 3 lines improvement; exact test for common odds ratio used for adjusted comparison

NLP, no light perception; LP, light perception; HM, hand motion vision; CF, count fingers visual acuity

Implications for research

The study of traumatic optic neuropathy cases is difficult due to the uncommon nature of the problem, the wide variety of exact injury to the nerve and thus natural history outcome and how this will affect results.

Implications for practice

The individual clinical situation is of course complex, and faced with a patient with severe visual loss and no clear guidance from the above studies as to which treatment is better, the clinician will have to decide how to proceed on the merits of each case.

References

1 Kline LB, Morawtz RB, Swaid SN. Indirect injury to the optic nerve. *Neurosurgery* 1984;**14**:756–64.
2 Steinsapir KD, Goldberg RA. Traumatic optic neuropathy. *Surv Ophthalmol* 1994;**38**:487–518.
3 Bilyk JR, Joseph MP. Traumatic optic neuropathy. *Semin Ophthalmol* 1994;**9**:200–11.
4 Turner JWA. Indirect injury to the optic nerves. *Brain* 1943;**66**:140–50.
5 Edmund J, Godtfredson E. Unilateral optic atrophy following head injury. Journal? 1963;**41**:693–7. Check on medline.
6 Kennerdell JS, Amsbaugh GA, Myers EN. Transantral ethmoidal decompression of optic canal fracture. *Arch Ophthalmol* 1976;**94**:1040–3.
7 Brandle K. Die posttraumatischen opticusschadigungen. *Confina Neurolog* 1955;**15**:169–208.
8 Matsuzaki H, Kunita M, Kawai K. Optic nerve damage in head trauma: clinical and experimental studies. *Jpn J Ophthalmol* 1982;**26**:447–61.
9 Levin LA, Beck RW, Joseph MP *et al*. The treatment of traumatic optic neuropathy: the international optic nerve trauma study. *Ophthalmology* 1999;**106**:1268–77.
10 Wang BH, Robertson BC, Girotto JA *et al*. Traumatic optic neuropathy: a review of 61 patients. *Plast Reconstr Surg* 2001;**107**:1655–64.
11 Agarwal A, Mahapatra AK. Visual outcome in optic nerve injury patients without initial light perception. *Ind J Ophthalmol* 1999;**47**:233–6.
12 Seiff SR. High dose corticosteroids for treatment of vision loss due to indirect injury to the optic nerve. *Ophthalmic Surg* 1990;**21**:389–95.
13 Elisevich KV, Ford RM, Anderson DP *et al*. Visual abnormalities with multiple trauma. *Surg Neurol* 1984;**22**:565–75.
14 Steinsapir KD, Goldberg RA. Traumatic optic neuropathies. In: Miller NR, Newman NJ, eds. *Walsh and Hoyt's Clinical Neuro-ophthalmology 5th edn*. Baltimore: Williams and Wilkins, 1998.
15 Lessell S. Indirect optic nerve trauma. *Arch Ophthalmol* 1989;**107**:382–6.

Section XII

Ophthalmic oncology

Arun D Singh, Editor

Ophthalmic oncology: mission statement

Ocular oncology is a small ophthalmic sub-specialty dealing with diagnosis and treatment of patients with ocular tumours and related disorders. Such specialist services are limited to a few large ophthalmic centres that can offer multi-specialty care involving oncologists, radiation oncologists, paediatricians, paediatric oncologists and genetic counsellors. As ocular tumours are rare, only few studies involving large numbers of patients have been conducted. Nevertheless, issues in ocular oncology are important as they not only impact visual outcome but also ocular salvage and life prognosis.

The aims of this section are to describe the available evidence from large case series, retrospective studies as well as even small case series to highlight important questions that have yet to be addressed. The section comprises three chapters delaing with common ocular tumours such as eyelid tymours, uveal melanoma and retinoblastoma.

50 Ocular adnexal and orbital tumours

Santosh G Honavar, Arun D Singh

Background

Malignant tumours of the eyelid, ocular adnexa and orbit constitute a significant proportion of cancers diagnosed and managed by an ocular oncologist.

Prevalence

Basal cell carcinoma, squamous cell carcinoma, and sebaceous gland carcinoma are the three common malignant tumours of the eyelids.[1] Basal cell carcinoma is the most common malignant tumour of the eyelid in the Caucasian population[2] while sebaceous gland carcinoma occurs more frequently in Asians.[3] Melanoma, lymphoma and ocular surface squamous neoplasia are the common malignant tumours of the conjunctiva.[4] Conjunctival melanoma and lymphoma are common in Europe and America[5] while ocular surface squamous neoplasia is predominant in Asia and Australia.[6,7] Common orbital malignancies include lymphoma, metastasis and lacrimal gland tumours.[8]

Treatment options

Although some of the basic principles of management are uniformly followed, there is wide variation in the overall management of a particular tumour between major clinical centres. In this chapter we have attempted to examine the evidence in support of some of the existing beliefs and treatment protocols in the management of these tumours.

Sebaceous gland carcinoma of the eyelid

Prevalence

Sebaceous gland carcinoma constitutes 1–3% of all malignant eyelid tumours.[9,10] The disease commonly affects the elderly population, and women more predominantly than men.[9,10] The tumour is relatively more common in the Asian population, constituting about 33% of all malignant eyelid tumours.[3]

Aetiology

The tumour arises from the meibomian glands in the tarsus, Zeis glands associated with the lashes, and rarely from the caruncle.[9,10] The clinical spectrum is broad and includes the typical nodular type, noduloulcerative type, ulcerative lesion and the diffuse pagetoid tumour.[9,10] While the nodular variant clinically simulates a common chalazion, the diffuse pagetoid type often presents as unilateral blepharoconjunctivitis (masquerade syndrome), leading to delayed diagnosis and inappropriate management.[9–11]

Treatment options

Wide surgical excision with histopathologically confirmed tumour-free margins is believed to be an effective treatment for sebaceous gland carcinoma.[9,10] Radiation is reserved for recurrences and inoperable cases.[9,10]

Prognosis

Between 9% and 36% of sebaceous gland carcinomas recur.[9] Recurrences may be local in the eyelid or orbit in 6–17% of cases, while regional lymph node metastasis occurs in 17% to 28%.[9] The mortality from sebaceous gland carcinoma is estimated to range from 6% to 30%.[9]

Several prognostic factors for local recurrence and tumour metastasis have been identified that include location and size of the tumour, its site of origin, duration of symptoms before excision and histological pattern and degree of cellular differentiation.[9,12,13] Poor prognosis is indicated by location of the tumour in the upper eyelid, size of 10 mm or more in diameter, origin from the meibomian glands or multicentricity, duration of symptoms for more than six months, infiltrative pattern of growth, invasion of lymphatic and vascular channels, and the orbit, and moderate to poor sebaceous differentiation.[9,12,13] From the literature, it is unclear whether intraepithelial invasion in sebaceous gland carcinoma indicates a poor prognosis although this is a prevalent clinical impression.

The evidence

Sebaceous gland carcinoma is such a rare tumour that it is not surprising that we did not find randomised controlled trials, systematic reviews, or meta-analyses addressing the issue.

Comment

Some retrospective studies suggest that cases of sebaceous gland carcinoma with intraepithelial neoplasia had a significantly greater mortality than cases without these changes. Boniuk and Zimmerman felt that the long delay in correct diagnosis and appropriate management probably contributes to 30% mortality in patients with intraepithelial neoplasia.[14] Rao and associates reported a five-year mortality rate of 43% in patients who had intraepithelial neoplasia, compared to 11% in patients who did not.[12,13] Doxanas and Green found that the mortality was not substantially influenced by the presence or absence of intraepithelial neoplasia.[15] In their series, tumour-related deaths occurred in 14% of patients with intraepithelial neoplasia and 18% in those without such involvement.[15] A recent retrospective case series by Chao and associates reported that patients with intraepithelial neoplasia carried a higher risk for orbital exenteration (36% v 7%), but comparable incidence of tumour metastasis.[16]

Implications for practice and research

Although there is a disagreement over the prognostic significance of intraepithelial neoplasia, the clinical significance of its early recognition cannot be overemphasised. The management of such tumours can be challenging. Conjunctival map biopsy may help delineate the extent of involvement.[17–19] Some authors have suggested observation of small areas of involvement while others have recommended surgical excision with clear margins, adjuvant cryotherapy, radiotherapy, or orbital exenteration depending on the nature and extent of involvement.

Basal cell carcinoma of the eyelid

Background

Basal cell carcinoma is the most common human malignancy and accounts for over 80% of all non-melanoma skin cancers.[20] It is the most common skin cancer of the eyelid (80–90%) in the Western population.[21–24] Most tumours arise from the lower eyelid or medial canthus.[25] These tumours rarely metastasise but can potentially cause mortality by extensive tissue destruction and direct invasion of the central nervous system.[26]

Treatment options

There are a variety of methods used to treat basal cell carcinomas.[25,26] The management strategy depends on the size, extent and location of the lesion.[25,26] Some of the modalities of management of basal cell carcinoma include electrodessication, cryotherapy, photodynamic therapy, local or systemic chemotherapy, surgical excision and radiation therapy.[25,26] Surgical excision is coupled with a suitable technique to determine the adequacy of the margins.[27–29] Mohs' micrographic technique is considered the most reliable surgical method for tumour extirpation.[30–34] It differs from the other methods of microscopic control in several respects. The tumour is excised in a layered manner, is carefully mapped and the entire surgical margin is examined microscopically.[34] Mohs' micrographic surgery is believed to have the lowest recurrence rate for both primary and recurrent tumours.[30–34]

In the past, ophthalmologists have traditionally tended toward surgical management for periocular basal cell carcinomas. However, the growing experience with radiotherapy and the improving success rate now make this modality an acceptable alternative in several cases.[26]

The evidence

We found no randomised controlled trial comparing the efficacy of the Mohs' micrographic procedure with radiation therapy in the management of periocular basal cell carcinoma.

Comment

We found several case series evaluating the two modalities individually and a systematic review article that gives an overview.[34] Five-year cure rates for Mohs' micrographic surgery in the treatment of small (<3 cm) primary periocular basal cell carcinomas have been reported by several authors to range from 97–99%.[35–42] The cure rate is high for smaller tumours and relatively low for larger tumours.[35–43] However, there was significantly more failure when the tumour size was 3 mm or larger (10%).[37–40] Callahan and associates report an impressive success (98%) in a group of 231 patients with large or recurrent tumours at an average follow up of four years.[44,45]

Radiation therapy for primary basal cell carcinoma carries a five-year cure rate ranging from 70–98%.[26,31,32,34,46–51] Five-year control rates of 95–98% in some series are comparable to the results of surgical therapy.[49] Basal cell carcinomas ≤ 2 cm in diameter are controlled with irradiation in more than 90% of cases.[26,34] Large tumours (>5 cm) are more likely to recur (>40%) than small tumours. There is evidence to suggest that morpheaform basal cell carcinoma may be more radio-resistant.[26,34]

Utilising modern techniques, both Mohs' surgery and radiotherapy would appear to offer good and nearly comparable control of periocular tumours.[34] The growing experience with radiotherapy and the improving success rate now makes this modality an acceptable alternative in several cases.[26,34]

Implications for practice and research

The choice between the two techniques for the management of basal cell carcinoma will depend on several factors including tumour location, size and extent; whether it is a primary or a recurrent tumour; the availability of a Mohs' surgeon, an oculoplastic surgeon, or a radiotherapist with experience in treating such tumours; the availability of tissue for reconstruction; and the potential functional consequences of treatment.[34] For small tumours Mohs' surgery is appropriate and reconstruction is fairly simple.[34] Although radiotherapy for such small tumours gives excellent results, it is less convenient, requiring multiple treatment sessions over several weeks, and probably offers little advantage over Mohs' surgery in most cases.[34] For medium-sized lesions, and for those that are very extensive and difficult to resect, radiotherapy offers a good alternative to surgery, yielding better cosmetic and functional results with only a marginally higher recurrence rate.[34] For all recurrent tumours, regardless of size, Mohs' surgery with histological control of margins is mandatory, and radiotherapy is not appropriate, unless the tumours are unresectable.[34]

Mohs' microsurgical technique and radiotherapy can be interchangeably used in most situations in patients with basal cell carcinoma. The nature, location, size and extent of the tumour, and the cosmetic and functional implications of a particular treatment modality help in deciding for a treatment option.

Ocular surface squamous neoplasia

Background

Ocular surface squamous neoplasia (OSSN) presents as a spectrum ranging from dysplasia to carcinoma *in situ* to invasive squamous cell carcinoma, involving the conjunctiva as well as the cornea.[52,53]

Prevalence

It is a relatively uncommon ocular tumour, with an incidence varying from 0·13 per 100 000 population in Africa[54] to 1·9 per 100 000 population in Australia.[55] Although the condition is predominant in Caucasians, darker skinned people in tropical climates closer to the equator do develop OSSN.[53] The disease preferentially occurs in older individuals.[52,53] The spectrum of histological severity of OSSN has been classified.[56,57]

Treatment options

Tumour excision with adequate margins is the most accepted method of treatment of OSSN.[52,53] Several variations in the surgical technique have been described.[52,53,58–60] Additional procedures may include cryotherapy to the excision edge and base, use of alcohol to remove the affected corneal epithelium, lamellar keratectomy and lamellar sclerectomy.[52,53,61]

Local recurrence rates following tumour excision range from 15–52%.[53] Inadequacy of excision margins has been identified as a major risk factor for recurrence.[57,62] Other modalities of treatment include radiotherapy, immunotherapy and chemotherapy.[52,53] These modalities are mostly advocated in situations where tumour excision is not feasible or optimal.[52,53] Recent attention has been given to the use of topical chemotherapy in the management of OSSN.[63–71] The topical chemotherapeutic agents that have been evaluated are mitomycin C and 5-fluorouracil (5-FU).[63–72]

Mitomycin C is an alkylating agent that induces cross-linkage of the DNA base pairs adenine and guanine and inhibits DNA synthesis in all phases of the cell cycle, in addition to causing breakage of single-stranded DNA.[72] The adjunctive use of mitomycin C is well established in trabeculectomy and recurrent pterygium surgery.[72]

Dermatologists have long used topical 5-FU in the treatment of premalignant and malignant epithelial diseases of the skin.[72] The drug has been evaluated for its antifibroblastic action in trabeculectomy. The mechanism of action of 5-FU is the inhibition of DNA formation by blocking the enzyme thymidylate synthetase.[72]

Question

Is there a role for primary topical chemotherapy in the management of ocular surface squamous neoplasia (OSSN)?

The evidence

We found no randomised controlled study evaluating the role of topical chemotherapeutic agents in the management of OSSN.

Comment

A review article by Majumdar and Epstein[72] summarises several small case series that have been published in peer-reviewed journals, which suggest a beneficial role of topical mitomycin C in the management of OSSN.[64–68] The role of 5-FU in the treatment of OSSN has been evaluated by several short case series, with moderate success.[63, 69–71] The available reports indicate that topical chemotherapy using mitomycin C or 5-FU drops may have a role in the management of OSSN.[63–73] However, the studies involve only a small number of cases and include a wide clinical spectrum.[63–73] It is difficult to define the indications and the dosage schedule clearly, based on the existing knowledge. The modality has been tried in a variety of indications, including primary therapy, as an adjuvant following surgical excision in cases with incompletely excised tumour or excision margin involvement detected on histopathology, and for recurrent tumour. The cases were mostly limited to dysplasia or carcinoma *in situ*. Only a few infiltrative squamous cell carcinomas have been treated with topical chemotherapy.[63–73] The minimum effective dosage needs to be established in further studies. Ocular toxicity of topical chemotherapeutic agents appears to be limited to the duration of treatment.[63–73] No major irreversible side effect has been reported.

Implications for practice and research

Surgical excision with margin control remains the standard of care in the management of localised OSSN. In patients with incompletely resected lesions, diffuse tumours where complete resection is not possible, or recurrent tumours, topical chemotherapy may be a viable option. It could also be used in patients who refuse, or are unable, to undergo surgical intervention.

Adenoid cystic carcinoma of the lacrimal gland

Background

A broad spectrum of neoplastic and inflammatory diseases can affect the lacrimal gland.[74] Lacrimal gland lesions constitute approximately 5–13% of orbital lesions that undergo biopsy.[75–77] Based primarily on Reese's clinicopathological survey of 112 consecutive lesions of the lacrimal gland, most authors report that approximately 50% of the lesions are epithelial in nature and 50% are non-epithelial in origin.[76] Of non-epithelial lesions, 50% are lymphoid tumours and 50% are infectious and inflammatory pseudotumours.[76] Among the epithelial tumours of the lacrimal gland, approximately 50% are benign pleomorphic adenomas, 25% adenoid cystic carcinoma, and the remainders are other types of carcinoma.[76]

Prognosis

Adenoid cystic carcinoma, the most common non-lymphoid malignant tumour of the lacrimal gland, affects younger patients and confers the worst prognosis.[74] Despite extensive surgery and radiation therapy, the prognosis for these patients remains grim, with survival of less than 50% at five years and 20% at 10 years.[75] Several studies document a recurrence rate of 55–88% within five years of diagnosis with standard local therapies.[78–83] The dismal cure rate and survival rate has been attributed to aggressive biological behaviour of the tumour and propensity to perineural, hematogenous and lymphatic invasion.[78–84] Radical orbitectomy for adenoid cystic carcinoma is advocated by many authorities.[85,86] This disfiguring surgery involves removing the orbital contents *en bloc* along with orbital bone.[85,86] Comparison of survival rates for radical versus eye-sparing procedures has failed to demonstrate improved survival with more radical procedures.[82–87] Complete surgical excision of adenoid cystic carcinoma of the lacrimal gland is difficult to achieve even with radical surgery.[84] In fact, the most common site of recurrence of the tumour is local.[82] Complex regional anatomy, an infiltrative growth pattern and perineural spread explain the apparent inability to remove every malignant cell surgically, regardless of the technique employed.[84] Because of the well-known limitations of surgery, nearly all patients undergoing resection of adenoid cystic carcinoma of the lacrimal gland receive postoperative radiotherapy.[84] However, the poor rate of local control and the tendency towards late metastasis suggest that radiotherapy is unable to alter the course of the disease favorably.[87]

Adenoid cystic carcinoma of the lacrimal gland has many similarities to malignant epithelial tumours of the parotid and salivary glands.[84] They share common morphology, embryogenesis and the biological potential for perineural invasion.[88,89] The prognosis of these tumours is equally dismal.[88,89] Chemotherapy is the treatment of choice for tumours that metastasise early and cannot be controlled locally with a combination of surgery and radiation therapy.[84] Some patients with adenoid cystic carcinoma of the salivary glands respond to chemotherapy.[90,91] Neoadjuvant chemotherapy with cisplatinum for adenoid cystic carcinoma of the salivary glands combined with surgery and radiation therapy has yielded some promising preliminary results.[90,91] There are efforts currently to evaluate neoadjuvant and adjuvant chemotherapy in the management of adenoid cystic carcinoma of the lacrimal gland.[92]

Question

Does chemotherapy in the management of adenoid cystic carcinoma of the lacrimal gland minimise local recurrence, metastasis and death?

The evidence

We found no randomised controlled trials relevant to this question.

Comment

The literature search identified only a case series in which two patients with locally advanced adenoid cystic carcinoma of the lacrimal gland were treated with a new chemotherapy protocol.[92] The regimen consisted of neoadjuvant preoperative cytoreductive intracarotid chemotherapy and postoperative intravenous chemotherapy as an adjunct to conventional orbital exenteration and radiation therapy.[92] Tumour shrinkage was radiographically documented following preoperative neoadjuvant chemotherapy, downstaging the disease in one case from an intracranial involvement to a respectable intraorbital tumour. Tumour necrosis was confirmed in the exenteration specimen. Systemic morbidity was minimal and both the patients were free of metastasis at 7·5 years and 9·5 years following treatment. Tse and Benedetto from the same group have since treated three additional patients.[74]

Adenoid cystic carcinoma of the lacrimal gland has a proclivity for microscopic perineural, soft tissue and bone infiltration, because of which complete tumour clearance may not be possible despite meticulous excision, exenteration, or even orbitectomy.[74,78,79,82–87] Adjuvant radiotherapy is a reasonable option but tissue penetration can be a limiting factor.[74] Not surprisingly, orbital exenteration, exenteration combined with radiation, and radical cranio-orbital resection have not resulted in improved survival.[74,78,82–87] Theoretically, chemotherapy has the best potential to eradicate occult metastatic disease.[74] Systemic chemotherapy often fails to deliver therapeutic concentration to the target area. In contrast, intra-arterial delivery achieves a higher drug concentration in the target area while minimising systemic side effects.[74,92] The new treatment protocol involving neoadjuvant preoperative intracarotid chemotherapy, orbital exenteration, postoperative radiation and postoperative adjuvant chemotherapy in the management of adenoid cystic carcinoma of the lacrimal gland has shown promising results.[74,92] However, the number of cases is small.

Implications for practice and research

There are indications that the new treatment protocol may improve the prognosis of adenoid cystic carcinoma of the lacrimal gland. To evaluate fully the beneficial effect of the new protocol over the conventional treatment of this rare disease, a multicentre randomised trail may be warranted.

References

1. Hornblass A. Clinical evaluation of tumors of the eye and adnexa. In: Hornblass A, Hanig CJ, eds. *Oculoplastic, Reconstructive, and Orbital Surgery, Volume 1, Eyelids.* Baltimore: Williams and Wilkins, 1988, pp. 193–206.
2. Margo CE, Waltz K. Basal cell carcinoma of the eyelid and periocular skin. *Surv Ophthalmol* 1993;**38**:169–92.
3. Ni C, Searl SS, Kuo PK *et al.* Sebaceous cell carcinomas of the ocular adnexa. *Int Ophthalmol Clin* 1982;**22**:23–61.
4. Shields JA, Shields CL. *Atlas of Eyelid and Conjunctival Tumors.* Philadelphia: Lippincott Williams and Wilkins, 1999.
5. Shields CL, Shields JA, Gunduz K *et al.* Conjunctival melanoma: risk factors for recurrence, exenteration, metastasis, and death in 150 consecutive patients. *Arch Ophthalmol* 2000;**118**:1497–507.
6. Shields CL, Shields JA, Carvaoho C *et al.* Conjunctival lymphoid tumors: clinical analysis of 117 cases and relationship to systemic lymphoma. *Ophthalmology* 2001;**108**:979–84.
7. Lee GA, Hirst LW. Ocular surface squamous neoplasia. *Surv Ophthalmol* 1995;**39**:429–50.
8. Shields JA. *Diagnosis and Management of Orbital Tumors.* Philadelphia: WB Saunders Company, 1989, pp. 20–7.
9. Kass LG, Hornblass A. Sebaceous carcinoma of the ocular adnexa. *Surv Ophthalmol* 1989;**33**:477–90.
10. Hornblass A. Clinical evaluation of tumors of the eye and adnexa. In: Hornblass A, Hanig CJ, eds. *Oculoplastic, Reconstructive, and Orbital Surgery, Volume 1, Eyelids.* Baltimore: William and Wilkins, 1988, pp. 232–8.
11. Honavar SG, Shields CL, Maus M *et al.* Primary intraepithelial sebaceous gland carcinoma of the palpebral conjunctiva. *Arch Ophthalmol* 2001;**119**:764–7.
12. Rao NA, McLean JW, Zimmerman LE. Sebaceous carcinoma of the eyelid and caruncle: correlation of clinicopathologic features with prognosis. In: Jacobiec FA, ed. *Ocular and Adnexal Tumors.* Birmingham: Aesculapuis, 1978, pp. 461–76.
13. Rao NA, Hidayat AA, McLean JW *et al.* Sebaceous carcinomas of the ocular adnexa: a clinicopathologic study of 104 cases with five year follow-up data. *Hum Pathol* 1982;**13**:113–22.
14. Boniuk M, Zimmerman LE. Sebaceous carcinoma of the eyelid, eyebrow, caruncle, and orbit. *Trans Am Acad Ophthalmol Otolaryngol* 1968;**72**:619–41.
15. Doxanas MT, Green WR. Sebaceous gland carcinoma: review of 40 cases. *Arch Ophthalmol* 1984;**102**:245–9.
16. Chao AN, Shields CL, Krema H *et al.* Outcome of patients with periocular sebaceous gland carcinoma with and without conjunctival intraepithelial invasion. *Ophthalmology* 2001;**108**:1877–83.
17. Wolfe JT III, Yeats RP, Wick MR *et al.* Sebaceous carcinoma of the eyelid. *Am J Surg Pathol* 1984;**8**:597–606.

18. Margo CE, Grossniklaus H. Intraepithelial sebaceous neoplasia without underlying invasive carcinoma. *Surv Ophthalmol* 1995;**39**: 293–301.

19. Putterman AM. Conjunctival map biopsy to determine pagetoid spread. *Am J Ophthalmol* 1986;**102**:87–90.

20. Scotto J, Fears TR, Fraumeni JF Jr. *Incidence of nonmelanoma skin cancer in the United States*. US Department of Health and Human Services NIH Publication, No. 83–2433, 1983.

21. Aurora AL, Blodi FC. Lesions of the eyelids: a clinicpathological study. *Surv Ophthalmol* 1970;**15**:94–104.

22. Aurora AL, Blodi FC. Reappraisal of basal cell carcinoma of the eyelids. *Am J Ophthalmol* 1970;**70**:329–36.

23. Kwitko ML, Boniuk M, Zimmerman LE. Eyelid tumors with reference to lesions confused with squamous cell carcinomas. I. Incidence and errors in diagnosis. *Arch Ophthalmol* 1963;693–7.

24. Lober CW, Fenske NA. Basal cell, squamous cell, and sebaceous gland carcinomas of the periorbital region. *J Am Acad Dermatol* 1991;**25**:685–90.

25. Shields CL. Basal cell carcinoma of the eyelids. *Int Ophthalmol Clin* 1993;**33**:1–4.

26. Margo CE, Waltz K. Basal cell carcinoma of the eyelid and periocular skin. *Surv Ophthalmol* 1993;**38**:169–92.

27. Chalfin J, Putterman AM. Frozen section control in the surgery of basal cell carcinoma of the eyelid. *Am J Ophthalmol* 1979;**87**:802–9.

28. Doxanas MT, Green WR, Iliff CE. Factors in the successful surgical management of basal cell carcinoma of the eyelid. *Am J Ophthalmol* 1981;**91**:729–36.

29. Vitaliano PP, Urbach F. The relative importance of risk factors in nonmelanoma carcinoma. *Arch Dermatol* 1980;**116**:454–6.

30. Mohs FE. Micrographic surgery for the microscopically controlled excision of eyelid cancers. *Arch Ophthalmol* 1986;**104**:901–9.

31. Rowe DE, Carroll R, Day DL Jr. Long-term recurrence rates in previously untreated (primary) basal cell carcinoma: implications for patient follow-up. *J Dermatol Surg Oncol* 1989;**15**:315–28.

32. Rowe DE, Carroll R, Day DL Jr. Mohs' surgery is the treatment of choice for recurrent (previously untreated) basal cell carcinoma. *J Dermatol Surg Oncol* 1989;**15**:425–31.

33. Swanson NA. Mohs' surgery: technique, indications, applications, and the future. *Arch Dermatol* 1983;**119**:761–73.

34. Dutton J, Slamovits T. Management of periocular basal cell carcinoma: Mohs' micrographic surgery versus radiotherapy. *Surv Ophthalmol* 1993;**38**:193–212.

35. Anderson RL, Ceilley RI. Multispecialty approach to excision and reconstruction of eyelid tumors. *Ophthalmology* 1978;**85**:1150–63.

36. Baylis HI, Cies WA. Indications of Mohs' chemosurgical excision of eyelid and canthal tumors. *Am J Ophthalmol* 1975;**80**:116–22.

37. Mohs FE. *Chemosurgery: Microscopically Controlled Surgery for Skin Cancer*. Springfield: Charles C Thomas, 1978.

38. Mohs FE. Chemosurgery: Microscopically controlled surgery for skin cancer: past, present, and future. *J Dermatol Surg Oncol* 1978;**4**:41–2.

39. Mohs FE. Mohs' micrographic surgery: a historical perspective. *Dermatol Clin* 1989;**7**:609–11.

40. Mohs FE. Micrographic surgery for the microscopically controlled excision of eyelid cancer: history and development. *Adv Ophthal Plast Reconstr Surg* 1986;**5**:381–408.

41. Robins P. Chemosurgery: my 15 years of experience. *Dermatol Surg Oncol* 1981;**7**:779–89.

42. Robins P, Rodriquez-Sains R, Rabinovitz H *et al*. Mohs' surgery for periocular basal cell carcinoma. *J Dermatol Surg Oncol* 1985;**11**:1203–7.

43. Anderson RL. Mohs' micrographic technique. *Arch Ophthalmol* 1986;**104**:818–19.

44. Callahan A, Monheit GD, Callahan MA. Cancer excision from eyelids and ocular adnexa: the Mohs' fresh tissue technique and reconstruction. *Cancer* 1982;**32**:322–9.

45. Callahan A. Mohs' technique. *Cancer* 1986;**36**:373–5.

46. Cobb GM, Thomson GA, Allt WEC. Treatment of basal cell carcinoma of the eyelids by radiotherapy. *Can Med Assoc J* 1964;**91**:743–8.

47. Fayos JV, Wildemuth O. Carcinoma of the skin of the eyelids. *Arch Ophthalmol* 1962;**67**:298–302.

48. Fitzpatrick PJ, Jamieson DM, Thompson GA *et al*. Tumors of the eyelids and their treatment by radiotherapy. *Radiology* 1972;**102**:661–5.

49. Fitzpatrick PJ, Thompson GA, Easterbrook WM *et al*. Basal and squamous cell carcinoma of the eyelids and their treatment by radiotherapy. *Int J Radiat Oncol Biol Phys* 1984;**10**:449–54.

50. Lederman M. Radiation treatment of cancer of the eyelids. *Br J Ophthalmol* 1976;**60**:794–805.

51. Nordman EM, Nordman LEO. Treatment of basal cell carcinoma of the eyelid. *Acta Ophthalmol* 1978;**56**:349–56.

52. Cha SB, Shields JA, Shields CL *et al*. Squamous cell carcinoma of the conjunctiva. *Int Ophthalmol Clin* 1993;**33**:19–24.

53. Lee GH, Hirst LW. Ocular surface squamous neoplasia. *Surv Ophthalmol* 1995;**39**:429–50.

54. Templeton AC. Tumors of the eye and adnexa in Africans of Uganda. *Cancer* 1967;**20**:1689–98.

55. Lee GA, Hirst LW. Incidence of ocular surface epithelial dysplasia in metropolitan Brisbane: a 10-year survey. *Arch Ophthalmol* 1992;**110**:525–7.

56. Grossniklaus HE, Green WR, Lukenback M *et al*. Conjunctival lesions in adults: a clinical and histopathologic review. *Cornea* 1987;**6**:78–116.

57. Pizzarello LD, Jakobiec FA. Bowen's disease of the conjunctiva: a misnomer. In: Jakobiec FA, ed. *Ocular and Adnexal Tumors*. Birmingham: Aesculapius, 1978, pp. 553–71.

58. Shields JA, Shields CL, De Potter P. Surgical management of conjunctival tumors. The 1994 Lynn B McMahan lecture. *Arch Ophthalmol* 1997;**115**:808–15.

59. Char DH, Crawford JB, Howes El *et al*. Resection of intraocular squamous cell carcinoma. *Br J Ophthalmol* 1992;**76**:123–5.

60. Freedman J, Rohm G. Surgical management and histopathology of invasive tumors of the cornea. *Br J Ophthalmol* 1979;**63**:632–5.

61. Zimmerman LE. The cancerous, precancerous, and pseudocancerous lesions of the cornea and conjunctiva: the Pocklington memorial lecture. In: Rycroft PV, ed. *Corneoplastic Surgery*. New York: Pergamon Press, 1969.

62. Erie JC, Campbell RJ, Liesegang J. Conjunctival and corneal intraepithelial and invasive neoplasia. *Ophthalmology* 1986;**93**: 176–83.

63. de Keizer RJW, de Wolff Rouendaal D, Van Delft JL. Topical application of 5-fluorouracil in premalignant lesions of the cornea, conjunctiva, and eyelid. *Doc Ophthalmol* 1986;**64**:31–42.

64. Frucht-Pery J, Rozenman Y. Mitomycin C therapy for corneal intraepithelial neoplasia. *Am J Ophthalmol* 1994;**117**:164–8.

65. Frucht-Pery J, Sugar J, Baum J *et al*. Mitomycin C treatment for conjunctival-corneal intraepithelial neoplasia. *Ophthalmology* 1997; **104**:2085–93.

66. Wilson MW, Hungerford JL, George SM, et al. Topical mitomycin C for the treatment of conjunctival and corneal epithelial neoplasia. *Am J Ophthalmol* 1997;**124**:303–11.

67. Heigle TJ, Stulting RD, Palay DA. Treatment of recurrent conjunctival intraepithelial neoplasia with topical mitomycin C. *Am J Ophthalmol* 1997;**124**:397–9.

68. Tseng S, Tsai Y, Chen F. Successful treatment of recurrent corneal intraepithelial neoplasia with topical mitomycin C. *Cornea* 1997;**16**:595–7.

69. Yeatts RP, Ford JG, Stanton CA *et al*. Topical 5-fluorouracil in treating epithelial neoplasia of the conjunctiva and cornea. *Ophthalmology* 1995;**102**:1338–44.

70. Midena E, Boccato P, Angeli C. Conjunctival squamous cell carcinoma treated with topical 5-fluorouracil: a case report. *Arch Ophthalmol* 1997;**15**:1600–1.

71. Midena E, Angeli CD, Valenti M *et al*. Treatment of conjunctival squamous cell carcinoma with topical 5-fluorouracil. *Br J Ophthalmol* 2000;**84**:268–72.

72. Majumdar PA, Epstein RJ. Antimetabolites in ocular surface neoplasia. *Curr Opin Ophthalmol* 1998;**9**:35–9.

73. Akpek EK, Ertoy D, Kalaysi D *et al*. Postoperative topical mitomycin C in conjunctival squamous cell neoplasia. *Cornea* 1999;**18**:59–62.

74. Tse DT, Neff AG. Recent developments in the evaluation and treatment of lacrimal gland tumors. *Ophthalmol Clin North Am* 2000;**13**:663–81.
75. Kennedy RE. An evaluation of 820 orbital cases. *Trans Am Ophthalmol Soc* 1984;**82**:134–57.
76. Reese AB. Expanding lesions of the orbit. *Trans Ophthalmol Soc UK* 1971;**91**:85–104.
77. Shields JA, Bakewell B, Augsburger JJ *et al.* Classification and incidence of space-occupying lesions of the orbit. A survey of 645 biopsies. *Arch Ophthalmol* 1984;**102**:1606–11.
78. Font RL, Gamel JW. Adenoid cystic carcinoma of the lacrimal gland. A clinicopathologic study of 79 cases. In: Nicholson DH, ed. *Ophthalmic Pathology Update.* New York: Masson Publishing, 1980.
79. Lee DA, Campbell RJ, Waller RR *et al.* A clinicopathologic study of primary adenoid cystic carcinoma of the lacrimal gland. *Ophthalmology* 1985;**92**:128–34.
80. Gamel JW, Font RL. Adenoid cystic carcinoma of the lacrimal gland: the clinical significance of a basaloid histologic pattern. *Hum Pathol* 1982;**13**:219–25.
81. Forrest AW. Pathologic criteria for effective management of epithelial lacrimal gland tumors. *Am J Ophthalmol* 1971;**71**:178–92.
82. Wright JE, Rose GE, Garner A. Primary malignant neoplasms of the lacrimal gland. *Br J Ophthalmol* 1992;**76**:401–7.
83. Henderson JW. Past, present and future surgical management of malignant epithelial neoplasms of the lacrimal gland. *Br J Ophthalmol* 1986;**70**:727–31.
84. Goldberg RA. Intra-arterial chemotherapy: a welcome new idea for the management of adenoid cystic carcinoma of the lacrimal gland. *Arch Ophthalmol* 1998;**116**:372–3.
85. Reese AB, Jones IS. Bone resection in the excision of epithelial tumors of the lacrimal gland. *Arch Ophthalmol* 1964;**71**:382–5.
86. Bartley GB, HarrisGJ. Adenoid cystic carcinoma of the lacrimal gland: is there a cure ... yet? *Ophthal Plast Reconstr Surg* 2002;**18**:315–18.
87. Polito E, Leccisotti A. Epithelial malignancies of the lacrimal gland: survival rates after extensive and conservative therapy. *Ann Ophthalmol* 1993;**25**:422–6.
88. Sakata K, Aoki Y, Karasawa K *et al.* Radiation therapy for patients with malignant salivary gland tumors with positive surgical margins. *Strahlenther Onkol* 1994;**170**:342–6.
89. Hemprich A, Schmidseder R. The adenoid cystic carcinoma: special aspects of its growth and therapy. *J Craniomaxillofac Surg* 1988;**16**:136–9.
90. Scheel JV, Schilling V, Kastenbauer E *et al.* Intraarterial cisplatin and sequential radiotherapy: long-term follow-up. *Laryngorhinootology* 1996;**75**:38–42.
91. Sessions RB, Lehane DE, Smith RJ *et al.* Intra-arterial cisplatin treatment of adenoid cystic carcinoma. *Arch Otolaryngol* 1982;**108**:221–4.
92. Meldrum ML, Tse DT, Benedetto P. Neoadjuvant intracarotid chemotherapy for treatment of advanced adenoid cystic carcinoma of the lacrimal gland. *Arch Ophthalmol* 1998;**116**:315–21.

51 Uveal melanoma

Arun D Singh, Paul A Rundle, Ian G Rennie

Background

Of all melanomas approximately 5% arise from the ocular and adnexal structures such as uvea, eyelids, conjunctiva and orbit.[1] The majority (85%) of ocular melanoma are uveal in origin whereas primary orbital melanoma is very rare.[1,2] Uveal melanoma is the most common primary intraocular malignant tumour.[3]

The diagnosis of uveal melanoma is made by clinical examination including slit lamp examination and indirect ophthalmoscopy, as well as ancillary studies such as fluorescein angiography and ultrasonography.[4] The accuracy of clinical diagnosis among Collaborative Ocular Melanoma Study (COMS) participants was reported to be greater than 99%.[5]

Incidence

A rising incidence of cutaneous melanoma has been observed in recent years.[1,6] With regards to uveal melanoma, there are only a few large population-based studies. Two studies from the United States have reported stability of incidence rate between 1950 and 1974 and between 1973 and 1997.[3,7] The reported incidence rate of uveal melanoma has ranged from 5·3 to 10·9 cases per million because of variations in inclusion and diagnostic criteria, and methodology used in calculating the incidence rate.

Treatment options

The traditional form of treatment, enucleation, has been challenged in recent years and alternative methods of treatment including radiotherapy (plaque radiotherapy, proton beam radiotherapy, helium ion radiotherapy), local resection and transpupillary thermotherapy have been used more frequently to manage posterior uveal melanoma.[4]

Prognosis

Approximately 40% of patients with posterior uveal melanoma develop metastatic melanoma to the liver within 10 years after initial diagnosis and treatment.[4,8] However, clinically evident metastatic disease at the time of initial presentation is uncommon, indicating early subclinical metastasis in the majority of cases.[8] Using conventional methods such as serum liver enzymes and liver scans, metastatic disease can be detected in only 1–2% of patients at the time of presentation.[9] Systemic screening protocols using physical examinations, liver function tests, chest *x* rays and liver imaging studies every six months to one year have been proposed but the effectiveness of the screening protocols remains to be established.[10]

Question

Is plaque radiotherapy associated with improved survival as compared with enucleation for management of uveal melanoma?

The evidence

We found only a single randomised controlled trial that compared these techniques.

Comment

The Collaborative Ocular Melanoma Study (COMS) is an ongoing prospective study investigating patient survival after treatment of choroidal melanoma.[11,12] The COMS consists of:

- a randomised trial of patients with medium choroidal melanoma treated with enucleation versus iodine-125 plaque irradiation
- a randomised trial of patients with large choroidal melanoma treated with enucleation only versus pre-enucleation external beam irradiation and enucleation
- a prospective observational study of patients with small choroidal melanoma.

Recently published initial results from the COMS indicate that for medium-sized melanomas, enucleation and iodine-125 brachytherapy offer similar survival rates. During the 12-year accrual period 1317 patients were enrolled. A total of 660 were assigned randomly to enucleation and 657 to iodine-125 brachytherapy. The estimated five-year

Table 51.1 Reported five-year mortality with uveal melanoma

Authors	Study	Treatment	Size	Method	Rate (%)
Diener-West et al., 1992[23]	Meta-analysis	Enucleation	Small	All cause mortality	16
			Medium	All cause mortality	32
			Large	All cause mortality	53
COMS, 1998[1]	COMS	Enucleation (with EBRT)	Large	All cause mortality	38
		Enucleation (without EBRT)	Large	All cause mortality	43
COMS, 2001[13]	COMS	Enucleation	Medium	All cause mortality	19
		Plaque	Medium	All cause mortality	18
Seregard, 1999[24]	Meta-analysis	Plaque	Small	Melanoma-related mortality	6
			Medium	Melanoma-related mortality	6
			Large	Melanoma-related mortality	26
Kroll et al., 1998[22]		Plaque and helium ion	–	Melanoma-related mortality	16
Seddon et al., 1990[20]		Proton beam irradiation	–	All cause mortality	19

COMS, Collaborative Ocular Melanoma Study; EBRT, external beam radiotherapy

cumulative mortality rates were 19% (95% CI 16–23%) for patients treated with enucleation and 18% (95% CI 15–21%) for patients treated with iodine-125 brachytherapy with a risk ratio of 0·93 (95% CI 0·76–1·14).

COMS is a landmark prospective randomised study enrolling a large cohort of patients. For medium-sized choroidal melanoma, iodine-125 brachytherapy can be offered to the patients without increasing the risk of mortality over the generally accepted standard therapy of enucleation. It is probable that these data can be equally extrapolated to other forms of plaque therapy such as ruthenium-106. Conversely, enucleation can also be recommended without fear of increasing mortality.

Question

Is proton beam radiotherapy, helium ion radiotherapy or local resection associated with improved survival as compared with enucleation for management of uveal melanoma?

The evidence

We did not find any randomised clinical trials comparing proton beam radiotherapy, helium ion radiotherapy or local resection with enucleation for management of uveal melanoma.

Comment

Several retrospective studies have evaluated different modalities of treatment in the management of uveal melanoma. Zimmerman and associates in 1979 reported their observations on the rise in the mortality rate a few years after enucleation. On the basis of 2300 case studies the postoperative mortality rate increased from the estimated pre-enucleation rate of 1% per year to a peak of 8% during the second year after enucleation and then decreased monotonically. The authors postulated that the procedure of enucleation had a detrimental effect on the expected natural course of the disease.

Others have subsequently shown that the excessive mortality after enucleation for uveal melanoma is not related to the enucleation but to an active phase of tumour progression that led to the diagnosis. However, since then many retrospective studies have shown that survival in patients with uveal melanoma is independent of the method of local treatment such as plaque radiotherapy, proton beam irradiation[20] or tumour resection (see Table 51.1).

Comparison of survival in patients treated with enucleation versus cobalt-60 plaque was performed on 237 patients with uveal melanoma. The eight-year survival estimates between the two groups was not statistically dissimilar (enucleation group 62%, plaque group 76%). In a larger study of 495 patients with uveal melanoma treated with enucleation and 556 patients treated with proton beam irradiation, the estimated five-year survival rate between the enucleation group and the proton beam group was similar (80% and 81% respectively). In a study of 731 cases that had been treated with helium ion and iodine-125 plaque radiotherapy, the estimated five-year survival rate was 76%, indicating similar survival to patients treated with enucleation.[22]

Implications for practice

For medium-sized choroidal melanoma, plaque radiotherapy can be offered to patients as an alternative to enucleation without compromising the overall patient survival.

Implications for research

Equal risk of metastasis with enucleation and plaque radiotherapy implies that the metastasis occurs prior to the diagnosis of uveal melanoma. Research into the role of prophylactic adjuvant systemic therapy to minimise the risk of metastasis should be considered.

References

1. Chang AE, Karnell LH, Menck HR. The National Cancer Data Base report on cutaneous and noncutaneous melanoma: a summary of 84,836 cases from the past decade. The American College of Surgeons Commission on Cancer and the American Cancer Society. *Cancer* 1998;**83**:1664–78.
2. Dutton JJ, Anderson RL, Schelper RL, Purcell JJ, Tse DT. Orbital malignant melanoma and oculodermal melanocytosis: report of two cases and review of the literature. *Ophthalmology* 1984;**91**:497–507.
3. Strickland D, Lee JA. Melanomas of eye: stability of rates. *Am J Epidemiol* 1981;**113**:700–2.
4. Shields JA, Shields CL, Donoso LA. Management of posterior uveal melanoma. *Surv Ophthalmol* 1991;**36**:161–95.
5. Anonymous. Accuracy of diagnosis of choroidal melanomas in the Collaborative Ocular Melanoma Study. COMS report no. 1. *Arch Ophthalmol* 1990;**108**:1268–73.
6. Rigel D, Carucci JA. Malignant melanoma: prevention, early detection, and treatment in the 21st century. *CA Cancer J Clin* 2000;**b**:215–36.
7. Singh AD, Topham A. Incidence of uveal melanoma in the United States: 1973–1997. *Ophthalmology* 2003;**110**:956–61.
8. Singh AD, Topham A. Survival rate with uveal melanoma in the United States: 1973–1997. *Ophthalmology* 2003;**110**:962–5.
9. Donoso LA, Folberg R, Naids R. Metastatic uveal melanoma. Hepatic metastasis identified by hybridoma-secreted monoclonal antibody Mab8-1H. *Arch Ophthalmol* 1985;**103**:799–801.
10. Eskelin S, Pyrhonen S, Summanen P *et al.* Screening for metastatic malignant melanoma of the uvea revisited. *Cancer* 1999;**85**:1151–9.
11. Collaborative Ocular Melanoma Study Group. The COMS randomized trial of iodine 125 brachytherapy for choroidal melanoma, III: initial mortality findings. COMS report no. 18. *Arch Ophthalmol* 2001;**119**:969–82.
12. Straatsma BR, Fine SL, Earle JD *et al.* Enucleation versus plaque irradiation for choroidal melanoma. *Ophthalmology* 1988;**95**:1000–4.
13. Collaborative Ocular Melanoma Study Group. The Collaborative Ocular Melanoma Study (COMS) randomized trial of pre-enucleation radiation of large choroidal melanoma II: initial mortality findings. COMS report no. 10. *Am J Ophthalmol* 1998;**125**:779–96.
14. The Collaborative Ocular Melanoma Study Group. Mortality in patients with small choroidal melanoma. COMS report no. 4. *Arch Ophthalmol* 1997;**115**:886–93.
15. Zimmerman LE, McLean IW, Foster WD. Does enucleation of the eye containing a malignant melanoma prevent or accelerate the dissemination of tumour cells? *Br J Ophthalmol* 1978;**62**:420–5.
16. Zimmerman LE, McLean IW. An evaluation of enucleation in the management of uveal melanomas. *Am J Ophthalmol* 1979;**87**:741–60.
17. Seigel D, Myers M, Ferris Fr, Steinhorn S. Survival rates after enucleation of eyes with malignant melanoma. *Am J Ophthalmol* 1979;**87**:761–5.
18. Augsburger JJ, Gamel JW, Lauritzen K, Brady LW. Cobalt-60 plaque radiotherapy *v* enucleation for posterior uveal melanoma. *Am J Ophthalmol* 1990;**109**:585–92.
19. Augsburger JJ, Schneider S, Freire J, Brady LW. Survival following enucleation versus plaque radiotherapy in statistically matched subgroups of patients with choroidal melanomas: results in patients treated between 1980 and 1987. *Graefe's Arch Clin Exp Ophthalmol* 1999;**237**:558–67.
20. Seddon JM, Gragoudas ES, Egan KM *et al.* Relative survival rates after alternative therapies for uveal melanoma. *Ophthalmology* 1990;**97**:769–77.
21. Augsburger JJ, Lauritzen K, Gamel JW *et al.* Matched group study of surgical resection versus cobalt-60 plaque radiotherapy for primary choroidal or ciliary body melanoma. *Ophthalmic Surg* 1990;**21**:682–8.
22. Kroll S, Char DH, Quivey J, Castro J. A comparison of cause-specific melanoma mortality and all-cause mortality in survival analyses after radiation treatment for uveal melanoma. *Ophthalmology* 1998;**105**:2035–45.
23. Diener-West M, Hawkins BS, Markowitz JA, Schachat AP. A review of mortality from choroidal melanoma. *Arch Ophthalmol* 1992;**110**:245–50.
24. Seregard S. Long-term survival after ruthenium plaque radiotherapy for uveal melanoma. A meta-analysis of studies including 1,066 patients. *Acta Ophthalmol Scand* 1999;**77**:414–17.

52 Retinoblastoma

Arun D Singh

Background

Retinoblastoma is the most common primary intraocular malignant tumour in children with an incidence of 1 in 15 000 live births.[1] The average annual incidence of retinoblastoma of 10·9 per million for children younger than five years in the United States has remained stable from 1974 to 1985.[2]

Aetiology and diagnosis

Retinoblastoma is a familial disorder with an autosomal dominant inheritance. Approximately 60% of the patients are considered sporadic and 40% are heritable. White pupillary reflex, or leukocoria, is the most common presentation.[3] Presence of intraocular calcium by ultrasonography or computed tomography is helpful in confirming the diagnosis.[4]

Retinoblastoma can be inherited as a familial tumour in which the affected child has a positive family history of retinoblastoma or as a non-familial (sporadic) tumour in which the family history is negative for retinoblastoma. Retinoblastoma can be classified in three different ways: familial or sporadic, bilateral or unilateral, and heritable or non-heritable (Table 52.1). Approximately 10% of newly diagnosed retinoblastoma cases are familial and 90% are sporadic.

Human retinoblastoma susceptibility gene (RB1) is located on chromosome 13 region 13–14. A review of published data indicates that mutations are distributed throughout the RB1 gene with no single mutational hotspot and are expected to alter pRB protein function.

Treatment options

In recent years there has been a trend away from enucleation,[8] with the increased use of alternative globe conserving methods of treatment including external beam radiotherapy,[9] plaque radiotherapy,[10] laser photocoagulation,[11] cryotherapy,[12] transpupillary thermotherapy[13] and chemotherapy.[14]

Since the 1990s chemoreduction has been increasingly used for the management of retinoblastoma to avoid external beam radiotherapy or enucleation.[15,16] Chemoreduction

Table 52.1 Classification of retinoblastoma

Variable	Extent	Type of retinoblastoma
Family history	Present	Familial (heritable)
	Absent	Sporadic (non-heritable)
Involvement	One eye	Unilateral (non-heritable)
	Both eyes	Bilateral (heritable)

implies usage of chemotherapy delivered intravenously to reduce the volume of intraocular retinoblastoma so as to make it amenable to focal therapy such as cryotherapy, thermotherapy or brachytherapy. Six-cycle chemoreduction using three agents (vincristine, etoposide and carboplatin) is generally prescribed.

Prognosis

Recent advances in the treatment of retinoblastoma have led to improved five-year survival rates of greater than 90% in the developed countries.[2,17] However, in developing countries retinoblastoma is still associated with high mortality because it tends to present at a much more advanced stage.

The metastasis in retinoblastoma usually occurs within one year of diagnosis of retinoblastoma. If there is no metastatic disease within five years of retinoblastoma diagnosis the child is usually considered cured.[18] Involvement of the central nervous system and hematogenous spread are the commonest sites of metastasis. Survival with metastatic retinoblastoma is generally limited to six months.[18,19]

Question

What is the role of chemoreduction in the management of retinoblastoma?

The evidence

We found no randomised controlled trials or meta-analyses relevant to this question.

Comment

Some small, uncontrolled prospective studies have reported the efficacy of chemoreduction in the management of retinoblastoma (Table 52.2). The extent of retinoblastoma is generally classified using a system proposed by Reese and Ellsworth.[20] The retinoblastoma is staged from group I to group V on the basis of number, size, and the location of the tumours. The Reese-Ellsworth (RE) classification predicts the visual prognosis. Murphree and associates reported tumour control in 10 eyes with RE group I–IV disease and failure in seven eyes with extensive subretinal seeding and 18 eyes with RE group V disease.[21] Kingston and associates were able to avoid enucleation in 12 of 20 eyes with RE group V, using chemoreduction and external beam radiotherapy.[22] In a large prospective (non-randomised study) involving 158 eyes of 103 patients, all eyes showed initial tumour regression.[23] About 50% of these eyes required external beam radiotherapy or enucleation. At five years, Reese-Ellsworth (RE) groups I–IV eyes showed better response than RE group V eyes. In RE group I–IV eyes, only 10% of the eyes required external beam radiotherapy and 15% necessitated enucleation, whereas in RE group V eyes almost 50% of the eyes failed therapy requiring external beam radiotherapy or enucleation.

Based on the available (non-comparative series) data it may be concluded that chemoreduction combined with adjuvant focal therapy offers about 50–90% probability of avoiding enucleation or external beam radiotherapy depending upon the severity of disease at initial presentation as judged by RE classification.

Chemoreduction is not without its problems, however. Recurrence of the neoplasm while on chemotherapy have been observed.[24] Immediate complications related to transient bone marrow suppression requiring hospital admissions and intravenous antibiotics with consequent delay in examinations under anaesthesia are frequent.[16,25] Risk of late complications such as drug-induced leukaemia have not yet been excluded.

Currently the choice of drug combinations, duration of chemotherapy and indications of chemoreduction are still under investigation. Therefore, it is recommended that chemoreduction therapy for retinoblastoma should only be offered as part of a clinical trial at a specialist centre. It is an arduous and prolonged task to monitor the progression of each tumour and access to all forms of focal adjuvant therapy should be available.

Despite recent advancement in retinoblastoma treatment, and the current trend in favour of measures to salvage the eye, enucleation is still a valid primary therapeutic option for advanced unilateral retinoblastoma.[8] Primary enucleation offers a high cure rate of 90–95%.[26] Metastasis may still develop in 5–10% of patients after primary enucleation for advanced unilateral retinoblastoma,[2,17] and at a much higher rate in the developing countries.[27,28] With the availability of effective chemotherapy regimens for intraocular retinoblastoma,[15,29] consideration of adjuvant chemotherapy to prevent metastasis in high-risk cases is appropriate. Nevertheless, the role of adjuvant post-enucleation chemotherapy in retinoblastoma has yet to be clearly defined.[30]

There is disagreement over the histopathological prognostic factors that define high risk for developing metastasis. Although no RCTs or meta-analyses exist, several studies (mostly retrospective) have addressed this issue. The reported occurrence of anterior chamber seeding (7%), choroidal infiltration (12–23%), invasion of optic nerve, scleral infiltration (1–8%) and extrascleral extension (2–13%) varies between series[18,31–35] It is now generally agreed, without strong evidence, that tumour invasion of the optic nerve at or beyond the lamina cribrosa, massive choroidal infiltration, scleral infiltration and extrascleral extension are risk factors predictive of metastasis[18,28,35,36] However, the role and significance of anterior chamber seeding and isolated iris or ciliary body infiltration as risk factors for metastatic retinoblastoma remains debatable.[18,28,35,36]

Question

What is the role of laser photocoagulation, cryotherapy, transpupillary thermotherapy and plaque radiotherapy in the management of retinoblastoma?

The evidence

We found no randomised controlled trial or meta-analysis comparing laser photocoagulation, cryotherapy, transpupillary thermotherapy and plaque radiotherapy in the management of retinoblastoma.

Comment

Retinoblastoma is a rare disease and it is not surprising that randomised trials comparing various treatment modalities are unavailable. The small case series are descriptive and provide information only on selected tumours that were specifically treated by a single modality. Such case series give information about the clinical situations where a given treatment would be indicated and the expected response rate.

Laser photocoagulation is an appropriate method of management in cases where the tumour is located posteriorly, the media is clear and the tumour is 3·0 mm or less in diameter and 2·0 mm or less in thickness without seeding into the adjacent vitreous.[37]

Table 52.2 Efficacy of chemoreduction in retinoblastoma

| Authors | No. of eyes | Treatment | | End-point | Results | |
		Chemotherapy	Adjuvant therapy		Response rate (%)	Good prognostic features
Murphree et al., 1996[21]	38	Carboplatin	Thermotherapy Cryotherapy	Avoid Enuc/EBRT	63	RE group I–II
	35	Vincristine Etoposide Carboplatin	Thermotherapy Cryotherapy Brachytherapy	Avoid Enuc/EBRT	29	RE group I–IV Absence of subretinal seeds
Kingston et al., 1996[22]	20	Vincristine Etoposide Carboplatin	External beam radiotherapy	Avoid Enuc	70	–
Gallie et al., 1996[29]	40	Vincristine Teniposide Carboplatin Ciclosporin	Thermotherapy Cryotherapy	Avoic EBRT	67–89	Absence of vitreous seeds
Shields et al., 2002[23]	158	Vincristine Etoposide Carboplatin	Thermotherapy Cryotherapy Brachytherapy	Avoid Enuc/EBRT	64–73	RE groups I–IV

Enuc, enucleation; EBRT, external beam radiotherapy; RE, Reese-Ellsworth

Table 52.3   **The role of adjuvant chemotherapy in preventing metastasis in high-risk retinoblastoma***

Authors	Study design	No. of treated cases	Selection criteria	No. of metastasis	Result
Howarth *et al.*, 1980[26]	Prospective	14	CHR, ON-RL, ON-TR ESE	1 (7%)	Effective
Wolff *et al.*, 1981,[42]	Prospective**	41	Unilateral RE-Group V	6 (12%)	Equivocal
Zelter *et al.*, 1991[43]	Retrospective	24	CHR, ON-RL, ON-TR, ESE	8 (33%)	Equivocal
Hungerford, 1993[45]	Retrospective	11	CHR, ON-RL	0	Effective
Khelfaoui *et al.*, 1996[35]	Retrospective	75	Variable	4 (6%)	Effective
Mustafa *et al.*, 1999[44]	Retrospective	27	CHR, ON-RL, ON-TR, ESE	5 (19%)	Ineffective
Uusitalo *et al.*, 2001[47]	Retrospective	11	ON-RL, ON-TR	1 (9%)	Effective
Honavar *et al.*, 2002[46]	Retrospective	46	AC, CB, CHR, ON-L, ON-RL, ON-TS, SCL, ECE	2 (4%)	Effective

*Only relevant and comparable data are tabulated.
**Randomised.
N, number of patients who received adjuvant chemotherapy; RE, Reese-Ellsworth; AC, anterior chamber seeding; iris, iris infiltration; CB, ciliary body infiltration; CHR, choroidal infiltration; ON-L, invasion of the optic nerve lamina cribrosa; ON-RL, invasion of the retrolaminar optic nerve; ON-TS, invasion of optic nerve transection; SCL, scleral infiltration; ESE, extrascleral extension

Cryotherapy is indicated for anteriorly located tumours with clear media. Cryotherapy is effective for the tumours less than 2·5 mm in diameter and less than 1·0 mm in thickness without seeding into the adjacent vitreous.[38] In a series of 138 tumours, 70% of tumours were cured with cryotherapy. There were few long-term ocular complications even with repeated cryotherapy.[39]

Transpupillary thermotherapy is generally used for relatively small tumours without associated vitreous or subretinal seeds and is used in conjunction with adjuvant chemotherapy. In a series of 188 tumours that had a mean tumour diameter of 3·0 mm and thickness of 2·0 mm, tumour regression was achieved in 86% with a recurrence rate of 14%. Larger tumours are at greater risk for complications such as focal iris atrophy and focal paraxial lens opacity because they require more intense therapy than smaller tumours.[40]

Plaque radiotherapy is highly effective in treating selected tumours with a high control rate. It can be used successfully even as a secondary treatment for tumours that have not been adequately controlled by other methods such as laser photocoagulation, cryotherpay or thermotherapy. In a series of 103 cases, for tumours with a mean diameter of 7 mm and the mean thickness of 4 mm, the control rate was 86%. The rate of tumour control was similar in the primary and secondary treatment groups.[41]

Question

Does post-enucleation adjuvant chemotherapy prevent metastasis in retinoblastoma?

The evidence

In the only prospective and randomised study by the Children's Cancer Study Group comprising 14 patients with high-risk retinoblastoma treated with adjuvant chemotherapy, no significant difference in survival was demonstrable in comparison to the control group.[42]

Comment

Various retrospective studies on adjuvant chemotherapy do not offer strong evidence about its efficacy (Table 52.3). Other studies have also suggested an equivocal benefit or lack of benefit.[43,44] On the other hand, several studies have indicated that adjuvant chemotherapy was beneficial.[26,35,45,46] In a recent study, Uusitalo and associates concluded that adjuvant chemotherapy is necessary for patients with tumour extending to the surgical margin of the optic nerve and is likely to be beneficial in preventing metastasis in patients with tumour extending beyond the lamina cribrosa.[47] Similarly, on the basis of retrospective data in patients with retinoblastoma manifesting histopathological high-risk characteristics, Honavar and associates reported a significant difference in the incidence of metastasis between the group that had received adjuvant chemotherapy (4%) and the group that had not (24%).[46]

Implications for research

It is evident that the major limitations of studies have been the rarity of the end-point (metastasis),[26,42] lack of comparable stratification for subgroup analysis,[26,35,43,48] and the absence of a control group.[26,43,44] A large randomised multi-centre prospective study is needed to identify specific high-risk characteristics in the presence of which post-enucleation adjuvant chemotherapy is needed.[46,47]

References

1. Bishop JO, Madsen EC. Retinoblastoma: Review of current status. *Surv Ophthalmol* 1975;**19**:342–66.
2. Tamboli A, Podgor MJ, Horm JW. The incidence of retinoblastoma in the United States: 1974 through 1985. *Arch Ophthalmol* 1990;**108**:128–32.
3. Abramson DH, Frank CM, Susman M *et al*. Presenting signs of retinoblastoma. *J Pediatr* 1998;**132**:505–8.
4. Shields CL, Shields JA. Recent developments in the management of retinoblastoma. *J Pediatr Ophthalmol Strabismus* 1999;**36**:8–18.
5. Friend SH, Bernards R, Rogelj S *et al*. A human DNA segment with properties of the gene that predisposes to retinoblastoma and osteosarcoma. *Nature* 1986;**323**:643–6.
6. Lee WH, Bookstein R, Hong F *et al*. Human retinoblastoma susceptibility gene: cloning, identification, and sequence. *Science* 1987;**235**:1394–9.
7. Harbour JW. Overview of RB gene mutations in patients with retinoblastoma. Implications for genetic screening. *Ophthalmology* 1998;**105**:1442–7.
8. Shields JA, Shields CL, Sivalingam V. Decreasing frequency of enucleation in patients with retinoblastoma. *Am J Ophthalmol* 1989;**108**:185–8.
9. Hernandez JC, Brady LW, Shields JA *et al*. External beam radiation for retinoblastoma: results, patterns of failure, and a proposal for treatment guidelines. *Intl J Rad Oncol Biol Phys* 1996;**35**:125–32.
10. Shields JA, Shields CL, De Potter P, Hernandez JC, Brady LW. Plaque radiotherapy for residual or recurrent retinoblastoma in 91 cases. *J Pediatr Ophthalmol Strabismus* 1994;**31**:242–5.
11. Shields JA, Shields CL, Parsons H, Giblin ME. The role of photocoagulation in the management of retinoblastoma. *Arch Ophthalmol* 1990;**108**:205–8.
12. Shields JA, Parsons H, Shields CL, Giblin ME. The role of cryotherapy in the management of retinoblastoma. *Am J Ophthalmol* 1989;**108**:260–4.
13. Shields CL, Santos MC, Diniz W *et al*. Thermotherapy for retinoblastoma. *Arch Ophthalmol* 1999;**117**:885–93.
14. Shields CL, Shields JA, Needle M *et al*. Combined chemoreduction and adjuvant treatment for intraocular retinoblastoma. *Ophthalmology* 1997;**104**:2101–11.
15. Ferris FL, Chew EY. A new era for the treatment of retinoblastoma. *Arch Ophthalmol* 1996;**114**:1412.
16. Friedman DL, Himelstein B, Shields CL *et al*. Chemoreduction and local ophthalmic therapy for intraocular retinoblastoma. *J Clin Oncol* 2000;**18**:12–17.
17. Anonymous. [National registry of retinoblastoma in Japan (1975–1982). The Committee for the National Registry of Retinoblastoma]. Nippon Ganka Gakkai Zasshi. *Acta Soc Ophthalmol Jpn* 1992;**96**:1433–42.
18. Kopelman JE, McLean IW, Rosenberg SH. Multivariate analysis of risk factors for metastasis in retinoblastoma treated by enucleation. *Ophthalmology* 1987;**94**:371–7.
19. McCay CJ, Abramson DH, Ellsworth RM. Metastatic patterns of retinoblastoma. *Arch Ophthalmol* 1984;**102**:391–6.
20. Reese AB. *Tumors of the eye*. Hagerstown: Harper & Row, 1976, pp. 90–132.
21. Murphree AL, Villablanca JG, Deegan WF 3rd *et al*. Chemotherapy plus local treatment in the management of intraocular retinoblastoma. *Arch Ophthalmol* 1996;**114**:1348–56.
22. Kingston JE, Hungerford JL, Madreperla SA, Plowman PN. Results of combined chemotherapy and radiotherapy for advanced intraocular retinoblastoma. *Arch Ophthalmol* 1996;**114**:1339–43.
23. Shields CL, Honavar SG, Meadows AT. Chemoreduction for retinoblastoma: factors predictive of failure and need for treatment with external beam radiotherapy or enucleation. *N Engl J Med* 2003;(in press).
24. Scott IU, Murray TG, Toledano S, O'Brien JM. New retinoblastoma tumors in children undergoing systemic chemotherapy. *Arch Ophthalmol* 1998;**12**:1685–6.
25. Benz MS, Scott UI, Murray TG *et al*. Complications of systemic chemotherapy as treatment of retinoblastoma. *Arch Ophthalmol* 2000;**118**:577–8.
26. Howarth C, Meyer D, Hustu HO, Johnson WW, Shanks E, Pratt C. Stage-related combined modality treatment of retinoblastoma. Results of a prospective study. *Cancer* 1980;**45**:851–8.
27. Ajaiyeoba IA, Akang EE, Campbell OB, Olurin IO, Aghadiuno PU. Retinoblastomas in Ibadan: treatment and prognosis. *West Afr J Med* 1993;**12**:223–7.
28. Singh AD, Shields CL, Shields JA. Prognostic factors in retinoblastoma. *J Pediatr Ophthalmol Strabismus* 2000;**37**:1–8.
29. Gallie BL, Budning A, DeBoer G *et al*. Chemotherapy with focal therapy can cure intraocular retinoblastoma without radiotherapy. *Arch Ophthalmol* 1996;**114**:1321–8.
30. White L. Chemotherapy for retinoblastoma: where do we go from here? *Ophthalmic Pediatr Genet* 1991;**12**:115–30.
31. Messmer EP, Heinrich T, Hopping W *et al*. Risk factors for metastases in patients with retinoblastoma. *Ophthalmology* 1991;**98**:136–41.
32. Magramm I, Abramson DH, Ellsworth RM. Optic nerve involvement in retinoblastoma. *Ophthalmology* 1989;**96**:217–22.
33. Shields CL, Shields JA, Baez KA *et al*. Choroidal invasion of retinoblastoma: Metastatic potential and clinical risk factors. *Br J Ophthalmol* 1993;**77**:544–8.
34. Shields CL, Shields JA, Baez KA *et al*. Optic nerve invasion in retinoblastoma. *Cancer* 1994;**73**:692–8.
35. Khelfaoui F, Validire P, Auperin A *et al*. Histopathologic risk factors in retinoblastoma: a retrospective study of 172 patients treated in a single institution. *Cancer* 1996;**77**:1206–13.
36. Chantada GL, de Silva MTG, Fandino A *et al*. Retinoblastoma with low risk for extraocular relapse. *Ophthalmic Genet* 1999;**20**:133–40.
37. Shields JA, Shields CL. Treatment of retinoblastoma with photocoagulation. *Transac PA Acad Ophthalmol Otolaryngol* 1990;**42**:951–4.
38. Shields JA, Shields CL. Treatment of retinoblastoma with cryotherapy. *Transac PA Acad Ophthalmol Otolaryngol* 1990;**42**:977–80.
39. Abramson DH, Ellsworth RM, Rozakis GW. Cryotherapy for retinoblastoma. *Arch Ophthalmol* 1982;**100**:1253–6.
40. Shields CL, Santos MC, Diniz W *et al*. Thermotherapy for retinoblastoma. *Arch Ophthalmol* 1999;**117**:885–93.
41. Shields CL, Shields JA, Cater J *et al*. Plaque radiotherapy for retinoblastoma: Long term tumor control and treatment complications in 208 tumors. *Ophthalmology* 2001;**108**:2116–21.
42. Wolff JA, Boesel CP, Dyment PG *et al*. Treatment of retinoblastoma: a preliminary report. *Int Congr Series (Amsterdam)* 1981;**570**:364–8.
43. Zelter M, Damel A, Gonzalez G, Schwartz L. A prospective study on the treatment of retinoblastoma in 72 patients. *Cancer* 1991;**68**:1685–90.
44. Mustafa MM, Jamshed A, Khafaga Y *et al*. Adjuvant chemotherapy with vincristine, doxorubicin, and cyclophosphamide in the treatment of postenucleation high risk retinoblastoma. *J Pediatr Hematol Oncol* 1999;**21**:364–9.
45. Hungerford J. Factors influencing metastasis in retinoblastoma. *Br J Ophthalmol* 1993;**77**:541.
46. Honavar SG, Singh AD, Shields CL *et al*. Post-enucleation adjuvant chemotherapy in high-risk retinoblastoma. *Arch Ophthalmol* 2002;**120**:923–31.
47. Uusitalo MS, van Quill KR, Scott IU *et al*. Evaluation of chemoprophylaxis in patients with unilateral retinoblastoma with high-risk features on histopathology examination. *Arch Ophthalmol* 2001;**119**:41–8.
48. Pratt CB, Crom DB, Howarth C. The use of chemotherapy in extraocular retinoblastoma. *Med Pediatr Oncol* 1985;**13**:330–3.

Section XIII

Rehabilitation

Gary Rubin, Editor

53 Vision rehabilitation

Gary Rubin

Background

Visual impairment is seldom life threatening. Nevertheless, it is among the most disabling of medical conditions and is more disabling than all chronic conditions except diabetes and cancer in older adults.[1] Visual impairment is strongly associated with disability and dependency in daily activities,[2–5] reduced physical activity,[6,7] social isolation,[8,9] and depression,[10] especially in older individuals. According to one study,[11] the quality of life of low-vision patients was significantly worse than that for age-matched controls and comparable to those with congestive heart failure or clinical depression.

Incidence and prevalence

The Royal National Institute for the Blind estimates that there are 1·7 million visually impaired individuals in the UK.[12] Approximately 35 000 people are registered as blind or partially sighted per year, and as the number of registrations underestimates the true incidence by a factor of two to three, the actual number of incident cases may be as high as 100 000. Incidence and prevalence statistics depend on the definition of visual impairment. Most epidemiological studies use a definition based on restrictions in visual acuity, visual fields, or both. However, recent data[2] suggest that other aspects of visual function, such as loss of contrast sensitivity or increased sensitivity to glare, independently contribute to visual disability. Were these other factors to be included in the definition of visual impairment then the numbers would be even greater.

Treatment options

Ninety per cent of visually impaired people are over 60 years of age[13] with over half the incidence attributable to age-related macular degeneration (AMD). As there is no cure for this disease and currently available treatments merely retard the rate of vision loss, macular degeneration patients and many others with visually disabling eye conditions must learn to make best use of their residual vision. That is the goal of vision rehabilitation. Although it has been estimated that over 150 000 low-vision consultations are offered annually in the UK at a cost of £21 million (plus the cost of low-vision aids) it is acknowledged that the availability of services is not adequate to meet the needs of the visually impaired population.[12] In addition, it was the consensus of a panel of service providers and patients that vision rehabilitation services need to be more comprehensive.[14] However, the evidence for the benefits of vision rehabilitation is limited. Surveys of patient satisfaction following vision rehabilitation have produced conflicting results ranging from 90% reporting that the service was sufficient to meet their needs[15] to 50% reporting dissatisfaction.[16] Similarly, there are wide discrepancies in the reported use of prescribed low-vision aids, such as magnifiers. Some studies find that 80–90% of patients find the devices useful for everyday activities,[17,18] while others report that the majority of patients stop using the devices within 18 months.[19] Without solid evidence as to the benefits of vision rehabilitation, it is difficult to argue for the expansion of rehabilitation services.

> ## Question
>
> What is the effectiveness of low-vision rehabilitation for visually impaired children or adults?

The evidence

We found no systematic reviews of randomised controlled trials of vision rehabilitation, although Cochrane reviews of low-vision devices and orientation and mobility training are currently underway. This review includes references from the Cochrance Eyes and Vision specialised register supplemented by an additional MEDLINE search. All controlled trials of visual rehabilitation were included, regardless of age of the participant, the type of intervention, location of the rehabilitation service (clinic or community), or cause of visual impairment. Studies that solely compared low-vision devices are not included.

We found eight randomised controlled trials, plus two trials that were controlled but not randomised. The ten studies are listed and summarised in Table 53.1. The total number of participants in the studies was 565. The smallest study included only 17 participants and the largest 226. Age-related macular degeneration was the most common cause of visual impairment, but half of the studies did not specify the diagnosis. The type of intervention varied greatly among the studies. There were three studies of orientation and mobility (O&M) training, three studies of other types of training, three studies based on the provision of specific low-vision devices, and one comparison of a conventional hospital-based low-vision service to an expanded service with home visits by a rehabilitation officer. The interventions were too different from each other to be synthesised into a single meta-analysis.

The three O&M studies included similar small numbers of participants, 35–40. Only one of the studies[20] showed a significant benefit of training. The trained group completed significantly more (86% *v* 82%) of the orientation, sighted guide, and independent travel activities correctly after 90 minutes per week for 10–12 weeks of O&M training. There was no significant change (61% *v* 60%) in the control group, who had a similar amount of physical exercise. One limitation of the study was that the pre- and post-training evaluations were carried out by O&M instructors who were not masked to the treatment assignment. Another concern was that the groups were not well matched for O&M skills prior to training. The other two studies[20,21] that found no benefit of O&M training attributed their null findings to problems with the outcome measures. In one case[20] the outcome was assessed by untrained volunteers whose assessments were not reliable. In the second case[21] it was argued that the outcome measures (walking speed and travel errors) were too narrowly defined to capture the benefits of O&M training.

The three other training studies all reported significant benefits for their respective interventions. In a study of 40 patients with AMD,[22] educational training in the use of low-vision aids that concentrated on eccentric viewing training improved patients' ability to do near, intermediate, and distance tasks, compared to an untrained group. For example, prior to training none of the patients were able to read newspaper text. With low-vision aids 100% of the trained group, but only 25% of the untrained group were able to read newsprint. Another study of AMD patients[10] evaluated the potential benefits of a self management training programme. Ninety-two patients were assigned to either six group sessions of behavioural skill training or no training. The trained group showed a significant improvement in mood and self-efficacy, compared to controls, but there was no difference on a generic quality of life scale. At the other end of the age spectrum, a study of 16 visually impaired children[23] found that dance instruction plus physical education improved the children's self concept of body position more than physical education alone. However, the two groups were not matched prior to the study. The dance instruction group had significantly worse position sense before training.

Three small studies of specific types of low-vision devices all reported a treatment benefit. One was a study of Fresnel prisms used to compensate for hemionopic visual field loss or visual neglect following stroke.[24] Forty patients were randomly assigned to prism or no prism. Patients who received prism showed greater improvement in visual perception tests at the four-week follow up than the control group. However, there was no difference between groups in activities of daily living or mobility function. Prisms were also used in a study of 30 patients with AMD to enhance the use of eccentric vision.[25] Visual acuity and self-reported function were assessed, although the methods used for the outcome assessment are not described. There was a trend towards more improvement in the prism group, but the results fell just short of statistical significance ($P = 0.06$). In the third study of low-vision devices, bioptic telescopes were prescribed to 17 low-vision patients with central vision loss caused by a variety of disorders. Half of the participants received O&M and driving training and half received no training. Outcomes were assessed for a wide variety of psychophysical tasks (such as peripheral letter recognition), functional tasks (such as visual memory), and driving simulator and on-the-road driving performance. The trained group showed significantly more improvement than the control group for half of the outcomes. There were no differences between groups for the remaining outcomes.

The largest and most thorough RCT of vision rehabilitation is a recent study of enhanced versus conventional low-vision services.[26] Two hundred and twenty-six patients with AMD were randomly assigned to one of three groups: conventional hospital-based vision rehabilitation, the conventional service plus three home visits by a trained rehabilitation officer, or the conventional service plus home visits by a volunteer community care worker. The third group was included as a control for the additional social contact by the rehabilitation officer. There was a wide range of outcome measures including generic and vision-specific quality of life, psychological adjustment and activity restriction questionnaires, measured performance on several reading tasks, and an assessment of low-vision device usage. Contrary to expectations, there were no benefits observed for the enhanced intervention group on any of the outcome measures.

Discussion

Despite the substantial number of people with visual impairment there have been only a few, mostly small, controlled trials of vision rehabilitation. Seven of the 10 studies reviewed here reported statistically significant benefit from the intervention, and one reported a marginal benefit. The studies used a wide variety of outcome

Table 53.1 Summary of controlled trials of vision rehabilitation

Study	Participants	Intervention	Control	Outcome	No. of subjects	Random allocation	Masked exam	Results
Chin, 1988[23]	Various, age 6–10 years	Dance instruction and physcal education	Physical education only	Test of positional concepts	8 (I) 8 (C)	Yes	No	Significant benefit
Rosenberg et al., 1989[25]	AMD	Prism relocation therapy	No therapy	Acuity and subjective function	19 (I) 11 (C)	Yes	?	Marginal benefit
Nilsson, 1990,[22]	AMD	Eccentric viewing training	No training	Reading acuity and speed, task success	20 (I) 20 (C)	Yes	?	Reported benefit for all tasks (no group statistics)
Rossi et al., 1990[24]	Stroke with hemianopia or visual neglect	Fresnel prism	No prism	Visual perception tasks, ADL scale	19 (I) 21 (C)	Yes	No	Significant benefit for visual perception tasks, no difference for ADL scale
Straw et al., 1991[28]	Legally blind, over age 60	O&M training	Physical exercise	Observed O&M skills	18 (I) 17 (C)	Yes	No	No benefit
Straw and Harley, 1991[20]	Legally blind, over age 60	O&M training	Physical exercise	Observed O&M skills	16 (I) 16 (C)	Yes	No	Significant benefit
Brody et al., 1999[10]	AMD	Group self-management training	No training	Mood, self-efficacy, and quality of life scales	44 (I) 48 (C)	Yes	?	Significant benefit for mood and self efficacy, no benefit for quality of well being
Szlyk et al., 2000[27]	Central vision loss age 16–78 years	Bioptic telescope and training	Bioptic telescope and no training	Skills assessment including driving	9 (I) 8 (C)	No?	?	Significant benefit
Soong et al., 2001[21]	Various, age 33–87 years	O&M training	No training	Walking speed and errors	19 (I), 18 (C)	No	Yes	No benefit of O&M
Russell et al., 2002[26]	AMD	Hospital-based vision rehab and home visits by rehab officer	Hospital-based vision rehab (C1), hospital rehab and generic home visit (C2)	Quality of life, psychological adjustment, self restriction, and low-vision device use	75 (I) 76 (C1) 75 (C2)	Yes	Yes	No benefit

AMD, age related macular degeneration; OKM, orientation and mobility; I, intervention; C, control

measures ranging from performance-based assessments to generic quality of life questionnaires. The statistical treatment of the outcomes also varied from one study to the next. None of the investigations reported relative risks comparing intervention with control. Given the heterogeneity of interventions and outcomes it is not possible to pool the results from multiple studies.

There are many additional studies of the effectiveness of vision rehabilitation that did not include a control group. These have not been included in this review. Two of the included studies did not use random assignment to treatment and control groups, but because the groups were matched for important covariates they have been incorporated. In the Soong *et al.* O&M study[21] the intervention group was recruited from an agency that provides O&M training while the control group was recruited from a university rehabilitation centre. The two groups were matched for age and level of impairment. Szlyk *et al.*'s study of bioptic telescope training[27] used intervention and control groups that were matched for age and visual function but were not randomly assigned.

Several of the studies did not control for placebo effects in the form of additional social contract for low-vision patients in the treatment group. The Straw and Harley[20] O&M studies and Straw *et al.*[28] and the Russell *et al.* study of enhanced low-vision services[26] are exceptions: Straw's control groups participated in physical exercise and Russell included a control group with visits by a volunteer community care worker.

Only two of the 10 studies appeared to use masked examiners. In the remaining eight studies those who administered the outcome assessment could have been aware of whether the participant was assigned to the treatment or control group.

Four of the reviewed trials used patients with AMD and two additional studies were limited to older participants, many of whom had some form of macular disease. While AMD accounts for half of those referred for vision rehabilitation services in the UK and North America[29,30] there is almost no evidence of the effectiveness of vision rehabilitation for children or adults of working age.

There have been no studies that compared conventional vision rehabilitation to no treatment. Given the widespread presumption that vision rehabilitation is beneficial, practitioners would be reticent to participate in a trial where their patients could be randomised to no treatment, and there are serious ethical concerns about designing such a study.

Implications for practice and research

Overall, the evidence of the effectiveness of vision rehabilitation is not strong. Larger trials are required and the diverse causes of visual impairment need to be considered.

More attention needs to be paid to the specification and statistical treatment of outcomes and the interpretation of potential benefits in terms of their impact on daily life.

References

1. Verbrugge LM, Patrick DL. Seven chronic conditions: their impact on US adults' activity levels and use of medical services. *Am J Public Health* 1995;**85**:173–82.
2. Rubin GS, Bandeen-Roche K, Huang GH *et al.* The association of multiple visual impairments with self-reported visual disability: SEE project. *Invest Ophthalmol Vis Sci* 2001;**42**:64–72.
3. Salive ME, Guralnik J, Glynn RJ, Christen W, Wallace RB, Ostfeld AM. Association of visual impairment with mobility and physical function. *J Am Geriatr Soc* 1994;**42**:287–92.
4. Appollonio I, Carabellese C, Magni E, Frattola L, Trabucchi M. Sensory impairments and morality in an elderly community population: A six-year follow-up study. *Age Ageing* 1995;**24**:30–6.
5. Jette AM, Branch LG. Impairment and disability in the aged. *J Chron Dis* 1985;**38**:59–65.
6. National Center for Health Statistics, Havlik RJ. Aging in the eighties. Impaired senses for sound and light in persons age 65 years and older. Preliminary data from the Supplement on Aging to the National Health Interview Survey, United States, January–June 1984. Advance data from Vital and Health Statistics. No. 125. DHHS Pub. No. (PHS) 86–1250. Hyattsville, MD: Public Health Service, September 19, 1986.
7. Hakkinen L. Vision in the elderly and its use in the social environment. *Scand J Soc Med* 1984;**35**(Suppl):5–60.
8. Rudberg MA, Furner SE, Dunn JE, Cassel CK. The relationship of visual and hearing impairments to disability: An analysis using the longitudinal study of aging. *J Gerontol* 1993;**48**:M261–5.
9. Thompson JR, Gibson JM, Jagger C. The association between visual impairment and mortality in elderly people. *Age Ageing* 1989;**18**:83–8.
10. Brody BL, Williams RA, Thomas RG, Kaplan RM, Chu RM, Brown SI. Age-related macular degeneration: a randomized clinical trial of a self-management intervention. *Ann Behav Med* 1999;**21**:322–9.
11. Scott IU, Smiddy WE, Schiffman J, Feuer WJ, Pappas CJ. Quality of life of low-vision patients and the impact of low-vision services. *Am J Ophthalmol* 1999;**128**:54–62.
12. Ryan B, Culham L. FRAGMENTED VISION – Survey of low vision services in the UK. London: Royal National Institute for the Blind, 1999.
13. Evans J. Causes of blindness and partial sight in England & Wales 1990–1991. *Studies on Medical and population subjects: No. 57.* London: HMSO, 1995.
14. Low Vision Consensus Group. *Low vision services: Recommendations for future service delivery in the UK.* London: Royal National Institute for the Blind, 1999.
15. Shuttleworth GN, Dunlop A, Collins JK, James CR. How effective is an integrated approach to low vision rehabilitation? Two year follow up results from south Devon. *Br J Ophthalmol* 1995;**79**:719–23.
16. McIlwaine GG, Bell JA, Dutton GN. Low vision aids – is our service cost effective? *Eye* 1991;**5**:607–11.
17. Leat SJ, Fryer A, Rumney NJ. Outcome of low vision aid provision: the effectiveness of a low vision clinic. *Optom Vis Sci* 1994;**71**:199–206.
18. D'Allura T, McInerney R, Horowitz A. An evaluation of low vision services. *J Vis Impair Blindness* 1995;**89**:487–493.
19. Humphry RC, Thompson GM. Low vision aids – evaluation in a general eye department. *Trans Ophthalmol Soc UK* 1986;**105**:296–303.
20. Straw LB, Harley RK. Assessments and training in orientation and mobility for older persons: Program development and testing. *J Vis Impair Blindness* 1991;**85**:291–6.
21. Soong GP, Lovie-Kitchin J, Brown B. Does mobility performance of visually impaired adults improve immediately after orientation and mobility training? *Optom Vis Sci* 2001;**78**:657–66.

22. Nilsson UL. Visual rehabilitation with and without educational training in the use of optical aids and residual vision. A prospective study of patients with advanced age-related macular degeneration. *Clin Vision Sci* 1990;**6**:3–10.

23. Chin DL. Dance movement instruction: Effects on spatial awareness in visually impaired elementary students. *J Vis Impair Blindness* 1988;**82**:188–92.

24. Rossi P, Kheyfets S, Reding M. Frensel prisms improve visual perception in stroke patients with homonymous hemianopia or unilateral visual neglect. *Neurology* 1990;**40**:1597–9.

25. Rosenberg R, Faye E, Fischer M, Budick D. Role of prism relocation in improving visual performance of patients with macular dysfunction. *Optom Vis Sci* 1989;**66**:747–50.

26. Russell W, Harper R, Reeves B, Waterman H, Henson D, McLeod D. Randomised controlled trial of an integrated versus an optometric low vision rehabilitation service for patients with age-related macular degeneration: study design and methodology. *Ophthalmic Physiol Opt* 2001;**21**:36–44.

27. Szlyk JP, Seiple W, Laderman DJ, Kelsch R, Stelmack J, McMahon T. Measuring the effectiveness of bioptic telescopes for persons with central vision loss. *J Rehabil Res Dev* 2000;**37**:101–8.

28. Straw LB, Harley RK, Zimmerman B. A program in orientation and mobility for visually impaired persons over age 60. *J Vis Impair Blindness* 1991;**85**:108–112.

29. Elliott DB, Strong JG, Pace R, Plotkin A, Bevers BA, Cassidy J. The demography of low vision in Ontario. *Optom Vis Sci* 1992;**69**:169.

30. Leat SJ, Rumney NJ. The experience of a university-based low vision clinic. *Ophthalmic Physiol Opt* 1990;**10**:8–15.

Index

Page numbers in *italics* refer to tables and boxes, those in **bold** refer to figures